Highlights of the

INSTRUCTIONAL COURSES

Volume 8, 1995

Highlights of the

INSTRUCTIONAL COURSES

Volume 8, 1995

Edited by

Frank E. Lucente, M.D.
Professor and Chairman
Department of Otolaryngology
State University of New York–Health Science Center at Brooklyn
Brooklyn, NY

with 269 *illustrations*

Mosby

St. Louis Baltimore Boston Carlsbad Chicago Naples New York Philadelphia Portland
London Madrid Mexico City Singapore Sydney Tokyo Toronto Wiesbaden

Mosby
Dedicated to Publishing Excellence

A Times Mirror
Company

Publisher: Anne Patterson
Editor: Robert Hurley
Developmental Editor: Lauranne Billus
Project Manager: John Rogers
Sr. Production Editor: Kathleen L. Teal
Design Coordinator: Renée Duenow
Manufacturing Manager: Theresa Fuchs

Printed in the United States of America
Composition by Clarinda Company
Printing/binding by Maple-Vail Book Mfg. Group

Mosby–Year Book, Inc.
11830 Westline Industrial Drive
St. Louis, Missouri 63146

International Standard Book Number 0-8151-0065-5

96 97 98 99 00 / 9 8 7 6 5 4 3 2 1

Contributors

KEDAR K. ADOUR, M.D.
Coordinator
Sir Charles Bell Society
Director of Research
Chairman
Cranial Nerve Clinic
Department of Head and Neck Surgery
Kaiser Permanente Medical Center
Oakland, California

JONATHAN E. AVIV, M.D.
Department of Otolaryngology
Columbia-Presbyterian Medical Center
New York, New York

MICHAEL S. BENNINGER, M.D.
Chairman
Department of Otolaryngology–Head and Neck Surgery
Henry Ford Hospital
Detroit, Michigan

ANDREW BLITZER, M.D., D.D.S.
Head and Neck Surgical Group
Department of Otolaryngology
St. Luke's-Roosevelt Medical Center
New York, New York

DENNIS I. BOJRAB, M.D.
EAR Consultants of Michigan
Assistant Clinical Professor
Wayne State University
Royal Oak, Michigan

C. RON CANNON, M.D., F.A.C.S.
Clinical Associate Professor
Departments of Surgery and Family Medicine
School of Medicine
Department of Diagnostic Sciences
School of Dentistry
University of Mississippi
Head & Neck Surgical Group
Jackson, Mississippi

JEAN-BERNARD CAUSSE, M.D.
Award Winner of the Faculty of Strasbourg
J. Causse Clinic
Colombiers, France

WILLIAM D. CLARK, M.D., D.D.S.
Department of Otolaryngology
Wilford Hall Medical Center
Lackland AFB, Texas

SHARON L. COLLINS, M.S., M.D., F.A.C.S.
Associate Professor
Department of Otoylaryngology–Head and Neck Surgery
Loyola University Medical Center
Maywood, Illinois

PETER D. COSTANTINO, M.D.
Associate Professor
Department of Otolaryngology–Head and Neck Surgery
Loyola University Medical School
Chief
Section of Head and Neck Surgical Oncology
Loyola University Cancer Center
Loyola University Medical Center
Maywood, Illinois

ROBIN T. COTTON, M.D., F.A.C.S., F.R.C.S.(C)
Professor
Department of Otolaryngology
University of Cincinnati College of Medicine
Director
Department of Pediatric Otolaryngology
Children's Hospital Medical Center
Cincinnati, Ohio

M. JENNIFER DEREBERY, M.D.
House Ear Clinic
House Ear Institute
Los Angeles, California

WILLIAM J. DICHTEL, Jr., M.D.
Associate Clinical Professor of Otolaryngology–Head and Neck Surgery
University of Virginia School of Medicine
Charlottesville, Virginia

WOLFGANG DILLMANN, M.D.
Professor
Department of Medicine
Division of Endocrinology
University of California, San Diego, School of Medicine
La Jolla, California

BARBARA JANE DIXON, B.S.
Clinical Staff
Floyd Medical Center
Rome, Georgia

HAMILTON S. DIXON, M.D.
Assistant Professor of Otolaryngology–Head and Neck Surgery
Vanderbilt University
Staff Physician
Floyd Medical Center
Rome Georgia

ISAAC ELIACHAR, M.D.
Department of Otolaryngology
Cleveland Clinic Foundation
Cleveland, Ohio

JACK L. GLUCKMAN, M.D.
Professor and Chairman
Department of Otolaryngology
University of Cincinnati Medical Center
The Barrett Center
Cincinnati, Ohio

JOEL A. GOEBEL, M.D., F.A.C.S.
Associate Professor
Washington University
St. Louis, Missouri

DONALD J. GRANDE, M.D.
Associate Clinical Professor of Dermatology
Harvard Medical School
Boston, Massachusetts
Chairman
Department of Dermatology
Lahey Clinic
Burlington, Massachusetts

JUDITH S. GRAVEL, Ph.D.
Associate Professor of Otolaryngology
Director of Audiology
Albert Einstein College of Medicine
Montefiore Medical Center
Bronx, New York

JOHN W. HOUSE, M.D.
House Ear Clinic
House Ear Institute
Los Angeles, California

GORDON B. HUGHES, M.D.
Director of Resident Education
Clinical Staff
Section of Otology-Neurotology
Department of Otolaryngology and Communicative Disorders
Cleveland Clinic Foundation
Cleveland, Ohio

ARNOLD E. KATZ, M.D., M.S., F.A.C.S.
Professor of Surgery (Otolaryngology)
State University of New York at Stony Brook
Chief
Division of Otolaryngology–Head and Neck Surgery
University Hospital
Health Sciences Center
Stony Brook, New York

DAVID W. KENNEDY, M.D.
Professor and Chair
Department of Otorhinolaryngology–Head and Neck Surgery
University of Pennsylvania
Hospital of the University of Pennsylvania
Philadelphia, Pennsylvania

JAMES A. KOUFMAN, M.D., F.A.C.S.
Director
Center for Voice Disorders of Wake Forest University
Professor of Otolaryngology
Bowman Gray School of Medicine
Wake Forest University Medical Center
Winston-Salem, North Carolina

HELEN F. KRAUSE, M.D., F.A.C.S.
Associate Clinical Professor
Departments of Otolaryngology
University of Pittsburgh School of Medicine
Pittsburgh, Pennsylvania
Pennsylvania State University College of Medicine
Hershey, Pennsylvania

YOSEF P. KRESPI, M.D.
Head and Neck Surgical Group
Department of Otolaryngology
St. Luke's-Roosevelt Medical Center
New York, New York

JED A. KWARTLER, M.D.
Ear Specialty Group
Springfield, New Jersey
Clinical Assistant Professor of Otolaryngology
University of Medicine and Dentistry of New Jersey
Newark, New Jersey

DONALD C. LANZA, M.D., F.A.C.S.
Assistant Professor
Department of Otorhinolaryngology–Head and Neck Surgery
University of Pennsylvania
Clinician Educator
University of Pennsylvania Medical Center
Philadelphia, Pennsylvania

BRUCE R. MADDERN, M.D., F.A.C.S., F.A.A.P.
Assistant Professor of Otolaryngology
Mayo Clinic
Chief of Otolaryngology
Nemours Children's Clinic
Wolfson Children's Hospital
Jacksonville, Florida

JANE R. MADELL, Ph.D.
Professor of Clinical Otolaryngology
State University of New York Health Science Center
Director
Division of Communicative Disorders
Long Island College Hospital
Brooklyn, New York

BRENT MEADOR, M.D.
Clinical Associate Professor
Department of Family Medicine
Instructor
Department of Psychiatry
University of Mississippi School of Medicine
Medical Director
Mississippi Baptist Chemical Dependency Unit
Jackson, Mississippi

FRED M.S. McCONNEL, M.D.
Clinical Professor of Surgery
Emory University
Northside Hospital
St. Joseph's Hospital
Scottish Rite Children's Medical Center
West Paces Medical Center
Atlanta, Georgia
Gwinnett Medical Center
Lawrenceville, Georgia
Eastside Medical Center
Snellville, Georgia
Veterans Administration Hospital
Decatur, Georgia

MARTINE MICHAT, M.D.
J. Causse Clinic
Colombiers, France

TOME MILHORN, M.D.
Professor
Department of Family Medicine
University of Mississippi School of Medicine
Jackson, Mississippi
Medical Director
Laurelwood Center Chemical Dependency Unit
Meridian, Mississippi

JOHN M. MOREHEAD, M.D.
Department of Otolaryngology
Wilford Hall Medical Center
Lackland AFB, Texas

RICHARD A. MOSCICKI, M.D.
Instructor in Medicine
Harvard University School of Medicine
Assistant Physician
Massachussetts General Hospital
Massachussetts Eye and Ear Infirmary
Boston, Massachussetts
Vice President
Clinical, Regulatory, and Medical Affairs
Genzyme Corporation
Cambridge, Massachussetts

Preface

Highlights of the Instructional Courses 1995 is a publication of manuscripts resulting from the Instruction Course Program which is held at the Annual Meeting of the American Academy of Otolaryngology–Head and Neck Surgery Foundation. The Instruction Course Program has become one of the most important educational activities of the Academy. Each year over 450 courses are given by practitioners for practitioners.

The program is assembled by the Instruction Course Advisory Committee on the basis of applications received from voluntary instructors and invitations issued to distinguished colleagues who bring special information, frequently from fields outside otolaryngology. The committee attempts to create a broad-based program which covers all aspects of clinical practice and relevant disciplines. Courses are grouped into the following categories: Allergy, Audiology, Basic Science, Computers, Facial Plastic and Reconstructive Surgery, General Otolaryngology, Head and Neck Surgery, Laryngology, Otology, Pediatric Otolaryngology, Practice Management, and Rhinology.

In order to assure that the most current and accurate information is presented, each course is updated annually and a new application is required every year. Courses are also reviewed intensively by the committee. Evaluations provided by everyone attending the courses are a critical part of the process of creating the best possible program. Each course is evaluated on the basis of several parameters and these scores are sent to the instructors, along with specific audience comments, within a month after the meeting. The instructors are urged to consider these scores and comments in preparing any future course proposals. The scores, comments, and attendance figures are also used by the committee in determining the acceptance or rejection of courses.

Numerous sources are consulted by the committee in preparing the annual program including the AAOHNS Board of Governors, various related AAOHNS committees and the leadership of other otolaryngologic societies and organizations. The goal is to provide the best possible educational service to the membership and to others who attend the Annual Meeting.

Each year the Instruction Course Advisory Committee reviews the entire program as well as the previous editions of Highlights and selects a group of instructors to be invited to submit manuscripts based on their courses. The manuscripts are thoroughly reviewed by the committee. Although the final publication is approved by the AAOHNS Foundation, it must be emphasized that the contents are the work and opinions of the author-instructors themselves and do not represent any official position of the Foundation.

Finally, I would like to thank the following: (a) the instructors who generously and promptly contributed their manuscripts to this publication, (b) all committee members who participated in the editorial review process, (c) Mr. Billy Tang who coordinated the entire project, (d) Mr. Robert Hurley, Lauranne Billus, Kathleen Teal, and Mia Carino at Mosby who guided the publication through its various stages, and (e) most importantly, all instruction course attendees who, by their active feedback, contribute to the creation of a continually improving Instruction Course Program.

Frank E. Lucente, MD, Coordinator
Instruction Course Program
American Academy of Otolaryngology–
Head and Neck Surgery Foundation, Inc.

PART FOUR LARYNGOLOGY

PART FIVE OTOLOGY

PART SIX PEDIATRIC

PART SEVEN RHINOLOGY

PART EIGHT ALLERGY

PART NINE PRACTICE MANAGEMENT

Highlights of the

INSTRUCTIONAL COURSES

Volume 8, 1995

1

Mandibular Fractures—What To Do When

Wm. D. Clark, M.D., D.D.S. and John M. Morehead, M.D.

In the 1970s treatment alternatives for the care of faciall fractures were quite limited. In the 1990s, we have many more therapeutic choices, and decision making has become much more complex. For any given fracture, there may be two or more acceptable treatment options. The factors that can influence the selection of a treatment plan are many and include considerations such as the surgeon's experience and the patient's desires.

In this course we emphasize choosing a proper treatment modality rather than the teaching of the details of surgical techniques. We will look at the problem from the perspective of the treatment options available and explore when to consider their application. Complications and their management are beyond the scope of this course.

We will be continually referring to stable and unstable fractures, and some clarification is needed in this regard. For our purposes, we define a stable fracture as one wherein the preinjury occlusion can be obtained and maintained with the application of mandibulo-maxillary fixation alone.

TRADITIONAL TECHNIQUES

By traditional techniques we mean those that were common before the popularization of rigid internal fixation. We will discuss each of them and decide when they might be applied.

Soft diet, observation, and possible physical therapy

There are a few mandibular fractures that require little in the way of specific treatment. Isolated fractures of the coronoid process are uncommon and require only that mandibular mobility be maintained while healing takes place. A soft diet is prescribed and advanced as tolerated. The surgeon should follow the patient to ensure that mandibular mobility is not compromised. Physical therapy is begun at the first sign of trismus. There are reports of late surgical excision of the coronoid process necessitated by severe trismus. We have no personal experience with that procedure. When there are other fractures of the mandible, treatment should be directed at their therapy with a heightened awareness of the need to prevent trismus.

Unilateral condylar area fractures in which the occlusion is normal, the fracture nondisplaced to minimally displaced, and the patient deemed reliable may be considered for noninvasive therapy. A liquid to soft diet is prescribed and weekly follow-up begun to access the maintenance of normal occlusion. Should the occlusion deteriorate, maxillomandibular fixation (MMF) will be needed. Patients meeting these criteria are usually young and it is suspected that the quality of the bone may be a major factor in producing this favorable situation.

Closed reduction with MMF

MMF is the usual therapy for unilateral condylar area fractures not meeting the above criteria (the majority do not). It is also required for all bilateral condylar area fractures. While there is no practical substitution for MMF in treating these condylar area fractures, it must be remembered that limitation of temporomandibular joint (TMJ) motion is a potential complication of both the injury and the treatment. Therefore, we must strive to balance the need for immobilization for fracture healing with the need to reduce the time in which the TMJ is immobilized. In children, the tendency for TMJ mobility problems is greater than that in adults. Fortunately, they also heal more rapidly. Our goal is to have children out of fixation in two to three weeks, using nighttime elastics for an additional week or two. In young, healthy adults three to four weeks of MMF combined with one to two weeks of nighttime elastics usually works well. Older and less healthy adults are treated with continuous MMF for four weeks and with nighttime elastics for an additional two.

MMF is a reasonable option for the stable body of mandible fractures when the dentition is adequate.[1] The minimum dental requirements are stable teeth on both sides of the fracture and enough teeth to support the hardware for MMF. Rigid fixation is also a choice for these fractures and will be discussed later. Recommended periods of immobilization are four weeks for children and six for adults. If a condylar area fracture is also present, full-time MMF is reduced to three weeks for children and four for adults, with two weeks of nighttime elastics added.

There are occasions when angle or symphyseal fractures may be stable enough to consider MMF as the sole treatment. These would represent exceptions to the general rule that treatment for fractures in those regions should include some form of internal fixation. The recommended periods of immobilization is four weeks for children and six for adults.

Open reduction with nonrigid fixation and MMF

This is the classic treatment for fractures of the mandibular angle and symphysis.[3] It is also an option for a mandibular body fracture when it cannot be reduced by closed techniques, the dentition is poor, and/or the fracture is unstable under MMF alone. Rigid internal fixation has enjoyed wide acceptance as the first-line treatment for these fractures and will be discussed later. Mandibular stability is indirectly proportional to the number of fractures present. Give consideration to using some form of internal fixation when stability is in doubt.

Supported MMF, with or without open reduction and nonrigid fixation

By supported MMF we mean techniques that stabilize and/or strengthen the fixation such as wiring arch bars to the facial skeleton and applying splints.

MMF may be unstable in several situations including the following:

1. Multiple missing teeth
2. Mobile teeth due to periodontal disease
3. Deciduous dentition
4. Mixed dentition

Wiring the MMF hardware (usually arch bars) to the facial skeleton does much to improve the stability in such cases. Three-point circummandibular wiring does the job for the mandibular hardware. For the maxilla, bilateral circumzygomatic wiring is combined with the surgeon's choice of pyriform aperture or anterior nasal spine wiring. The application of these simple measures in the event of the unfavorable states listed will often make the difference between success and failure. Dental splints can also be used as stabilizing measures.

Dental splints

Properly designed, splints can do the following:

1. Resist separation of the bodies of the mandible when there is loss of anterior continuity
2. Resist rotation of a segment about the long axis of the body of the mandible
3. Resist inferior rotation of an anterior segment of the mandible ("bucket-handle" effect)
4. Replace missing teeth to provide stops and locks with opposing teeth
5. Stabilize teeth loosened by periodontal disease or trauma
6. Severe as the sole therapy for selected body of mandible fractures in young children

Fabrication of splints requires special equipment and experience in handling dental materials. Fortunately, many dental labs can do much of the specialized work if provided good impressions of the dental arches. General anesthesia is often required to obtain impressions, especially when there are mobile fragments or the patient is a young child. If alginate or similar water-based impression materials are used, the impressions should be wrapped in moist paper towels and placed in a water-tight container until the casts are poured.

Plaster casts are made from the impressions. When occluded, the malocclusion produced by the fracture will be evident (Fig. 1-1). The fractures are duplicated in the mandibular cast. Then it is possible to occlude the fragments of the cast with the maxilla and reproduce the preinjury occlusion (Fig. 1-2). The cast fragments are temporarily joined (dental "sticky wax" works well). Permanent repair of the cast is made with plaster of Paris (Fig. 1-3).

The repaired cast then becomes the template for constructing the splint of self-curing polymethymethlacrylate.[5] Our favorite design is a lingual splint modified to replace any missing posterior teeth (Fig. 1-4). An alternative design incorporates both a lingual splint and an occlusal wafer.

The splint described above can be used as the sole treatment of selected body of mandible fractures in young children. The splint is attached by three-point circummandibular wiring and the child allowed to take a diet as tolerated. Since TMJ mobility is not an issue and nighttime elastics are not an option, these splints are routinely left in place for six weeks.

Dentures as splints. In effect, dentures are facio-occlusio-lingual splints. When fractured, they are quickly and easily repaired by a dental lab. To use as Gunning splints, they simply need to be fixed to the facial skeleton

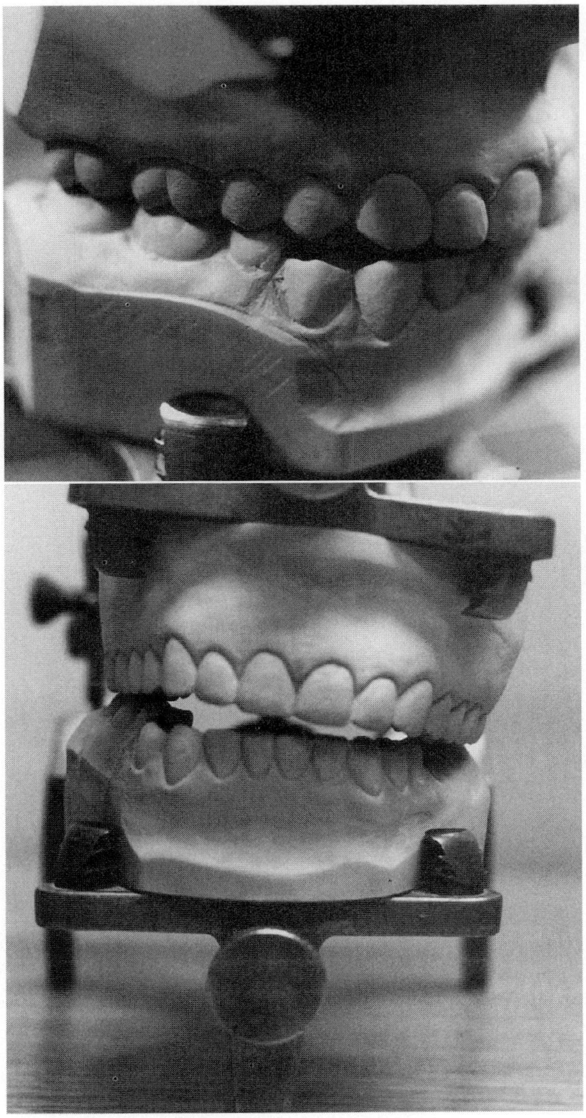

A

B

FIG 1-1
Plaster cast shows malocclusion.

(we prefer the same wiring described for supported MMF) and attached to one another. There are many acceptable ways to provide the interconnection between the dentures. Our choice for modifying dentures for MMF is as follows:

1. Remove the mandibular central incisors to provide space for alimentation, clearing of secretions, and egress of vomitus (Fig. 1-5)
2. Drill holes in the interdental papillae between each posterior tooth and on both sides of the canine teeth (Fig. 1-6)
3. Attach Erich arch bars, in segments, to the two dentures (Fig. 1-7)[2]

All modifications to the dentures are done before the patient is anesthetized. It is then a simple matter to attach the dentures to the patient and then to each other. We prefer a few dental elastics for the first two days and stainless steel wire thereafter. The elastics provide a margin of safety should postoperative vomiting occur, while the wires are more hygienic and durable for the duration of the MMF.

Gunning splints. The fabrication of high-quality Gunning splints requires a good deal more than impressions and availability of a dental laboratory. Also required is the ability to register centric occlusion and determine appropriate intermaxillary distance, skills that most non-dentists lack. A dental consultant's help should be obtained in cases needing Gunning splints.

These splints may be used to provide MMF in the following circumstances:

1. Edentulous patient with one or both dentures missing
2. One dentured arch and one edentulous arch with no denture available

External fixation

Widespread popularity of rigid internal fixation has contributed to the decline in popularity of external fixation. However, this technique still has some applications and should be kept in one's armamentarium.[1] The following remain strong indications for external fixation:

1. Trauma to mandible involving loss of large amounts of bone (gunshot wound is the classic example)
2. Fractures of the edentulous mandible with no dentures available and insufficient space for compression plate placement

BEYOND TRADITIONAL TECHNIQUES

Rigid internal fixation

In recent years, rigid internal fixation has become the standard against which other treatments of facial fractures are measured. There are three general classes of these devices.

Lag screws. There are at least three indications for lag screws in the treatment of mandibular fractures:

1. To secure fragments when there is sufficient obliquity of the fracture such that the length of the overlap equals two or more times the thickness of the mandible
2. Treatment of angle fractures by intraoral placement (see Niederdellman.[6] Farris[4])

A 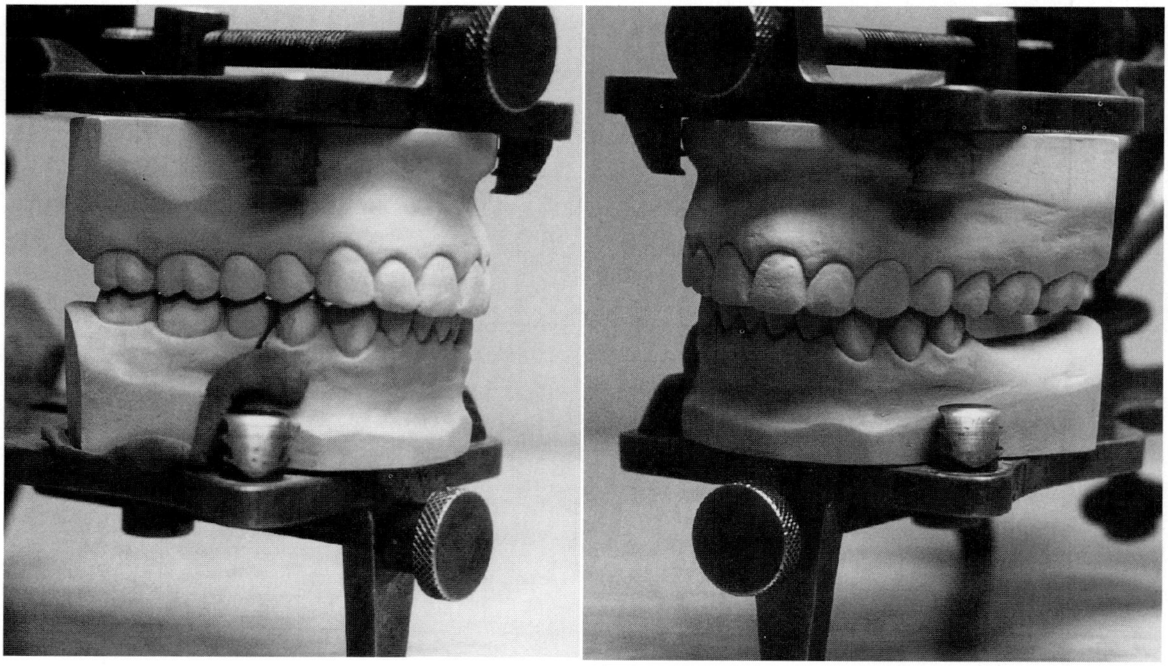 B

FIG 1-2
After the fracture(s) are reproduced in plaster, the fragments may be occluded against the maxillary cast. This should reproduce the pre-injury occlusion.

A 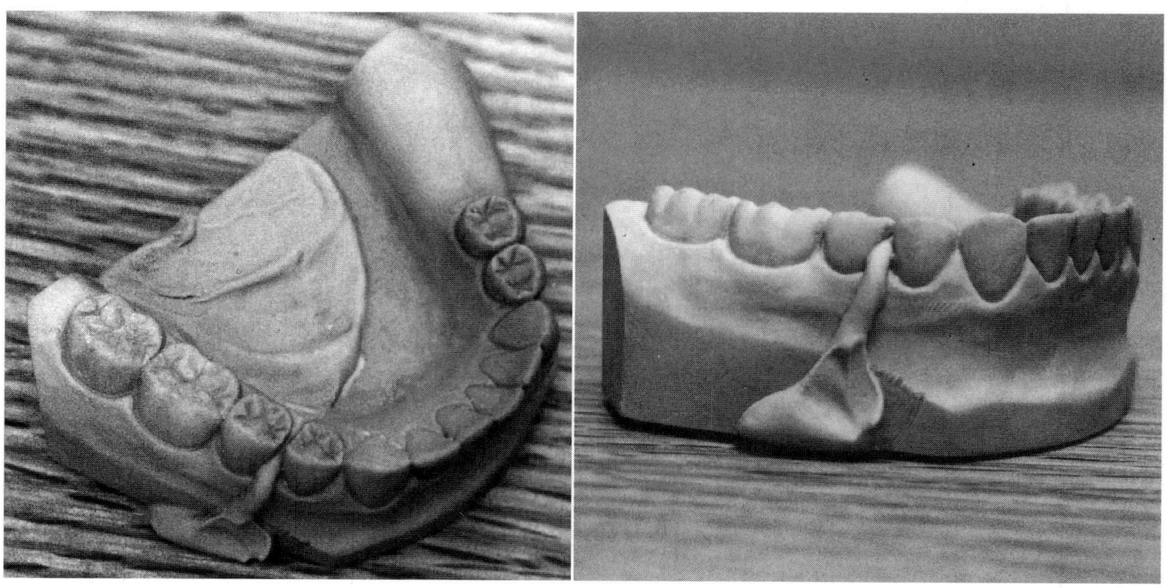 B

FIG 1-3
The mandibular cast has been repaired with plaster.

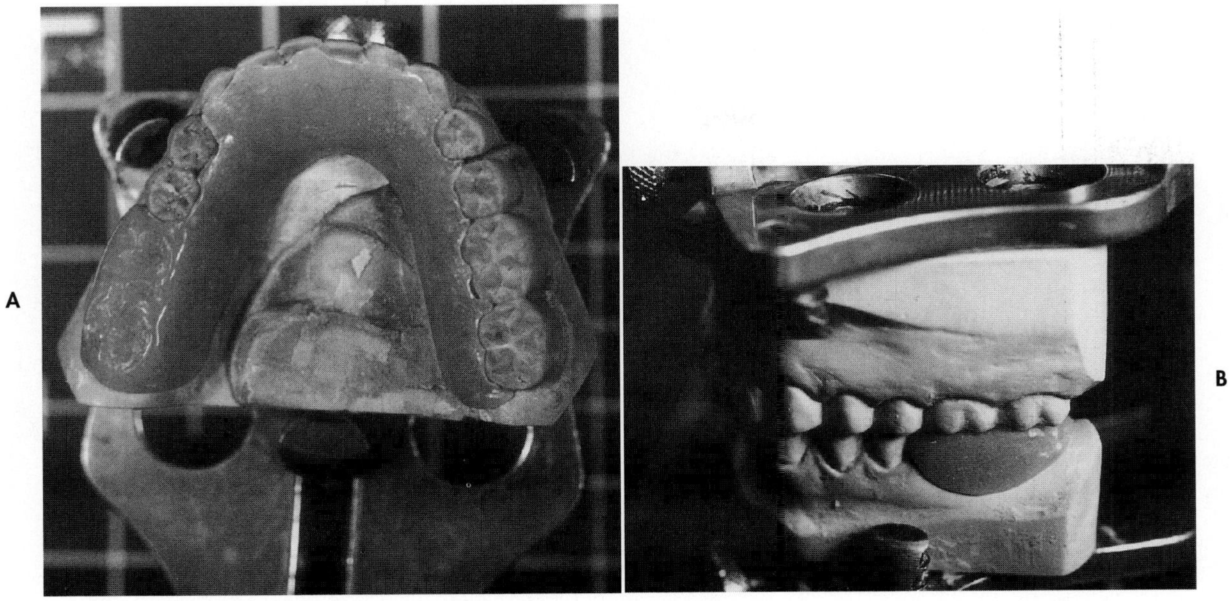

FIG 1-4
A splint is made of self-curing polymethylmethacrylate using the repaired mandibular cast as a template. Any missing posterior teeth are replaced by the splint to provide occlusal stops and locks.

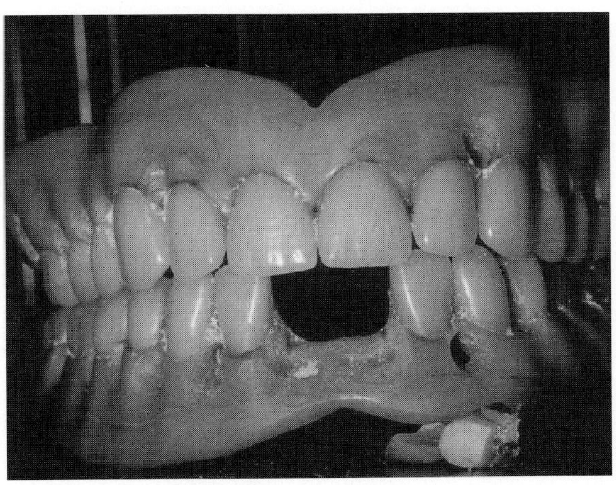

FIG 1-5
Mandibular central incisors are removed from the denture to allow for alimentation, clearing of secretions and egress of vomitus.

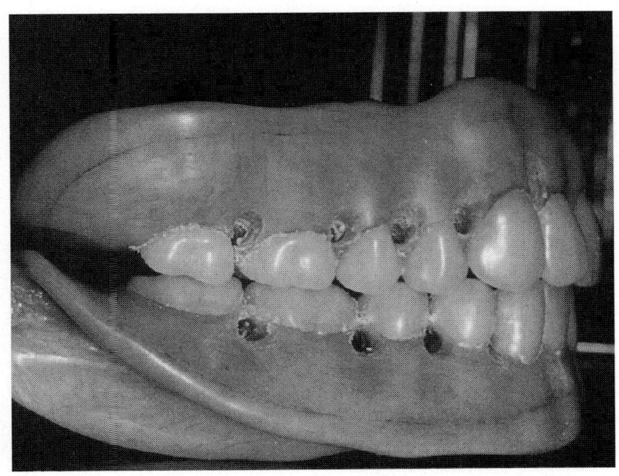

FIG 1-6
Drill holes are placed in the interdental papillae between each posterior tooth and on both sides of the canines.

3. Treatment of symphyseal fractures (two screws placed from opposite sides of the fracture)

Dynamic compression plates. This class includes the most useful of the rigid devices. The list of claimed advantages of these devices over traditional treatment is impressive[7]:

1. Improved patient comfort
2. Maintenance TMJ mobility
3. Ease of oral hygiene
4. Lack of airway concerns
5. Ease of clearance of secretions and vomitus
6. Lower rates of infection, delayed union and nonunion

A

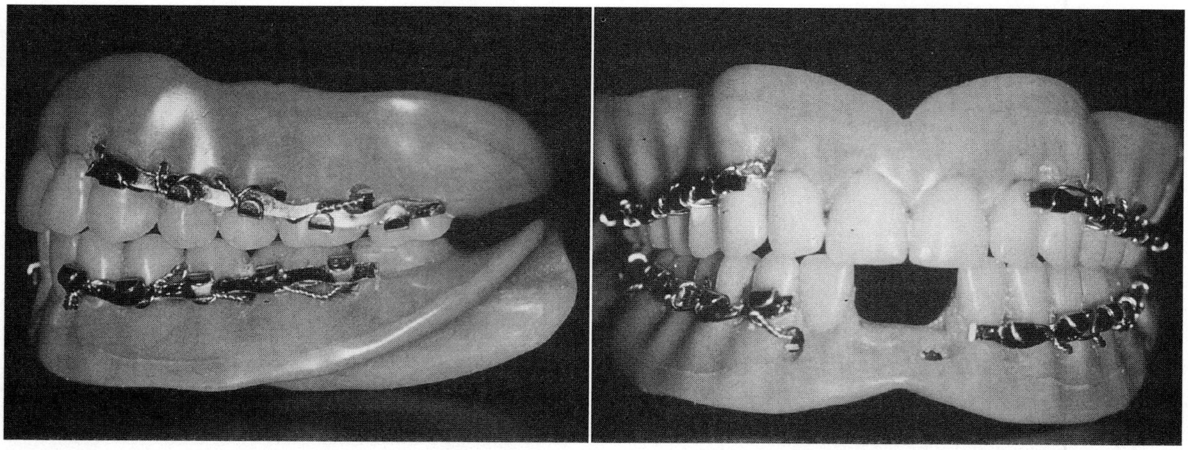

B

FIG 1-7
Arch bars are attached in segments to aid in cosmesis.

The first five of these claims are indisputable and there is accumulating evidence supporting the last group of claims. Where there are advantages, there will usually be disadvantages. The following are the disadvantages of dynamic compression plates (DCP):

1. Need for wide exposure
2. Larger amounts of implanted foreign material
3. Possible need for removal of hardware
   Infection
   Cold intolerance
   The question of possible long-term effects from metallic components of the hardware
4. Longer operating times with associated higher costs
5. Need for expensive, specialized instruments and supplies
6. No possibility of dynamic improvement in fracture reduction

There are several specific indications for DCP's over non-rigid forms of treatment:

1. Poorly controlled seizures when the need for MMF would be eliminated
2. Mandibular fractures combined with LeFort fractures
3. Patient intolerance of MMF
4. Inability to stabilize the fracture(s) with nonrigid means

The types of mandibular fractures that can be treated with DCP's include the following:

1. Body
2. Angle
3. Symphyseal area
4. Multiple fractures that include one or more of the above (note that even if a concomitant condylar fracture dictates a period of MMF, the use of rigid fixation at the other fracture sites allows early removal of the MMF)

Many patients with isolated body of mandible fractures can be treated with either closed reduction combined with MMF or rigid internal fixation with a compression plate. When one technique is not clearly indicated over the other, it seems legitimate to have the patient choose his or her treatment. Some will be happy to suffer the inconvenience of MMF to avoid open surgery, while others will eagerly accept the alternative.

When compression plates are placed at the inferior border of the mandible, distracting forces are produced at the alveolar surface. There are two ways to counteract this: Tension banding may be used in the form of arch bars, tension splints, or tension band plates. An alternative is the use of an eccentric dynamic compression plate (EDCP). EDCP's have an extra set of holes that direct forces superiorly, thus compressing both the inferior and superior borders of the mandible.

Another technical point in using compression plates is the need to slightly over contour them to avoid distracting forces on the lingual side. Three to five degrees of over contouring produces the desired results.

Placement of DCP's requires exacting technique as there is little margin for error. Traditional techniques are much more forgiving and should be mastered first by the inexperienced maxillofacial surgeon.

Pitfalls with compression plating.—The following pitfalls are to be avoided when using DCP's:

1. Failure to provide compression at the superior surface of the mandible
2. Failure to over contour plates, thus allowing splaying on the lingual surface of the mandible
3. Failure to avoid tooth sockets, tooth buds, or the mandibular canal with drill holes
4. Failure to extend plate far enough on either side of the fracture line to allow sufficient screws
5. Failure to ensure security of each screw placed (e.g., failure to use an oversized screw when the hole is stripped)
6. Failure to achieve anatomic reduction/preinjury occlusion before placement of rigid device (temporary placement of MMF is the usual means of accomplishing this goal)

Reconstruction plates.—These devices are an excellent choice for bridging gaps and securing multiple fragments. In the latter application they are unsurpassed.

LOOSE ENDS

Favorable versus unfavorable fracture lines

The vector of force applied by the internal pterygoid muscle is the key to understanding whether a fracture line is favorable or unfavorable. This muscle pulls the angle of the mandible anterially, superiorly, and medially. If a fracture line would be separated by such a force, it is unfavorable. If a fracture line would be compressed by such a force, it is favorable.

A source of considerable confusion has been classifying favorability in regard to vertical versus horizontal. The correct terminology is favorable or unfavorable about the horizontal or vertical axis. Therefore, it is not whether the fragment moves horizontally or vertically but whether the rotation of the posterior fragment is about the horizontal axis (a line through the two mandibular condyles) or vertical axis (a line from superior to inferior through the condyle of the side in question).

Special fractures

Fractures of the alveolar process make up a small percentage of mandibular fractures. However, they can be difficult to treat. We know of no cookbook approach to these fractures. It is necessary to do what is needed to reduce them and to do what is needed to hold the reduction until the fracture is well headed. Techniques to hold them in place include arch bars, dental wiring, interosseous wiring, circummandibular wiring with MMF, and miniplate application. The caution with these fractures is not to underestimate their difficulty.

Condylar area fractures are common. They can usually be treated by simple MMF. There has long been a debate about when open reduction is indicated in the management of these fractures. Some find many indications to open these fractures, while others question if they should ever be opened. We agree with Zide and Kent[8] regarding the absolute indications for opening condylar fractures:

1. Displacement of the condyle into the middle cranial fossa
2. Foreign body embedded in the fracture site
3. Lateral extracapsular displacement of the head of the condyle
4. No other way to reduce the fracture

The same authors present relative indications that we find somewhat confusing, repetitious, and less than convincing.

The tooth in the fracture line

Past teaching was to always extract teeth in fracture lines. In recent years there has been a trend toward conserving teeth when it seems reasonable.[8] Probably, the routine use of antibiotics has contributed to the successful retention of many teeth. In general, teeth associated with periapical or periodontal pathology are extracted. Those that are very mobile are not saved. When the tooth itself has sustained a class III fracture (exposed pulp), it is extracted. Rarely, the presence of a tooth will prevent reduction of a fracture due to a crush deformity of the empty portion of the socket. When this occurs, the crush deformity must be corrected or the tooth extracted. Otherwise, healthy appearing teeth are not condemned simply because of being in a fracture line.

REFERENCES

1. Clark WD, Bailey BJ: Management of fractures of the mandible. In Mathog RH, editor: *Maxillofacial trauma.* Baltimore, 1984, Williams & Wilkins.
2. Clark WD: Management of mandibular fractures. *Amer J of Otolaryng* 13:125, 1992.
3. Dingman RO, Natvig P: *Surgery of facial fractures.* Philadelphia, 1964, WB Saunders.
4. Farris PE, Dierks EJ: Single oblique lag screw fixation of mandibular angle fractures. *Laryngoscope* 102:1070, 1992.
5. Miller RH, editor: *The surgical atlas of airway and facial trauma.* New York, 1983, Grune & Stratton.
6. Niederdellman H, Shetty V: Solitary lag screw osteosynthesis in the treatment of fractures of the angle of the mandible: a retrospective study. *Plast Reconstr Surg,* 80:68, 1987.
7. Spiessl B: Internal Fixation. In Mathog RH, editor: *Maxillofacial trauma.* Baltimore, 1984, Williams & Wilkins.
8. Zide MF, Kent JN: Indications for open reduction of mandibular condyle fractures. *J Oral Maxillofac Surg* 41:89, 1983.

2

Reconstruction of Large Facial Defects after Mohs Surgery

Arnold E. Katz, M.D., M.S., F.A.C.S. and Donald J. Grande, M.D.

Although there are now only a few medical centers that don't include the services of a fellowship-trained dermatologic surgeon for the treatment of extensive and/or recurrent basal cell carcinomas, Frederic E. Mohs' technique of microscopically controlled excision of skin malignancies still has detractors. Indeed, the technique is expensive, time-consuming, and probably over-used. Mohs surgeons are often accused of making larger defects than are necessary. In all likelihood, the opposite is true. The technique has been modified, and today microscopically controlled excision (MCE) of basal cell carcinoma is a method of fresh tissue surgical removal of tumor[12] that allows for microscopic examination of the entire undersurface and peripheral margins of the surgical specimen. Multiple random biopsies do not accomplish this result. Mohs surgery not only produces the highest cure rate of any available skin cancer treatment,[15] but it also provides for the maximal conservation of normal surrounding tissue.[11]

One need not treat all basal cell carcinomas with Mohs surgery. Specific locations of the face, especially around the eyes, nose, lips, and ears, are areas of high recurrence rates and may benefit from this technique.[10] Large, greater than 2 cm in diameter, and/or recurrent tumors,[1] especially of the morpheoform type, should also be treated by this method. Immunocompromised patients, young patients, patients exposed to therapeutic doses of x-ray or ultraviolet light, or those patients with basal cell nevus syndrome should be strongly considered for Mohs micrographic surgery (see box on p. 12).

While most basal cell carcinomas are highly curable, some are extremely difficult to treat; and indeed, some patients present with lesions for which there is no effective therapy (Fig. 2-1, *A* and *B*). Perineural spread[7] and metastatic spread[1] of basal cell carcinoma have been reported. "Anyone who thinks there are no problem cases of basal cell carcinoma has either not seen very many patients with these tumors or does not do an adequate follow-up."[1]

PREOPERATIVE PLANNING

Most defects after Mohs excision can and should be closed primarily and immediately. For example, in patients with excessive lower lid and glabellar laxity (Fig. 2-2, *A*), primary closure will yield excellent results in the medial canthal area (Fig. 2-2, *B*). Many defects can yield excellent cosmetic results when allowed to heal by secondary intention.[14] When, however, it is felt that collaboration with a facial plastic surgeon is a likely possibility, preoperative consultation is indicated. During the preoperative evaluation, the patient must be informed that the size of the defect following excision cannot always be accurately predicted. Reconstructive techniques should be described in as comforting and reassuring a manner as possible. Photographs of similar lesions of different sizes from previous patients are extremely helpful during these consultations. Patients must be told that although appearance will be "OK" weeks after surgery, the reconstruction will require months for the scars to mature and become much less noticeable. While secondary procedures, scar revisions, and dermabrasion should also be discussed, it is our experience that they are rarely required.

Because most of the patients are elderly, complete history and physical examination is necessary prior to Mohs excision of the malignancy. Silent cardiac abnormalities and other general medical problems should be evaluated, so that these issues will not arise encountered during or after the Mohs excision and prevent the reconstruction from proceeding as planned.

This course will discuss the facial reconstructive techniques that have been most useful for us in dealing with large and/or difficult defects most often encountered after Mohs surgery. Some of the more common reconstructive

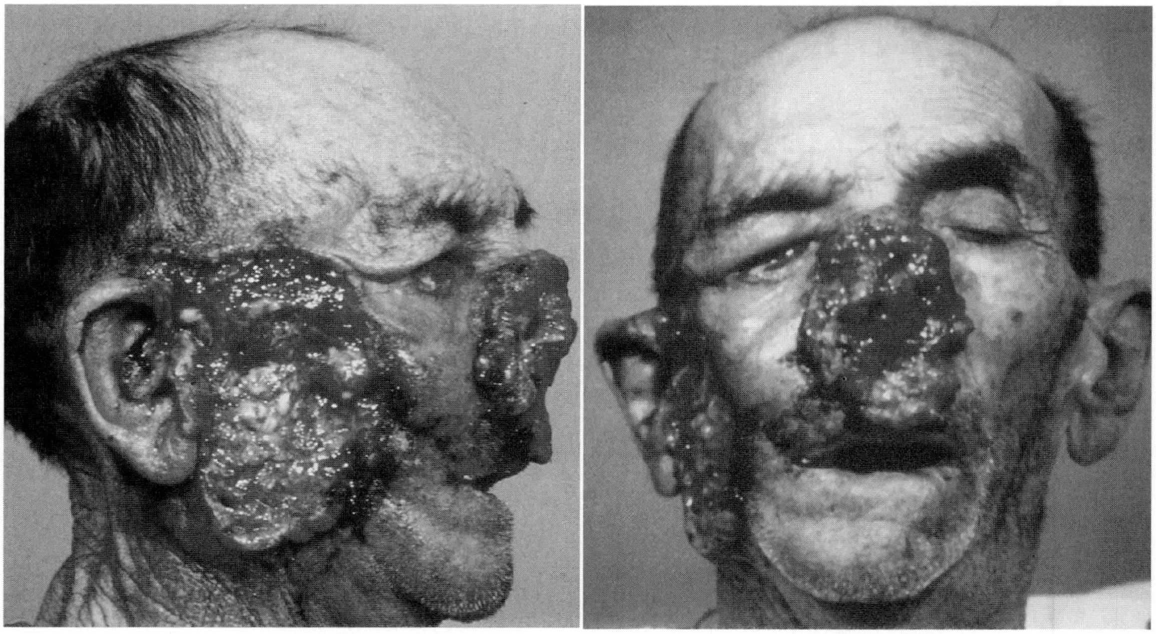

FIG 2-1
A, Lateral view of a patient with advanced disease for which there is no effective therapy. **B,** Frontal view of same patient

> **Indications for Micrographic Surgery**
>
> High recurrence areas (near the eyes, nose, lips, and ears)
> Recurrent tumors
> Morpheoform tumors
> Tumors greater than 2 cm in diameter
> Immunocompromised patients
> Young patients
> Previous history of x-ray or ultraviolet light treatment for acne
> Basal cell nevus syndrome

complications will also be discussed, with special emphasis on their prevention and management.

ADVANCEMENT-ROTATION FLAPS

We have found these flaps to be extremely helpful in the one-stage reconstruction of large defects of the midface.[8] They are relatively easy to design, if one keeps the basic parameters in mind. The arc of the flap should be four times the diameter of the defect to assure closure of the donor site, without the necessity of additional flaps and/or grafts (Fig. 2-3). We have found these flaps extremely hearty and versatile for closure of defects involving the nose, cheek, lower eye lid, medial canthal area, temple, and combina-tions of the above.[3] The following examples demonstrate principles to be considered when employing this technique:

Case 1

The defect after removal of a basal cell carcinoma measured 3.5 × 3.0 cm (Fig. 2-4, *A*) and was easily closed with an advancement-rotation flap, trimming the standing-cone deformity in the nasolabial groove as a single-stage procedure (Fig. 2-4, *B*). While the result was satisfactory, with no distortion of the lower lid or upper lip, the horizontal scar across the upper cheek was noticeable (Fig. 2-4, *C*). As the next two cases will demonstrate, raising a larger flap than is necessary for closure, will yield a more favorable result.

Cases 2 and 3

A similarly placed defect resulted in a more acceptable result by carrying the incision gently but directly into an infraorbital crease, continuing into a lateral canthal wrinkle, a preauricular crease, and, finally, a prominent wrinkle in the neck (Fig. 2-5, *A* and *B*). Even larger defects in this area are favorably reconstructed with this design (Fig. 2-6, *A* and *B*).

Case 4

It is extremely important for the reconstructive surgeon to examine the patient and document findings after

A

B

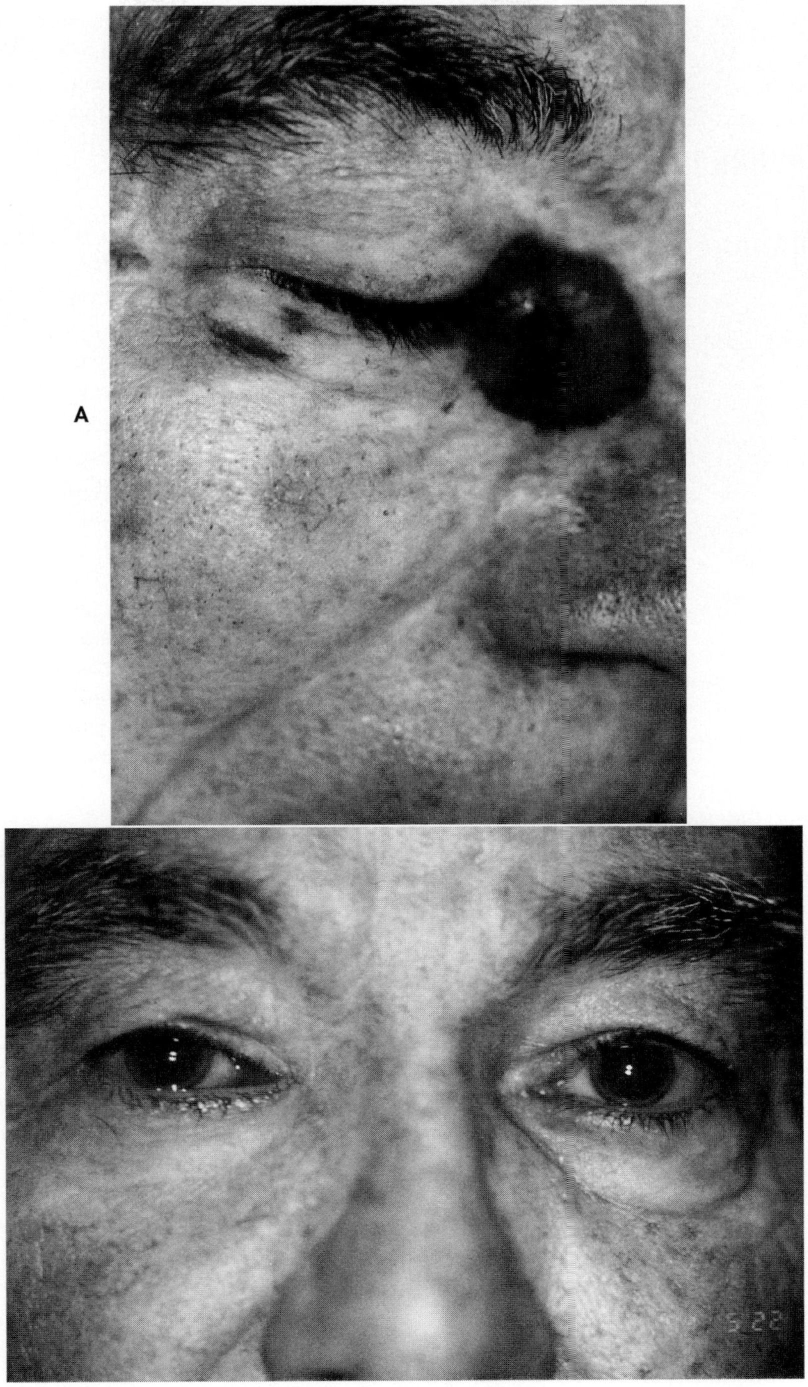

FIG 2-2
A, Patient with lower lid and glabellar laxity. **B,** Excellent result with primary closure and the removal of Burrow's triangles.

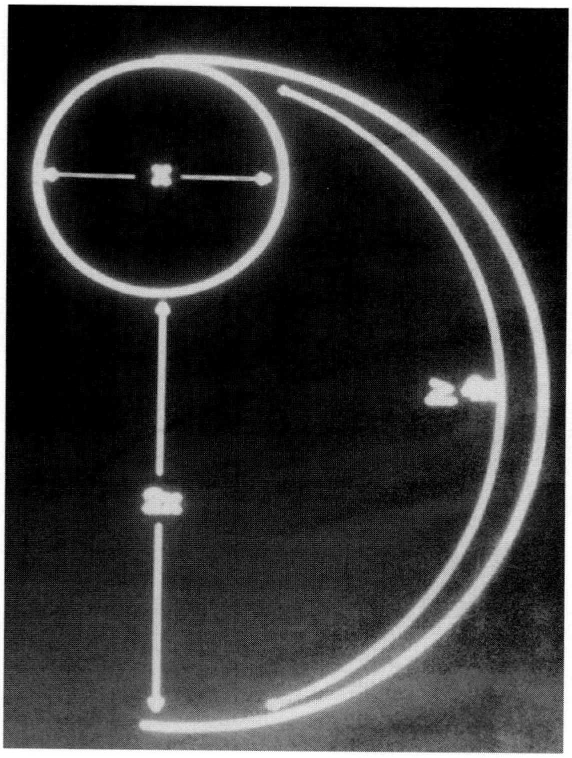

FIG 2-3
In advancement-rotation flaps, closure is easily accomplished when the arc is four times the diameter of the defect.

Mohs surgery, but before the reconstruction. When one examines any patient with a defect around the eye, function of the lid should always be noted (Fig. 2-7, *A* and *B*). Even after reconstruction with a cheek-neck advancement-rotation flap designed as described above, weakness of the lower lid and the accompanying Bell's phenomenon was obvious (Fig. 2-7, *C*). Since the weakness was present preoperatively, it was decided not to explore the facial branches which were at risk during the reconstruction. A satisfactory result with full spontaneous recovery of the facial nerve was noted several months postoperative (Fig. 2-7, *D* and *E*).

Cases 5 and 6

When multiple lesions are present in relatively close proximity, the Mohs surgeon should be encouraged to excise these neoplasms simultaneously. If this is not done, it is conceivable that the flaps designed for the reconstruction could inadvertently involve the second lesion and thereby spread tumor. The advancement-rotation flap can be used to reconstruct multiple defects simultaneously (Fig. 2-8, *A-C*) or in combination with other techniques, such as primary closure (Fig. 2-9, *A-C*).

Case 7

RS presented with a 20-year history of recurrent basal cell carcinoma despite treatment with surgery and radiation therapy (Fig. 2-10, *A*). Treatment with Mohs surgery resulted in a defect of the nose, lower lid, medial canthus, and cheek, measuring 6.5 × 5.5 cm (Fig. 2-10, *B*). Reconstruction with a cheek-neck advancement-rotation flap (Fig. 2-10, *C*) yielded a satisfactory result, without the necessity of tissue expanders or grafts (Fig. 2-10, *D*).

Case 8

After having a recurrent basal cell carcinoma treated with Mohs surgery, MG was told that there was tumor extending along the infraorbital nerve and into the periorbital fat (Fig. 2-11, *A*). An orbital exenteration with a partial maxillectomy was recommended and completed (Fig. 2-11, *B*). Reconstruction was accomplished with an advancement-rotation flap lined with a split-thickness skin graft (Fig. 2-11, *C*) with an acceptable result (Fig. 2-11, *D*); however, the pathologist reported that there was no tumor seen in the specimen. It was only after the Mohs surgeon pointed out to the pathologist where the tumor was to be found that it could be documented along the infraorbital nerve (Fig. 2-11, *E*). Random biopsies, even done with the complete specimen in hand, is not as accurate in following basal cell carcinoma as with horizontally oriented sectioning as described by Frederic E. Mohs. Multiple random biopsies should not be described as Mohs surgery.

Cases 9 and 10

Although the cheek-neck advancement-rotation flap is not frequently recommended for lip reconstruction, it can be very helpful in preventing superolateral tension on the upper lip with upward distortion of the vermillion boarder in those patients, in which one might recommend cheek advancement (Fig. 2-12, *A*)). After elevating the flap (Fig. 2-12, *B*), all the tension should be controlled with suturing the flap to the nasal ala and allowing the remaining portion of the flap to "fall into place," thereby reconstructing the upper lip without any tension or distortion of the vermillion boarder (Fig. 2-12, *C*). This technique is especially of value when a large portion of the cheek is removed along with the lip. An excellent result was achieved in reconstructing an 8.3 × 7.6 cm combined defect of the cheek and lip, even after some early postoperative cyanosis resolved spontaneously (Fig. 2-13, *A-C*).

Case 11

It is not uncommon for a flap, which may appear cyanotic either during or shortly after the procedure, to survive after the cessation of anesthesia. It is uncommon for a "good-looking" flap to die in the postoperative period, un-

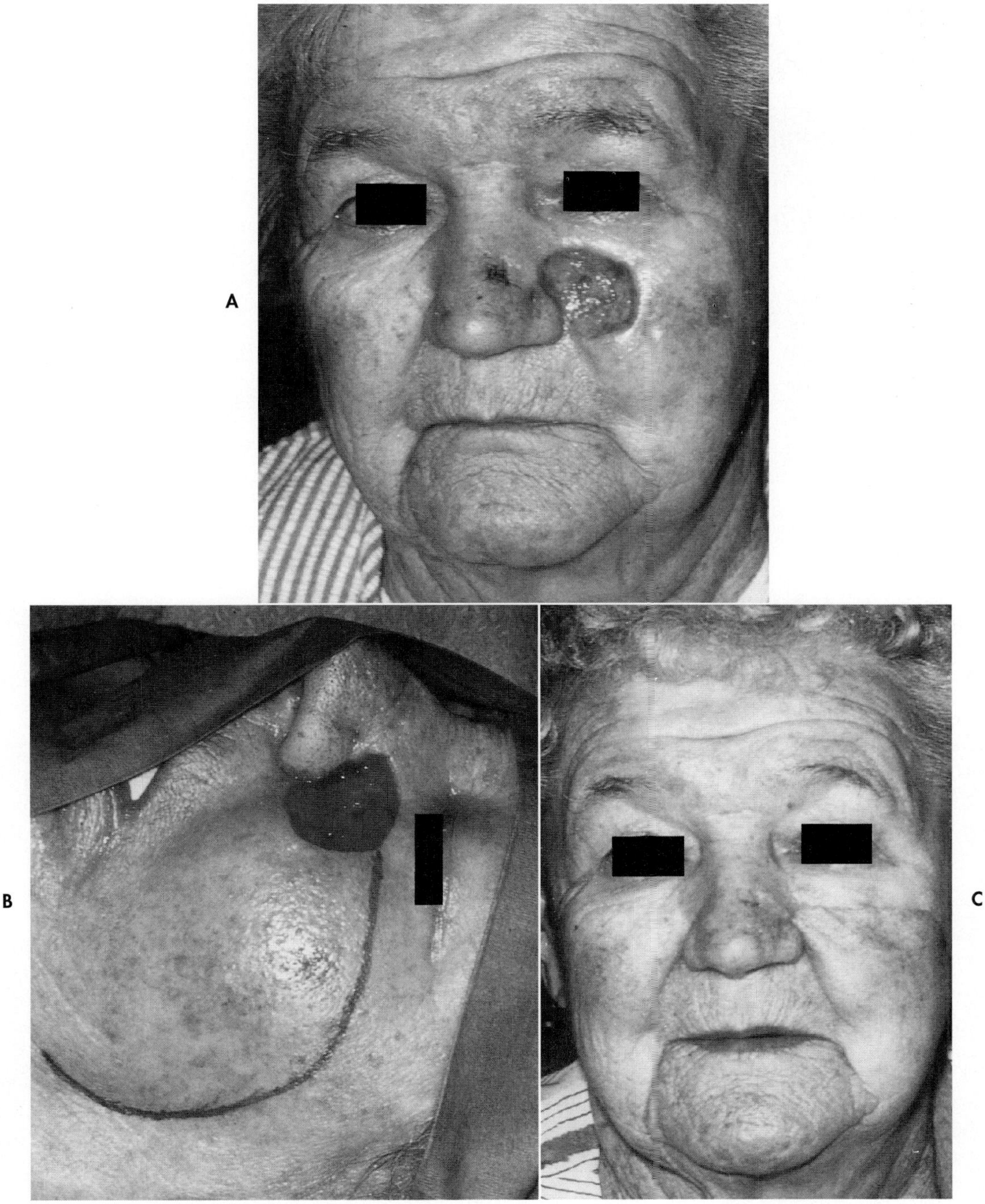

FIG 2-4
Case 1. **A,** Facial defect after excision of basal cell carcinoma, measuring 3.5 × 3.0 cm. **B,** Design of advancement-rotation flap. **C,** Horizontal scar across cheek is less than ideal.

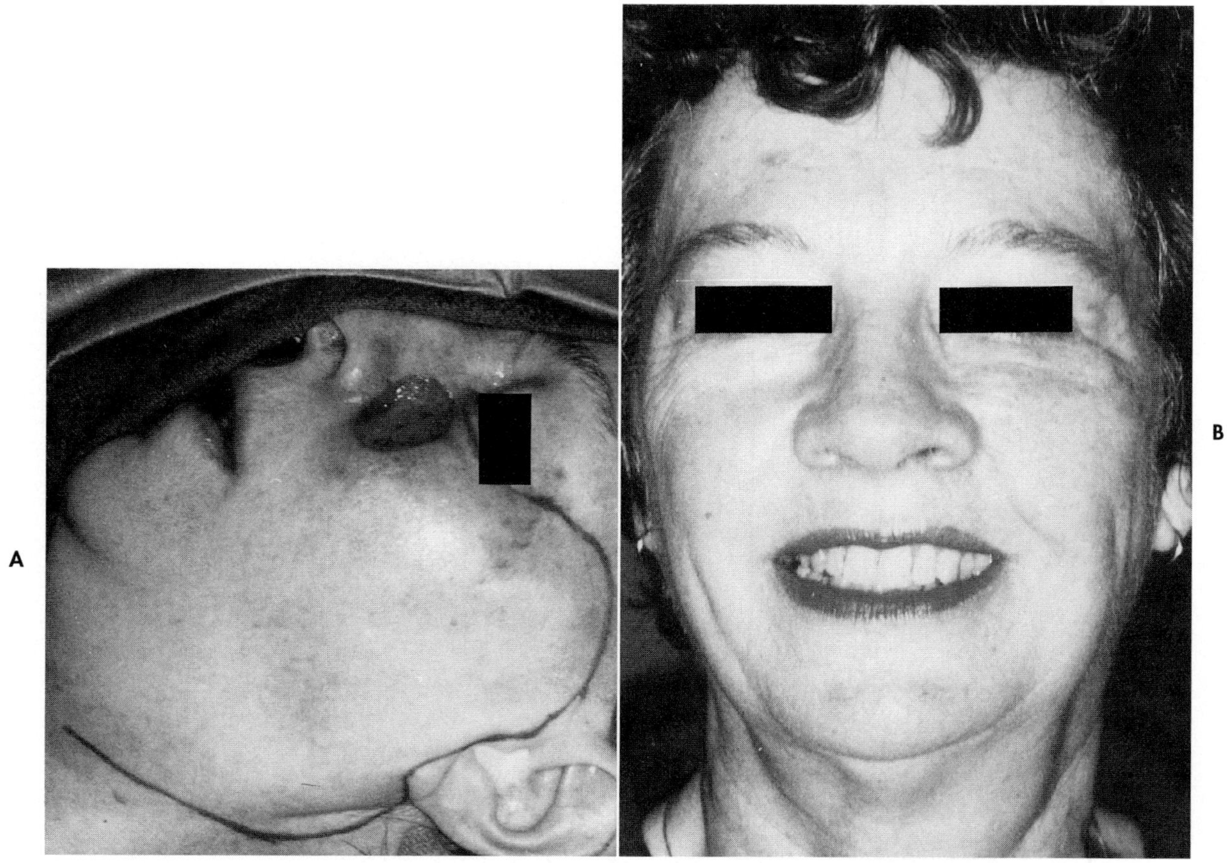

FIG 2-5
Case 2. **A,** More appropriate design of advancement-rotation flap utilizing infraorbital crease. **B,** Horizontal incision is less obvious.

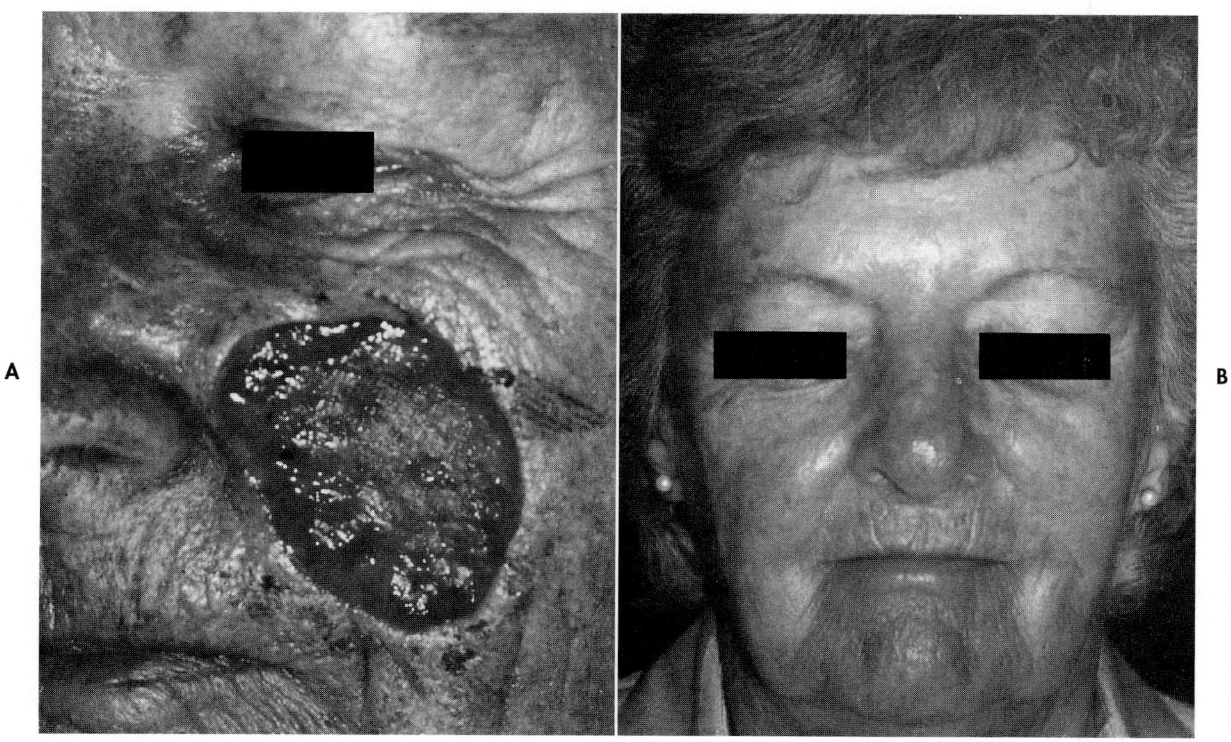

FIG 2-6
Case 3. **A,** Large defect of cheek after Mohs surgery. **B,** Result 6 months postoperatively.

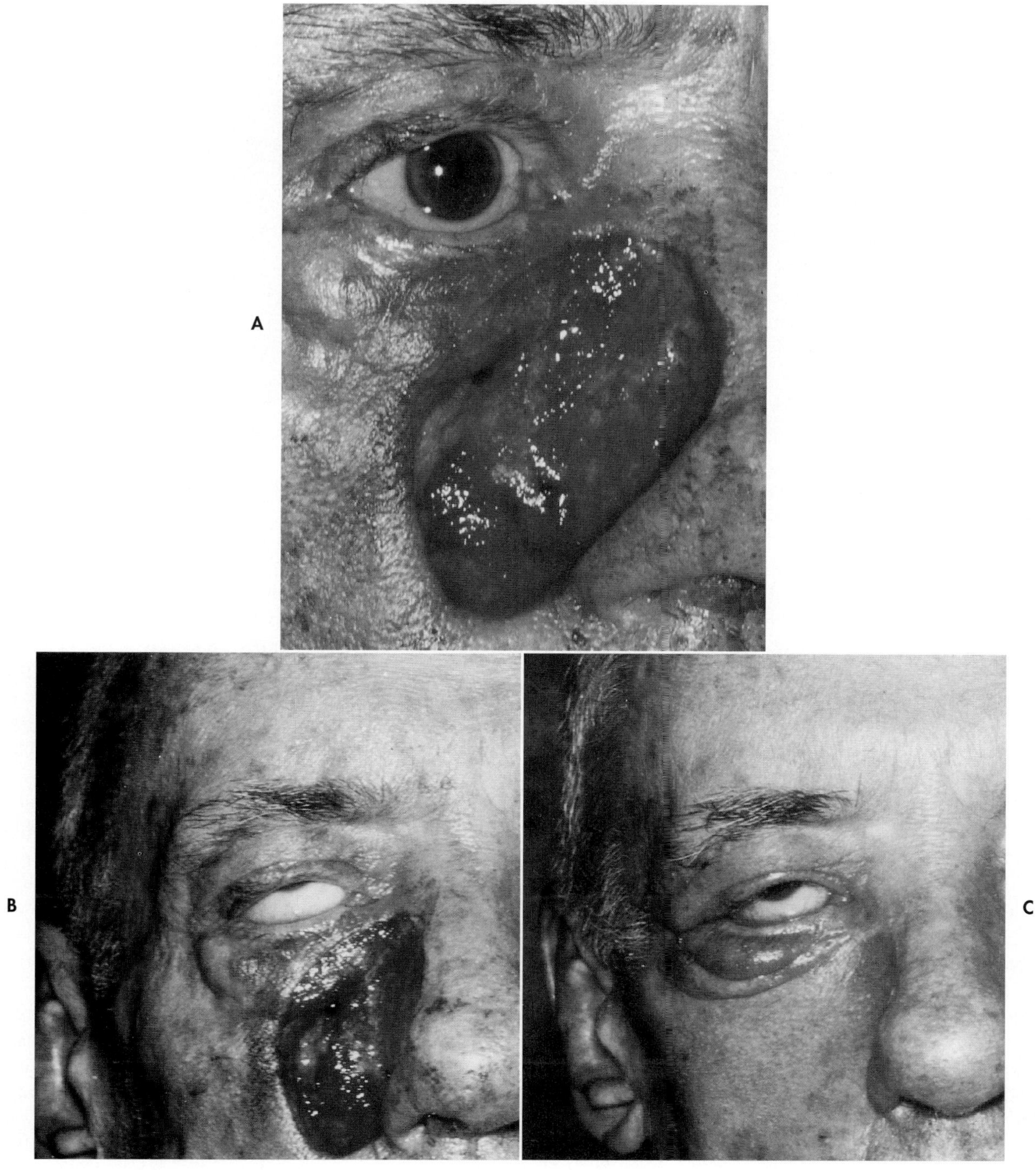

FIG 2-7
Case 4. **A,** Defect of nose, eyelid, and cheek after Mohs surgery. **B,** Weakness of lower lid documented before reconstruction. **C,** Weakness persists after reconstruction with advancement-rotation flap.

D 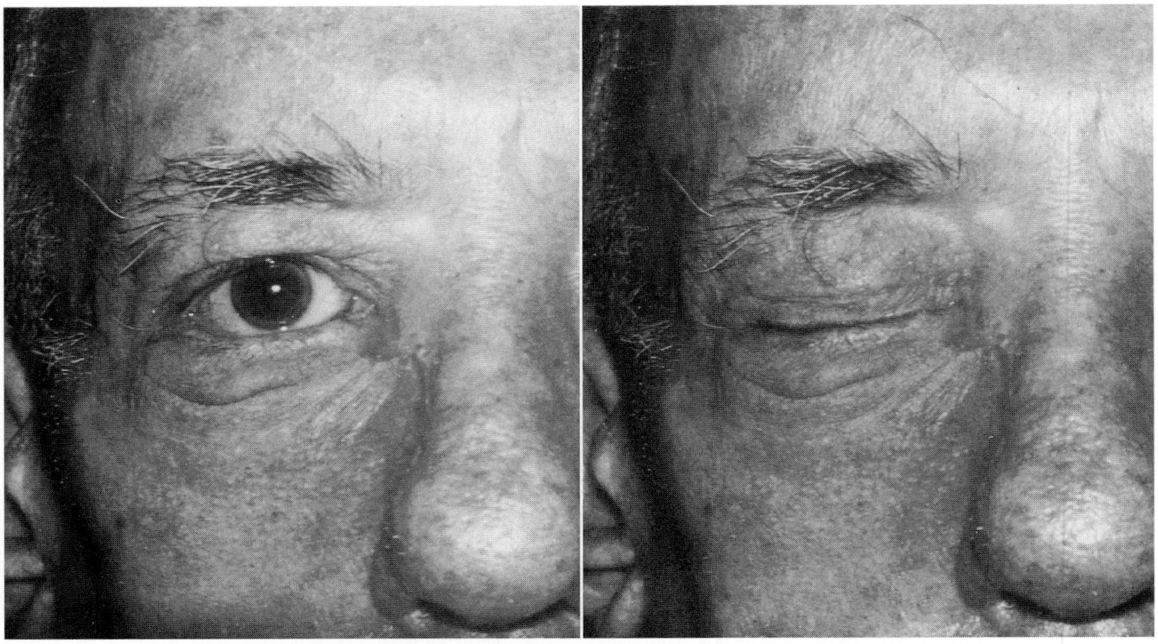 E

FIG 2-7, cont'd
D, Excellent result 6 months postoperative. **E,** Spontaneous recovery of seventh nerve.

less there is a postoperative technical misadventure or the host is a smoker. LW was left with a 4.4 × 3.7 cm defect of the cheek (Fig. 2-14, *A*) and was reconstructed with an advancement-rotation flap as described as above (Fig. 2-14, *B*). Before the flap was elevated it was liberally injected with local anesthesia with epinephrine at 1:100,000 concentration. The patient was a heavy smoker and the flap died (Fig. 2-14, *C*). The wound was treated with debridement only of the dry crusted debris without grafting or additional tissue transfer. The patient cleaned the wound with one-half strength hydrogen peroxide three times a day and applied a thin coat of bacitracin ointment. He was followed closely as an outpatient and given a great deal of support and encouragement. The defect healed quite satisfactorily by secondary intention (Fig. 2-14, *D*, and *E*). Presently, we do not use any epinephrine in our local anesthesia or inject preoperatively when general anesthesia is employed to assist with hemostasis. We advise all of our patients to stop smoking for one week preoperative and at least one week postoperative. When flaps or parts of flaps do not survive, they are treated conservatively as described above with surprisingly good results.

GRAFTING

Grafting can be quite helpful in the repair of certain defects of the temple, forehead, and nose. One must, however, make every attempt to avoid the two most common pitfalls of grafting: poor color and/or texture match and the "step-off" deformity (Fig. 2-15).

Full-thickness skin grafts frequently result in a more desirable outcome than split-thickness grafts. Grafts from the post-auricular area are usually not a good match for the nose, and skin from the chest, abdomen, or extremities should not be grafted to the face if at all possible. One should always attempt to select a donor sight as close to the defect as possible. Preauricular, nasolabial, and supraclavicular skin are often available and are usually an excellent match for defects about the face.

The "step-off" deformity can be avoided by allowing a deep wound to granulate for two to three weeks, by suturing the edges of the defect to the bed, or by utilizing the purse-string subcuticular partial closure before grafting.[5]

The purse-string suture[9] makes it possible to decrease the size of most facial defects by about 50%.[4] Decreasing the size of a defect allows for the harvesting of a smaller graft, which may be more easily obtainable from a favorable donor sight. The technique is quite simple and usually utilizes a 3-0 or 4-0 Proline suture. The entry point should be about 5 mm from the edge of the defect (Fig. 2-16, *A*). In a subcuticular fashion, the suture is placed until a 90 degree arc has been traversed. At that point, the suture is brought through the skin 5 mm from the edge of the defect (Fig. 2-16, *B*). Before reentering the wound, a pull-through suture of different color is placed to help stabilize the purse-

A

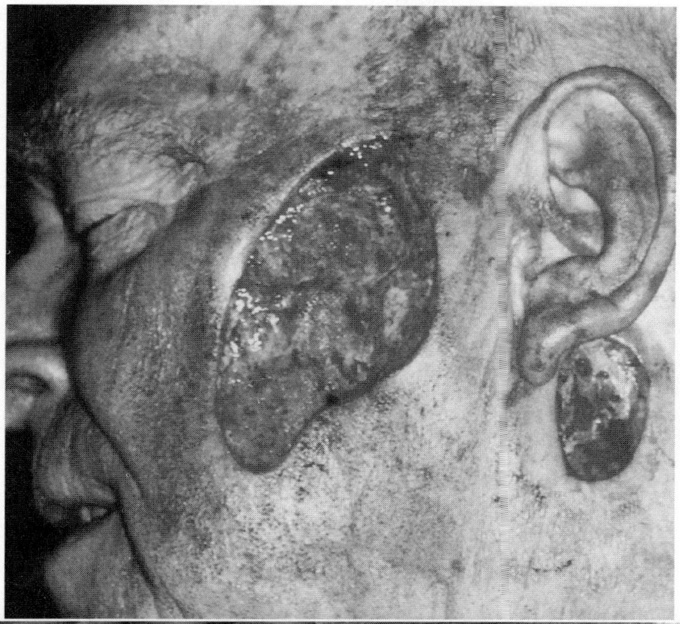

B

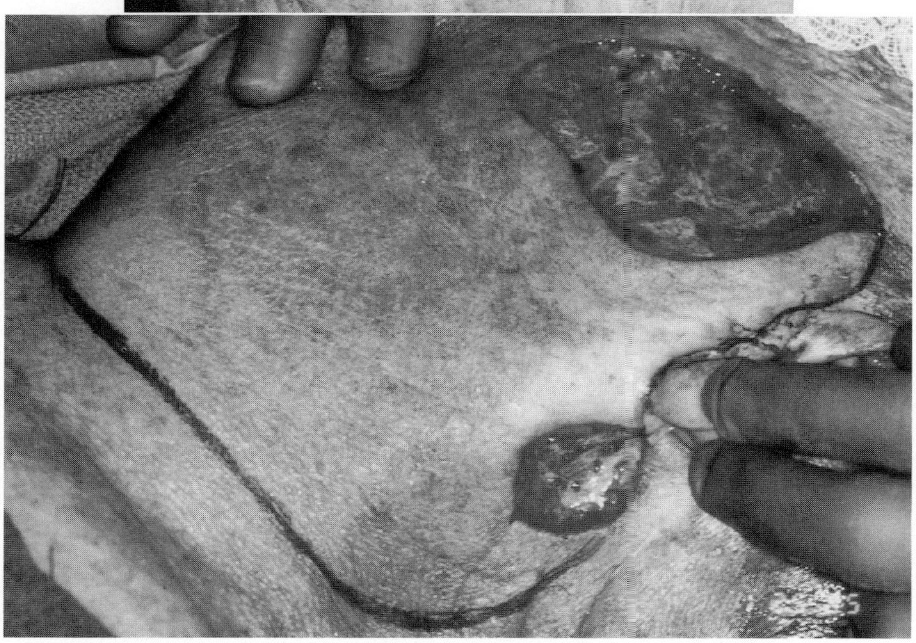

FIG 2-8
Case 5. **A,** Multiple basal cell carcinomas removed simultaneously. **B,** Design of advancement-rotation flap incorporating both defects.

C

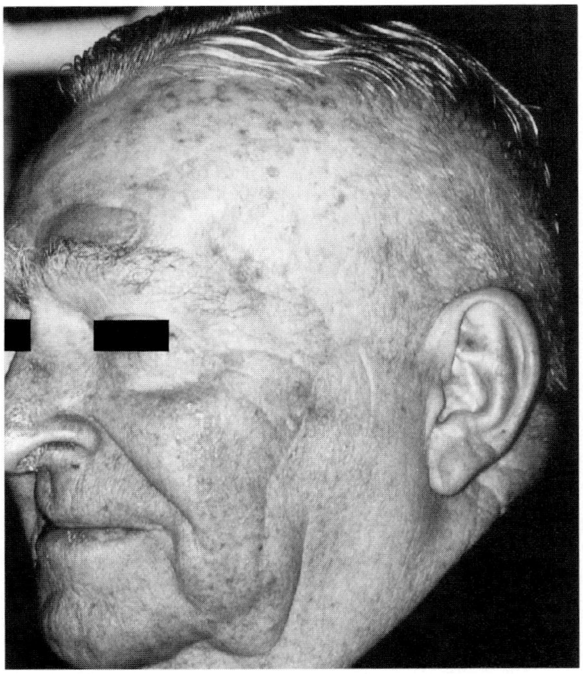

FIG 2-8, cont'd
C, Satisfactory result with single-stage procedure.

string suture and to provide for easy access at the time of suture removal. This procedure is repeated until the purse-string suture traverses the 360 degrees and is then tied with care so as not to distort adjacent structures (Fig. 2-16, *C*).

Case 12

The "step-off" deformity can be prevented by allowing a wound to granulate before grafting. Three weeks after excision, the edges are rolled and the depth of the wound has filled in with granulation tissue (Fig. 2-17, *A*). After the edges have been freshened and a supraclavicular full-thickness skin graft has taken, the results are quite acceptable, without any distortion of the brow or lower lid (Fig. 2-17, *B*). We rarely use this option at present, however, because of the great inconvenience of caring for the wound for this extended period of time. As will be described later, the purse-string subcuticular suture accomplishes the desired result much more conveniently for the patient.

Case 13

When the defect is not deep and the skin of the nose is quite thin (Fig. 2-18, *A*), immediate grafting with a full-thickness supraclavicular graft can provide excellent results. In this situation, a flap would most likely have been too thick, resulting in a loss of the fine tip features, which have been preserved with this full-thickness skin graft (Fig. 2-18, *B*).

Case 14

Grafting can and should be combined with local flaps when both techniques are indicated. A 56-year-old female sustained a 2.0 × 2.0 cm defect involving the upper third of the columella, the nasal tip, and the right alar rim (Fig. 2-19, *A*). Before suturing a full-thickness supraclavicular graft, advancement flaps of the right nasal ala and the columella were raised and turned in place. An excellent result can be observed at one year postoperative (Fig. 2-19, *B* and *C*).

Case 15

The "step-off" deformity can also be minimized by suturing the edges of the defect to the bed of the wound. A 15.0 × 9.5 cm defect of the forehead and temporal area resulted from the removal of a morpheoform basal cell carcinoma (Fig. 2-20, *A*) and was reconstructed with a split-thickness skin graft after tacking the edges of the wound to the bed under tension. This not only decreased the area to be covered but also helped eliminate the "step-off" deformity. After the antibiotic impregnated cotton batten bolster dressing (Fig. 2-20, *B*) was removed, the potential deformity could easily be appreciated (Fig. 2-20, *C*). Without any additional surgery, the above described technique resulted in complete elimination of the "step-off" as demonstrated several years later (Fig. 2-20, *D*).

Cases 16 and 17

The purse-string suture as described above is a convenient way to eliminate the "step-off" deformity and reduce the size of the defect by about 50%. It has proved to be extremely valuable in reconstructing the preauricular and glabellar areas. An 8.0 × 5.5 cm preauricular defect (Fig. 2-21, *A*) was converted to a 5.0 × 4.0 cm area, leading to partial closure with normal hair-bearing skin (Fig. 2-21, *B*). A 5.6 × 5.0 glabellar defect involving the medial aspects of both upper and lower eye lids (Fig. 2-22, *A*) was reconstructed with a purse-string suture and a full thickness skin graft in a single-stage procedure (Fig. 2-22, *B*).

Case 18 and 19

The purse-string suture is particularly well suited for midline defects of the nose, especially in patients with a generous, drooping tip (Fig. 2-23, *A*). The tip is refined and raised (Fig. 2-23, *B*) so that the graft completes the appearance of a more youthful-looking nose (Fig. 2-23, *C*). When the lesion is off midline (Fig. 2-24, *A*), resulting in an asymmetric defect (Fig. 2-24, *B*), the remaining skin of the nose should be harvested (Fig. 2-24, *C*). In most cases, this nasal skin will provide sufficient tissue for grafting after the purse-string suture has decreased the size of the original de-

Text continued on p. 25.

A

B

C

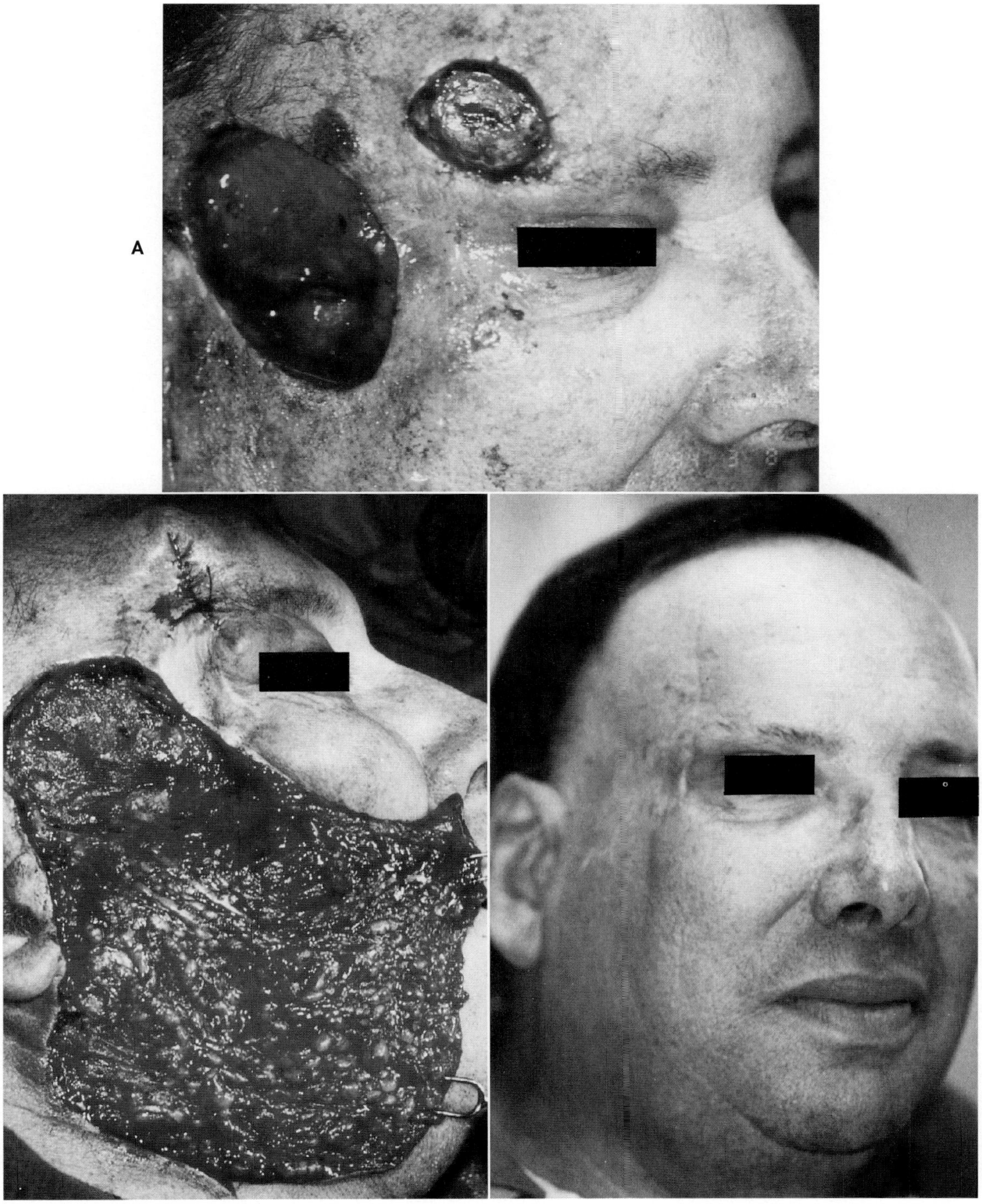

FIG 2-9
Case 6. **A and B,** Basal cell carcinomas removed simultaneously. **C,** Lesions closed separately with primary closure (forehead) and advancement-rotation flap (temple).

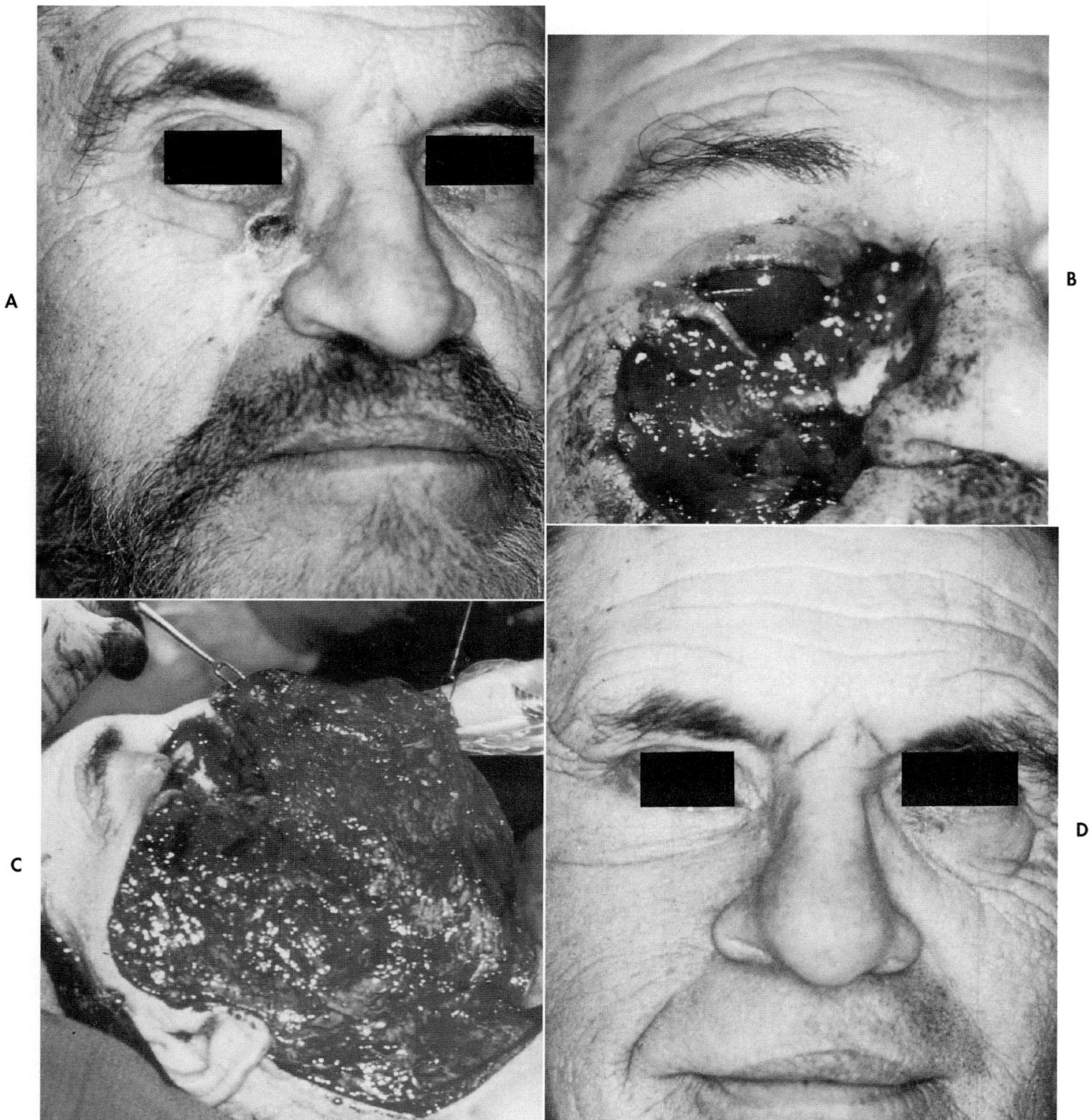

FIG 2-10
Case 7. **A,** Recurrent basal cell carcinoma. **B,** Defect after Mohs excision measuring 6.5 × 5.5 cm. **C,** Design of advancement-rotation flap. **D,** Result of single-stage repair 6 months postoperative.

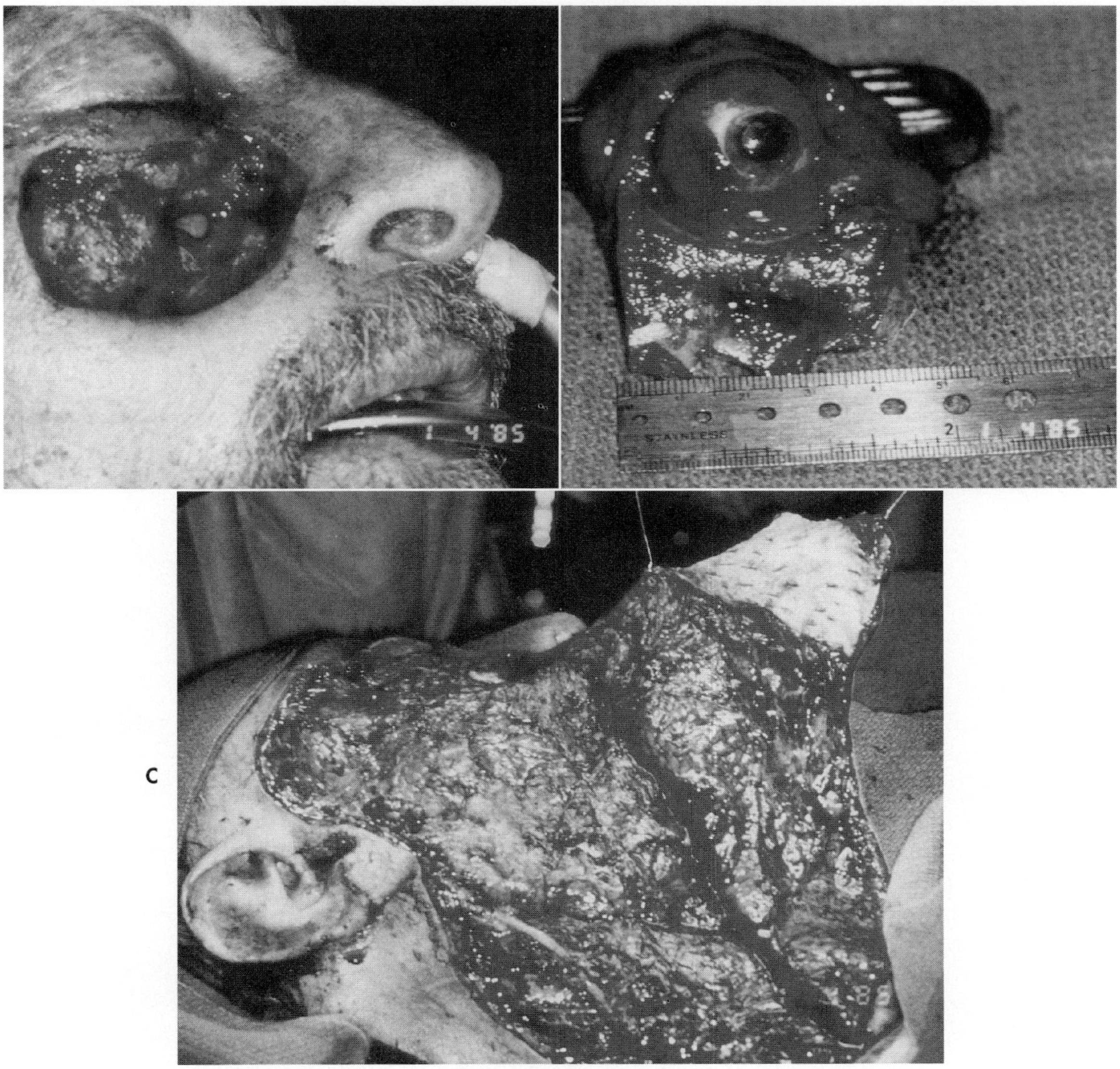

FIG 2-11
Case 8. **A,** Defect with residual basal cell carcinoma reported along infraorbital nerve. **B,** Orbital exenteration with partial maxillectomy. **C,** Reconstruction with advancement-rotation flap, lined with split-thickness skin graft.

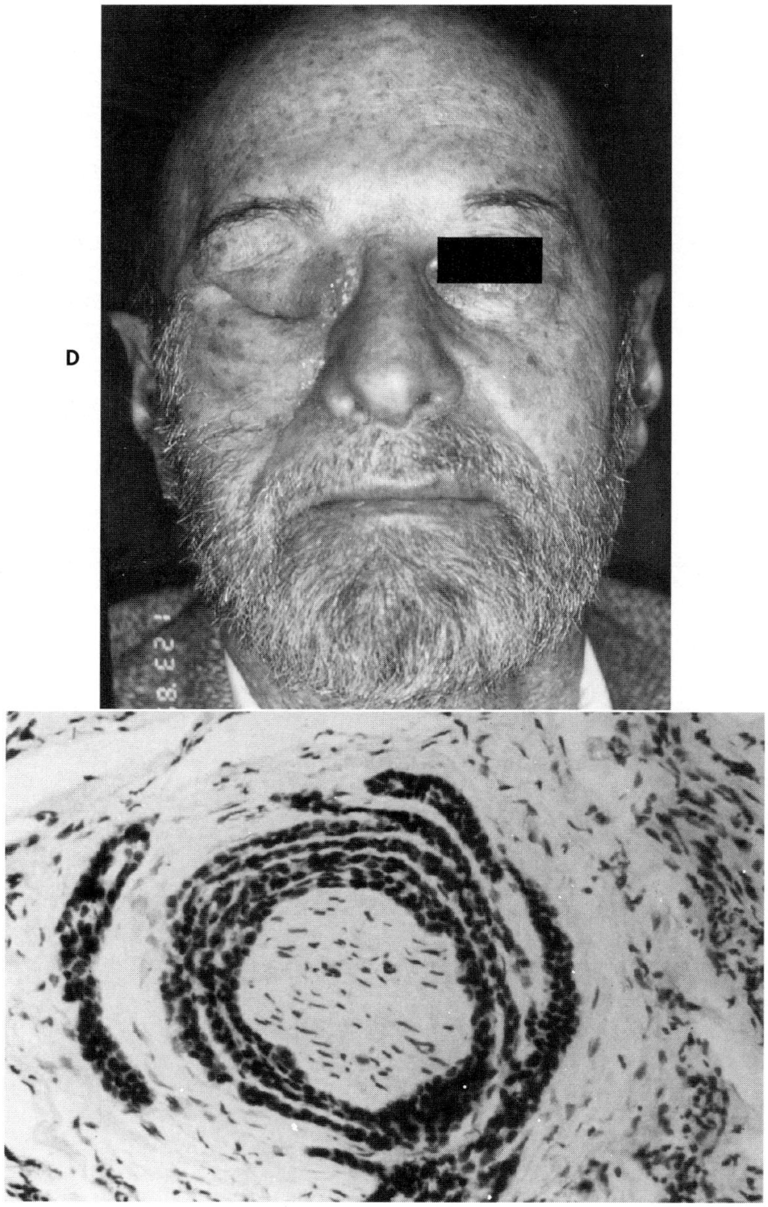

FIG 2-11, cont'd
D, Postoperative result at 3 weeks. **E,** Tumor documented along infraorbital nerve.

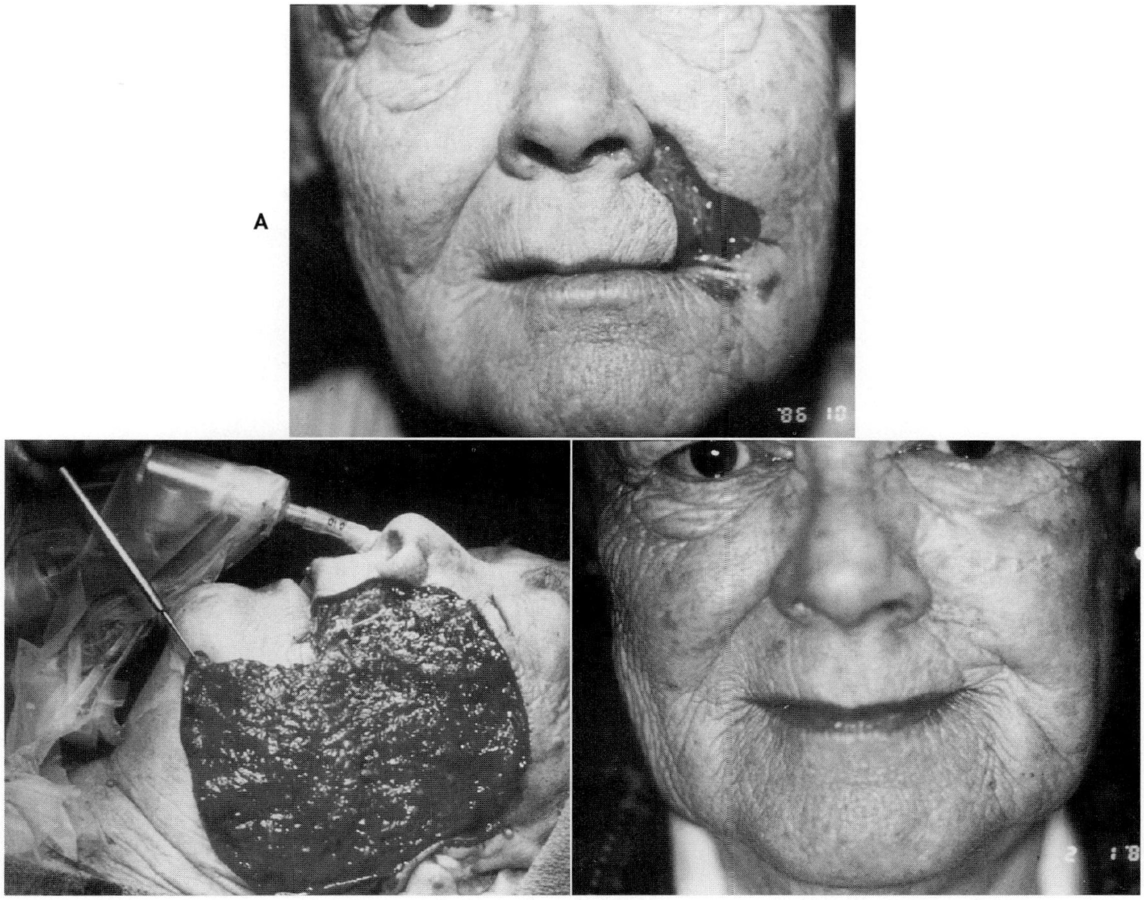

FIG 2-12
Case 9. **A,** Defect of lip after Mohs surgery. **B,** Design of advancement rotation flap. **C,** Result 2 months postoperative with no distortion of vermillion border.

fect. This case also demonstrates the improved appearance of the nose when compared to the bulbousity and drooping of the tip that was present before the lesion was removed (Fig. 2-24, *D* and *E*).

TRANSPOSITION FLAPS

For most lateral defects of the nose, bilobe or nasolabial transposition flaps provide a simple single-stage reconstruction with quite acceptable results. Grafting lateral defects of the nose leads to distortion and asymmetrical elevation of the ipsilateral nasal ala.

Case 20

While it is usually possible to utilize either the bilobe or the nasolabial for smaller defects of the nose, the reconstruction for each patient should be individualized. After the patient is anesthetized, consider several options (Fig. 2-25, *A*) and determine which procedure will result in the least secondary distortion and/or scarring (Fig. 2-25, *B*). If the entire cosmetic unit is undermined, it is possible to avoid the "pin-cushioning," which can result when the recipient bed contracts with the normal scarring process (Fig. 2-25, *C*).

Cases 21 and 22

For larger defects of the lateral nasal wall (Fig. 2-26, *A*), the nasolabial flap (Fig. 2-26, *B*) is often useful. With through-and-through 3-0 chromic quilting sutures, it is even possible to create the illusion of an alar crease (Fig. 2-26, *C*), which does help to camouflage the reconstruction over time (Fig. 2-26, *D*). This is possible even for full-thickness defects of the lateral wall of the nose (Fig. 2-27, *A-D*).

MULTIPLE FLAPS

One should be prepared to consider the possibility of utilizing multiple flaps, instead of attempting to search for the single flap to solve the reconstructive problem at hand. Although a well-designed single flap usually solves most reconstructive problems, at times multiple flaps may yield a

Text continued on p. 35.

A

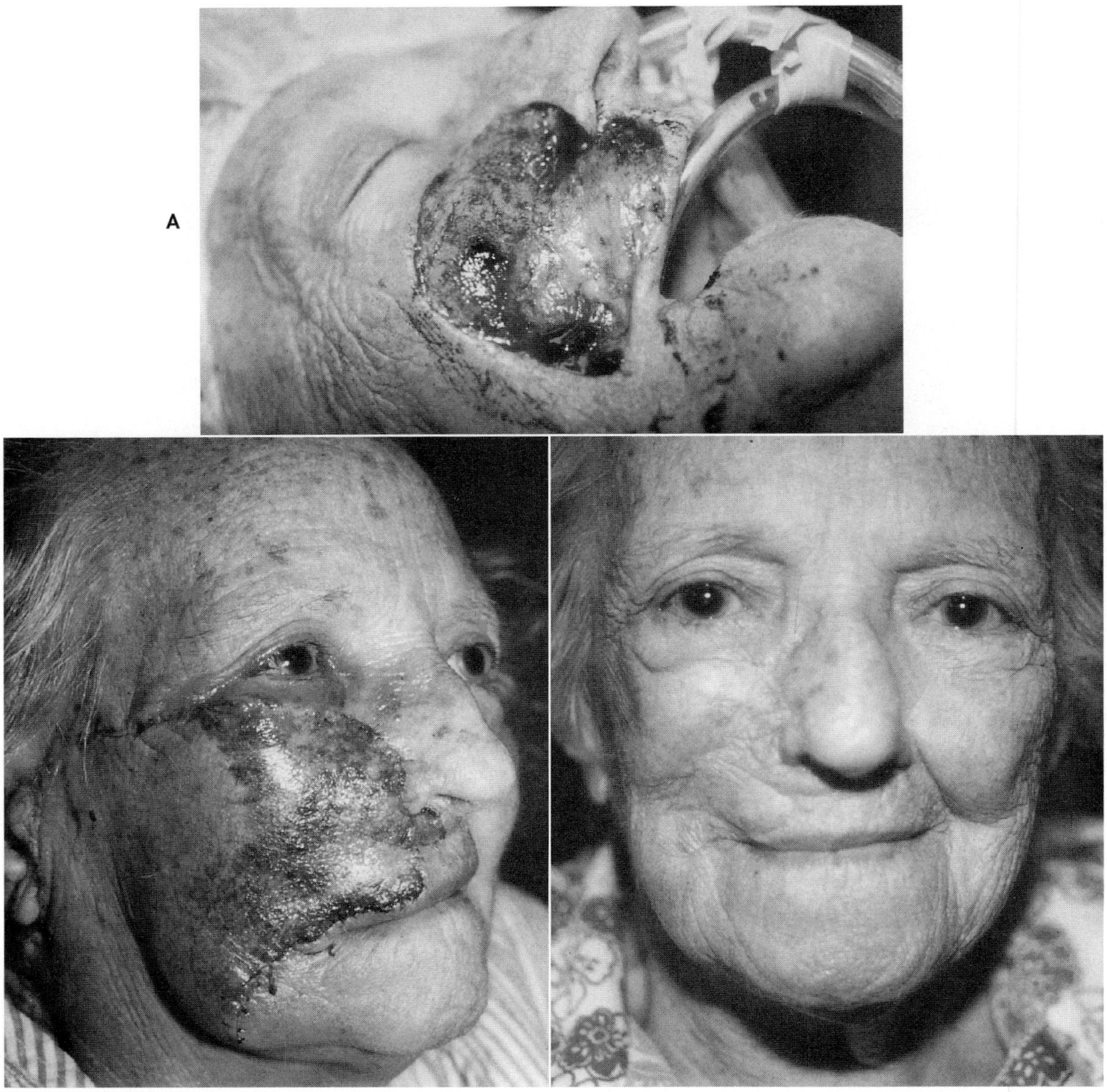

B

C

FIG 2-13
Case 10. **A,** Defect of cheek and lip measuring 8.3 × 7.6 cm. **B,** Cyanosis noted on fourth postoperative day. **C,** Result at 5 months postoperative. (From Katz AE and Grande DJ: Defects after Mohs surgery. In AAO-HNS: Instructional Courses, vol. 2, 1989, Mosby.)

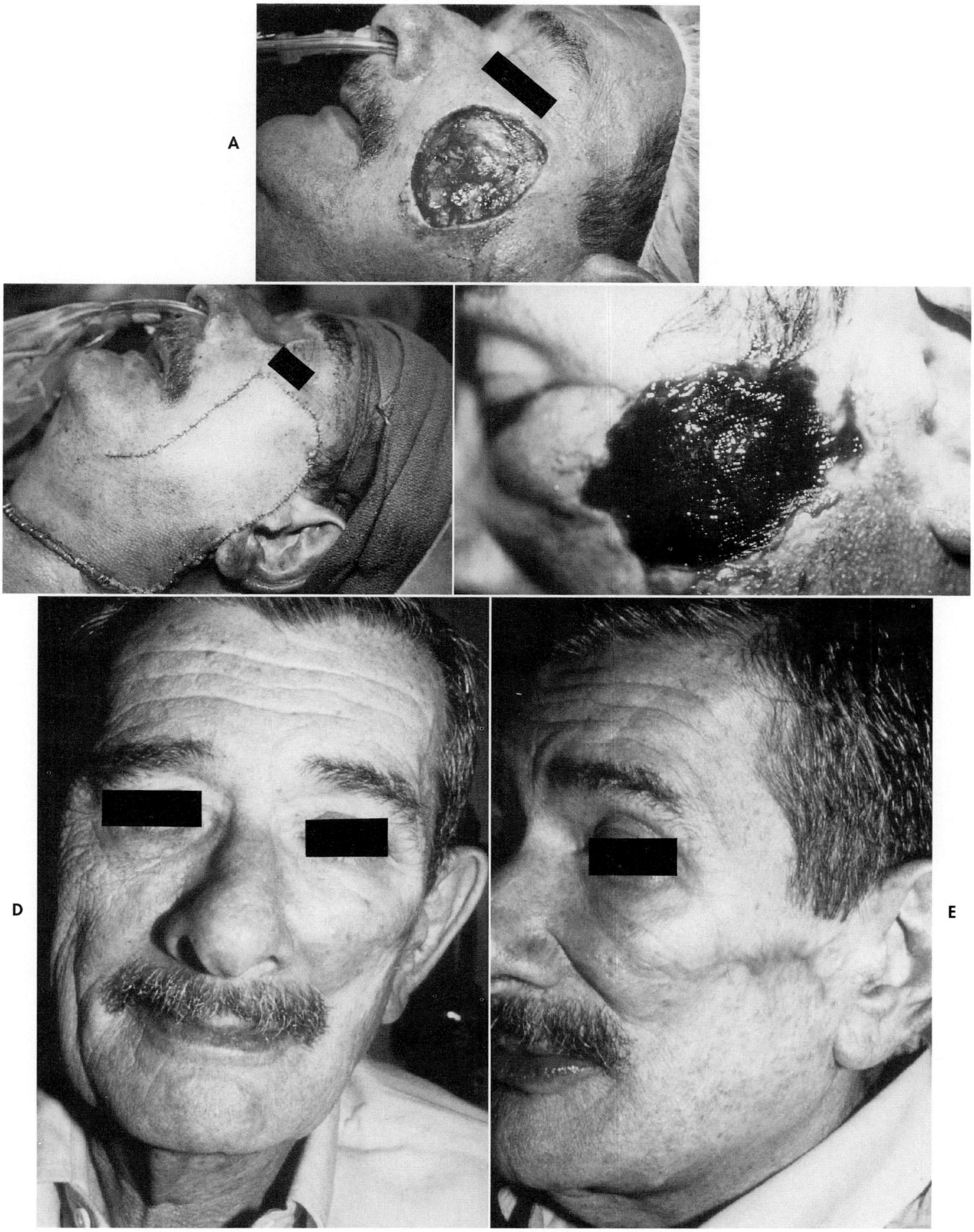

FIG 2-14
Case 11. **A,** Defect of cheek after Mohs surgery measuring 4.4 × 3.7 cm. **B,** Reconstruction with advancement-rotation flap. **C,** Flap necrosis. **D,** Frontal view. **E,** Lateral view of satisfactory healing by secondary intention.

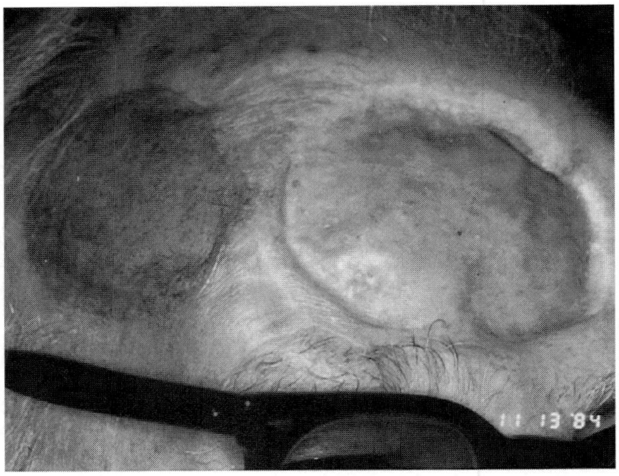

FIG 2-15
Poor color match and "step-off" deformity sometimes seen with grafting. (From Katz AE and Grande DJ: Defects after Mohs surgery. In AAO-HNS: Instructional Courses, vol. 2, 1989, Mosby.)

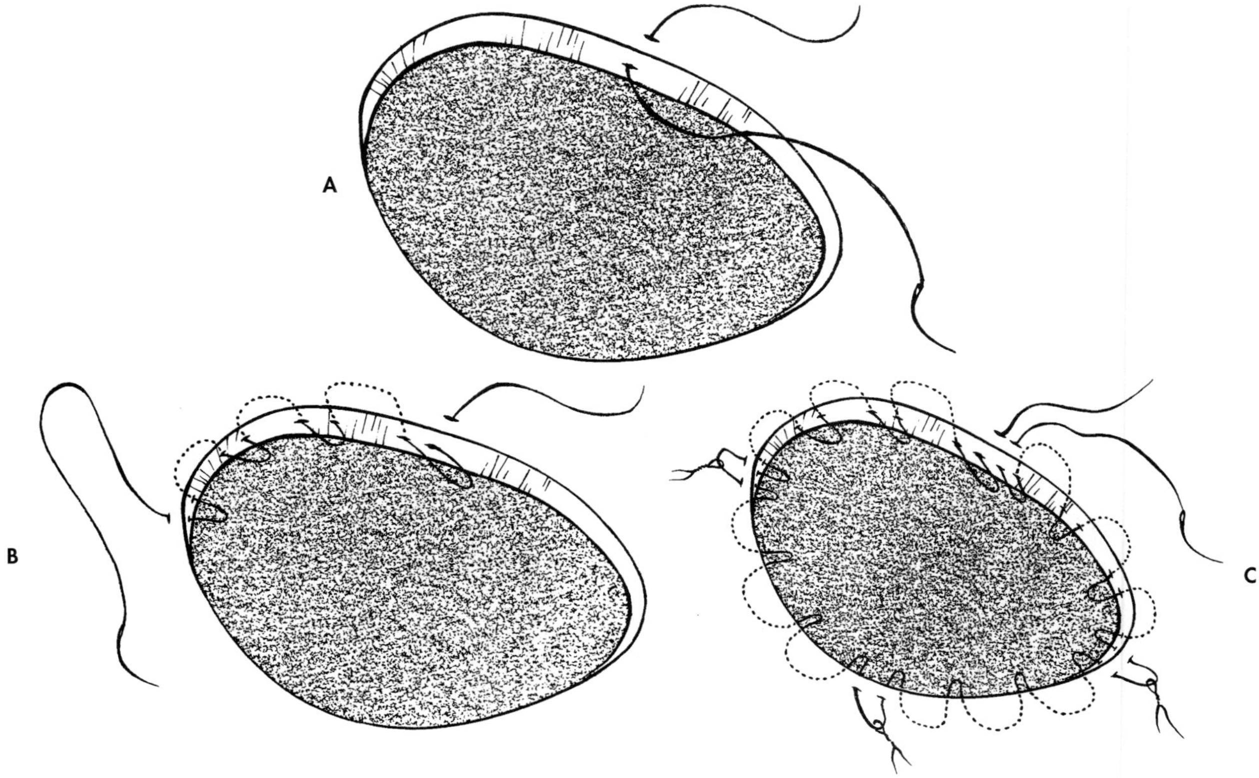

FIG 2-16
A, Purse-string suture should enter wound 5 mm from edge of defect. **B,** At 90 degrees, suture is brought through skin in preparation for placing of pull-suture. **C,** Purse-string suture in place prior to tightening. (From Katz AE and Grande DJ: Defects after Mohs surgery. In AAO-HNS: Instructional Courses, vol. 2, 1989, Mosby.)

A

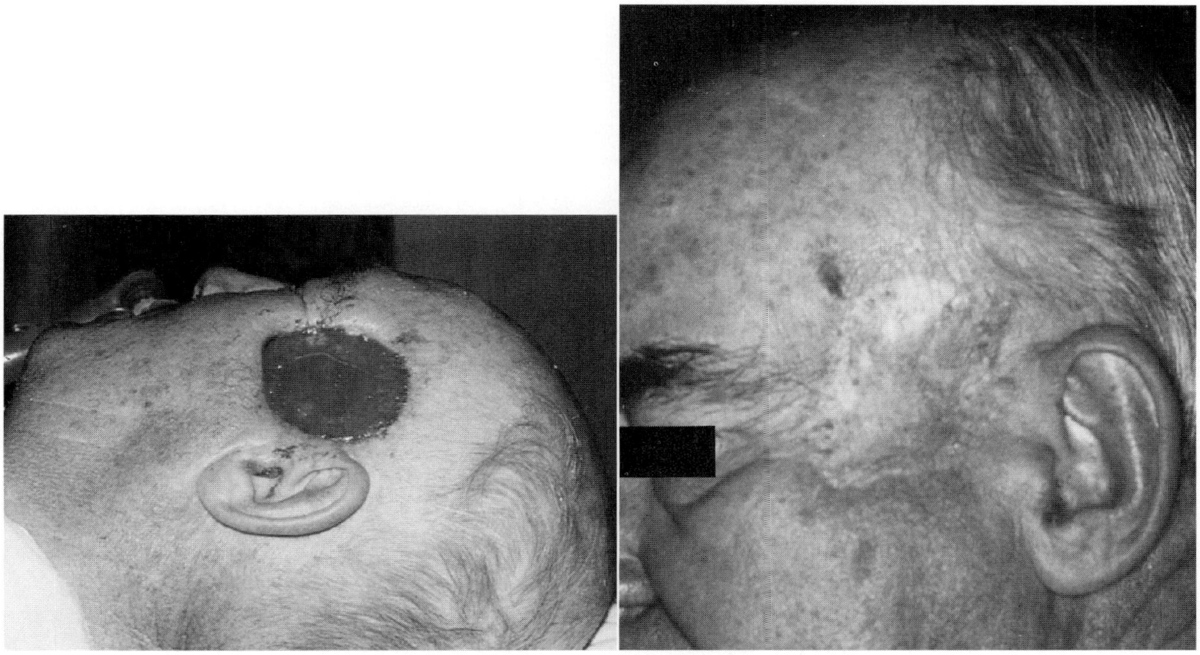

B

FIG 2-17
Case 12. **A,** Deep wound after 3 weeks of healing. **B,** "Step-off" avoided by grafting over a bed of granulation tissue.

A

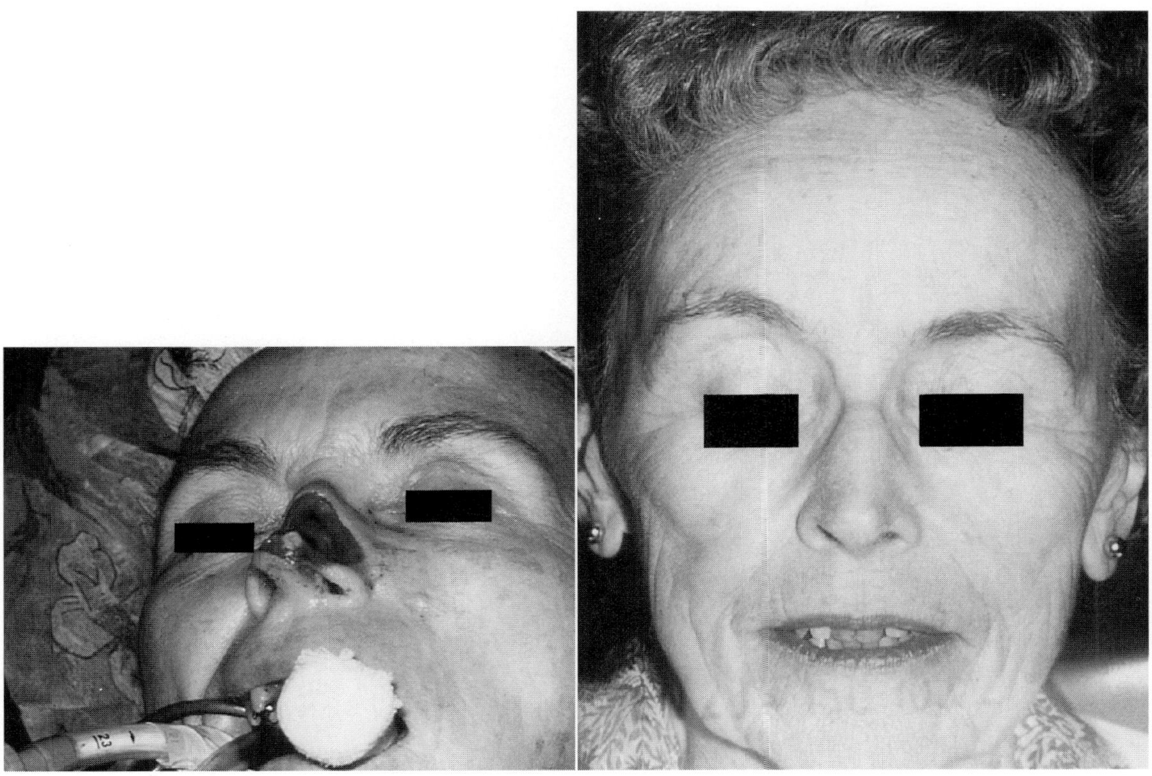

B

FIG 2-18
Case 13. **A,** Nasal defect after excision of basal cell carcinoma. **B,** Maintenance of fine detail of nasal tip with supraclavicular full-thickness skin graft.

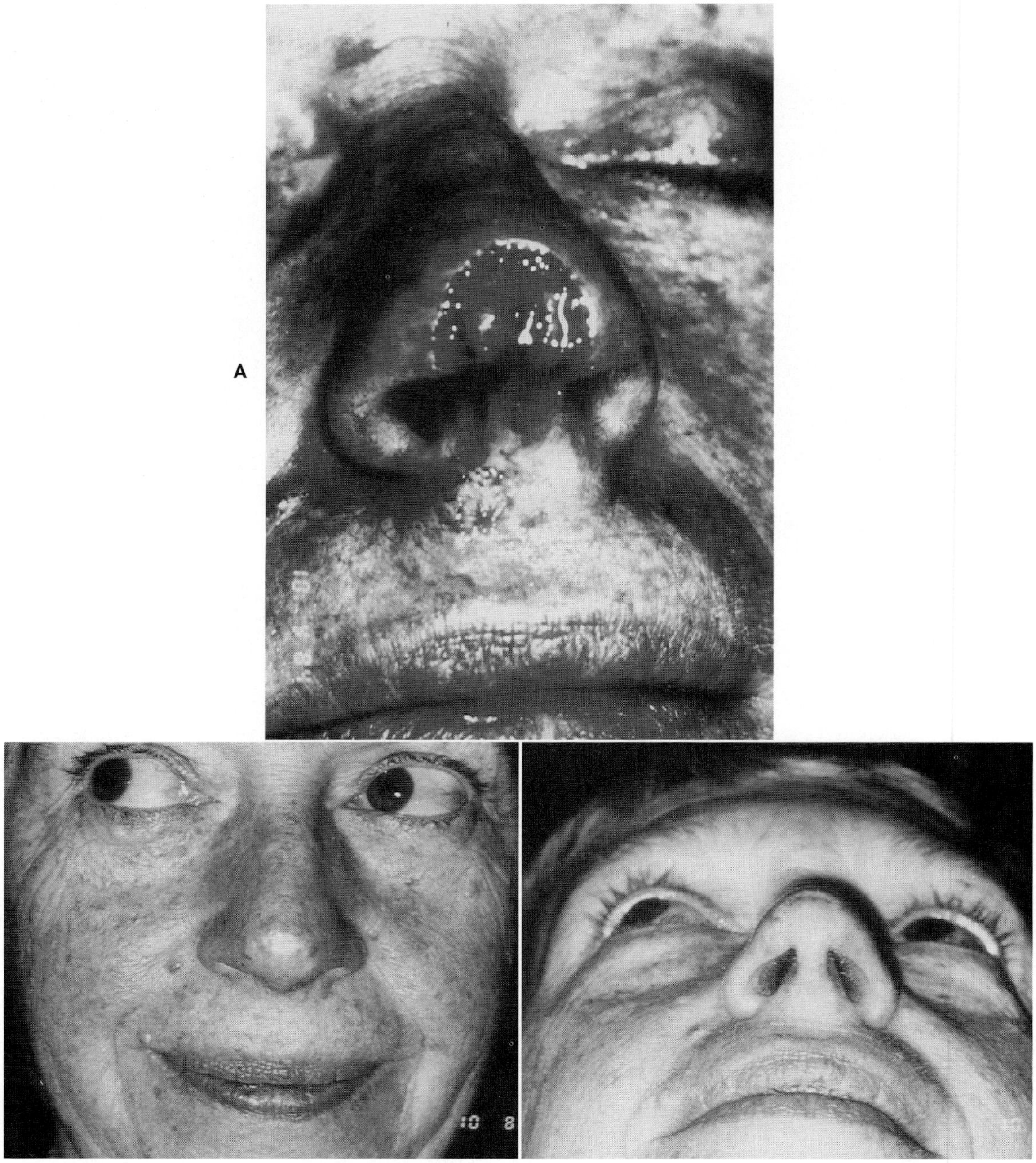

A B C

FIG 2-19
Case 14. **A,** Defect of nasal tip, columella, and right alar rim measuring 2.0 × 2.0 cm. **B,** Full-thickness skin graft. **C,** Advancement flaps of columella and right nasal ala.

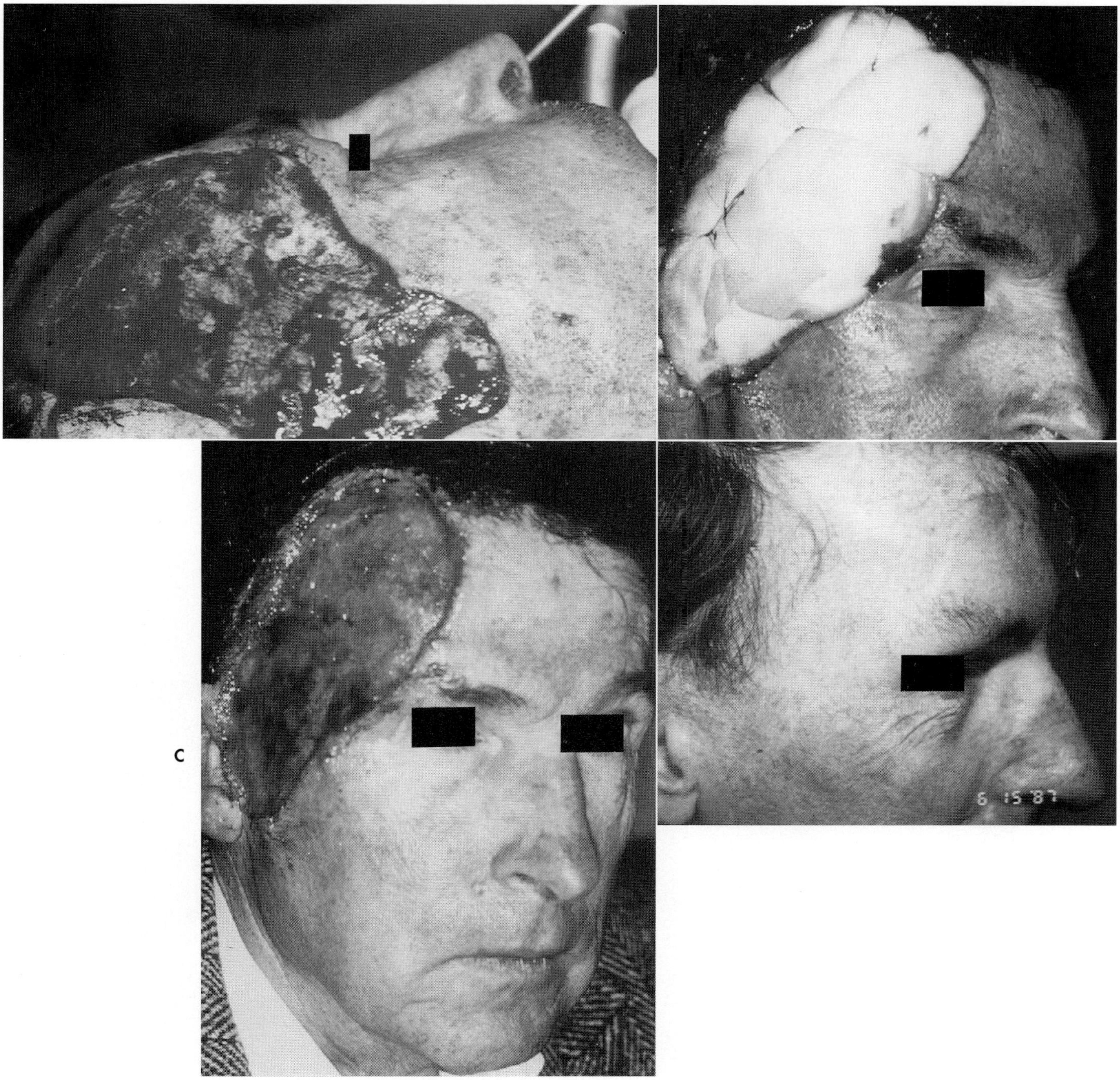

FIG 2-20
Case 15. **A,** Defect of forehead, measuring 15.0 × 9.5 cm. **B,** Cotton bolster dressing impregnated with antibiotic ointment. **C,** Potential "step-off" deformity immediately after removal of bolster dressing. **D,** Elimination of "step-off" deformity.

A 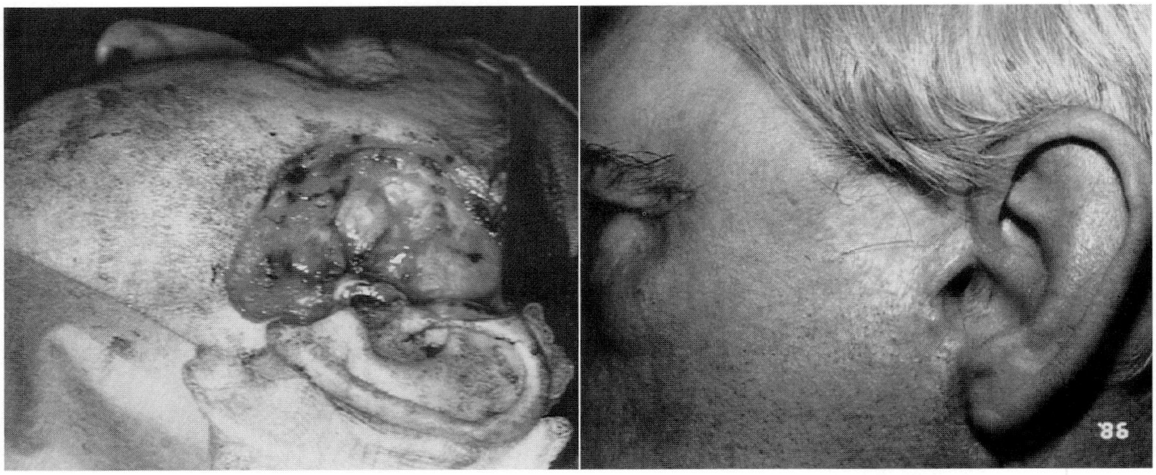 B

FIG 2-21
Case 16. **A,** Preauricular defect measuring 8.0 × 5.5 cm. **B,** Result 5 months postoperative. (From Katz AE and Grande DJ: Defects after Mohs surgery. In AAO-HNS: Instructional Courses, vol. 2, 1989, Mosby.)

A 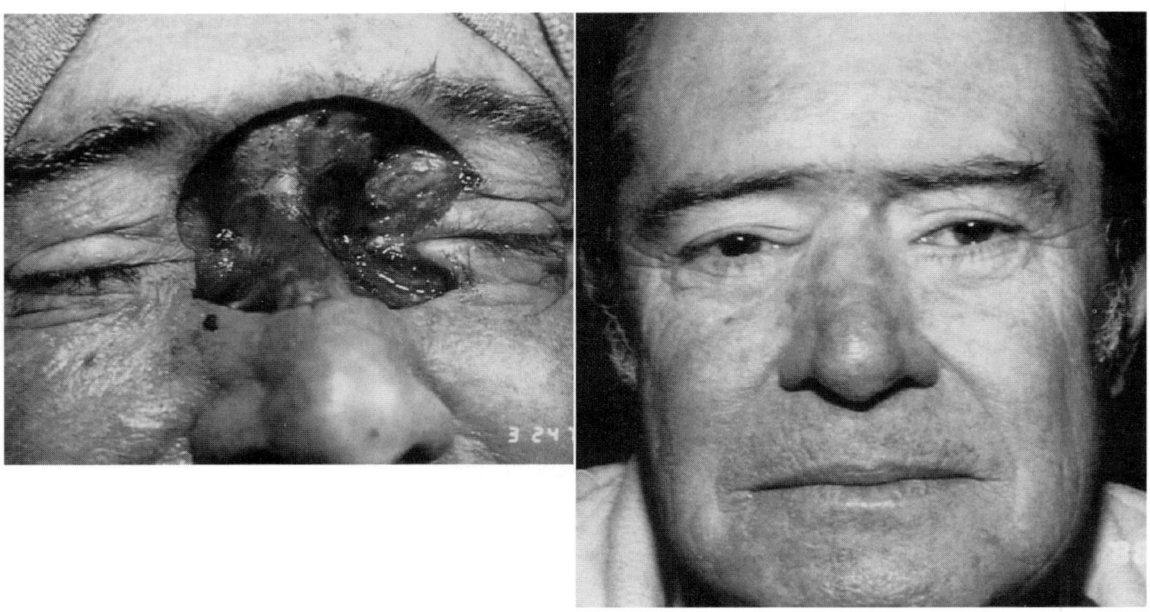 B

FIG 2-22
Case 17. **A,** Defect of midface measuring 5.6 × 5.0 cm. **B,** Result at 6 months after partial closure with purse-string suture and full-thickness skin grafting. (From Katz AE and Grande DJ: Defects after Mohs surgery. In AAO-HNS: Instructional Courses, vol. 2, 1989, Mosby.)

A

B

C

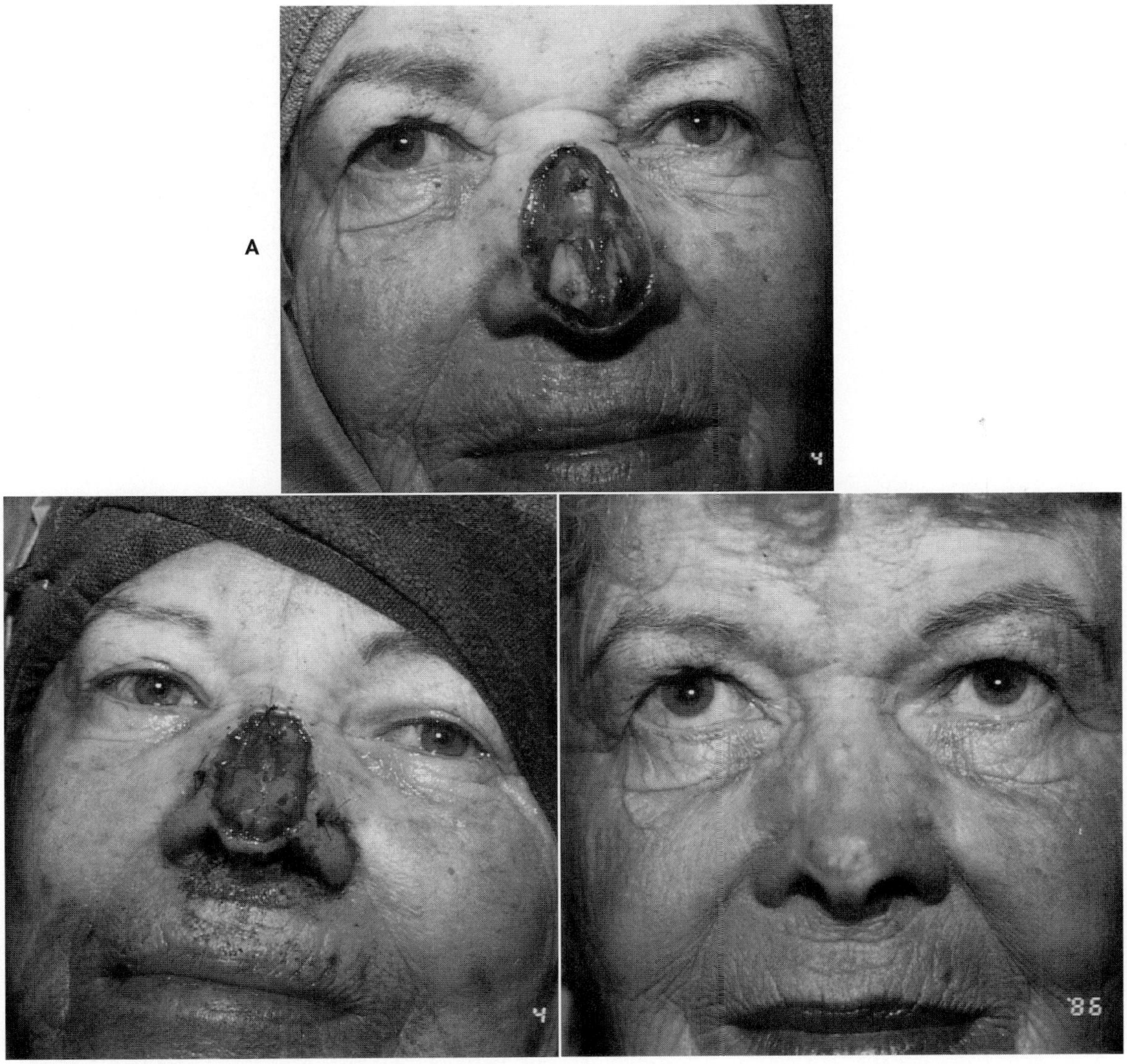

FIG 2-23
Case 18. **A,** Defect of nose measuring 5.0 × 4.0 cm. **B,** Partial closure of defect to 3.5 × 2.5 cm. **C,** Result at 6 months postoperative. (From Katz AE and Grande DJ: Defects after Mohs surgery. In AAO-HNS: Instructional Courses, vol. 2, 1989, Mosby.)

A

B

C

D

E

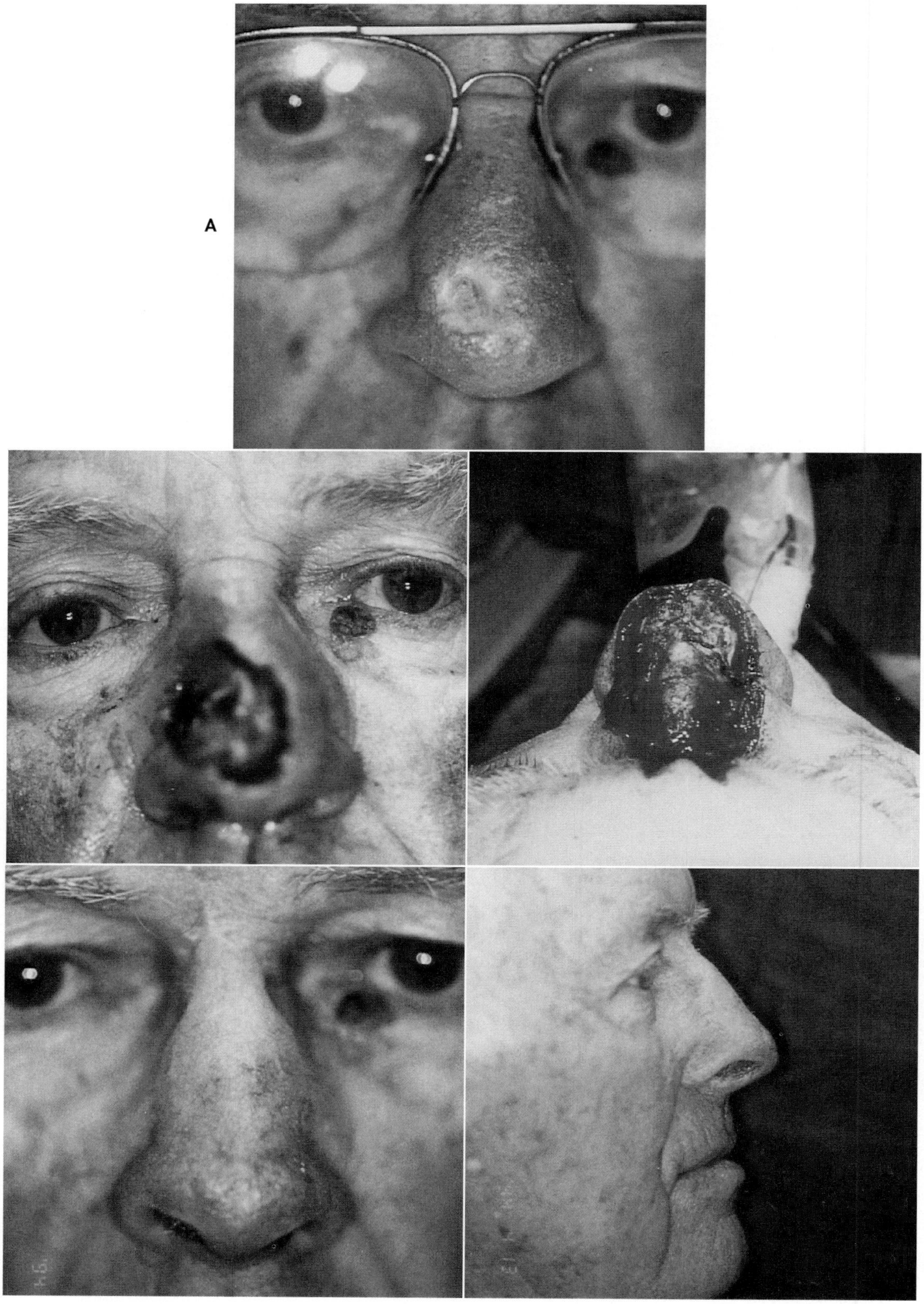

FIG 2-24

Case 19. **A,** Basal cell carcinoma to the right of midline. **B,** Asymmetric defect after Mohs surgery. **C,** Remaining skin of nasal dorsum harvested to complete cosmetic unit. **D,** Nasal tip raised and refined. **E,** Profile demonstrating pleasing appearance of nasal-labial angle.

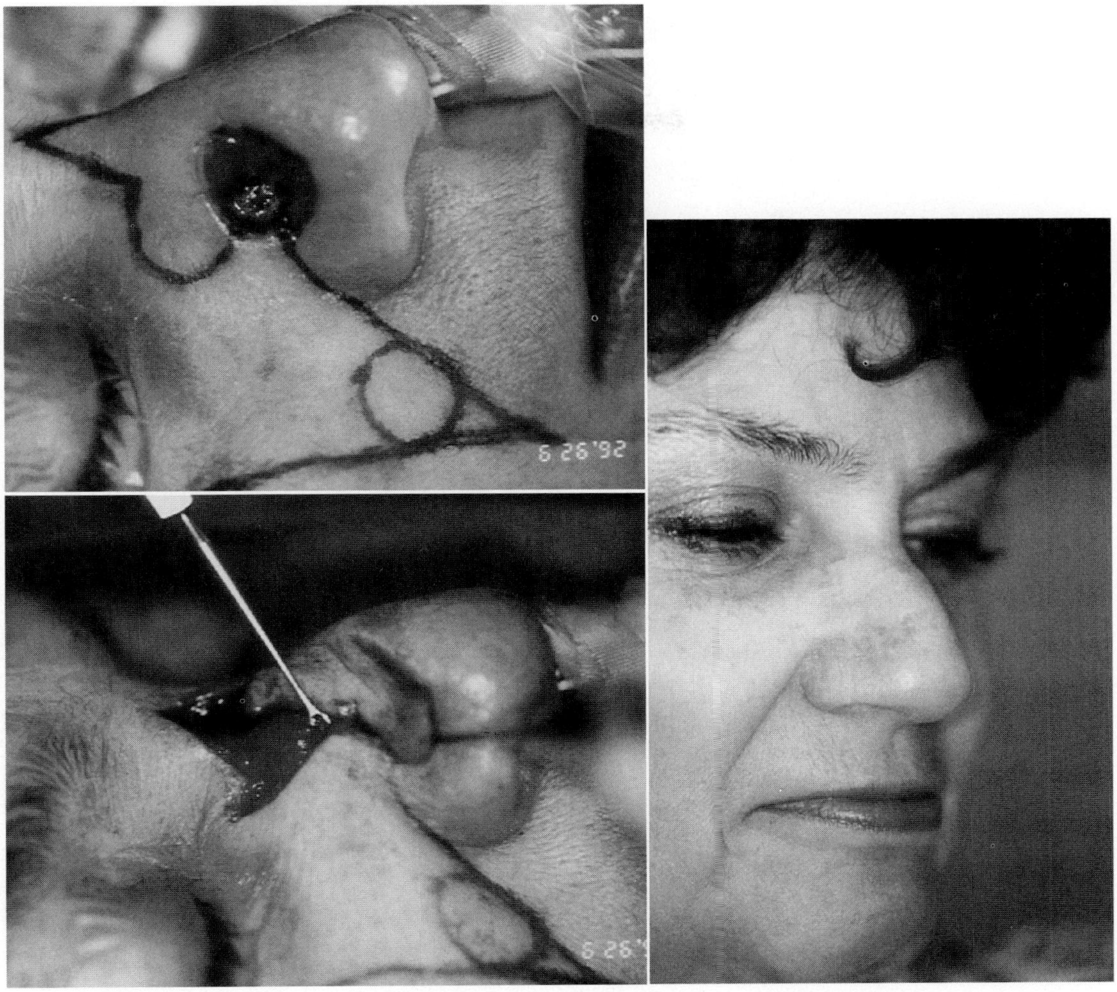

FIG 2-25
Case 20. **A,** Lateral defect of nose. **B,** Bilobe transposition flap. **C,** Result at 14 months postoperative.

better functional and cosmetic result as demonstrated by the following selected examples:

Case 23

A recurrent basal cell carcinoma resulted in retraction of the upper lip and prevented closure of the mouth, leaving the patient with a constant snarl (Fig. 2-28, *A*). The excision crossed the midline, involved the nasal sill, and extended into the oral commissure (Fig. 2-28, *B* and *C*). Bilateral advancement flaps with the excision crescentic perialar triangles allowed the patient to achieve full closure with complete oral competence (Fig. 2-28, *D*).

Case 24

After excision of a deeply infiltrating basal cell carcinoma, a full-thickness defect of the left side of the nose resulted (Fig. 2-29, *A*). A mucoperichondrial flap for the septum was designed for the inner layer (Fig. 2-29, *B*), while an extended nasolabial flap was planned for the outer layer (Fig. 2-29, *C*). After closing the donor defect with a cheek rotation flap, the result of this single-stage procedure was quite acceptable, with no distortion of the eye lid or upper lip (Fig. 2-29, *D*).

Case 25

Multiple flaps were required to repair a large defect of the upper lip, nose, and cheek. It is important to leave dentures in place at the time of reconstruction, so as not to be misled at the time of surgery concerning the competence of the oral commissure (Fig. 2-30, *A*). A perialar crescentic triangle[13] was removed on the right before reversed Karapandzic flaps[2] were utilized to reconstruct the upper lip (Fig. 2-30, *B*). A cheek advancement-rotation flap was then used to close the cheek and nasal defects on the left

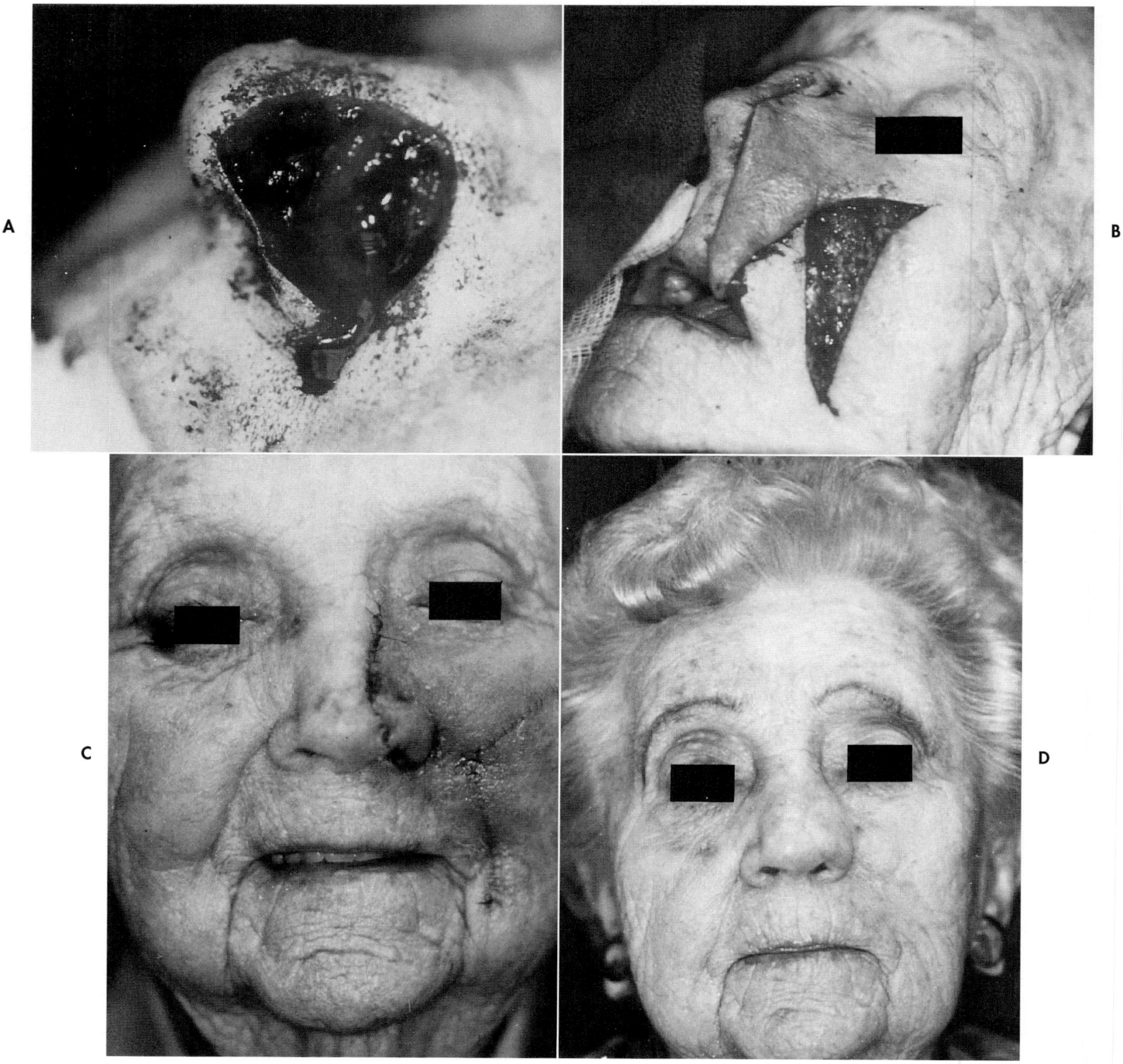

FIG 2-26
Case 21. **A,** Lateral defect of nose. **B,** Nasolabial transposition flap. **C,** Through-and-through quilting sutures to create an alar crease. **D,** Result at 4 months postoperative.

A

B

C

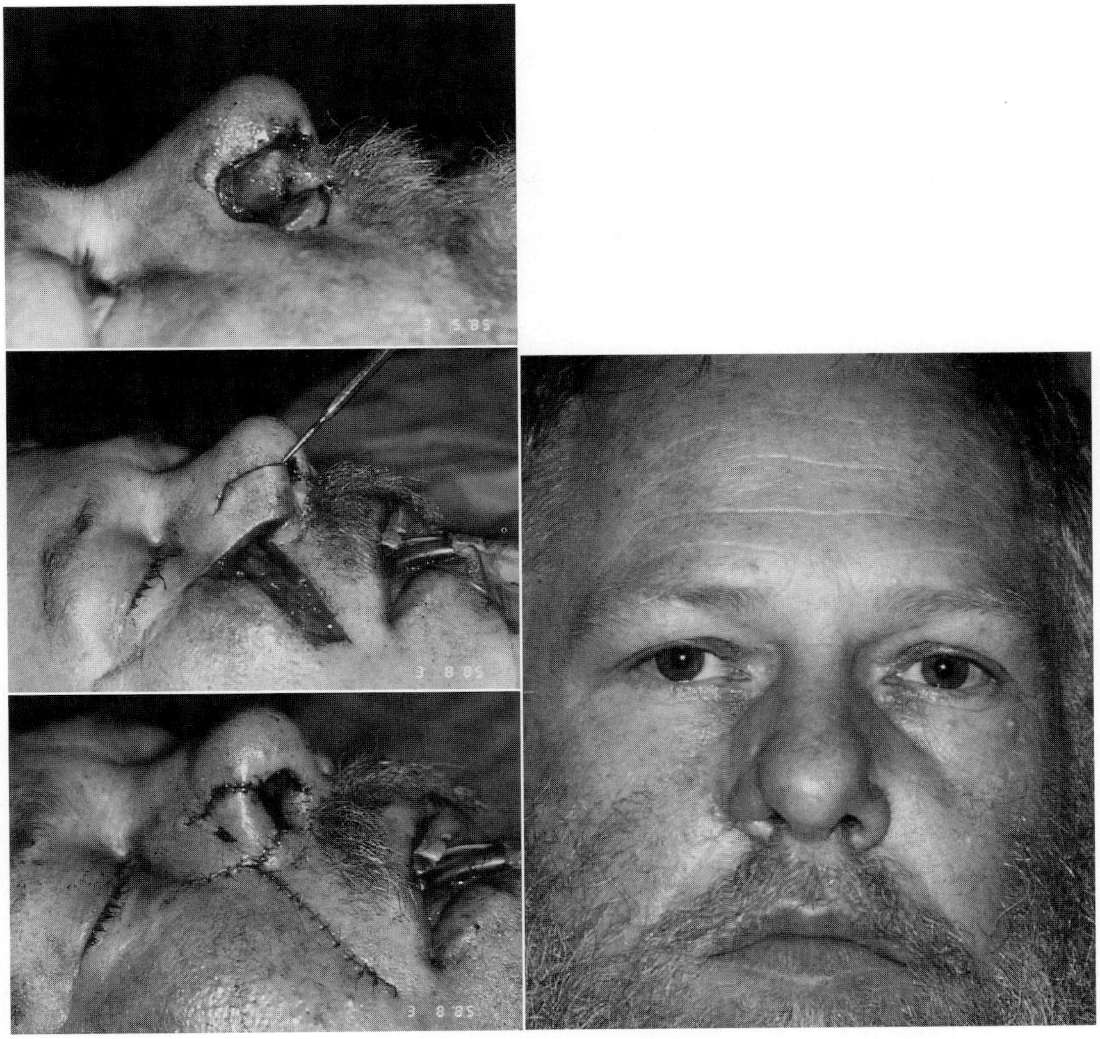

D

FIG 2-27
Case 22. **A,** Full-thickness defect measuring 2.5 × 2.0 cm. **B,** The nasolabial flap is raised, turned, and sutured into place. **C,** A through-and-through quilting suture creates the illusion of an ala. **D,** Result 3 months postoperative. (From Katz AE and Grande DJ: Defects after Mohs surgery. In AAO-HNS: Instructional Courses, vol. 2, 1989, Mosby.)

(Fig. 2-30, *C*). Although microstomia was present in the immediate postoperative period, the patient was soon able touse dentures without difficulty, without any additional procedures (Fig. 2-30, *D*).

CONCLUSIONS

Although this course is not designed to present an exhaustive discussion of all types of flaps and grafts that can be used in facial reconstruction, the techniques presented are the ones that are most frequently used for the reconstruction of patients suffering from large defects after Mohs surgery. After re-examining the past several hundred cases in which we have been involved, it was noted that about 30% were repaired with a cheek or cheek-neck advancement-rotation flaps. An additional 30% required grafting, while transposition flaps played a major role in about 25% of the cases. Various techniques were employed for the remaining 15% of patients treated, including primary closure, forehead flaps, and even healing by secondary intention for those patients who were too unstable medically to withstand additional surgery.

Each patient must evaluated individually, because each patient presents with unique challenges. One must keep an open mind and allow the patient's defect and skin color and elasticity to "speak" and to suggest the most appropriate reconstructive technique. There can be no greater challenge and no greater joy derived from successfully reconstructing a face.

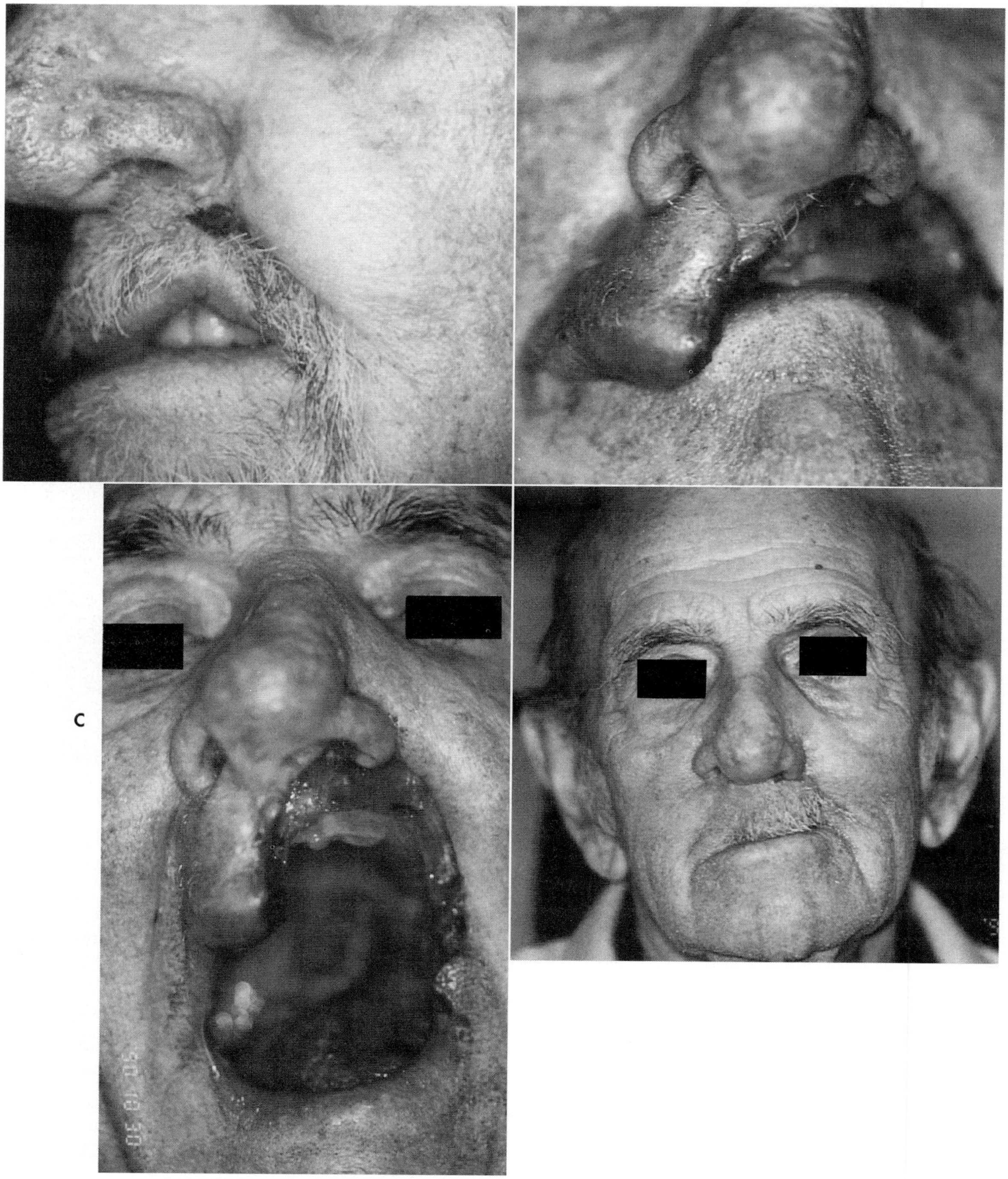

FIG 2-28
Case 23. **A,** Recurrent basal cell carcinoma with a constant snarl. **B,** Defect of lip after excision with Mohs surgery. **C,** Defect also involved nasal sill and oral commissure. **D,** Result one month postoperative after reconstruction with bilateral advancement flaps.

A B C D

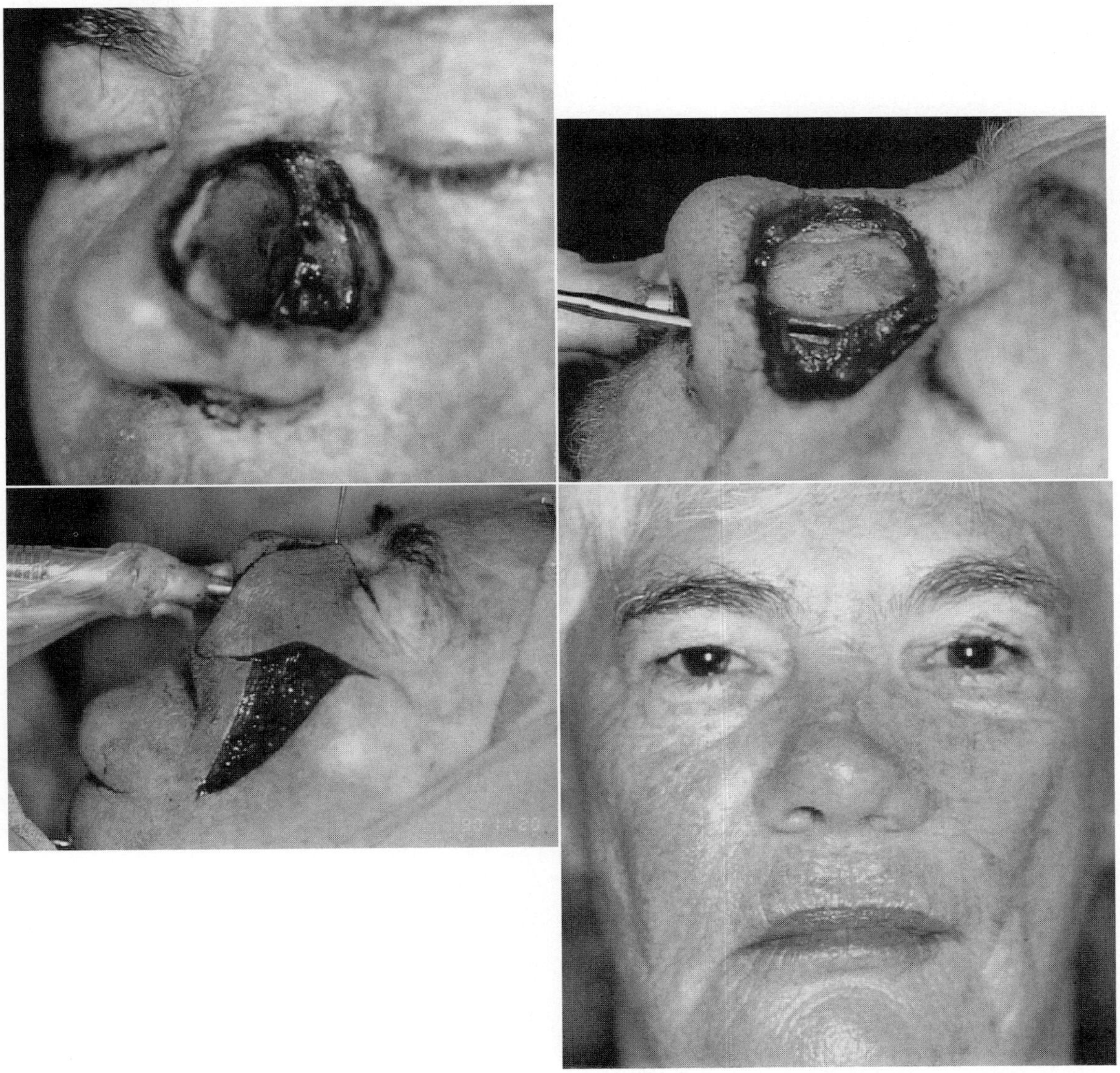

FIG 2-29
Case 24. **A,** Full-thickness defect of left side of nose. **B,** Raising of septal mucoperichondrial flap for inner lining. **C,** Nasolabial flap for external lining. **D,** Result 6 months postoperative. (From Katz AE and Grande DJ: Defects after Mohs surgery. In AAO-HNS: Instructional Courses, vol. 2, 1989, Mosby.)

A B C D

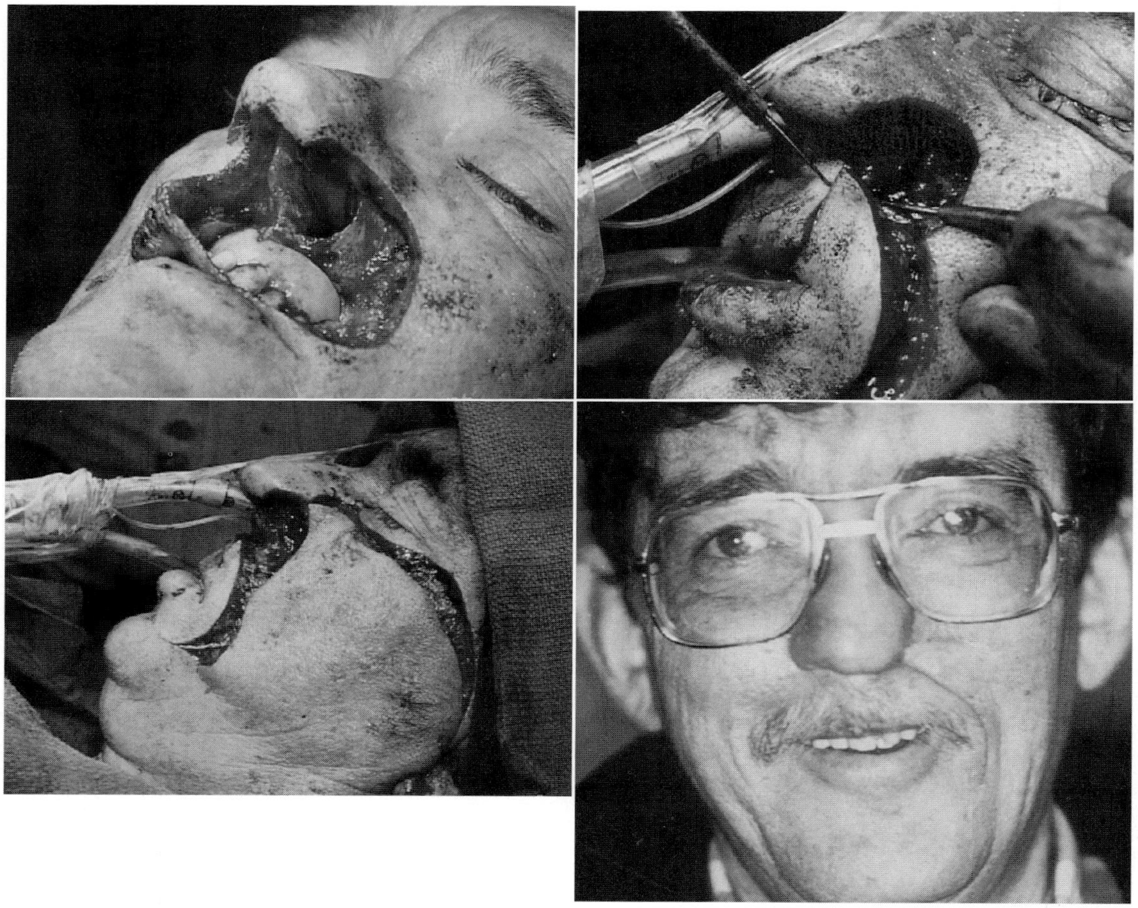

FIG 2-30
Case 25. **A,** Defect of upper lip, nose, and cheek, measuring 6.0 × 4.0 cm. Note dentures in place. **B,** Perialar crescentic triangle removed prior to turning reversed Karapandzic flaps. **C,** Cheek advancement-rotation flap used to close cheek and nasal defects. **D,** Result 11 months postoperative. (From Katz AE and Grande DJ: Defects after Mohs surgery. In AAO-HNS: Instructional Courses, vol. 2, 1989, Mosby.)

REFERENCES

1. Jackson R and Adams RH: Horrifying basal cell carcinoma: a study of 33 cases and a comparison with 435 non-donor cases and a report on four metastatic cases. *J Surg Oncol* 5:431-463, 1973.
2. Karapandzic M: Reconstruction of lip defects by local arterial flaps. *Br J Plast Surg* 27:93-97, 1974.
3. Katz AE and Grande DJ: Cheek-neck advancement-rotation flaps following Mohs excision of skin malignancies. *J Dermatol Surg Oncol* 12:949-955, 1986.
4. Katz AE and Grande DJ: Delayed reconstruction of large facial defects after Mohs surgery. In Johnson JT, Blitzer A, Ossoff R, and Thomas JR, editors: Instructional Courses, vol 2, American Academy of Otolaryngology—Head and Neck Surgery. St. Louis, 1989, The CV Mosby Company, pp 165-190.
5. Katz AE and Grande DJ: Purse-string closure of defects. *Operative Tech Otol-Head Neck Surg* 4:71-75, 1993.
6. Mohs FE: Chemosurgery: microscopically controlled surgery for skin cancer. Springfield, Ill, 1978, Charles C Thomas, Publisher.
7. Morris, JGL and Joffe R: Perineural spread of cutaneous basal and squamous cell carcinomas. *Arch Neurol* 40:424-429, 1983.
8. Mustarde JC: The use of flaps in the orbital region. *Plastic Reconst Surg* 45:146-150, 1970.
9. Peled IJ, Zagher U, and Wexler MR: Purse-string suture for reduction and closure of skin defects. *Ann Plast Surg* 14:465-469, 1985.
10. Stanley RB, Burres SA, Jacobs JR, and Mathog RH: Hazards encountered in management of basal cell carcinomas of the mid-face. *Laryngoscope* 94:378-385, 1984.
11. Swanson NA, Grekin RC, and Baker SR: Mohs surgery: techniques, indications and application in head and neck surgery. *Head Neck Surg* 6:683-692, 1983.
12. Tromovitch TA and Steyman SJ: Microscopically controlled excision of skin tumors: chemosurgery (Mohs): fresh tissue technique. *Arch Dermatol* 110:231-232, 1974.
13. Webster JP: Crescentic perialar cheek excision for upper lip flap advancement with a short history of upper lip repair. *Plast Reconst Surg* 16:434-464, 1955.
14. Zitelli JA: Wound healing by secondary intention: a cosmetic appraisal. *J Am Acad Dermatol* 9:407-415, 1983.
15. Zitelli JA: Mohs surgery: concepts and misconceptions. *Int J Derm* 24:541-548, 1985.

3

Functional Tongue Reconstruction—A Systematic Approach

Mark L. Urken M.D. and Jonathan E. Aviv M.D.

The choices available to the head and neck surgeon in reconstructing defects of the tongue range from healing by secondary intention to the use of local, regional, or free flaps. The consequences of ablative cancer surgery of the tongue involve not only loss of motor function but loss of sensory function as well. Both of these factors greatly effect a patient's ability to recover useful deglutition and articulation. Since it is currently impossible to restore a functioning motor unit to resected tongue tissue, the thrust of current reconstructive efforts is to maximize the function of the tongue remnant. This can be accomplished with tissue design modifications and/or the use of sensate cutaneous free flaps, in which a microneural repair is performed between a cutaneous sensory nerve supplying the flap and a recipient nerve in the head and neck.

The purpose of this course is to develop a systematic approach which will allow one to consider and implement an array of reconstructive techniques based on extent of defect and its functional consequences. This course will address the following:

1. The functional problems resulting from both impaired motor function and lack of sensation in the tongue and its specific impact on deglutition
2. Local, regional, and free flap design modifications, tailored to the size and location of a variety of tongue defects

Before discussing the details of tongue reconstruction a brief review of tongue anatomy and its relevance to deglutition will be made. In addition, the proposed mechanisms of sensory nerve regeneration will be outlined.

Tongue musculature can be broadly divided into extrinsic and intrinsic muscles. The extrinsic muscles are the genioglossus, hyoglossus, styloglossus, and palatoglossus muscles. These muscles have their origin along the mental spine, hyoid bone, or styloid process and insert either into the hyoid bone or into other extrinsic or intrinsic tongue muscles. The primary actions of the extrinsic tongue muscles are to pull the tongue forward, backward, upward, and downward.[9] The intrinsic tongue muscles are bundles of interlacing fibers containing connective tissue septa. These muscles originate in the tongue submucosa and insert into each other and into the extrinsic tongue muscles in various locations throughout the tongue. The primary action of the intrinsic muscles are to produce changes in the shape of the tongue during articulation and deglutition. One can realize from the complexity of origins and insertions of these muscles that to physiologically reproduce these intertwining muscular actions is impossible. Therefore, our direction in tongue reconstruction is to attempt to maximize function of the tongue remnant so that its primary tasks of assisting in speaking, swallowing, and airway protection can be maintained.

Deglutition can be divided into four stages: oral preparatory, oral, pharyngeal, and esophageal. Normal tongue movement is essential for both the oral and pharyngeal stages of swallowing. McConnel described swallowing as a pressure-generation mechanism powered by a two-pump system. He called these pumps the oropharyngeal propulsion pump (OPP) and the hypopharyngeal suction pump (HSP).[12] While several factors may affect the OPP, any condition that primarily affects the anterior two thirds of the tongue will necessarily affect the OPP. In addition, the tongue base also plays an important role in the generation of forces that propel a food bolus posteriorly. Without a tongue base tongue-palate contact cannot be made and bolus propulsion becomes impaired. Clearly, maintenance or restoration of tongue mobility is critical to functional tongue reconstruction. While there are many reconstructive options, for progressively larger tongue defects most standard methods of restoring or maintaining functioning tongue tissue are insufficient in attaining a functional reconstruction.

While restoring new motor function to the tongue is not yet a reconstructive possibility, restoring sensation to the reconstructed tongue is. Why bother restoring sensation? It has been shown that increasing areas of anesthesia in the oral cavity severely impairs articulation and deglutition.[10] It has also been shown that one can reliably restore sensory innervation to tissue provided that a Schwann cell pathway is available to guide the transected axons back to a receptor organ.[8] This has been demonstrated both in transplanted skin grafts and, more to our point here, in transplanted, reinnervated free flaps. The actual mechanism of sensory innervation is divided into two broad categories. In one situation, particularly in skin grafts, there has been documentation of sensory nerve ingrowth from surrounding tissues.[4] With sensate free flaps, a microneural repair between a sensory nerve supplying the free flap and a recipient nerve in the head and neck results in direct sensory nerve reinnervation. This reinnervation depends on various factors. These include the condition of the donor and recipient nerves, the type and quantity of sensory end organs in the transferred tissue and sensory reeducation. Because of the types of reconstruction otolaryngologist–head and neck surgeons perform, we have a built-in sensory reeducation system simply as a result of the area we are reconstructing. One must use the tongue as an integral part of daily survival; the same is not true of one's hands. In our experience it is the cortical representation of the RECIPIENT nerve which determines where a patient will localize sensory stimuli after a microneural repair.

We are attempting to restore tongue sensation. However, before restoring a sensory deficit, it would help us define our goals if we knew what normal tongue sensation is, whether or not there were age-related changes in oral sensation, and whether or not radiation therapy affected tongue sensory discrimination. To answer these questions we modified the Mackinnon-Dellon Disc-criminator for use in the oral cavity and found out the following: For both static and moving two-point discrimination, the tongue tip was the most sensitive area, followed by the lateral dorsal tongue, lateral ventral tongue, and floor of mouth. We noted age-related changes in sensory discrimination as well, with people less than 40 in general having a statistically significant more sensitive two-point discrimination level.[1] We also found that radiation therapy significantly impairs sensory discrimination of the tongue relative to controls. Previously existing neurohistologic data supports our clinical findings.[7]

Sensate potential free skin flaps have been demonstrated with the lateral arm,[1] lateral thigh,[3] dorsalis pedis, and radial forearm free flaps.[16] We have been using the radial forearm free flap as a thin, pliable sensate piece of tissue as our workhorse flap in reconstructing large tongue defects. The following summarizes our approach to reconstructing a variety of tongue defects. For our purposes tongue defects will be divided into one quarter glossectomy, hemiglossectomy, resection of the entire mobile tongue, or the entire tongue base and total glossectomy.

ONE QUARTER GLOSSECTOMY

The definition of a one quarter glossectomy, or limited glossectomy, is a resection of the tongue that involves one fourth or less of the mobile tongue or tongue base. These defects can be reconstructed with primary closure. However, if the defect extends to the mucosa of the floor of the mouth then split-thickness skin grafts are utilized to maintain mobility of the tongue and to prevent tethering of the tongue to the floor of the mouth or to mucoperiosteum of the mandible.

A variety of tongue flaps have been used to close small tongue defects.[6] However, as the defect of the tongue increases, the amount of manipulation of the residual tongue increases. This manipulation leads to greater disturbances in tongue function and it is our philosophy to avoid the use of tongue flaps except in the most unusual circumstances.

Small defects of the base of the tongue are best managed by primary closure or by advancement of the end of the tongue posteriorly.[6] However, if posterior rotation of the tongue leads to distortion of the mobile tongue than additional tissue must be introduced. The type of tissue that can be introduced under these circumstances is either a sensate radial forearm free flap which provides bulk and sensation to the tongue base or, for patients in whom free tissue transfers is not suitable, a pedicled flap from the chest wall or trunk may be considered.

HEMIGLOSSECTOMY

When one half or greater of the tongue is resected, significant oral function impairments ensue. The critical consideration is the existence of a residual segment of mobile tongue that has an intact motor supply. If there is even a small mobile tongue remnant that remains, then one should make every effort to restore shape and a portion of the volume of the tongue as well as to reestablish sensation. This is achieved by separating the reconstruction of the mobile tongue from the reconstruction of the floor of mouth. The greater the redundancy of tissue in the neotongue the less tethering of the mobile tongue will take place. With this basic principle established, the more likely the remnant of motorized tongue will be able to power the reconstructed tissue along with its typical movements. Our flap of choice for achieving this is the radial forearm free flap with the bilobe design (Fig. 3-1).[2,14] This flap design takes advantage of the vascularity of the forearm skin as well as thinness, pliability and ability to deliver sensory potential. The essence of this design is to create two lobes of tissue separated by an approximate 30° to 45° angle which allows com-

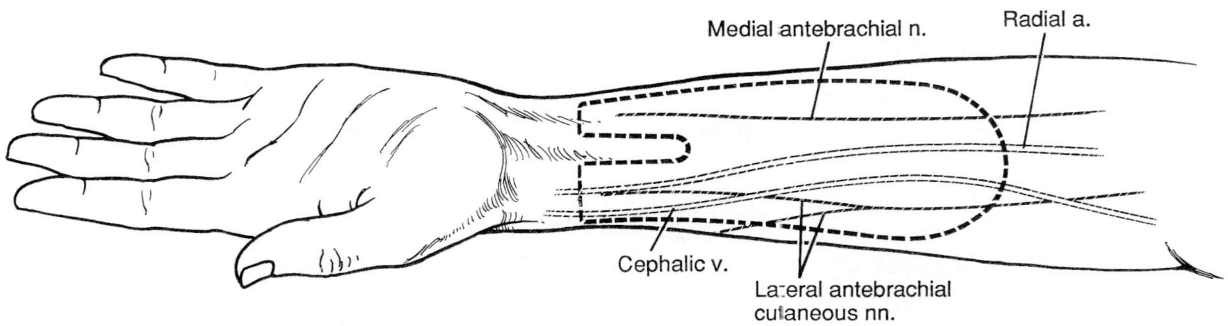

FIG 3-1
Bi-lobed radial forearm free flap.

plete freedom of movement of both the reconstructed tongue and the floor of mouth. If bulk is necessary, bulk can be added to the mobile tongue or tongue base by harvesting additional subcutaneous tissue extension flaps that can be buried underneath the epithelial surface of the neo tongue. We first introduced the use of the sensate radial forearm free flap for pharyngeal reconstruction in 1989.[16] Our continued enthusiasm for the use of this donor site is based on the quality of the tissue that is thin, well vascularized, and pliable. Furthermore, one is able to harvest this flap with a two-team approach. In addition, the length and caliber of its nutrient vessels and sensory nerves makes this flap particularly appealing.

Other donor sites for sensate free flaps include the lateral arm, lateral thigh, and the dorsum of the foot. Invariably these flaps lack the versatility, ease of harvest, and low morbidity of the radial forearm free flap.

RESECTION OF THE ENTIRE MOBILE TONGUE OR ENTIRE TONGUE BASE

When near total glossectomies result in defects of the entire mobile tongue with preservation of the tongue base or resection of the tongue base with preservation of the mobile tongue, reconstruction requires tissue that provides both bulk and sensation (Fig. 3-2). Bulk is essential for mobile tongue defects to provide contact between the neotongue and the palate. In the tongue base, functional reconstruction requires bulk to achieve contact with the pharyngeal walls and soft palate. Again, to achieve these reconstructions a radial forearm free flap with a bilobed design in conjunction with harvesting of considerable amounts of additional vascularized subcutaneous fat will provide both the necessary bulk and the sensation for customized reconstruction of both the mobile tongue and the tongue base[15] (Fig. 3-3 and 3-4).

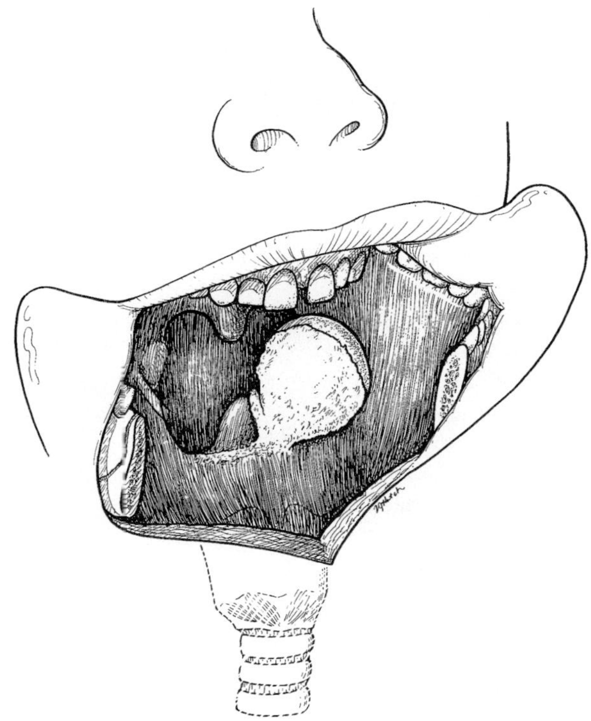

FIG 3-2
Schematic of near-total glossectomy defect.

TOTAL GLOSSECTOMIES DEFECTS

In general, total glossectomy defects require bulky tissue to assist in articulation and deglutition. Regional myocutaneous flaps tend to sag over time because of the gravitational pull on the vascular pedicle. Free myocutaneous flaps such as rectus abdominus and latissimus dorsi have a muscle component that can be sutured directly to the mandible to support the position of the overlying fat and skin, thus greatly eliminating the problem of sagging and pulling toward the origin of the vascular pedicles. The key component of total glossectomy reconstruction, however, is prevention of aspiration. The technique that we like to use is a epiglottic laryngoplasty first described by Biller, et al, in 1983.[5] In this type of laryngoplasty the mucosa of the epiglottis and aryepiglottic folds is bivalved and a two-layer closure is performed leaving a mucosa-lined opening at the apex of the epiglottis. This allows one to produce voice with minimal risk of aspiration.

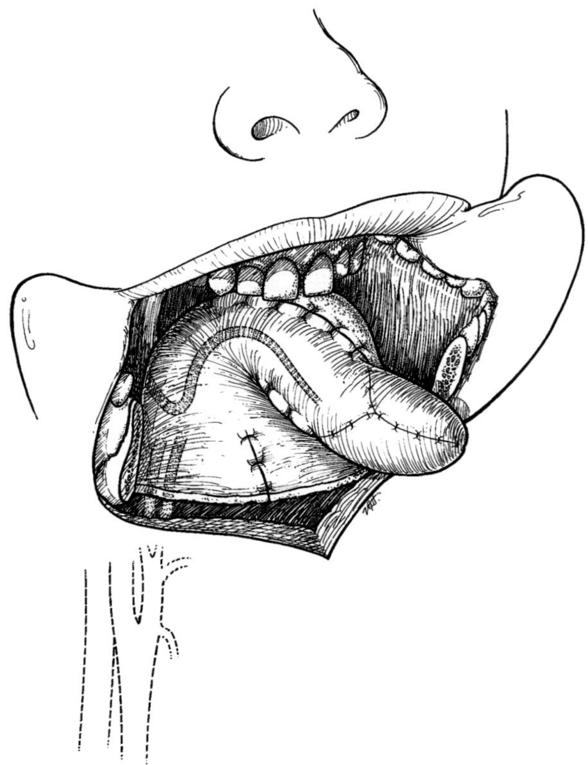

FIG 3-3
Insetting of a bilobed radial forearm free flap to reconstruct a near total glossectomy defect.

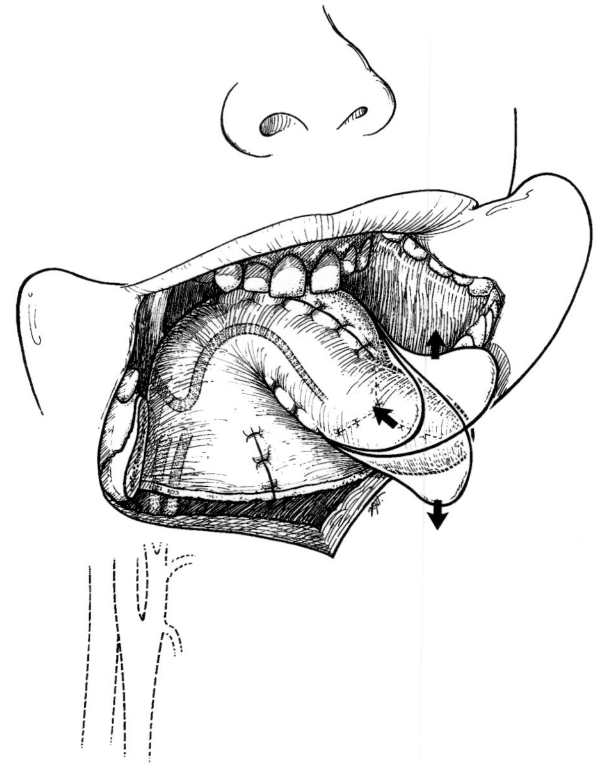

FIG 3-4
Schematic of potential tongue range of motion that could take place following a bilobed tongue reconstruction.

HEMIGLOSSECTOMY WITH SEGMENTAL MANDIBULECTOMY

When there is a combination of significant glossectomy defect with a segmental mandibulectomy defect, the choices for reconstruction must not only include the soft tissue component but the bony component as well. There is no single composite flap that provides bone of sufficient dimension to achieve functional mandibular reconstruction and a mobile sensate soft tissue flap with the freedom of customized design that has been outlined previously. Our preference for vascularized bone is the iliac crest because of the large stock of bone that can be harvested.[17] We have successfully combined the radial forearm and iliac crest flaps in series of patients with complex composite defects of the tongue and mandible.[18] In select cases of composite defects involving the posterior mandible, a titanium reconstruction plate is often suitable to serve as a spacer.

TOTAL MOBILE TONGUE DEFECTS WITH SEGMENTAL DEFECTS OF ANTERIOR MANDIBLE

For total mobile tongue defects with segmental mandibular defects, Salibian[13] introduced the use of a horizontally placed iliac crest platform to restore the form of the anterior mandibular arch and to provide long-term structural support to the overlying soft tissues used to create the neotongue. Although, this technique does not provide sensate soft tissue, it is a reliable one-flap reconstruction of this difficult composite defect.

Total glossectomy with lateral segmental mandibulectomy can be reconstructed using the soft tissue flaps previously described in conjunction with a mandibular reconstruction plate as a spacer for the bony defect. However, when the mandibular defect involves the mandibular arch, we do employ free tissue transfer with an iliac crest osteocutaneous flap with the bone again being placed in a horizontal position to support the overlying skin paddle that is used to resurface the oral cavity.

For larger soft tissue defects of the pharynx as well as tongue, we have combined a separate radial forearm with iliac bone flap placed in a horizontal position.[18]

CONCLUSION

Customized tongue reconstruction represents a systematic functional approach to the management of different glossectomy defects based on their sizes and location. One must remember, however, that innovations in tongue reconstruction must be tempered by the prognosis of this disease process. However, if the quality of life of these patients can be improved, this will prove to be a worthwhile endeavor.

REFERENCES

1. Aviv JE, Hecht C, Weinberg H: Surface sensibility of the floor of mouth and tongue in healthy controls and in radiated patients. *Otol Head Neck Surg* 107:418-423, 1992.
2. Aviv JE, Keen MS, Rodriguez HP, et al: Bilobed radial forearm free flap for functional reconstruction of near total glossectomy defects. *Laryngoscope* 104:893-900, 1994.
3. Baek S: Two new cutaneous free flaps: The medial and lateral thigh flaps. *Plast Reconstr Surg* 71:354-363, 1983.
4. Berger A, Meisse G: Innervated skin grafts and flaps for restoration of sensation to anesthetic areas. *Chir Plast (Berl)* 3:33-37, 1975.
5. Biller HF, Lawson W, Baek S: Total glossectomy. *Arch Otol.* 109:69-73, 1983.
6. Chicarilli Z: Sliding posterior tongue flap. *Plast Reconstr Surg* 79:697-700, 1987.
7. Dixon AD: The position, incidence and origin of sensory nerve terminations in the oral mucous membrane. *Arch Oral Biol* 7:39-48, 1962.
8. Dykes, RW: Recovery of sensory function following skin flaps in humans. *Plast Reconstr Surg* 79:434-435, 1987.
9. Hollinshead, WH: Anatomy for Surgeons: Volume I. *The head and neck,* ed. 3, Harper & Row, Philadelphia, 1982, pp. 367-371.
10. Kapur K, Garret N, Fisher E: Effect of oral anesthesia on food manipulation during mastication. *Arch Oral Biol* 35:397-403, 1990.
11. Katsaros J, Schusterman M, Beppu M, et al: The lateral upper arm flap: anatomy and clinical applications. *Ann Plast Surg* 12:489-500, 1984.
12. McConnel FM, Logemann J: Diagnosis in treatment of swallowing disorders. In Cummings C, Frederickson J, Krause C, et al, editors: *Otol head and neck surg, update* Vol 2. St. Louis, 1990, Mosby–Year Book.
13. Salibian A, Rappaport I, Allison G: Functional oral mandibular reconstruction with a microvascular composite growing flap. *Plast Reconstr Surg* 76:819-825, 1985.
14. Urken ML, Biller HF: A new design for the sensate radial forearm free flap to preserve tongue mobility following significant total glossectomy. *Arch Otol Head and Neck Surg* 120:26-31, 1994.
15. Urken ML, Moscoso JF, Lawson W, Biller HF: A systematic approach to functional reconstruction of the oral cavity following partial and total glossectomy. *Arch Otolaryngol Head Neck Surg* 120:589-601, 1994.
16. Urken ML, Vickery C, Weinberg H, Biller HF: The neurofasciocutaneous radial forearm flap in head and neck reconstruction: a preliminary report. *Laryngoscope* 100:161-173, 1990.
17. Urken ML, Vickery K, Weinberg H, et al: The internal oblique iliac crest osteomyocutaneous microvascular free flap in head and neck reconstruction. *J Reconst Micro Surg* 5:203-214, 1989.
18. Urken ML, Weinberg H, Vickery C, et al: The combined sensate radial forearm and iliac crest free flaps for reconstruction of significant glossectomy mandibulectomy defects. *Laryngoscope* 102:543-558, 1992.

Part Two

General

4

Nicotine Addiction and Cure: A Head and Neck Perspective

C. Ron Cannon, M.D., F.A.C.S., Brent Meador, M.D. and Tom Milhorn, M.D.

In both cigarette and smokeless forms, tobacco has been implicated as a prime etiologic factor in the development of squamous cell carcinoma of the upper aerodigestive tract. In an addictive society, tobacco remains the most common form of drug abuse. The neoplastic aspects of tobacco are well recognized, but its basic pathophysiology and addiction aspects are much less appreciated. The otolaryngologist–head and neck surgeon has the unique responsibility to patients with nicotine addiction, as the primary caretaker of patients with head and neck cancer and as a medical specialist who is responsible for the general well–being of their patient.

In this chapter a basic review of tobacco with its history and economic implications as well as its neoplastic potential is presented. Basic pathophysiology and effects of tobacco and nicotine on various organ systems are reviewed. Another portion of the chapter will deal with the addictive aspects of tobacco. The final section will aid the otolaryngologist–head and neck surgeon in formulating a treatment plan for the nicotine-addicted patient.

Ben Franklin once said: "An ounce of prevention is worth a pound of cure." This is very true for tobacco use. We must shift our emphasis from a third order of treatment (management of an established disease) or second order of treatment (early diagnosis or treatment when the disease is curable) to a first-order treatment plan, i.e., *prevention.* Tobacco is currently used more than any drug in the world. A tobacco year (TY) is defined as daily consumption of 20 cigarettes, 4 cigars, or 5 pipes for one year. Who, then, are the patients currently smoking? Smoking is very prevalent in our society simply because of the diverse base of people who use tobacco. The men who smoke currently are generally blue collar workers, laborers, or craftsmen. Women who now smoke are generally those in the higher income groups. In terms of ethnic groups who smoke, Hispanics smoke more frequently than other ethnic groups. Also divorced or separated men and women smoke more than their married counterparts. The prevalence of men who smoke has decreased from 52.5% in 1935 to only 32% in 1985. The percentage of women who smoke, however, has increased from 18.1% in 1935 to 29% in 1985.

The use of smokeless tobacco in this country is growing at an alarming rate. This form of tobacco use became popular in the 1970s. This group is primarily young men, mostly athletes. Its use has been popularized by baseball players who are seen chewing tobacco. There are twelve million users of smokeless tobacco in this country. The sales of smokeless tobacco have increased by 11% per year since the early 1970s. The use of smokeless tobacco is the fastest growing form of nicotine addiction in this country. Eighty percent of those who use smokeless tobacco have "experimented" with it before age 15.

ECONOMICS

The tobacco industry employs 2.3 million Americans, making up 2.5% of our nation's work force. The tobacco industry generates 60 billion dollars per year, making up 2.5% of our gross national product. The American public spends 42 billion dollars per year in buying cigarettes, while the tobacco industry spends 2.5 billion per year in advertising. Tobacco is the number one agricultural crop in the states of Virginia, South Carolina, Kentucky, and North Carolina. In terms of annual tobacco production, China is the number one country producing tobacco (2 million in metric tons), while the United States is second (700 thousand metric tons).

The cultivated tobacco plant is an annual plant in that it lives only one growing season. The average tobacco plant is 4 to 6 feet tall and produces about 20 leaves. A mature plant can produce up to a million seeds during a year. Enough to plant about 100 acres of tobacco.

The tax revenues generated from tobacco on a federal,

state, and local level were 6.2 billion dollars in 1977. The United States Federal Inspectors examine tobacco before it is sold and grade it according to the governmental standards. It is also interesting that the government has price supports that guarantee the seller a certain price for his tobacco.

Health care costs

What are the health care costs from the use of tobacco? The total cost of smoking-related health care and loss of productivity is approximately 65 billion dollars per year. In those who smoke one pack per day, there is a 50% increased chance of being ill—requiring hospitalization or absenteeism from work as compared with a nonsmoking employee. The loss of productivity from smoking-related illnesses approaches 24 billion dollars per year. It is also interesting that 25% of deaths from fires occur in people who smoke in bed.

Cigarette smoking is accountable for 350,000 deaths per year. This is six times as many Americans each year as were killed during the entire Vietnam war. Cigarette smoking is the largest single preventable cause of death and disability in this country.

HISTORICAL REVIEW

Tobacco use is said to have begun some 5,000 years before Christ by an evil and powerful sorcerer known as Acayatl. Tobacco use began with the Central American Indians and was taken back to Europe after discovery of this part of the world by Columbus. Subsequently it was popularized in this country hundreds of years later. The word tobacco derives from the Y-shaped tabago pipes used by these Central American Indians. Each one of the forks of the Y was inserted into the nostril when smoking.

Harry S. Truman once said that, "Columbus brought syphilis to the Indians and they gave him tobacco, it is doubtful which is worse." In 1492, Columbus discovered the Americas. Two of his sailors, Rodrigo de Jerez and Luis de Torres were reportedly the first Europeans to smoke. In fact, de Jerez so frightened people by the smoke coming from his nose and mouth, that the Spanish Inquisition imprisoned him for demonic possession.

In 1560, Jean Nicot served as ambassador to France for the Portuguese King, Sebastion. Nicot treated a stomach ailment of Catherine de Medici, the queen of France. She was so pleased with his treatment that she subsequently named the tobacco plant after him, "nicotiana." It was later latinized to *nicotina tabacum*. About this time, tobacco was used for medicinal purposes and was sold only in apothecary shops. It was used as a treatment for sores, fistula, abscesses, and basal cell carcinomas among other things. In all, it had about sixteen different uses.

With time the use of tobacco spread to other European countries. Sir Walter Raleigh of England persuaded Queen Bess to try a silver pipe full of tobacco. She liked the pipe and pipe smoking subsequently became popular in the upper level of society in this country. The King of England, James I, initially outlawed tobacco but then relented and allowed merchants to be licensed to import tobacco. By popular legend, the first time Sir Walter Raleigh lit up his pipe at home, his servant poured water on him falsely assuming that his master was on fire. King James I's differences with Sir Walter Raleigh over tobacco and other issues led ultimately to Sir Walter Raleigh being beheaded.

In this country the first commercial tobacco crop was planned in Jamestown, Virginia, in 1612 by John Rolfe, the husband of the Indian princess, Pocohontas.

In 1760, Pierre Lorillard, a French Huguenot immigrant set up a snuff mill in New York. Some of the ingredients and blends that Lorillard used may have actually come from George Washington's plantation where tobacco was grown. In 1787 the earliest known tobacco advertising campaign was launched by Peter and George Lorillard.

In 1827 an Englishman by the name of John Walker developed a friction match. This was important as it allowed smoking to be done anywhere, thus contributing to the spread of cigarette smoking. In 1852, Johan Lundstrom developed the safety match by including chlorate potash over a red morphus phosphorous. Another important development which led to the spread of cigarette smoking was the development of a cigarette-rolling machine by John Bonsack of Richmond, Virginia, in 1884. Previously, Russian immigrants to the United States and women were hired to hand roll cigarettes. This manual production allowed the production of 2500 to 3000 cigarettes per day. Hand-rolled cigarettes were thus more expensive and generally bought only by the upper class. The new cigarette-rolling machines could roll 200 cigarettes per minute, 120,000 a day. This made the price of cigarettes lower and thus available to the lower economic classes.

Washington Duke, a Civil War soldier, was captured during the Civil War, and, after release from the Union prison, was forced to sell his land. He and his four sons bagged and sold tobacco and obtained a hold on the tobacco industry. J. B. Duke, a descendant, commenced large scale production of cigarettes and in 1890 the American Tobacco Company was formed, using Powhatan, the father of Pocohontas, as its symbol. In 1911, due to antitrust legislation, the American Tobacco Company was broken into five smaller companies. The Reynolds Company developed Camel cigarettes, a combination of a Turkish and seasoned barley tobacco. The American Tobacco Company produced Lucky Strike, Lorillard produced Old Gold cigarettes, and Liggett and Myers produced Chesterfield cigarettes.

One of the first to recognize the deleterious effects of tobacco was Effie Tylacote. This English physician reported in the medical journal, The Lancet, in 1927, that in almost every case of lung cancer, the patient smoked. Alton Oschner also reported a relationship between cigarette smoking and lung cancer in the 1930s. A critic at that time noted that the sale of nylon stockings like the sale of tobacco, paralleled the increased incidence of lung cancer. Medical journals used to accept cigarette advertisements. JAMA started cigarette advertising in 1934 and continued to do so until shortly after a 1953 landmark report by Wynder and Graham demonstrating the relationship between lung cancer and smoking. During the 1960s when scientists established that smoking was indeed harmful, some cigarette manufacturers reacted to these medical findings by reducing the tar and nicotine content of the cigarettes. For example, the tar content before this time for each cigarette was approximately 38 mm and was reduced to 12 mm. The nicotine content was reduced from 2.3 mg to 1.2 mg.

At a White House conference on May 23, 1961, President John Kennedy was asked what could be done about smoking and health. He promised to investigate this matter and appointed a panel of eight physicians, a chemist, and a statistician. The first Surgeon General's report regarding cigarette smoking was released by Dr. Luther Terry on January 11, 1964. In 1966 the legislative branch of the Federal government required that cigarettes be labeled hazardous to your health. In 1967 the Federal Communication Commission ruled that the "fairness doctrine" required equal time in regard to cigarette advertising. The responses by the American Cancer Society and others were so effective that the tobacco industry subsequently ceased television and radio advertising. In 1971, Congress banded radio and TV commercials advertising cigarettes. In 1973, airlines were required to separate smokers and nonsmokers.

PATHOPHYSIOLOGY

Tobacco smoking is a very complex process which involves the inhalation of cigarette smoke and pyrolates products through the cigarette. Main stream smoke is that smoke which is actually inhaled by the smoker. Side stream is that smoke which is released directly into the environment. Most scientists consider that side stream smoke is more dangerous to non-smokers than main stream smoke which is filtered through the smoker's lungs. Exhaled main stream smoke is released into the environment at a rate of about ten puffs per cigarette. Side stream smoke is produced during the entire 5 to 10 minutes the cigarette is burning. Some of the toxic content products from cigarette smoke may stay in the environment for several hours.

Cigarette smoke contains approximately 4,000 chemical components, 43 of which are known to be carcinogens. This tobacco smoke is composed of cigarette constituents consisting of organic matter, nicotinic alkaloids, and additives. The pyrolate products are carbon dioxide, carbon monoxide, and tar.

IMPORTANCE TO THE OTOLARYNGOLOGIST–HEAD AND NECK SURGEON

The effects of tobacco use in terms of development of head and neck cancer are well known. Some of the products in cigarette smoke which are carcinogens are polycyclic hydrocarbons, nitrosamines, and indole carbazole. Some of these carcinogens may act as both initiators and promoters. An *initiator* has its effect after a single brief exposure. Its effects are irreversible. The effect of initiator on a given cell is inheritable by that cell's progeny and probably works by a genetic mutation of the DNA. *Promoters* act in a more gradual process and may be partially reversible. There are two phases, a proliferative phase and a progressive phase. The length of the time for induction of a carcinoma can vary from less than ten years for initiators to several decades for promoters.

There are approximately 30 to 50 thousand new cases of head and neck cancer in this country each year. Other sites in which tobacco use has been implicated in cancer development are those of the esophagus, lung, pancreas, kidney, bladder, and possibly the uterus.

Cigarette smoke has the effect of paralyzing the cilia of the upper aerodigestive tract. The smoke from cigarettes can paralyze the cilia for a period of 12 to 24 hours. The importance of second-hand smoke in causing cancer has been recognized since the early 1990s. It is felt that second-hand smoke may be a causative factor as many as 5,000 deaths per year. In fact, nonsmokers exposed to cigarette smoke in the work place demonstrate impaired pulmonary functions consistent with those who smoke one half pack cigarettes per day. The importance of second-hand smoke is seen in the pediatric age group in terms of increased incidence of otitis media with effusion as well as sinusitis. Other generalized effects of cigarette smoking are depression of the sense of smell and taste.

There are effects on other organ systems of which the otolaryngologist should be aware (box on p 52). Cardiovascular system disorders include exercise-induced angina, coronary artery disease, myocardial infarction, sudden death, development of aortic aneurysm, peripheral vascular disease, and Buerger's disease. (Also known is thromboangiitis obliterans, which are nonatheromatous plaques involving the smaller arteries of the hands and feet leading to nonhealing ulcers and gangrene.) Effects on the lung are those of COPD, bronchitis, and cough, as well as carcinoma. In children this can lead to exacerbation of asthma, bronchiolitis, as well as decreased growth. Miscellaneous effects are those of peptic ulcer disease, development of polycythemia vera, decreased sperm counts, increased accident rates, and esophageal reflux. Perinatal effects are those of an increased fetal mortality, low birth weight, increased rate of spontaneous abortion, development of congenital abnormalities, as well as hyperactivity. Effects on dentition are those of discoloration of the teeth, abrasion of the enamel of the teeth, loss of teeth, gum recession and increased rates of periodontal disease.

If one is able to stop smoking, the risk of development of cancer is reduced in a parallel fashion to that for lung cancer. After smoking cessation, the risks of developing oral cavity cancer are decreased by 60% after five years' cessation. After 15 years the risk is reduced greater than 90%.

Effects of Smoking on Various Organ Systems

Cardiovascular

Exercise-induced angina
Coronary artery disease
Sudden death
Aortic aneurysm
Peripheral vascular disease
Buerger's disease

Pulmonary

COPD
Bronchitis
Cough
Carcinoma
Asthma
Bronchiolitis

Miscellaneous

Peptic ulcer disease
Polycythemia vera
Esophageal reflux
Decreased sperm counts
Increased accident rates

Perinatal

Increased fetal mortality
Low birth weight
Increased spontaneous abortion
Hyperactivity

Dental

Discoloration
Enamel Abrasion
Gum recession
Loss of dentition
Increased periodontal disease

From Adour K: Bell's palsy: Contemporary Perspectives on Etiology and Management. In *UC Otolaryngology Update: 1994*, November 3-5, 1994, San Francisco.

ADDICTION

In his initial report on smoking in 1964, the Surgeon General did not define smoking as an addiction. This report did not stop investigators from studying nicotine as the dependency-inducing agent in cigarette smoke. By 1988, the Surgeon General's report did address nicotine as the addicting agent in tobacco. The Diagnostic and Statistical Manual of Mental Disorders lists criteria for nicotine dependence. These include:

1. Persistent desire, or unsuccessful attempts to quit
2. Major portion of income spent in obtaining the substance
3. Continued use despite the acknowledgment of a health problem
4. Discomfort, even upon brief withdrawal, leading to continuous attempts at relief of craving

Nicotine dependence can be recognized by observing smokers. Smokers will adjust their smoking behavior to maintain a given level of nicotine. For example, the higher the concentration of nicotine in a delivery system, the lower the rate of smoking or the shallower the inhalation. The converse is also true. The lower the concentration of nicotine in a delivery system, the faster the rate of smoking or the deeper the inhalation.

Smokers tend to maintain nicotine levels between 30 and 40 ng/ml of plasma. It has also been observed that smokers will increase their smoking rate and/or their depth of inhalation of mecamylamine, a centrally acting cholinergic blocking agent used to block nicotine effects.

Tolerance is generally associated with chemicals that are addictive. It basically refers to an acquired resistance to the effects of any drug. Chronic tolerance has been shown in animals but has not been definitely shown in humans. The DSM-IV describes nicotine tolerance as the absence of nausea and dizziness commonly associated with the first use of tobacco products.

The major type of negative reinforcement for individuals addicted to alcohol, barbiturates, and heroin is withdrawal relief. This is the same for smokers. Schacter has suggested that the sole purpose for nicotine seeking is for withdrawal relief. Nicotine replacement in smokers who have been deprived of nicotine relieves the withdrawal symptoms of irritability and discomfort.

Nicotine is absorbed from practically any anatomic site, including the lungs and buccal and nasal mucosa. It enters the bloodstream and is metabolized in the liver to continine and nicotine-n-oxide which are nth associated with dependency. Inhalation provides the quickest, most effective and most addictive route to the brain. Nicotine has been shown to bind to certain areas of rat brain with a high affinity. Areas known to be important for reinforcement, the substantia nigra and the ventral tegmental area, are high affinity sites. The projections from ventral tegmental area to the nucleus accumbens are important in reward medication and are also high affinity sites. The neurotransmitters involved are dopamine and serotonin. The effects of nicotine in the central nervous system are most likely responsible for reward and reinforcement. The nicotine effects are similar to the stimulants cocaine and amphetamines. Nicotine, as with many other psychoactive substances, has a defined withdrawal syndrome. The need to avoid withdrawal symptoms is a major reason that only 5% of smokers are successful in unaided attempts to quit smoking. The DSM-IV lists the diagnostic criteria for nicotine withdrawal. These include; dysphoric or depressed mood, insomnia, irritability, frustration, anger, anxiety, difficulty concentrating, restlessness, decreased heart rate, and increased appetite or weight gain. Withdrawal symptoms are also associated with a slowing of the EEG, decreases in catecholamine and cortisol levels, REM changes, decreased performance on neuropsychological testing, and decreased metabolic rate. These withdrawal symptoms can appear within a few hours of cessation, peak in 1 to 4 days, and can last for 3 to 4 weeks.

While there has been much debate about the addictive properties of nicotine, there is no doubt that it meets the criteria for an addictive drug. The American Medical Association, the American Psychiatric Association, and the American Society of Addiction Medicine all recognize nicotine as an addicting mood-altering substance. Perhaps the greatest tragedy is that nicotine users continue to use their nicotine-containing products with full knowledge of the medical problems that are associated with their use. This adds to the increased cost of health care considering the extreme morbidity and mortality associated with nicotine use.

TREATMENT

Your patient makes a conscious decision to quite smoking when three factors are present: (1) a perceived risk from continuing to smoke, (2) a net value in stopping, and (3) a belief that smoking cessation can be achieved. You can make an important contribution to your patients' health by helping them arrive at this point and by taking advantage of it once they do.

Immediate benefits

Some of the immediate benefits of smoking cessation include improved ability to breathe, less coughing, regained sense of taste and smell, fresher breath, improved exercise tolerance, no more burn holes in clothing, no more tobacco stains on teeth and fingers, no ashtrays to empty, better insurance status, decreased risk of passive smoking damage to family members and others, and financial savings. You can use these benefits as early, positive reinforcement.

Stages of quitting

Investigators have identified five stages in the smoking cessation process:

1. *Precontemplation.* In this stage, patients are unlikely to be responsive to direct intervention. They have little concern about the negative aspects of smoking, and heavy-handed messages may increase their resistance to quitting. A calm, factual presentation of the risks, delivered in a low-key fashion, is the best approach.
2. *Contemplation.* In this stage, patients are much more receptive to information about the dangers of smoking. They will often ask for help.
3. *Action.* This is the stage of quitting tobacco use.
4. *Maintenance.* This is the most difficult stage. It involves remaining abstinent.
5. *Relapse.* A return to smoking occurs so often in patients attempting to give up cigarettes that it has to be considered part of the quitting process.

A practical approach to quitting

The 1987 Surgeon General's report concluded that the pharmacologic and behavioral processes that determine tobacco addiction are similar to those that determine addiction to drugs such as heroin and cocaine. Given this fact, the approach to the treatment of nicotine addiction should be similar to that of addiction to other drugs of abuse; that is, it should be composed of two elements; (1) detoxification and (2) behavior modification.

Detoxification

Two agents for detoxification from nicotine have been approved by the Food and Drug Administration: (1) nicotine gum and (2) nicotine transdermal patches. The use of these agents is sometimes call nicotine-substitution therapy.

Nicotine gum. Each piece of nicotine gum (Nicorette) contains 2 mg of nicotine bound to an ion-exchange resin in a gum base. Instructions are given to chew the gum for 20 to 30 minutes when an urge to smoke occurs, up to a total of 30 pieces per day. Patients should be advised to chew gently and slowly until they experience a taste or tingling, then to pause until the sensation disappears before starting to chew again. Most people chew 10 to 15 pieces of gum per day. Chewing too few may result in inadequate nicotine blood levels and therapeutic failure. The gum is typically used for three months, with gradual tapering after that. Unfortunately, about 10% of nicotine gum users have difficulty giving up the gum.

The most common adverse effects of nicotine gum are sore mouth or throat, hiccups, tired jaws, nausea or other gastrointestinal symptoms, palpitations, and mouth ulcers.

Nicotine gum should be used only after smoking has ceased.

Nicotine transdermal patches. Nicotine patches, for practical purposes, have replaced nicotine gum as a detoxification agent. The patches contain nicotine that is released gradually from a gel-matrix reservoir (Habitrol, Nicotrol, Prostep) or across a rate-limiting membrane (Nicoderm).

A new patch is applied to a different area of skin daily, rotating on a weekly basis. Every few weeks, the patch size (nicotine dose) is reduced so that the nicotine blood level is tapered gradually. Habitrol and Nicoderm are supplied in three sizes (21 mg/hr, 14 mg/hr, 7 mg/hr), as is Nicotrol (15 mg/hr, 10 mg/hr, 5 mg/hr). Prostep is supplied in two sizes (22 mg/hr and 11 mg/hr).

Nicotine gum can be used when necessary to taper individuals off the patches or to prevent relapse from nicotine craving once the course of patches has been completed.

Contraindications to nicotine patches include recent myocardial infarction, life-threatening arrhythmias, unstable angina, and pregnancy. The maximum-strength patch probably should not be used in individuals with significant coronary artery disease.

A number of myocardial infarctions have occurred in individuals who continued to smoke while wearing the patch. Patients should be warned of this danger.

The most common side effect of nicotine transdermal patches is skin irritation.

Behavior modification

Behavioral techniques that may be useful include: (1) self-control strategies, (2) stimulus-control strategies, (3) coping skills, and (4) contingency management.

Self-control strategies include continually reminding oneself of reasons to stop smoking and smoking in the least pleasurable way possible (for example, not smoking immediately after meals, always smoking alone, and using the least preferred brand of cigarettes).

Stimulus-control strategies include limiting the number of cues for smoking and reducing the ability of cues to evoke the desire for a cigarette. The latter phenomenon is called cue extinction. The first step is identifying the cues, which may include specific times, places, emotions, or social settings. Environmental cues include cigarette lighters, ashtrays, pipes, and other smoking paraphernalia. Specific activities that often trigger a desire to smoke include completing a meal, drinking a cocktail, or talking on the telephone. Situations that may provoke relapse include social pressures, stress, anger, frustration, or depression.

Once the cues are identified, a plan for dealing with them individually must be developed and put into action.

The following approach is helpful in cue extinction: Seven to ten days before quitting, the smoker selects three cues he or she has identified as being the most difficult to endure without a cigarette. During this time, the smoker continues to smoke, but not in response to the selected cues. This usually involves waiting at least ten minutes after the cue has passed before lighting a cigarette.

Coping skills include using stress reduction and stress relaxation techniques, as well as seeking out nonsmoking environments and social support. Useful techniques involve thinking of the negative aspects of smoking and the positive aspects of not smoking, using self-encouragement, avoiding situations in which the temptation to smoke will be particularly strong, and substituting low-calorie food, beverages, or gum for cigarettes. Thinking of not smoking one day at a time is a particularly helpful tool.

Contingency management involves arranging for a reward contingent on not smoking during a specified period following cessation. This may be accomplished through a written contract with friends, the family, or a physician. Reward for abstaining is more effective than punishment for smoking. The reward does not have to be large but it should be frequent.

Five-step program

The following five-step program is a useful approach to smoking cessation by busy physicians:

Step 1. *Review the patient's smoking status and take a brief smoking history.* The smoking history should include: age smoking initiated, length of time smoked, average number of cigarettes per day smoked, tar content of cigarettes, family members who smoke, smoking-related illnesses, family history of smoking-related illnesses, attempts to quit (how many attempts made, longest period of abstinence, withdrawal symptoms experienced, methods used to quit, what stimulated relapse), current motivation to quit, history of other substance abuse, and workplace smoking policy.

Providing health-risk information about continued smoking is an integral part of this step. Medical findings should be personalized whenever possible. The effects of passive smoking on the health of the patient's spouse, children, and co-workers should be included in this discussion.

Step 2. *Assess the patient's interest in quitting.* The patient's readiness to stop smoking, level of motivation, and confidence in success should be determined. If the patient is in the "precontemplation" stage and is not ready to make an attempt to stop smoking, recommendations and materials can be supplied that may influence the patient later. The patient should be encouraged to reduce the number of cigarettes smoked. If the patient is determined to be in the "contemplation" stage, you should determine the main reason he or she is considering quitting. This reason can be used to reinforce the quitting effort. If the patient expresses a desire to quit smoking, proceed to the following step.

Step 3. *Set a target quit date.* The patient, with your help, chooses a target quit date. He or she may be asked to sign a contract acknowledging that a date has been set and promising to stop smoking entirely on that date. Studies have shown that quitting on a predetermined quit date is more effective than gradually tapering and quitting.

You may wish to prescribe a nicotine patch at this time, with the instructions that the patient is to put on the first patch just prior to bedtime the night before the quit date. At this time, all remaining cigarettes are to be disposed of and cigarette lighters and ashtrays eliminated from the environment.

Step 4. *Suggest Smoking Cessation Strategies.* This step is usually the most difficulty for physicians because there are so many options. You may choose to: (1) provide the patient with self-help material, (2) work personally with the patient using material from one of a number of organizations, or (3) refer the patient to a community smoking cessation program.

Selected sources of materials for patients and physicians include the American Academy of Family Physicians, American Cancer Society, American Lung Association, American Health Association, Doctors Ought to Care (DOC), National Cancer Institute, National Heart, Lung, and Blood Institute, and the Office on Smoking and Health.

Strategies that can be used prior to the quit date include having patients: (1) sign a no smoking contract, (2) list reasons for wanting to quit: they can then repeat a different one of these several times nightly to reinforce the desire to quit. (3) buy cigarettes by the single pack only, (4) give up smoking in the car, (5) smoke the least pleasurable brand, (6) cut down to a pack per day if more than that is being smoked, (7) think about quitting one day at a time rather than the rest of their lives, and (8) make a list of the times, places, and situations in which the urge to smoke is the greatest. In addition, you can recommend stress relaxation techniques (including a relaxing audiotape), discuss expected withdrawal symptoms, and encourage the patient to begin an exercise program to help prevent possible weight gain.

Strategies that can be used after the quit date include having patients: (1) take five deep breaths and exhale slowly after an urge to smoke occurs, (2) play with a pen to occupy the hand that usually has a cigarette in it, (3) suck air through a cut-off soda straw when the urge to smoke is particularly strong, (4) rub the patch gently and say "This is all the nicotine I need" in response to craving a cigarette, (5) play a relaxation tape if one tends to smoke when anxious, (6) avoid the times, places, and situations in which the urge to smoke is known to occur if at all possible. Put into play the predetermined strategies for dealing with the above when they cannot be avoided.

Step 5. *Schedule follow-up appointments and telephone calls.* Follow-up serves three purposes: (1) it allows tapering of the nicotine patch size, (2) provides support, and (3) allows determination of patient adherence. Should relapse occur, you can support the patient in learning from the experience and beginning over again. Many patients have to attempt smoking cessation a number of times before finally achieving success.

SUMMARY

The otolaryngologist–head and neck surgeon is uniquely qualified to interface with patients who have tobacco induced inflammatory and neoplastic diseases. This chapter has reviewed tobacco's history, as well as a pathophysiology and addictive aspects. Using the treatment strategies advocated in this text, the physician can positively impact the patient with nicotine addiction.

SUGGESTED READING

1. American Psychiatric Association; Diagnostic and Statistical Manual of Mental Disorders, ed. 3, Revised, Washington, D.C., 1987, APA.
2. Ca: A Cancer Journal for Clinicians: *Cigarette Smoking: The Need for Action* 38(4): 194-212, 1988.
3. Charlton A: *Children and Passive Smoking: A Review.* J Fam Prac 38:267-273, 1994.
4. Chesebro MJ: *Passive Smoking.* Am Fam Phys 37:212-218, 1988.
5. Cocores, JT: *The Clinical Management of Nicotine Dependence.* New York, 1991, Springer Verlag.
6. Cox JL: *How to Help Your Patients Stop Smoking.* J Am Acad Phys Assist 3:600-608, 1990.
7. Davis RM: *Current Trends in Cigarette Advertising and Marketing.* N Engl J Med 316:725-732, 1987.
8. Gritz ER: *Cigarette Smoking: The Need for Action by Health Professionals.* Cancer 38:194-212, 1988.
9. Henningfield JE, Nemeth-Coslett R: *Nicotine Dependence. Interface Between Tobacco and Tobacco-related Disease. Chest* 93 (suppl 2):37S-55S, 1988.
10. Hoffman D, Hecht SS: *Nicotine-derived N-nitrosamines and Tobacco-related Cancer. Cancer Res* 45:2285, 1985.
11. Holt GR: *Toxicology of Upper Aerodigestive Tract Pollutants.* Otolaryngology–Head and Neck Surgery, Vol. 106, Number 6.
12. Hughes JR, Higgins ST, Hatsukami D: *Effects of Abstinence from Tobacco: A Critical Review.* In Kozlowski LT, Annis H, Cappel HD, et al, editors: *Research Advances in Alcohol and Drug Problems.* New York, 1990, Plenum Press, pp. 317-398.
13. Husten CG, Manley MW: *How to Help Your Patients Stop Smoking.* J Am Acad Fam Pract 42:1072-1126, 1990.
14. Kellar KJ, Schwartz RD, Martino AM: *Nicotine Cholinergic Receptor Recognition Sites in the Brain.* In Martin WR, Van Loon GR, Iwamoto ET, Davis LT, editors: *Tobacco Smoking and Nicotine. A Neurobiological Approach.* New York, 1987, Plenum Press, pp. 467-480.
15. Kottke TE, Battista RN, DeFriese GH, et al: *Attributes of Successful Smoking Cessation Interventions in Medical Practice: A Meta-Analysis of 39 Controlled Trials.* JAMA 259(1a):2883-2889, 1988.
16. Kozlowski LT, Ferrence RG, Corbit T: *Tobacco Use: A Perspective for Alcohol and Drug Researchers.* Br J Addict 85:243, 1990.
17. Kozlowski LT, Jarvik ME, Gritz ER: *Nicotine Regulation and Cigarette Smoking.* Clin Pharmacol Ther 17:93-97, 1975.
18. Krogh D: *Smoking: The Artificial Passion.* New York, 1991, W.H. Freeman and Company.
19. Milhorn HT: *Nicotine Dependence.* J Am Acad Fam Pract 39:214-224, 1989.
20. Pomerleau CS, Pomerleau OF, Majchrzak MJ: *Mecamylamine Pretreatment Increases Subsequent Nicotine Self-Administration as Indicated by Changes in Plasma Nicotine Level.* Psychopharmacology 9:391-393, 1987.
21. Rose JE, Jarvik ME, Rose KD: *Transdermal Administration of Nicotine. Drug Alcohol Dependence.* 13:209-213, 1984.
22. Russell MA: *Nicotine Intake and Its Regulation. J Psychosom Research* 24(5):253-264, 1980.
23. Schacter S: *Regulation, Withdrawal and Nicotine Addiction.* In Krasnegor NA, editor: *Cigarette Smoking as a Dependent Process.* Rockville, MD, 1979, National Institute of Drug Abuse.
24. Schmiterlow CG, Hansson E, Andersson G, et al: *Distribution of Nicotine in the Central Nervous System.* In Murphree HB, editor: *The Effects of Nicotine and Smoking on the Central Nervous System.* New York, 1967, Annals of the New York Academy of Sciences.
25. Schneider NG, Jarvik ME: *Nicotine Gum Versus Placebo Gum: Comparison of Withdrawal Symptoms and Success Rates.* Nat Inst Drug Abuse Res Mongr Ser 53:83-101, 1988.
26. Stolerman IP, Dunker P, Jarvik ME: *Nicotine Tolerance in Rats: Role of Dose and Dose Interval.* Psychopharmacologia 34:317-324, 1974.
27. U.S. Department of Health, Education and Welfare: A Report to the Surgeon General, Public Health Service, Washington, D.C., 1964, Government Printing Office.
28. U.S. Department of Health and Human Services: The Health Consequences of Smoking. A Report to the Surgeon General, Washington, D.C., 1988, Government Printing Office.

5

The Otolaryngologic Manifestations of Gastroesophageal (Laryngopharyngeal) Reflux Disease

James A. Koufman

It has been estimated that approximately half of otolaryngology (ORL) patients with laryngeal and voice disorders have gastroesophageal reflux disease (GER, GERD) as the primary cause or as a significant etiologic cofactor.[12] In addition, in these patients the available data confirm that refluxed gastric contents actually come in direct contact with laryngopharyngeal structures.[2,10,11,27] Thus, GER in ORL patients should be more accurately termed ***laryngopharyngeal reflux disease (LPR, LPRD).*** LPRD appears to be associated with a variety of diverse clinical manifestations. The box on p. 58 lists the most common symptoms and diagnoses that have been reported (in otolaryngology) to be reflux related.

It now appears that LPR may be the single most common cause of laryngeal and voice disorders. However, this discovery is somewhat controversial and still not accepted (or recognized) by all otolaryngologists. Even among otolaryngologists who have a relatively high index of suspicion for laryngopharyngeal reflux, it appears that LPR is still often underdiagnosed and undertreated. There appears to be a four-part explanation for this phenomenon:

1. ***ORL patients with LPR usually do not have heartburn.*** Less than half of ORL patients with LPR (documented by pH monitoring) complain of heartburn or regurgitation, symptoms that clinicians have traditionally felt must be present in order to diagnose GER.[10,11,17,24,27] Generally, ORL patients with LPR do not have esophagitis, and, thus, they do not suffer from its principal symptom, heartburn. This appears to be due to the fact that the mechanism of LPR in ORL patients is rather different from that seen in typical gastroenterology GER patients.
2. ***Most ORL patients with LPR do not have "red" larynges.*** The most common finding in reflux laryngitis is edema and not erythema. Traditionally, otolaryngologists have looked for the findings termed "posterior laryngitis" (piled up interarytenoid mucosa and red arytenoids) as the diagnostic *sine qua non* for "reflux laryngitis." Indeed, laryngeal edema is the far more common finding and it may be diffuse or it may create the illusion of "sulcus vocalis," an appearance that is the result of subglottic edema in Reinke's space.[11]
3. ***Traditional diagnostic tests are often falsely negative in LPR patients.*** The diagnosis of LPR may be confounded by false negative diagnostic tests. Barium esophagography, radionuclide scanning, the Bernstein acid-perfusion test, and esophagoscopy with biopsy are all usually negative in the ORL patient with LPR.[10,11,17,27] Again, this is probably because the mechanism of LPR in ORL patients is different from that in gastroenterology patients with GER—the latter usually have esophagitis, while LPR patients do not.[10,27] In addition, LPR is frequently intermittent, and exacerbations may depend to some extent upon ever-changing dietary and life style factors.[10]

Recently, in our laboratory, using double-probe pH monitoring (pH-metry), we demonstrated that as

Symptoms and Laryngeal Conditions Associated With Reflux Symptoms

Chronic dysphonia
Intermittent dysphonia
Vocal fatigue
Voice breaks
Chronic throat clearing
Excessive throat mucus
"Postnasal drip"
Chronic cough
Dysphagia
Globus

Conditions associated with reflux as the cause or as a causative cofactor

Reflux laryngitis
Subglottic stenosis
Carcinoma of the larynx
Endotracheal intubation injury
Contact ulcers and granulomas
Vocal nodules and cysts
Posterior glottic stenosis
Unilateral or bilateral arytenoid fixation
Paroxysmal laryngospasm
Globus pharyngeus
Polypoid degeneration
Laryngomalacia
Pachydermia laryngis
Recurrent leukoplakia

many as one-third of patients with LPR would be falsely assumed to be "normal" had it not been for the presence of the second (pharyngeal) probe to document the LPR. In other words, even single-probe esophageal pH-metry is relatively insensitive to LPR.[11] At present, double-probe pH-metry is the "gold standard" test for the diagnosis of LPR. Even so, false negative studies may sometimes occur with pH-metry, particularly in the intermittent or "life style" LPR patient.

4. ***ORL patients with LPR often fail to respond to a therapeutic trial using traditional antireflux therapy.*** The "traditional" treatment of GER with dietary and life style modifications, as well as with H2-blocker medications (e.g., cimetidine, ranitidine, famotidine), fails in approximately 35% of ORL patients with LPR.[10] This is because the larynx is very sensitive to reflux-induced injury and because H2-blocker therapy produces only partial suppression of gastric acid production.

   In addition, in many cases, the intensity of the attempted treatment is inadequate, and the duration of the therapeutic trial may be too short as well. Some clinicians mistakenly assume that a therapeutic trial of antireflux therapy of several weeks' duration is adequate, but that is not the case.

   Patients with long-standing LPR often require months of "optimal" treatment with complete acid suppression (using omeprazole 20 mg twice daily) to resolve symptoms.[10,11,24] (Unquestionably, the drug omeprazole has revolutionized the treatment of LPR, and, until it became available, a therapeutic trial had little meaning as a diagnostic test.)

WHAT MAKES THE LPR PATIENT DIFFERENT?

In 1981, a clergyman presented to the author with a recurrent granuloma on the laryngeal surface of the epiglottis; it had been removed three times previously. I removed the lesion a fourth time and it recurred. Then, I performed a laser epiglottectomy, but granulation tissue formed at the operative site on the tongue base. Despite the fact that the patient had no typical reflux symptoms and a normal barium esophagogram, I placed him on stringent antireflux treatment and, eventually, his granuloma healed.

This was the first time that I had encountered a patient with laryngopharyngeal reflux who denied any of the symptoms considered typical for GER. Indeed, this case opened my eyes to the possibility that LPR in ORL patients might be quite different in terms of its symptoms, its mechanism, and its sequelae, compared with gastroenterology patients with esophagitis. Indeed, the clinical pattern of LPR in ORL patients is quite different, and this observation remains at the root of the current controversy surrounding the diagnosis and treatment of LPR.

In 1986, Wiener *et al*[27] from our institution published a land-mark study. They studied 32 consecutive patients with hoarseness by double-probe pH-metry, as well as by esophagoscopy with biopsy and by Bernstein acid-perfusion test. Three-fourths of the patients had documented reflux disease by pH-metry; however, 75% had normal esophagoscopy and biopsy and 100% had normal Bernstein tests.[27] On the basis of that study, we postulated: (1) that occult (silent) and sometimes intermittent LPR could be associated with the development of inflammatory and neoplastic conditions of the upper aerodigestive tract and (2) that the symptoms and mechanism of LPR are different from those seen in "typical" GER patients.

Subsequently, we have had an opportunity to study almost a thousand LPR patients with double-probe pH-metry. At this point, we now can add some pieces to the puzzle, although why LPR patients are so different from gastroenterology (GI) patients has not been fully elucidated.

As a generalization, GI patients have poor esophageal motility and poor lower esophageal sphincter (LES) function, whereas LPR patients generally have relatively good esophageal motor and LES function but faulty upper esophageal sphincter (UES) function.[10,11] GI patients with GER usually experience abnormal supine nocturnal reflux but only uncommonly experience daytime upright reflux (LPR). In contrast, LPR patients most often experience ab-

TABLE 5-1
Differences between the typical gastroenterology patient with esophagitis and the typical otolaryngology patient with laryngopharyngeal reflux

	Gastroenterology	Otolaryngology
Symptoms		
Heartburn and/or regurgitation	Yes	No
Hoarseness, dysphagia, globus throat clearing, cough, etc.	No	Yes
Findings		
Endoscopic esophagitis	Yes	No
Laryngeal inflammation	No	Yes
Diagnostic yield (abnormality)		
Esophageal biopsy (inflammation)	Yes	No
Abnormal esophageal radiography	Yes	Sometimes
Esophageal pH monitoring	Yes	Yes
Pharyngeal pH monitoring	No	Yes
Pattern of reflux		
Supine (nocturnal)	Yes	Sometimes
Upright (awake)	Sometimes	Yes
Response to Treatment		
Dietary/life style modification	Yes	Sometimes
Rate of success with H2-blockers*	85%	65%
Rate of success with omeprazole*	99%	99%

*Assuming adequate dosage and duration of therapy.
Table data adapted from Koufman JA: The otolaryngologic manifestations of gastroesophageal reflux disease. Laryngoscope 101:(Suppl 53):1-78, 1991.[2]

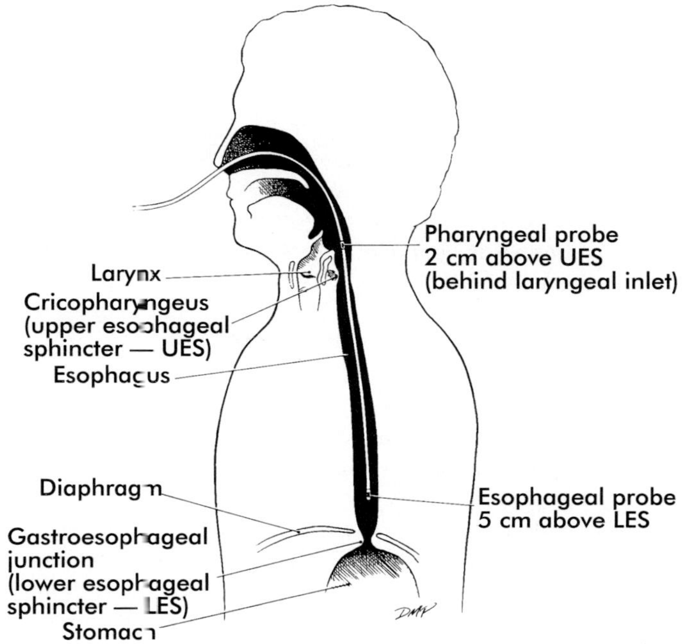

FIG 5-1
Technique of ambulatory 24-hour double-probe pH monitoring. (From The Otolaryngologic Manifestations of Gastroesophageal Reflux Disease, In *Larynogoscope* 101:April, 1991.)

normal daytime upright (and laryngopharyngeal) reflux but uncommonly experience supine nocturnal reflux. Not surprisingly, esophageal motility is much more frequently abnormal in GI patients than in ORL patients with LPR.[10,11,27]

In addition, it has been shown experimentally that instilling acid in the distal esophagus of normal subjects and in patients with esophagitis usually results in a prompt increase in resting tone of the UES.[2] This does not appear to be the case in LPR patients, in whom our studies have shown that the UES does not serve as an effective barrier to prevent LPR.[10,11] Thus, it appears that significant differences in esophageal motility and in upper esophageal sphincter function may explain some of the clinical differences in the two patient populations. **Table 5-1** summarizes these differences.

DIAGNOSIS OF LARYNGOPHARYNGEAL REFLUX

When a patient presents with dysphonia, globus, dysphagia, chronic throat clearing and cough, or "too much mucus in the throat," symptoms that suggest the possibility of LPR, the clinician should perform a complete otolaryngologic examination and then consider performing a "reflux work-up." For over a decade now, it has been our routine to complete a "patient profile (reflux) data sheet" (see Appendix A) and to perform a complete otolaryngologic examination on all new patients with laryngeal and voice disorders. If LPR is suspected, based upon the patient's symptoms or laryngeal findings, then the following studies are performed: (1) videoendoscopic examination; (2) 24-hour double-probe pH-metry; and (3) barium esophagography.

Fig. 5-1 shows the technique (probe positioning) of double-probe pH-metry. It is important to recognize that the second (pharyngeal) probe must be placed above the upper esophageal sphincter (UES). Double-probe pH-metry has tremendous advantages over any other diagnostic method, because it is both highly sensitive and specific for LPR.[10,20] Furthermore, pH-metry reveals the pattern of reflux, so that subsequent treatment can be custom tailored for each patient. For example, if the patient does not have supine nocturnal reflux then elevation of the head of the bed need not be recommended.

For many years, pH-metry has been available and standards (normal values) have been established in many laboratories.[10,20,21] In general, the most important parameter is considered to be the percentage of time that the pH is less than 4, and this measurement is usually recorded for time in the *upright position,* time in the *supine position,* and the *total time* of the study. For the upright period, the upper limit of normal is approximately 8.0% and for the supine, approximately 2.5%.[21]

Why the pharyngeal probe is essential in the ORL patient

Positive pharyngeal (double-probe) pH monitoring, with the second probe being placed behind the larynx just above the cricopharyngeus, is virtually diagnostic of LPR. (No normal control [n = 40] has ever had a documented pharyngeal reflux episode.) Therefore, it must be concluded that even a single pharyngeal reflux event should be considered diagnostic of reflux as a cause in patients with upper aerodigestive symptoms.[10,20] Fig. 5-2 shows an example of an abnormal double-probe pH study—reflux is seen in both the esophageal and the pharyngeal probes.

Double-probe pH-metry is particularly important in ORL patients with LPR because the correct diagnosis might otherwise be missed. Recently, it was shown that 23% (28/122) of a consecutive series of ORL patients with pH-documented LPR had normal total acid exposure times in the esophageal probe.[11] In other words, were it not for the positive pharyngeal probe findings, these 28 patients would have been falsely presumed not to have LPR. Pharyngeal probe monitoring is necessary in ORL patients because it increases the diagnostic yield using pH-metry from 39% to 62% (abnormal).[11]

Barium esophagography

It is also advisable to obtain a barium swallow/esophagogram in ORL patients with LPR, because this test allows the otolaryngologist to assess the integrity of the esophageal lining.[18] Although barium study is not a sensitive test for diagnosing LPR or GER, it may demonstrate significant abnormalities that might otherwise be missed.[10] In a series of 128 patients, the results of barium study revealed that 18% had esophagitis, 14% had a lower esophageal ring, and 3% had a peptic stricture.[10]

CLINICAL MANIFESTATIONS

In a large series of LPR patients, dysphonia (hoarseness) was found to be the most common symptom (92%),[10] and its pattern was either chronic or intermittent. Patients with intermittent dysphonia often complain that they suffer from "laryngitis" that lasts for days or weeks, several times a year.

Additional symptoms were experienced by the majority of the patients: chronic throat clearing (50%), chronic cough (44%), globus (33%), and dysphagia (27%). Half of the patients denied having any heartburn whatsoever; 13% had two or fewer episodes per week, 27% had two to four episodes per week, and only 10% complained of more frequent or daily heartburn.[10]

Although most patients with LPR present with mild to moderate dysphonia as the primary symptom, some suffer from more serious, even life-threatening, conditions. Less common laryngeal manifestations of LPR include laryngospasm, arytenoid fixation, laryngeal stenosis, and carcinoma. LPR is also associated with the development of polypoid degeneration (Reinke's edema), vocal nodules, and other functional voice disorders.

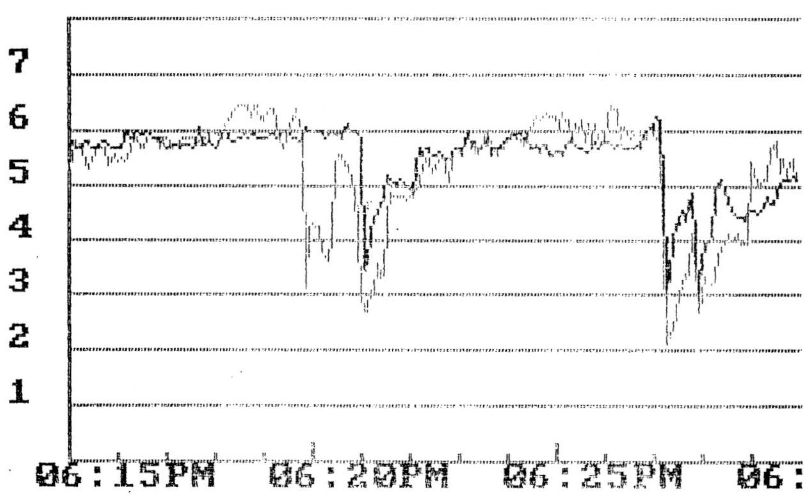

FIG 5-2
Example of an abnormal double-probe pH study. (The lighter line represents the esophageal pH tracing and the darker line represents the pharyngeal pH tracing.) For a pharyngeal reflux event to be considered "positive," a precipitous pH drop (below 4.0) in the esophageal probe must be seen, immediately followed by a similar precipitous drop in pH in the pharyngeal probe. On the tracing shown, three significant laryngopharyngeal reflux events are demonstrated, occurring at approximately 6:21 P.M., 6:27 P.M., and 6:28 P.M.

The clinical manifestations of LPR can be divided into three groups, based upon severity—*minor, major, and life threatening*. This subgrouping system (Table 5-2) is not arbitrary, and it influences the clinician's approach to the diagnosis and treatment of each of the three patient groups; each group is managed differently. Patients with airway obstruction and malignant neoplasia are considered to have "life-threatening" LPR. Those with other, less severe symptoms and findings are subgrouped into the "minor" or "major" groups, based not only upon the severity of the clinical situation but also taking into account the vocal needs and occupation of the patient.

Reflux and functional voice disorders

The term *functional voice disorder (FVD)* applies to a variety of vocal abuse/misuse/overuse syndromes. Within the last few years, based upon the findings, these conditions have also been termed *muscle tension dysphonias (MTDs),* because transnasal fiberoptic laryngoscopy (TFL) usually shows abnormal laryngeal biomechanics. The most commonly observed pattern is *supraglottic contraction,* either anteroposterior contraction (foreshortening of the vocal cords), or false vocal cord approximation.[13]

The FVD group of conditions is often associated with the secondary development of histopathologic changes of vocal cords, which include hematomas, nodules, ulcers, granulomas, and Reinke's edema. With the availability of pH-metry, data now suggest that the majority of patients with these functional lesions have LPR in addition to abnormal (or altered) laryngeal biomechanics.[11] In many cases, it is likely that the LPR has precipitated the problem.[9]

TABLE 5-2
Relative severity of symptoms and sequelae related to laryngopharyngeal reflux

Minor	Major	Life-threatening*
Dysphonia† (in the "nonvocal professions")	Dysphonia† (in a vocalist or professional voice user)	Subglottic stenosis
Ulcer/granuloma† (in the "nonvocal professions")	Ulcer/granuloma† (in a vocalist or professional voice user)	Posterior laryngeal stenosis
Globus	Leukoplakia	Arytenoid fixation
Dysphagia	Pachydermia	Carcinoma (especially in the nonsmoker)
Chronic throat clearing	Dysplasia	Laryngospasm
Chronic cough	Chronic cough‡	

*The "life-threatening" group is defined by either *airway obstruction* or *malignancy*.
†The purpose of establishing a "difference" between the "severity" (of the same symptom) in the vocalist and the nonvocalist is to emphasize that economic and emotional consequences of a voice disorder depend on the vocal needs and demands of each patient. When a well-known professional vocalist (a "star"), for example, develops a voice disorder, this may have profound consequences, and, thus, effective treatment must be maximized (see text).
‡On occasion, this symptom may be so severe that the patient is relatively incapacitated.

As part of the evaluation of each patient with an FVD, the clinician should elicit a "reflux history." In addition, patients who have posterior laryngeal erythema, edema, or thick mucus in the endolarynx should be suspected of having LPR. This is not to say that treatment of LPR alone will resolve most FVDs, however, that is the case in some patients. On the other hand, failure to treat LPR when it is present may doom what otherwise would be an effective therapeutic intervention.[8,9,13]

The laryngeal findings may be subtle. The appearance of a (subglottic) groove giving each of the vocal folds the appearance of a sulcus (a "pseudosulcus") should alert the clinician to the possibility of LPR. Mucus in the endolarynx is not usually the result of infection or "postnasal drip" but is probably the result of a local tissue (inflammatory) response to chronic irritation, i.e., LPR. Likewise, ulceration and granulation may be seen in non-LPR patients; however, most such patients do have LPR.

Vocal process granulomas

The etiology and treatment of granulomas of the vocal process remain controversial; however, LPR should always be suspected. Granulomas usually result from the combination of acute mucosal ulceration of the vocal process, LPR, and chronic vocal trauma due to throat clearing and/or a hard glottal attack.[8] Even without LPR, chronic vocal trauma can lead to vocal cord ulcers or granulomas; however, in the majority of cases, LPR is a causative factor. The clinician should, in each case, consider each of the possible contributing etiologic factors and correct each if therapy is to be effective. In the case of granulomas, effective antireflux therapy (namely, twice-daily omeprazole) is sufficient to allow healing in the majority of patients, as long as they are able to refrain from vocally abusive behaviors.

Surgical removal of vocal process granulomas is often an exercise in futility, since they usually recur. The majority of these lesions resolve within six months with antireflux (omeprazole) therapy with good vocal hygiene. Surgical removal of granulomas is, however, indicated in three situations.[8]

1. *When granulomas cause airway obstruction.* Airway obstruction from granulomas is uncommon but occurs sometimes. This provides a rather obvious indication for surgical removal.
2. *When carcinoma is suspected (for biopsy).* The majority of vocal process granulomas appear as smooth, shiny, bilobed grey-white masses on the arytenoids. When a granuloma appears to "spread" anterior to the vocal process or takes on a ragged

"keratotic" appearance, the possibility of carcinoma must be entertained, and excisional biopsy is indicated.

3. *When the granuloma matures and becomes a fibroepithelial polyp.* On occasion, after an extensive period of treatment, a granuloma may take on the appearance of a mature, pedunculated fibroepithelial polyp. When this occurs, additional medical treatment will fail to eradicate the lesion and it should be excised.

Paroxysmal laryngospasm

Laryngospasm is an uncommon complaint, but patients who experience this frightening symptom are usually able to describe "events" in vivid detail. If the clinician mimics severe inspiratory stridor, the patient will confirm that his or her breathing during an "attack" does indeed sound similar.

Laryngospasm is often paroxysmal, and it usually occurs without warning. For some patients, the attacks awake them from sleep, and for others the attacks occur during the day. In some cases, the attacks may have a predictable pattern, e.g., postcibal or during exercise, and some patients are aware of a relationship between LPR and the attacks (others are not).

Of eleven patients who presented to the author with recurrent paroxysmal laryngospasm within the last three years, ten had documented LPR by pH-metry and all eleven responded to treatment with omeprazole by a complete cessation of the laryngospasm episodes (unpublished data, 1994).

Polypoid degeneration (Reinke's edema)

Polypoid degeneration results from chronic laryngeal irritation over a period of many years. It is almost always bilateral and occurs most frequently in elderly female smokers. Nevertheless, it is seen is nonsmoking patients with LPR and/or hypothyroidism.

Polypoid degeneration may improve with antireflux therapy and cessation of smoking, but most patients with these lesions require surgical treatment as well. It is interesting to note that this group of patients has been reported to have a very high incidence (41%) of prolonged postoperative dysphonia (defined as more than 4 weeks).[14] This, in retrospect, may be due to continued LPR after surgery.

Most patients with polypoid degeneration have abnormal pH-metry.[11] Consequently, LPR should be considered in the differential diagnosis, and, at the very least, patients undergoing vocal cord surgery for this condition should receive antireflux treatment during the perioperative period.

Laryngeal stenosis

Except for trauma, LPR is the primary cause of laryngeal stenosis, including subglottic stenosis and posterior laryngeal stenosis[5,10,11,15]; pH-metry documented LPR has been found in 92% of cases.[10] Treatment with omeprazole or fundoplication will result in subsequent decannulation of the vast majority of patients with stenosis, in some cases without surgery.[11]

The traditional dichotomy between mature and immature stenoses probably represents an oversimplification. *Immature* implies that massive edema and granulation tissue are present and that the inflammatory process is on-going; *mature* implies that acute inflammation has resolved and that the stenosis is composed of mature fibrous tissue with thin (normal) overlying epithelium.

Surgical attempts to correct immature stenoses usually fail unless the LPR is controlled. Conversely, mature stenoses usually can be corrected. In reality, many cases are neither mature nor immature, but somewhere in between. The same also may be true of many acquired laryngeal webs.

pH-metry and antireflux therapy are routinely indicated in all cases of laryngeal stenosis. As the data base grows, this admonition will probably become less controversial. In the meanwhile, the author has found that omeprazole or fundoplication are essential adjuncts to surgery.

Carcinoma of the larynx

The risk factors for the development of laryngeal carcinoma include GER.[10,16,25] The author has reported a series of 31 consecutive cases of laryngeal carcinoma in which abnormal reflux was documented in 84% but only 58% were active smokers.[10] The relationship between LPR and malignant degeneration remains to be proved, but the available pH-metry data suggest that most patients who develop laryngeal malignancy both smoke and have LPR.[10,11] In addition, apparently premalignant lesions may resolve with appropriate antireflux therapy.[10,11]

The previously identified risk factors for laryngeal carcinoma, tobacco and ethanol, also strongly predispose one to reflux. Tobacco and alcohol adversely influence almost all of the body's antireflux mechanisms; they delay gastric emptying, decrease lower esophageal sphincter pressure and esophageal motility, decrease mucosal resistance, and increase gastric acid secretion.[10] Routine pH-metry, followed by omeprazole treatment, is recommended for all patients with laryngeal neoplasia, with or without other risk factors for the development of carcinoma of the larynx.

SPECIAL CONSIDERATIONS

LPR in pediatric patients

Pediatric patients also suffer from laryngopharyngeal reflux. Dysphonia, laryngospasm, laryngomalacia, central apnea, and pulmonary disorders, such as asthma, have been shown to be related to LPR in infants and children.[1,4,16,19] Recent experimental data also suggest that the sudden infant death syndrome (SIDS) also may be LPR related.[23,26] Diagnostic double-probe pH-metry is especially useful in pediatric patients because they seldom complain of symptoms and because so little is known about LPR in the pediatric population.

The treatment algorithms presented below still apply to infants and children. However, omeprazole is usually not prescribed for pediatric patients under 16 years of age. Therefore, H2-blockers are the mainstay of medical treatment. As a consequence, patients with *major* or *life-threatening* LPR need to be monitored carefully. If there is evidence of medical treatment failure, the patient should be retested while on treatment; and, if the pH-metry is still abnormal, fundoplication may be indicated.

Xerostomia, LPRD, and GERD

Xerostomia is commonly encountered in otolaryngologic practice and is a major risk factor for the development of abnormal reflux.[22] This is because salivary bicarbonate is needed to restore the intraluminal esophageal pH after a reflux episode; without normal saliva, the esophageal pH remains very low for an extended period of time.

Esophageal acid clearance is a two-stage process, with volume clearance of the acid bolus being necessary before the intraluminal pH can be restored.[3] In patients with esophageal dysmotility, volume clearance is delayed; however, this is not a common problem in ORL patients with LPR.

Spontaneous "physiologic" reflux events occur frequently, almost universally, after meals. When any reflux event occurs, the intraesophageal pH drops precipitously. Before the intraluminal pH can begin to be normalized, the volume of the refluxed bolus must be cleared. This is usually accomplished by the next swallow.

Once volume clearance is achieved, the intraluminal pH remains very low until neutralized in a step-wise fashion by salivary bicarbonate, delivered by a series of subsequent swallows. In normal people, this process takes several swallows (3-5 minutes).[3] In patients with xerostomia, each reflux episode (physiologic or otherwise) is associated with a prolonged period of esophageal acid exposure, regardless of esophageal motor function.

Rosman et al.[22] studied seven ORL patients with head and neck irradiation, all with normal esophageal motility; however, six of the seven had abnormal esophageal acid clearance and abnormal pH-metry. In addition to radiation, xerostomia is commonly seen with sicca syndrome, Sjorgren's syndrome, scleroderma and most other collagen vascular diseases, cystic fibrosis, and with many medications (e.g., anticholinergics, antihypertensives, antihistamines).

The timing of microlaryngeal surgery

Few patients with vocal cord lesions, such as Reinke's edema, vocal nodules, and cysts require "emergency" surgery. In view of the fact that many patients with these lesions also have LPR, it behooves the otolaryngologist to correct the LPR prior to surgery, if possible. In general, antireflux therapy should be instituted three to six months prior to surgery and should be continued postoperatively.

TREATMENT

There are three levels of antireflux therapy: level I—dietary and life-style modification plus antacids; level II—level I plus use of an H2-blocker (such as cimetidine, ranitidine, or famotidine); and level III—antireflux surgery (e.g., fundoplication) or omeprazole therapy. The elements of the three levels of antireflux therapy are shown in the box below.

Clinical experience in ORL patients with LPR seems to indicate that treatment must be individualized, with the level of treatment depending on the severity of the patient's condition. For patients with *"minor" reflux,* level I or II treatment is appropriate initial therapy, however, treatment

Treatment ("levels") for laryngopharyngeal GERD

Level I—antireflux therapy [ART]

Dietary modification
- No eating or drinking within 3 hours of bedtime
- Avoid overeating or reclining right after meals
- No fried food; low fat diet
- Avoid coffee, tea, chocolate, mints, and soda pop
- Avoid all caffeine-containing foods and drinks
- Avoid alcohol, especially in the evening
- Avoid any other food that causes problems

Life-style modification
- Elevate the head of the bed 4-6 inches
- Avoid wearing tight-fitting clothing or belts
- If you use tobacco, quit!

Liquid antacids q.i.d.
- (1 tablespoon 1 hour after each meal and at bedtime)

Level II—medication [plus ART]

As level I above

Initial treatment
- Ranitidine 150 mg bid
- Or an equivalent dose of another H2-blocker
- Prokinetic agents (e.g., cisapride) may be used as an adjunct

Escalation for treatment failures
- Ranitidine 150 mg qid up to 300 mg qid
- Or an equivalent dose of another H2-blocker

Level III—proton pump inhibitor or antireflux surgery

As level I above or as below

Omeprazole 20 mg b.i.d. (1st thing in the morning and at 5 P.M.) The duration of "initial" treatment should be six months and large patients may require larger doses

Fundoplication

failure can be expected in approximately 35%.[10] If level II treatment fails, level III treatment with omeprazole may be indicated.

The problem with H2-blockers is that pepsin, which is the actual injurious agent in the refluxate, is acid activated and, at pH 4.5, 70% of peptic activity remains.[10] Therefore, since the patient's intragastric pH is less than 4 at the therapeutic nadir (several times each day), activated pepsin is present several times each day and can produce significant laryngeal injury. In other words, for patients with LPR, in whom even infrequent reflux may cause significant damage, H2-blockers leave them "uncovered" for several hours each day.

The medication *omeprazole* has revolutionized antireflux treatment.[7,28] Unlike the H2-blockers, omeprazole is a proton pump inhibitor. In the parietal cell, the last step in acid production is the exchange of a hydrogen ion for a potassium ion. This step requires the participation of an enzyme that is inhibited by omeprazole.[28] Omeprazole, in a dose of 20 mg twice daily, produces complete acid suppression in most patients and, hence, spectacular treatment results when compared with those of H2-blockers.[7,28]

It is interesting to note that in patients with LPR, symptoms do not resolve in a matter of days or weeks and often it takes several months for complete resolution to occur. The duration of initial therapy with omeprazole therefore should be six months. Follow-up data reveal that half of the patients so treated are completely well (all symptoms and findings resolved) by 3 months and virtually all by 6 months of treatment.[10,11]

Omeprazole therapy is especially useful in difficult-to-diagnose cases. Until its availability, a trial of antireflux therapy had no validity as a diagnostic test. On the other hand, in selected cases, a therapeutic trial of omeprazole therapy may be used as a diagnostic test. With such treatment, it is important not to underdose or to treat for too short a period of time.

For patients with *major* or *life-threatening LPR*, omeprazole (20 mg twice daily, occasionally three times daily) is the obvious initial treatment of choice. A "minimum" of twice-daily dosing is necessary (in most patients) to prevent significant acid production around the clock. Ideally, the medication should be taken when the patient arises in the morning and late in the afternoon, prior to the evening meal.

Fundoplication as a surgical antireflux treatment is also highly effective; however, it does appear to require special technical expertise. Surgical antireflux procedures are a real therapeutic option for some patients, particularly young patients with severe reflux. Fundoplication is often recommended for patients with subglottic and tracheal stenosis, since this group appears to have a very high failure rate with medical treatment (and a high likelihood of developing recurrent airway problems later on if medical treatment subsequently fails).

Three therapeutic algorithms

Chronic, intermittent, or chronic-intermittent LPR can cause, or indefinitely perpetuate, a laryngeal disorder. Using a canine model, it has been shown that intermittent (three times per week only) applications of acid and pepsin to the subglottic region following mucosal injury results in nonhealing, ulceration of the cricoid, and even subglottic stenosis.[10,15]

The larynx is far more susceptible to injury from reflux compared with the esophagus. The larynx has no acid-clearance mechanism, as does the esophagus, and, furthermore, its mucosa is thinner and less well adapted to reflux. Optimal treatment of LPR therefore requires complete cessation of acid/pepsin injury if healing is to occur.

H2-blockers may be effective treatment for most GI patients with esophagitis because they reduce the total acid exposure time; however, merely "turning the acid down" is not sufficient treatment for many patients with laryngeal conditions—the acid must be "turned off." Omeprazole is the only medication that effectively accomplishes this goal.

Table 5-2 suggests that there are three categories of severity of LPR in ORL patients. Clearly, the otolaryngologist has fewer options in treating patients with *major* or *life-threatening* LPR than in patients with *"minor" reflux*. It is therefore reasonable to propose three treatment algorithms for LPR. In creating these treatment algorithms, consideration must be given not only to short-term "initial" treatment but also to long-range therapy (years). Hence, the age and the occupation of the patient must also be considered in formulating treatment algorithms.

Treatment of "life-threatening" LPR. Ideally, all patients with laryngeal carcinoma and airway obstruction (due to acquired webs and stenoses, laryngospasm, etc.) should undergo pH-metry before treatment is started, but this is not always possible, particularly if the patient requires emergency surgical treatment such as tracheotomy. Nevertheless, every effort should be made to obtain pH-metry prior to treatment in this group of patients because: (1) it establishes the diagnosis, (2) it determines the severity of the LPR (and establishes a baseline), (3) it allows treatment to be individualized, and (4) it justifies "unconventional" treatment. For similar reasons, a barium study should be obtained, but this study may be performed after initiation of treatment since the early treatment phase is unlikely to alter the radiographic findings, e.g., stricture.

Initial treatment of LPR in these patients should be with omeprazole 20 mg twice or three times daily, as well as with dietary and life style modification. (The three times daily dose is used for some patients weighing over 200 pounds). In the event that the patient is unable to take an orally administered medicine, an intravenous ranitidine drip should be employed, and the gastric contents should be neutralized using antacids and/or continuous enteral alimentation (through a feeding tube) as well.

In selected cases, those with the most severe form of LPR, particularly young patients (under 40 years of age), Nissen fundoplication should be considered as an alternative early on. If, for example, a young person presents with laryngeal airway obstruction, no prior history of trauma or intubation, and pH evidence of severe LPR with a very low LES pressure (less than 6 mm Hg) on manometry, then fundoplication is probably the first and best antireflux treatment. While this situation is uncommon, it does occur.

For most patients, omeprazole is the treatment of choice for at least the first six months or until such time as the clinical situation that prompted the intervention has resolved. For example, it is injudicious to stop the omeprazole in patients with the laryngeal stenosis still being treated for the stenosis. Since some of these patients present with airway obstruction severe enough to require tracheotomy, omeprazole treatment should be continued until the patient has been successfully decannulated and it is clear that the LPR is under control, the latter being confirmed by repeat pH-metry.

In practice, most patients with stenosis will require either chronic omeprazole therapy or fundoplication. The same is true for many patients with carcinoma of the larynx, especially, nonsmokers who develop carcinoma. In this group, the risk of the patient developing new malignant vocal cord lesions exceeds the risks of long-term antireflux treatment with a proton pump inhibitor.

When omeprazole was introduced in the United States in 1989, the Food and Drug Administration recommended that it be used in a dose of 20 mg per day for only six to eight weeks. This overconservative recommendation was made because omeprazole in large doses for a prolonged period had been shown to produce carcinoid tumors in laboratory animals.[28] It was soon clear that this regimen was woefully inadequate to treat LPR.[10,11] Fortunately, long-term omeprazole therapy has been used extensively in Europe without evidence of any malignant potential, and it is now believed that the drug is safe and that it must be employed in larger doses and for prolonged periods if it is to be of optimal benefit.[7]

Therefore, in patients with life-threatening LPR over the age of 60 years, "chronic," "long-term," twice-daily omeprazole treatment is recommended. On the other hand, if the patient has only supine or upright reflux disease, not both, a single daily dose may suffice for maintenance after the acute phase of the illness has resolved.

For patients under 40 years of age, fundoplication is usually recommended. For patients between the ages of 40 and 60 years, treatment is selected on an individual basis. In the latter situation, the severity of the LPR and of the underlying ORL condition is considered, as well as the preferences of the patient and his or her overall medical condition.

Treatment of "major" LPR. The initial part of the treatment algorithm for patients in this group is similar to that outlined above, except that fundoplication is rarely considered. As a rule, the first six months of treatment should consist of omeprazole therapy and a program that optimally manages the patient's diet, weight, and life-style: (1) smoking cessation (if the patient smokes), (2) weight reduction (if the patient is overweight), (3) avoidance of overeating and night eating, (4) a low fat diet, and (5) avoidance of known "refluxogenic" foods, such as coffee, chocolate, mints, and soda pop.

The initial phase of antireflux therapy has two simultaneous goals: to arrest the inflammatory process in the larynx by abolishing gastric acid and, if possible, to reconstitute the body's normal antireflux defenses.[6] The causes of LPR are multifactorial, and many patients can reduce or eliminate reflux effectively, while others have irreversible esophageal dysfunction so that life style and dietary management by itself is never sufficient "therapy." The initial six-month period, while the patient is taking omeprazole, should therefore be used to optimize those "reversible" factors that are within the patient's control. Some patients report, for example, that the LPR seems to cease or decrease significantly when their weight is close to ideal.

After six months of therapy, assuming that the patient's voice symptoms have returned to normal and assuming good patient compliance, the omeprazole dose should be tapered and the patient started on an H2-blocker. This regimen usually is accomplished by reducing the dose of omeprazole to an every morning schedule and adding ranitidine 300 mg every night (or an equivalent dose of another H2-blocker) for one week. Thereafter, ranitidine is prescribed in a dose of 300 mg twice daily or 150 mg four times daily. In addition, patients should be warned that they may experience a "rebound" or obvious worsening of the reflux for a few days following cessation of the omeprazole. The patient should be followed closely during this period of transition.

After the patient has been taking the H2-blocker for six to eight weeks, the otolaryngologist should reexamine the patient. If the patient complains of recurrent symptoms or there are findings that suggest a recrudescence of LPR, then the dose of H2-blocker may be increased in a step-wise fashion over a period of weeks or months to ranitidine 300 mg four times daily.

If the patient appears to be failing medical treatment on this 1,200 mg per day total dose, repeat pH-metry should be obtained while the patient is continuing to take the medication (during the study). In this way, medical treatment failure can be objectively documented. When this situation is encountered, the otolaryngologist must consider other therapeutic options, e.g., level III.

In addition to chronic omeprazole therapy and fundoplication, a third alternative therapeutic program, so-called "pulsed therapy," may be utilized in selected patients. This consists of alternately prescribing omeprazole and an H2-blocker every six months. When such a program is employed, patients may complain that during the six-month period on the H2-blocker regimen they have to be much more careful of their "life style" (diet, alcohol intake, etc.) and that they generally "don't do as well" as when they are taking omeprazole. Pulsed therapy can be further individualized on a patient-to-patient basis. For example, in the professional vocalist with reflux laryngitis, omeprazole may be used before and during periods of a heavy performance schedule (particularly if this schedule is seasonal or intermittent). Pulsed therapy has the "advantage" of allowing parietal cell "recovery" during the H2-blocker phase of treatment. In view of the fact that malignant degeneration does not appear to occur in humans, the true potential advantage of pulsed therapy (as opposed to "chronic" omeprazole therapy) may be only theoretical.

Treatment of "minor" (common) LPR. For many otolaryngologists, this "minor" reflux group comprises the majority of patients with reflux laryngitis. Minor reflux patients typically have symptoms of intermittent dysphonia, chronic throat clearing, globus pharyngeus, and dysphagia and findings such as laryngeal edema and "posterior laryngitis." It is both appropriate and prudent for the otolaryngologist to adopt a less aggressive and more conventional approach to the management of patients in this group. Clearly, it is not essential to obtain pH-metry in all of these patients prior to treatment. Furthermore, conventional (level I or II) antireflux therapy is sufficient for many patients in this group.

Patients who fall into the minor group, based upon the symptoms and findings, should be managed conservatively if they do not have "lesions" for which surgery is contemplated. In my opinion, all "surgical patients" should be treated with omeprazole prior to and after surgery, until healing is complete and "complete resolution" has occurred (i.e., normal stroboscopy has returned). In other words, the routine use of perioperative omeprazole appears to decrease postoperative complications of laryngeal surgery and to enhance the results.

Even with patients in the minor reflux group, initial treatment should probably be *level II,* i.e., include the use of an H2-blocker. Clinical experience suggests that relatively few ORL patients with true LPR respond to life-style/dietary modification and antacid treatment alone.

If initial level II therapy fails, the dose of ranitidine should be escalated in a step-wise fashion—150 mg up to 300 mg four times daily (or an equivalent dose of another H2-blocker may be used). If the patient still appears to be failing medical treatment at this higher dose, pH-metry should be obtained with the patient on treatment. Such patients may be treated with omeprazole. Medical treatment failure with H2-blockers, regardless of dose, is encountered rather frequently in patients with LPR.

Regardless of the level of treatment, it should be continued for a minimum of six months. If the patient becomes asymptomatic after this interval, medication may be subsequently discontinued. However, it is important to counsel patients prior to terminating treatment that LPR is frequently chronic-intermittent. Indeed, many patients have disease-free intervals of months or years, but many eventually suffer recurrences of LPR with similar, or sometimes new, laryngeal symptoms and manifestations.

This chronic-intermittent pattern of LPR often requires the clinician to individualize treatment over the long term, and suggests that many "asymptomatic" ORL patients with LPR, especially professional vocalists, may need long-term "intermittent" follow-up to prevent the development of significant recurrent symptoms, because early intervention for recurrences is a desirable goal.

SUMMARY

LPR is an illusive, ubiquitous, and pernicious cause of laryngeal inflammatory and neoplastic disorders. Frequently underdiagnosed and undertreated, LPR is believed to be an etiologic factor in approximately half of patients with laryngeal and voice disorders. The pervasive and potentially serious nature of LPR demands that clinicians caring for patients with laryngeal disorders consider the diagnosis in every case. The most important advance in the diagnosis of LPR is ambulatory 24-hour double-probe pH monitoring, and the medication omeprazole has revolutionized the treatment of LPR in ORL patients.

REFERENCES

1. Andze GO, Brandt ML, Blanchard H. Diagnosis and treatment of gastroesophageal reflux in 500 children with respiratory symptoms: the value of pH monitoring. *J Pediatr Surg* 26:295-300, 1991.
2. Gerhardt DC, Schuck TJ, Bordeaux EA, et al: Human upper esophageal sphincter response to volume, osmotic, and acid stimuli. *Gastroenterol* 75:268-274, 1978.
3. Helm JF, Dodds WJ, Riedel DR, et al: Determinants of esophageal acid clearance in normal subjects. *Gastroenterol* 85:607-612, 1983.
4. Herbst JJ, Minton SD, Book LS. Gastroesophageal reflux causing respiratory distress and apnea in newborn infants. *J Pediatr* 95:763-768, 1979.
5. Jindal JR, Milbrath MM, Hogan WJ, et al: Gastroesophageal reflux disease as a likely cause of "idiopathic" subglottic stenosis. *Ann Otol Rhinol Laryngol* 103:186-191, 1994.
6. Katz PO, Knuff TE, Benjamin SB, et al: Abnormal esophageal pressures in reflux esophagitis: Cause or effect? *Am J Gastroenterol* 81:744-746, 1986.
7. Klinkenberg-Knol EC. *Recent advances in the diagnosis and management of gastro-oesophageal reflux disease: The role of omeprazole in clinical practice.* Amsterdam, 1990, VU University Press.
8. Koufman JA: Contact ulcer and granuloma of the larynx. In Gates GA, editor: *Current Therapy in Otolaryngology—Head and Neck Surgery.* ed 5, St. Louis, 1993, Mosby.
9. Koufman JA: Medicine in the vocal arts. *North Carolina Med J* 54:79-85, 1993.
10. Koufman JA: The otolaryngologic manifestations of gastroesophageal reflux disease. *Laryngoscope* 101:(Suppl 53)1-78, 1991.
11. Koufman JA: pH Monitoring in otolaryngology patients with gastroesophageal reflux disease: Why the pharyngeal probe is essential. (Unpublished data, 1994.)
12. Koufman JA: Voice disorders. *Visible Voice* 1:2-3; 16-19, 1992.
13. Koufman JA, Blalock PD: Functional voice disorders. *Oto Clin N A* 24:1059-1073, 1991.

14. Koufman JA, Blalock PD: Is voice rest never indicated? *J Voice* 3:87-91, 1989.
15. Little FB, Koufman JA, Kohut RI, et al: Effect of gastric acid on the pathogenesis of subglottic stenosis. *Ann Otol Rhinol Laryngol* 94:516-519, 1985.
16. Morrison MD: Is chronic gastroesophageal reflux a causative factor in glottic carcinoma? *Otolaryngol Head Neck Surg* 99:370-373, 1988.
17. Ossakow SJ, Elta G, Colturi T, et al: Esophageal reflux and dysmotility as the basis for persistent cervical symptoms. *Ann Otol Rhinol Laryngol* 96:387-392, 1987.
18. Ott DJ, Cowan RJ, Gelfand DW, et al: The role of diagnostic imaging in evaluating gastroesophageal reflux disease. *Postgrad Radiol* 6:3-14, 1986.
19. Ramenofsky ML, Leape LL. Continuous upper oesophageal pH monitoring in infants and children with GER, pneumonia, and apneic spells. *J Pediatr Surg* 16:374-378, 1981.
20. Richter JE, Ed. *Ambulatory Esophageal pH Monitoring: Practical Approach and Clinical Applications.* Tokyo, 1991, Igaku-Shoin.
21. Richter JE, Bradley LA, DeMeester TR, Wu WC, et al: Normal 24-hour pH values: Influence of study center, pH electrode, age, and gender. *Dig Dis Sci* 37:849-856, 1992.
22. Rosman AS, Goldberg H, Federman Q, et al: Chronic xerostomia alters 23-hour pH and is associated with esophageal inflammation. *Gastroenterol* 94:A387, 1988 (Abst.).
23. Shatz A, Hiss J, Arenberg B: Basement-membrane thickening of the vocal cords in sudden infant death syndrome. *Laryngoscope* 101:484-486, 1991.
24. Toohill RJ, Mushtag E, Grossman TW, et al: Pharyngeal, laryngeal and tracheobronchial manifestations of gastroesophageal reflux. *Proceedings of the XXIV World Congress of Otolaryngology-Head and Neck Surgery.* Berkeley, Calif, Kugler and Ghendini Publishing.
25. Ward PH, Hanson DG: Reflux as an etiological factor of carcinoma of the laryngopharynx. *Laryngoscope* 98:1195-1199, 1988.
26. Wetmore RF: Effect of acid on the maturing rabbit and their possible significance to sudden infant death syndrome. *Laryngoscope* 103: 1242-1254, 1993.
27. Wiener GJ, Copper JB, Wu WC, et al: Is hoarseness an atypical manifestation of gastroesophageal reflux (GER)? An ambulatory 24-hour pH study. *Gastroenterol* 90A:1691, 1986 (Abst.).
28. Wolfe MM, Soll AH. The physiology of gastric acid secretion. *N Engl J Med* 319:1707-1715, 1988.

APPENDIX A
Data Flow Sheet: Ambulatory 24-Hour pH Monitoring

(1) Series #: ______________

Patient Name: ______________________________ Unit Number: ______________

Telephone Number: (H) ______________ (W) ______________ Date: ______________

(2) Presumptive Dx(s): ______________________________

(3) Age: ________ (4) Sex: /1/ Male /2/ Female

(5) Race: /1/ Caucasian /2/ Black /3/ Oriental /4/ Other: ______________

(6) pH probe:
- /1/ Single Probe
- /2/ Double Probe
- /3/ Other: ______________

(7) /1/ Diagnostic
- /2/ On Treatment
- /3/ Call-Back
- /4/ Other: ______________

(8) Cohort
- /1/ Carcinoma
- /2/ Stenosis
- /3/ Laryngitis
- /4/ Globus
- /5/ Dysphagia
- /6/ Chr. Cough
- /7/ Other: ______________

(9) Study Number: /1/ First /2/ Second /3/ Third

HISTORY

(10) Never Used Tobacco

Tobacco Consumption

(11) Cigarettes	(12) PPD: _____	(13) Pack years: _____
(14) Ex-Smoker	(15) Pack years: _____	(16) Years ago quit: _____
(17) Smokeless	(18) Hours/day: _____	(19) Years: _____
(20) Cigar	(21) Cigars/day: _____	(22) Years: _____
(23) Pipe	(24) Bowls/day: _____	(25) Years: _____

Alcohol Consumption

(26) None

(27) Social

(28) Social binger

(29) Moderate

(30) Heavy

(31) Medication History
- /1/ Med's associated with GI symptoms
- /2/ Med's not associated with GI symptoms
- /3/ Other: ______________________________

____

____

Past Medical Hx

(32) Ulcer hx: /1/ no /2/ yes (year: _____)

(33) Previous UGI tract surgery: /1/ no /2/ yes

(34) Diabetes: ______________________________

(35) ASCVD: ______________________________

(36) Other: ______________________________

Dietary Hx

(37) Coffee:	/1/ None	/2/ 1-3 cups/day	/3/ $\geq$4 cups/day
(38) Tea:	/1/ None	/2/ 1-3 cups/day	/3/ $\geq$4 cups/day
(39) Soda:	/1/ None	/2/ 1-3 cans/day	/3/ $\geq$4 cans/day
(40) Chocolate:	/1/ None	/2/ $\geq 4 \times$ /wk	/3/ daily
(41) Mints:	/1/ None	/2/ $\geq 4 \times$ /wk	/3/ daily
(42) Fried Food:	/1/ None	/2/ $\geq 4 \times$ /wk	/3/ daily

(43) Dietary Score (Total of items 37-42): ________

SYMPTOMS

(44) **Heartburn or Regurgitation**
/1/ None
/2/ 0-1 episodes per week
/3/ 2-4 episodes per week
/4/ Frequently (daily)
/5/ Most of the time

OTHER SYMPTOMS

(45) Intermittent hoarseness
(46) Chronic hoarseness
(47) Globus
(48) Dysphagia
(49) Throat clearing
(50) Chronic cough

(51) Use Tums, Rolaids, or other antacids: /1/ no /2/ yes

FINDINGS

(52) Height (in.): ________________ (53) Weight (lbs.): ________________
(54) **Laryngeal Examination:** /1/ not done /2/ normal /3/ abnormal
(55) Mild edema (58) Posterior erythema (61) Granulation (64) Carcinoma
(56) Moderate edema (59) Diffuse erythema (62) Leukoplakia (65) Other: ___
(57) Severe edema (60) Ulceration (63) Stenosis ________________
(66) **Barium Swallow:** /1/ Not done /2/ Normal /3/ Abnormal
(67) Hiatal hernia (72) Dysmotility
(68) Stricture (73) Achalasia
(69) Radiological reflux (74) Ring
(70) Esophagitis (75) Other: ____
(71) Esophagitis w/erosions
(76) **Endoscopy:** /1/ Not done /2/ Normal /3/ Abnormal
(77) Erythema/mild esophagitis (80) Stricture
(78) Esophagitis w/erosions (81) Cancer
(79) Barrett's esophagitis (82) Other: ____
(83) **Manometry:** /1/ Not done /2/ Normal /3/ Abnormal
(84) Achalasia (87) Nonspecific motility disorder
(85) "Nutcracker" esophagus (88) Other: ____
(86) Diffuse spasm (DES)

PH MONITORING RESULTS	ESOPH	NORMAL	PHARYNX
% Time pH ≤4, upright _____	(89) _____	≤5.85	(92) _____
% Time pH ≤4, supine _____	(90) _____	≤1.81	(93) _____
% Time pH ≤4, total _____	(91) _____	≤4.39	(94) _____

(95) **pH Probe Interpretation**
/1/ Normal
/2/ Abnormal esophagus
/3/ Abnormal pharynx
/4/ Both abnormal
/5/ Pseudo pharynx reflux
/6/ Other: ____

(96) **Medical Treatment**
/1/ None /3/ ART & H_2: ____
/2/ ART /4/ Other: ____

(97) Duration of Rx (months): _____ (98) Follow Up (months): ____

(99) **Outcome:** /1/ Resolved
/2/ Relapses
/3/ Persistent Sx
/4/ Dead
/5/ Lost to Follow Up
/6/ Other: __________________________

(100) Fundoplication: ____

COMMENTS ____
____
____

6

Evaluation of Dysphagia

Fred M.S. McConnel, M.D.

In evaluation of dysphagia, the history and physical examination with careful characterization of the symptoms will usually yield the diagnosis. The remaining work up may only confirm the diagnosis made by history and physical examination. This work-up will consist of barium swallow and endoscopy, cultures, biopsies, and manometry when indicated. With oral and pharyngeal dysphagia, determining the functional alteration of the swallowing mechanism, however, does require further work up with modified barium swallow and possible pharyngeal manometry with fluoroscopy (manofluorography). Treatment is focused upon the etiology and aiding the patient to compensate for the alteration of the swallowing mechanism. In some instances, the etiology can be treated, such as with Zenker's diverticulum, infections, or esophageal reflux, and the dysphagia resolved. However, in other cases such as those with postcancer resections and neurologic etiologies, the patient's dysphagia is not cured. In these cases, the patient's compensatory mechanism must be supported by swallowing therapy and, in rare instances, surgery, prosthesis, or medication. In dysphagia secondary to cancer, the reconstruction should be designed to give the best functional results.

HISTORY

The two major symptoms to characterize are dysphagia (difficult swallowing) and/or odynophagia (painful swallowing). Odynophagia is most common with acute disorders such as bacterial, viral, and fungal pharyngitis, tonsillitis, and foreign bodies. A typical symptom pattern will be given by the patient. For any adult who presents with pain on swallowing for over one month with no other significant history, a malignancy must be a ruled out. Unilateral pain, referred otalgia, increased pain on swallowing, change in voice quality, weight loss, and blood in the sputum are all symptoms suggestive of malignancy. The history of odynophagia is often accompanied by complaints of dysphagia. Solid food dysphagia is a significant pathologic symptom. This symptom can be secondary to a neurologic problem, a pharyngeal esophageal segment (PES) opening dysfunction, stenosis, or a cancer. Even in the event of a negative physical examination and barium swallow, direct laryngoscopy and esophagoscopy should be performed when any of the above symptoms are associated with dysphagia of unknown etiology.

Chronic odynophagia can also result from fungal infections, e.g., monilia as seen in AIDS patients or in patients undergoing chemotherapy. Pharyngitis secondary to chronic gastric reflux is another possible cause for chronic dysphagia and/or odynophagia. The classical presentation of this disorder is a patient awaking with the symptom in the morning with improvement throughout the day. A history of heart burn (pyrosis), especially following large meals, is also suggestive of this diagnosis. However, heart burn occurs approximately once a month in one third of the normal population. The barium swallow may or may not show gastric reflux and/or hiatal hernia. Often, continuous pH monitoring of the esophagus is required to document the occurrence of gastric reflux. However, a trial of a acid suppression drug and conservative measure such as elevating the head of the bed, decreasing the size of meals, and weight loss can be tried if pH monitoring for reflux is not an alternative or practical for the patient.

A neurologic or degenerative disease may present as a sudden onset or as a slowly progressive chronic dysphagia. Connective tissue disorders and muscular dystrophies usually present with a dysphagia which increases over a number of years. The disorders in this group may be misdiagnosed initially as "globus hystericus." Box on p. 72 shows a differential diagnosis of dysphagia.

THE PHYSICAL EXAMINATION

The physical examination consists of mirror examination, fiber optic examination, and manual palpation of the oral cavity, the tongue base, and the neck. With acute bacterial and viral infections, typical physical findings are expected. Fungal infections are associated with milder ery-

Differential Diagnosis of Dysphagia

I. Central nervous system neurologic problems
   A. Cerebrovascular accidents
   B. Head injury
   C. Spinal cord injury
   D. Polio
   E. Cerebral palsy
   F. Infections
   G. Guillain-Barré syndrome

II. Cranial nerve deficits
   A. Glossopharyngeal nerve
   B. Vagus nerve
   C. Hypoglossal nerve

III. Degenerative disease
   A. Parkinson's disease
   B. Amyotrophic lateral sclerosis
   C. Motor neuron disease
   D. Myasthenia gravis
   E. Multiple sclerosis
   F. Alzheimer's disease
   G. Dementia
   H. Huntington's disease
   I. Progressive cerebellar degeneration
   J. Syringobulbia

IV. Muscle and connective tissue disorders
   A. Oculopharyngeal muscular dystrophy
   B. Muscular dystrophy
   C. Dermatomyositis
   D. Polymyositis
   E. Scleroderma
   F. Systemic lupus erythematosus

V. Cancer resections
   A. Lip
   B. Floor of mouth
   C. Tongue
   D. Palate
   E. Total glossectomy
   F. Vertical laryngectomy
   G. Horizontal laryngectomy
   H. Total laryngectomy
   I. Total laryngopharyngectomy

VI. Esophageal disease
   A. GE reflux
   B. Infections
      1. Bacteria
      2. Fungal
      3. Viral
      4. Tuberculosis
      5. Syphilis
      6. Actinomycosis
   C. Esophagitis
      1. Acute chemical
      2. Drug induced (iron, potassium, quinidine, antiinflammatory drugs, antibiotics)
      3. Pemphigus
      4. Epidermolysis bullosa dystrophica
      5. Lichen planus
      6. Stevens-Johnson syndrome
      7. Uremia
      8. Behçet's syndrome
   D. Dysmotility
      1. Diffuse esophageal spasm
      2. Nutcracker esophagus
      3. Achalasia
      4. Nonspecific motility disorders
   E. Structural problems
      1. Stenosis, strictures, rings, and webs
      2. Diverticulum
      3. Extrinsic compression
      4. Hiatal hernia
      5. Lacerations (Mallory-Weiss syndrome)
      6. Perforations
      7. Varices
   F. Connective tissue diseases
      1. Scleroderma
      2. Not defined
   G. Cancer

VII. Specific swallowing disorders
   A. Globus hystericus
   B. Pharyngoesophageal segment opening dysfunction
   C. Zenker's diverticulum

From McConnel FMS: Dysphagia. In Gates, GA, editor: *Current Therapy in Otolaryngology—Head and Neck Surgery* ed. 5, St. Louis, 1994. (With permission.)

thema which affects the oral cavity and pharynx. Increased amount of saliva in the pharynx is a helpful sign of the presence of a foreign body, if the object itself is not seen in the pharynx. Saliva pooling in the pyriform sinuses indicates impaired pharyngeal clearance. Assessment of the range, rate and coordination of lip and tongue function is necessary, as is examination of laryngeal function, especially vocal fold and vestibular closure and degree of elevation. Neurological assessment of cranial nerves IX, X, XI, and XII are imperative.

Observing the patient chew and swallow should be a part of the physical examination and can be very revealing. Through this process, the degree of oral control and the mastication ability can be assessed. The degree of impairment of the pharyngeal swallow and esophageal problems are more difficult to evaluate from the physical examination. The major concern in evaluating the state of the pharyngeal swallow is the degree of aspiration and its etiology. The presence of coughing is suggestive of aspiration. However, the absence of coughing does not reliably indicate that the patient's swallow is free of aspiration. As many as 30% of dysphagic patients aspirate without coughing. A modified barium swallow is the preferred method to detect the presence of aspiration and determine its etiology.

DIAGNOSTIC TESTS

Barium swallow

The barium swallow is the most common test ordered. Structural abnormalities can be seen such as cancer, stenosis, webs, diverticulum, paralysis, and esophageal pathology. The functional impairments of the pharynx are more difficult to diagnose with this study. Barium swallow also may not accurately identify esophageal reflux.

Direct laryngoscopy and esophagoscopy

Direct laryngoscopy and esophagoscopy are the mainstays of the otolaryngologic diagnostic work-up. If no positive findings are found on fiber optic examination, laryngoscopy, and esophagoscopy, direct endoscopy should still be performed. Fiber optic laryngoscopy does not replace direct laryngoscopy if one suspects a possible malignancy. The tongue base, laryngeal surface of the epiglottis, postcricoid region, and pyriform sinuses cannot be completely examined with the fiber optic scope. An equally important aspect of direct endoscopy is the bimanual palpation of the oral cavity, tongue base, pharynx, and neck. This can best be performed under general anesthesia. Fiber optic laryngoscopy is very helpful, particularly in observing vocal cord motion, which cannot be done with direct endoscopy. Many times, mirror examination does not allow time to study vocal cord motion. The best evaluation of vocal cord motion is by fiber optic video laryngoscopy with strobe. A very helpful procedure which enhances fiber optic laryngoscopy is the "pudding swallow." The patient swallows thick pudding with the flexible fiber optic laryngoscopy in the pharynx. One can see residual pudding in impaired functional region of the pharynx and note aspiration in the larynx and trachea. The addition of the pudding swallow can give very helpful clinical information for evaluation of pharyngeal swallowing.

The modified barium swallow

The modified barium swallow procedure has been developed to examine the oral preparatory, oral, and pharyngeal aspects of deglutition radiographically. This procedure involves studying the patient's deglutition under normal physiologic conditions. Therefore, the patient is examined while he or she is seated upright and swallows a variety of food consistencies. Because patients with dysphagia often complain of difficulty swallowing particular food consistencies, each patient is initially given a small amount (⅓ teaspoon) of liquid, paste, or pudding and a chewable material (usually a quarter of a small cookie). The limited amount of material prevents significant aspiration and facilitates detailed observation of the anatomy and physiology of the oral cavity and pharynx. The patient is initially viewed in the lateral plane. The lateral view permits accurate measurement of oral and pharyngeal transit times, as well as accurate observation of the movement patterns of structures in the oral cavity, pharynx, and larynx and of any aspiration that may occur. If the patient is viewed in the anterior/posterior plane, the trachea and the esophagus overlap so that assessing aspiration is difficult. After small (1 ml) swallows of material are examined, larger calibrated amounts (3 ml, 5 ml, 10 ml) may be introduced if the patient does not aspirate on the smaller amounts. Oropharyngeal swallow physiology changes as bolus size increases, so that patients may have more or less difficulty with larger bolus sizes. When swallows of each food consistency and various bolus sizes have been examined in the lateral plane, the patient is turned and viewed in the anterior/posterior plane in order to assess the symmetry of oral and pharyngeal control during the swallow. Then techniques to improve the patient's swallow, particularly postural changes, are usually attempted and assessed radiographically. At the end of this diagnostic procedure, the clinician writes a report describing the patient's swallowing disorder, the amount and etiology of any aspiration that has occurred on any swallows, treatment recommendations, and recommendations regarding the potential for oral feeding. The patient's attending physician then uses this information in decisions regarding the patient's nutritional management.

Types of swallowing impairments observed during the modified barium swallow. Anatomic or physiologic swallowing disorders may occur in any phase of the swallow.[1-5] In the oral preparatory phase, swallowing disorders include: (1) incomplete lip closure, (2) reduction in tension in cheek musculature due to surgical or neurologic damage, (3) reduction in motion of the lower jaw, usually from surgical or traumatic damage, and (4) reduction in range or coordination of tongue movement, which may be neurologic, surgical, or traumatic in origin.[7,8]

Disorders in the oral stage of the swallow are similar to those in the oral preparatory phase. However, damage to tongue function may affect only one particular direction of movement, such as elevation of the tongue or anterior/posterior motion of the tongue. Both directions of tongue movement are necessary to perform the upward and backward propulsion of the bolus to initiate the swallow.

Disorders in the pharyngeal phase of the swallow may include: (1) a delayed or absent triggering of the pharyngeal swallow, resulting in food falling into the pharynx without any of the four neuromotor aspects of the pharyngeal phase occurring; (2) reduction in velopharyngeal closure, resulting in reflux of material into the nasal cavity; (3) damage to the pharyngeal stripping wave, either unilateral or bilateral, so that the squeezing action of the pharyngeal constrictors is inadequate to clear the entire bolus through the pharynx and some food is left behind in the pharyngeal recesses after the swallow; (4) damage to the elevation of the larynx which tucks it under the base of the tongue to divert material away from the top of the airway, resulting in some residue of food at the top of the airway after the swallow; (5) damage to laryngeal adduction or airway closure, so that food can leak through the larynx into the airway during the swallow; and (6) damage to the cricopharyngeal region or laryngeal elevation, so that the cricopharyngeal region cannot open in a timely fashion or sufficiently to allow the bolus to pass into the esophagus, leaving food in the pyriform sinuses after the swallow.[3-5,6,7]

A number of these swallowing disorders in each aspect or stage of deglutition may cause aspiration or the entry of food into the airway below the true vocal cords. Aspiration can occur before, during, or after the pharyngeal swallow. Before the swallow, aspiration can occur if the patient loses control of food with his or her tongue during oral preparation, causing the food to drip into the pharynx before he or she can initiate a pharyngeal swallow. Aspiration can also occur before the swallow because of a delayed triggering of the pharyngeal swallow, causing food to fall into the pharynx while the airway is still open. Aspiration can occur during the swallow when food slips through the larynx, which has not closed sufficiently. After the swallow, aspiration can occur when food remains in the pharynx for any of the reasons described and is inhaled or falls into the airway as the patient takes a breath following the swallow.

TABLE 6-1
Manometric classification of primary esophageal motility disorders

Manometric diagnosis	Major manometric findings
Achalasia	Absent peristalsis Increased les pressure Incomplete les relaxation
Diffuse esophageal spasm (DES)	Simultaneous contractions Intermittent normal Peristalsis
Nutcracker esophagus	Increased amplitude of peristalsis
Hypertensive lower esophageal sphincter (LES)	Elevated les pressure Normal les relaxation
Nonspecific esophageal motility disorders (NEMD)	Assorted abnormalities

From Castell, D.O.: Treatment of esophageal motility disorders. Second Symposium on Dysphagia (March 10-11, 1988). Baltimore, MD, The Johns Hopkins Swallowing Center.

Manometry

Manometry is useful for evaluation of motility impairment of the esophagus. Table 6-1 shows manometric finding for different esophageal dysfunctions. Most clinical manometry labs use water infusion manometers which are adequate for esophageal pressures but are not adequate for the rapid changing pressure and motion of the pharynx. The measurement of intra bolus forces, which requires simultaneous fluoroscopy and solid state manometry (manofluorography), is required for the best evaluation of pharyngeal function.

Manofluorography

Unlike the pressures in other regions of the gastrointestinal tract, pharyngeal pressures have a number of pressure-generating sources: the tongue, the palate, the larynx, and the pharyngeal walls. Only manofluorography allows quantitative analysis of the amount of pressure each structure generates and what portion of this pressure is applied to the bolus to establish a pressure gradient. It is of considerable clinical significance to be able to determine if the dysfunction is caused by the tongue, the pharyngeal walls, the larynx, or a combination. With this type of analysis, surgical reconstruction and treatment of pharyngeal dysphagia can be placed on a more rational basis. Manofluorography simultaneously records pressure, anatomic events, and bolus transit on a single video tape along with timing numbers. The anatomic events and bolus location are determined by lateral view fluoroscopy. This is recorded on the left ⅔ of the video screen. The pressure events are measured by four solid state, computerized manometers with the display of

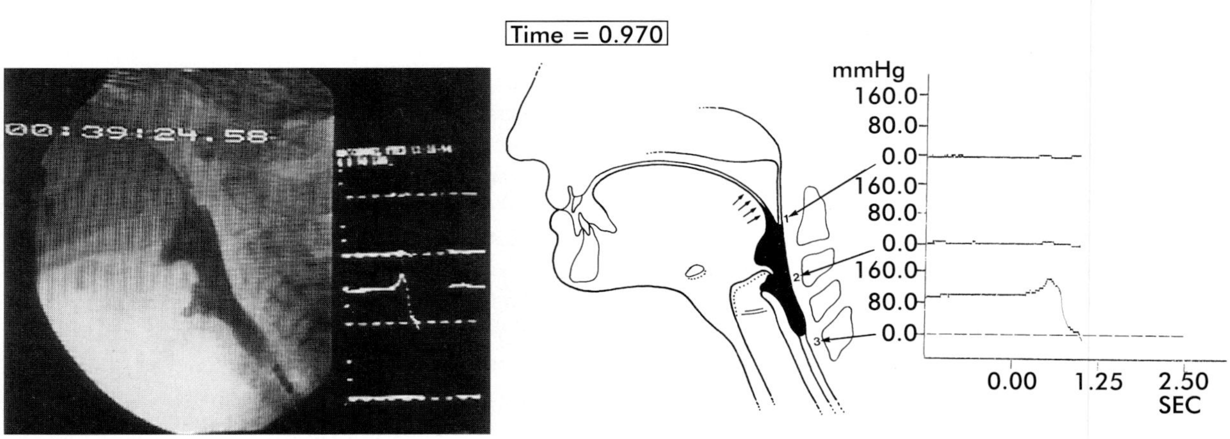

FIG 6-1
McConnel evaluation of Dysphagia.

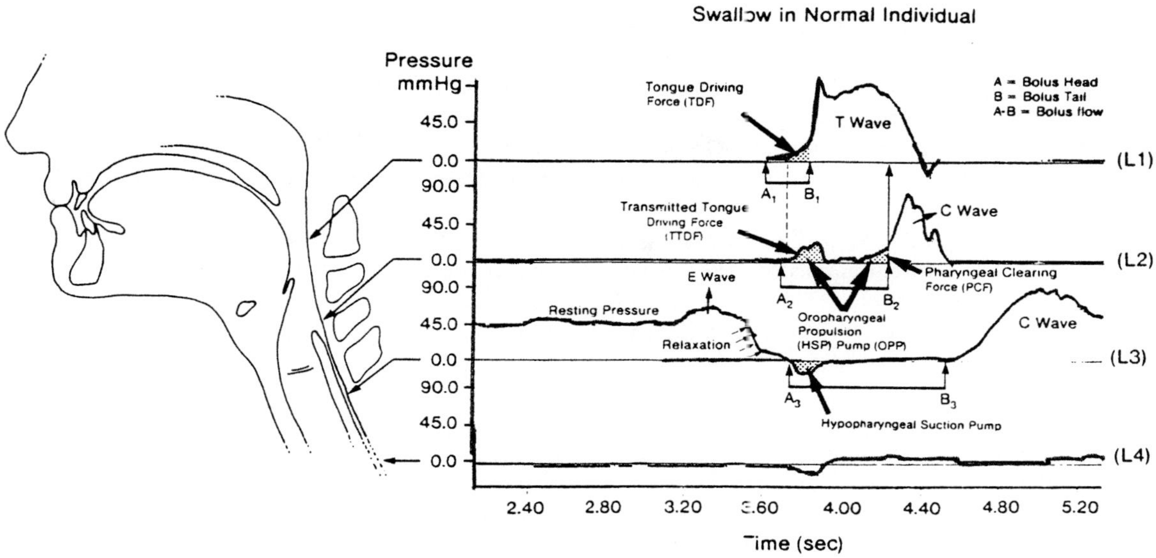

FIG 6-2
A manofluorogram of a normal swallow. The normal pressure pattern form all four leads (L1 to L4) are shown. Pressures exerted onto the bolus over time (forces) are indicated by shading.

TABLE 6-2
Manofluorogram quantitative data: types of dysphagia

Parameters	Normal	Wallenberg's syndrome	Guillain-Barré syndrome	Oculopharyngeal muscular dystrophy	Irradiation fibrosis	Dermatomyositis	Pharyngeal dysphagia
Tongue driving force	1.5	13.7	0	0	0	*	*
Oropharyngeal propulsion pump	3.3	23.8	0	0	0	21.2	7.8
Hypopharyngeal suction pump	−2.1	−0.5	−2.7	−2.2	−0.7	−0.7	−0.1
Pharyngeal transit time	835 msec	1160 msec	>1 min	>1 min	>1 min	950 msec	804 msec
Bolus residue	0	25%	100%	100%	75%	30%	0
Aspiration	0	0	++	+	+++	0	0

*Parameter was not measurable.
From McConnel FMS et al: Laryngoscope 98:705, 1988. (With permission.)

the pressure waves on the right ⅓ of the video screen. The still-framed composite presentation of both is called the manofluorograph and is shown on Fig. 6-1. With still framing of the video tape, the determination of pressure recorded during the time of bolus passage by a sensor is determined. With this analysis, a manofluorogram (Fig. 6-2) for the determination of intrabolus force is constructed. Intrabolus forces are the most sensitive method for determining pharyngeal dysfunction. When a patient complains of dysphagia and other tests are negative, intrabolus force determination can diagnose dysfunction. A patient with significant bolus residual in the pharynx after the swallow as seen on x-ray, it is difficult to know if the problem is due to a lack of PE segment opening or decrease propulsive force due to impairment of tongue or pharyngeal wall contraction. The measurement of intrabolus forces with the manofluorogram provides measurement of these separate forces (box on p. below).

Conceptually, the pressure generation mechanism can be best understood as a two-pump system. The tongue and up

Intrabolus Forces	
TDF	Tongue driving force
OPPF	Oropharyngeal propulsion pump force
TTDF	Transmitted tongue drive force
PCF	Pharyngeal clearing force
HSP	Hypopharyngeal subatmospheric pressure

per pharynx form a propulsion pump with the tongue being the piston and the pharyngeal wall being the chamber. This pump is called the oropharyngeal propulsion pump. The other pump is formed by the larynx and hypopharynx. With anterior superior motion of the larynx, the PE segment is opened lowering the prebolus pressure. This pump is called the hypopharyngeal subatomospheric pressure pump.

The oropharyngeal propulsion pump (OPP in Fig. 6-2) is formed by the sum of two forces applied directly to the bolus, transmitted tongue driving force (TTDF in Fig. 6-2) and the pharyngeal wall contraction (PCF in Fig. 6-2). The output of this pump (oropharyngeal propulsion pump) is best measured at the level of the pharynx just above the arytenoids. The oropharyngeal propulsive pump value is effected by both the upper pharynx and hypopharynx. A decrease in tongue driving pressure results in decreased oropharyngeal propulsive pump. Any pathology which decreases the tongue mobility, such as surgical resection, C.N. XII nerve paralysis, neuromuscular disorder, or a degenerative neurologic disease will decrease the tongue driving force. One can also have a chamber defect such as a palate resection, pharyngeal wall resection, paralysis, or muscular

TABLE 6-3
Modified barium swallow (MBS), fluoroscopic and manofluorogram (MFG) results

Fluoroscopic bolus problems based on MBS	Fluoroscopic anatomic findings	MFG findings
Oral cavity		
Poor ant. bolus Control bolus Residual possible Bolus leakage Between lips	Impaired tongue Motion and/or lip Incompetence and/or mandibular arch loss	Reduced TDF and TTDF with mandibular anterior arch loss, HSP may be reduced.
Poor posterior Bolus control with nasopharynx reflux and/or spillage of bolus into pharynx, poor bolus clearance with residual	Tongue base and/or palate defect and/or impaired motion	Reduced TDF and TTDF
Oropharynx		
Nasopharynx-pharyngeal bolus reflux	Soft palate, and/or pharyngeal wall impairment and/or pharyngeal obstruction or dysmotility	Decreased OPPF and/or HSP with obstruction of pharynx, an increased OPPF may be recorded
Oropharynx wall bolus residual	(1) Impairment of tongue, palate or pharyngeal wall or (2) Pes opening dysfunction	(1) Decreased TDF, with decreased TTDF and/or PCF or (2) Decreased HSP with increased OPPF (TTDF + PCF) and TDF
Vallecular bolus residual	(1) Impaired tongue base impairment and/or (2) Decreased laryngeal anterior elevation	Decreased TDF and TTDF and/or (2) Decreased HSP with increased OPPF and TDF
Hypopharynx		
Hypopharyngeal wall bolus residual	(1) Impaired pharyngeal wall movement and/or (2) Decreased PES opening	(1) Decreased PCF, TTDF or (2) Decrease HSP with increased TTDF and PCF depending on degree of PES opening
Aspiration before swallow	Impaired tongue motion, control or mass.	Decreased TDF, TTDF and/or PCF and/or timing impairment
Aspiration during the swallow	Poor tongue function, decrease laryngeal elevation, absence of supraglottic structure or vocal cord removal and/or paralysis or timing problem	Decreased TDF, TTDF or PCF and/or timing impairment
Aspiration after the swallow	Decreased pharyngeal wall motion or decrease PES opening	Decrease or absence HSP with increased OPPF

dystrophy which can affect the pharyngeal clearing force (PCF) component of the oropharyngeal propulsion pump.

The oropharyngeal propulsion pump is also affected by PE segment opening. If the opening of the PE segment is obstructed, an increased pump pressure will be measured. With laryngeal elevation, a negative pressure is measured before the bolus head arrives in the PE segment. The HSP is the term for the subatmospheric pressure generated in the PES. In swallowing disorders with impaired anterior elevation of the larynx which decreases the PE segment opening or in inferior constrictor muscle relaxation problems, an increased oropharyngeal propulsion pump (OPP) value will be measured. Though a decrease in the hypopharyngeal subatmospheric pressure (HSP) will also be measured, the oropharyngeal propulsive pump value is increased more significantly. Table 6-2 shows examples of alterations of these parameters in a number of different types of dysphagia. Table 6-3 shows anatomic fluoroscopic finds, with possible modified barium swallow results and manofluorogram results.

REFERENCES

1. Aguilar N, Olson M, Shedd D: Rehabilitation of deglutition problems in patients with head and neck cancer, *Am J Surg* 138:501, 1979.
2. Blonsky E, Logemann J, Bosches B, Fisher H: Comparison of speech and swallowing function in patients with tremor disorders and in normal geriatric patients: a cinefluorographic study, *J Gerontol* 30:299, 1975.
3. Calcaterra T, Kadell B, Ward O: Dysphagia secondary to cricopharyngeal muscle dysfunction, *Arch Otolaryngol* 101:726, 1975.
4. Curtis D, Hudson T: Laryngotracheal aspiration: analysis of specific neuromuscular factors, Radiology 149:517, 1983.
5. Donner M, Silbiger M: Cinefluorographic analysis of pharyngeal swallowing in neuromuscular disorders, *Sem Roentgenol* 9:273, 1974.
6. Hurwitz A, Nelson J, Haddad J: Oropharyngeal dysphagia: manmetric and cine esophagraphic findings, *Dig Dis* 20:313, 1975.
7. Logemann J: *Evaluation and treatment of swallowing disorders,* San Diego, 1983, College Hill Press Inc.
8. Logemann J: *A manual for fluoroscopic examination of swallowing.* San Diego, 1986, College Hill Press Inc.
9. McConnel FMS: Dysphagia 499-498. In Gates G, editor: *Current therapy in otolaryngology head and neck surgery,* ed 5 St. Louis, 1994, Mosby.

7

Diagnosis and Management of Cerebrospinal Fluid Leaks*

Daniel W. Nuss, M.D. and Peter D. Constantino, M.D.

The modern era of skull base surgery has ushered in a number of advances that have expanded the role of the otolaryngologist in both diagnosis and treatment of cerebrospinal fluid (CSF) leaks, which were previously regarded as primarily neurosurgical problems. Despite the fact that CSF leaks are relatively uncommon, a thorough understanding of their management is of major importance because of their potentially devastating clinical sequelae.

The basic pathology common to virtually all CSF fistulas encountered by otolaryngologists is a defect in the dura overlying the base of the skull. Such defects allow CSF to find its way out of the intracranial compartment and into the extracranial spaces by way of associated or pre-existing defects in the frontal, ethmoid, sphenoid, or temporal bones. Conceptually, at least, this would seem to represent a straightforward problem. In actual practice, however, diagnosis and treatment of CSF leaks can be extremely challenging for a variety of reasons.

In this review, the problem of CSF leakage will be detailed, with emphasis placed on the otolaryngologist's perspective. In so doing, the clinical importance of CSF leaks will be discussed and normal CSF physiology and pathophysiologic considerations contributing to the development and persistence of fistulas presented. Diagnostic strategies for clinical detection of CSF leaks, laboratory confirmation of CSF in suspect fluids, and anatomic localization of fistula site will be examined, and the various treatment options will be outlined. The special problem of CSF leakage that arises during or after endoscopic sinus surgery will also be discussed.

*The authors wish to very gratefully acknowledge Ms. Dorothy Hoolahan of the Department of Otolaryngology, Louisiana State University School of Medicine, for her kind assistance in the preparation and organization of this manuscript.

THE CLINICAL IMPORTANCE OF CSF LEAKS

If one could ignore the threat of meningitis, CSF fistulas would be no more than a nuisance, perhaps causing only a runny nose or stuffy ear. In reality, however, the threat of meningitis in patients with CSF leakage is substantial, because when CSF can find its way out of the meningeal envelope, microbes can find their way in. The actual risk of an individual patient developing meningitis depends on the clinical situation, but the incidence in various series published on the subject ranges from 4% to as high as 50%.[2,13,15]

With early diagnosis and aggressive antibiotic therapy alone, some cases of meningitis can be managed successfully, i.e., without neurologic complications. On the other hand, the consequences of even a single episode of meningitis can be neurologically devastating. In the short term, meningitis can be associated with brain abscess, seizures, coma, or death. If the patient survives, long-term sequelae, such as deafness, hydrocephalus, and cognitive and intellectual deficits often follow.

In view of these observations, it might seem that patients with CSF fistulas should be routinely placed on prophylactic antibiotics. However, according to two prospectively studied series of patients with CSF leaks, the overall incidence of meningitis as well as the morbidity and mortality rates associated with its occurrence are not significantly different when comparing patients who receive prophylactic antibiotics and those who do not.[13,15] In other words, antibiotics are generally *not* effective in preventing the very serious intracranial consequences of CSF leakage. This implies that when considering the significant risk of meningitis and postmeningitic sequelae, as well as the lack of efficacy of prophylactic antibiotics when spontaneous closure fails to occur, the *only* effective treatment for persisting CSF leaks is surgical closure.

CSF DYNAMICS

In order to successfully manage patients with CSF leaks, it is important to understand the dynamics of CSF production and reabsorption and the various problems that can predispose to the development and/or recurrence of CSF fistulization.

CSF is produced in the choroid plexus of the lateral, third, and fourth ventricles of the brain. After passing through these sites, it flows out of the ventricular system into the basal cisterns via the foramina of Magendie and Luschka, near the foramen magnum. From there, the fluid circulates within the subarachnoid space, passing downward around the spinal cord and upward around the cerebral and cerebellar hemispheres. Eventually it comes into contact with the arachnoid villi, which protrude into the great dural venous sinuses (Fig. 7-1). These villi essentially act as glomeruli, allowing the CSF to be reabsorbed into the blood within the venous sinuses.

In adults, about 450 ml CSF are produced daily, while the total volume of the normal subarachnoid space, cisterns, and ventricular system is only about 125 to 150 ml. Thus, the entire volume of CSF is replaced several times in a day. The function of CSF has been compared with that of lymph in other parts of the body, and this continuous recirculation of the fluid supports that comparison. Because the central nervous system has few if any lymphatic channels,[40] CSF probably acts as an interface between the brain and the blood for the exchange of electrolytes, impurities, and other substances. This exchange is highly selective and governed mainly by the specialized epithelial cells of the choroid plexus (blood-brain barrier).

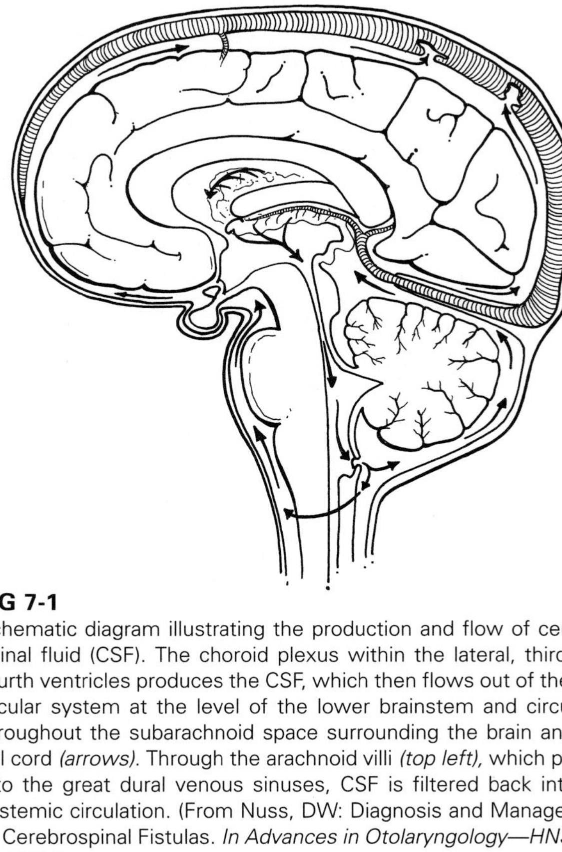

FIG 7-1
Schematic diagram illustrating the production and flow of cerebrospinal fluid (CSF). The choroid plexus within the lateral, third, and fourth ventricles produces the CSF, which then flows out of the ventricular system at the level of the lower brainstem and circulates throughout the subarachnoid space surrounding the brain and spinal cord *(arrows)*. Through the arachnoid villi *(top left)*, which project into the great dural venous sinuses, CSF is filtered back into the systemic circulation. (From Nuss, DW: Diagnosis and Management of Cerebrospinal Fistulas. *In Advances in Otolaryngology—HNS*, vol. 8, 1994.)

The normal balance of CSF production and reabsorption can be upset by a number of pathologic situations. Reabsorption of CSF may be substantially impaired after any intracranial event that evokes an inflammatory response, such as head trauma, intracranial surgery, sudden intracranial bleeding, or meningitis. When CSF reabsorption is impaired, intracranial pressure (ICP) usually becomes elevated. Meningitis is a particularly important cause of impaired CSF reabsorption, because many patients with untreated CSF leaks have already had meningitis at some point before the leak is recognized. If a CSF fistula is repaired in such patients, the early result may be good, only to have the leak recur some time later because of persistent increased ICP that results from impaired reabsorption. Therefore, impaired CSF reabsorption and its effect on ICP must be taken into account in the treatment and long-term follow-up of patients with CSF leakage, especially those who have had meningitis.

TRAUMATIC VS NONTRAUMATIC LEAKS

When considering CSF leaks, it is helpful to classify them as either traumatic or nontraumatic.[30] The distinction between these two groups is important because the clinical features and the prognostic implications are different for each.

Traumatic CSF fistulas are by definition those that develop after some form of trauma. Head injury ("open" or "closed") is certainly the most frequent cause, responsible for leaks in up to 3% of all head trauma patients and in 5% to 11% of patients with basilar skull fractures.[22] Surgical procedures may also be responsible for traumatic (iatrogenic) CSF leaks. Such procedures include such obvious examples as craniotomy, skull base tumor resections, and trans-sphenoidal hypophysectomy, but they may also include certain other procedures in which the cranial vault is inadvertently penetrated, as during endoscopic sinus surgery, mastoidectomy, or even septorhinoplasty. It is therefore imperative for all clinicians to bear in mind that many of the procedures commonly performed in the nose or ear carry a small *but not negligible* risk of intracranial injury.

Most patients with traumatic CSF fistulas experience definite leakage within 48 hours after the trauma (although certain traumatic leaks may not become apparent until a considerable time later). Traumatic leaks are usually abrupt in onset, and the volume of drainage, while variable, is generally low. When the mechanism of injury is closed head trauma, up to 80% of patients can be anosmic, because the blow that causes the CSF leak also generates sufficient force to shear the olfactory nerve filaments at their points of exit through the cribiform plate. The trauma in these patients can also be severe enough that about 20% of patients have a pneumatocele (intracranial air) at diagnosis. Additionally, approximately 25% to 50% of patients with traumatic CSF leaks develop meningitis. Surprisingly, headache may not be a predominant complaint in patients with traumatic CSF leaks despite the occurrence of head injury. This is not so in patients who have nontraumatic leaks. Traumatic leaks may resolve without surgical intervention in some patients, although the majority require repair. Once these leaks are closed, the incidence of recurrence is quite low.

Nontraumatic CSF fistulas are those that occur in the absence of trauma. This group has previously been referred to as having "spontaneous" CSF leaks. As Ommaya[31] has stated, however, the term "spontaneous" means literally without cause, and no CSF leak is ever without an etiology. Most authors have abandoned this term in favor of "nontraumatic," with the understanding that leaks occurring in the absence of trauma must be thoroughly investigated until the cause is identified, since only then can the appropriate treatment be instituted.

Causes of nontraumatic CSF leaks include intracranial tumors (which may lead to fistula formation by elevating intracranial pressure and/or eroding the skull base), osteomyelitis of the skull base, hydrocephalus, congenital anomalies, arachnoidoceles (especially those involving the pituitary fossa—the so-called "empty sella syndrome"), and others.[30] Several factors are known to contribute to the development of nontraumatic CSF fistulas. They are represented by the mnemonic "four P's of fistula formation." These physiologic and anatomic features include intracranial *pressure,* brain *pulsation,* cranial base *pneumatization,* and arachnoid *pits.*

As discussed above, *intracranial pressure* has a direct influence on the egress of CSF when a fistulous tract (or a potential tract) is present. In patients with elevated intracranial pressure (ICP), the meningeal sac may be gradually distended, favoring the development of meningoceles that protrude through congenital defects or through natural avenues of least resistance, such as the sella. Eventually the meninges break down and CSF begins to flow. In these cases, the fistula acts as a kind of pressure relief valve, and leakage in these patients is very difficult to control by any means until ICP is restored to normal.

Brain *pulsation* is a normal physiologic event that contributes to fistula formation in concert with other factors. Over time, pulsation may lead to thinning and erosion of bone along some parts of the skull base. Alternatively, pulsation (like elevated ICP) may promote herniation of meninges and/or brain through congenital or traumatic defects in the skull, eventually leading to meningeal rupture with subsequent CSF leakage.

The extent of *pneumatization* of the cranial base is another important factor because in well-pneumatized skulls, the bone over the paranasal sinuses and the temporal bone is often extremely thin. The presence of this very thin bone creates a path of least resistance for a developing fistula (Fig. 7-2).

The distribution of *arachnoid pits* along the cranial base is a likely causative factor in some nontraumatic CSF leaks. Arachnoid villi are mostly found along the convexity of the brain, in communication with the major dural venous sinuses near the calvarium. In some skulls, however, they also occur along the cranial base, where they relate to the basal meningeal veins.[12] In these basal locations, the arachnoid villi protrude and cause "pitting" of the cranial floor. If the pits occur over a pneumatized area such as the sphenoid sinus, for example, they may transmit brain pulsations that eventually erode the bone with subsequent fistula formation (Fig. 7-3).

The clinical features of non-traumatic CSF leaks differ from those of traumatic origin. Non-traumatic leaks are quite uncommon. Usually they begin insidiously, with initial drainage so scant that it is often mistaken for allergic rhinitis. Eventually, the drainage increases steadily and often becomes profuse. Anosmia and pneumatocele are rare among patients with non-traumatic leaks. It appears that the risk of meningitis is actually somewhat lower in these patients than in those with traumatic fistulas, but it is difficult to estimate just how much lower. (This apparent lower risk

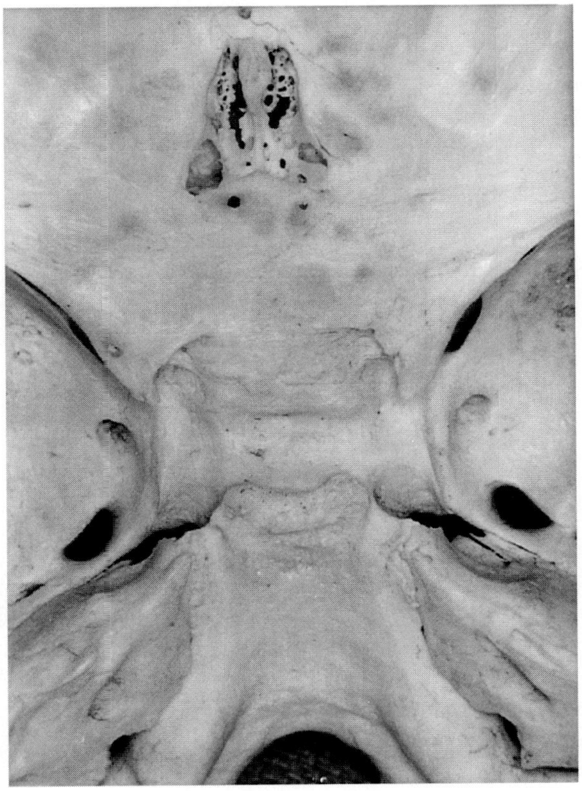

FIG 7-2
Photograph of well-pneumatized skull, showing extremely thin bone overlying the ethmoid and sphenoid sinuses. Such areas of thin bone are often the sites of CSF fistulization.

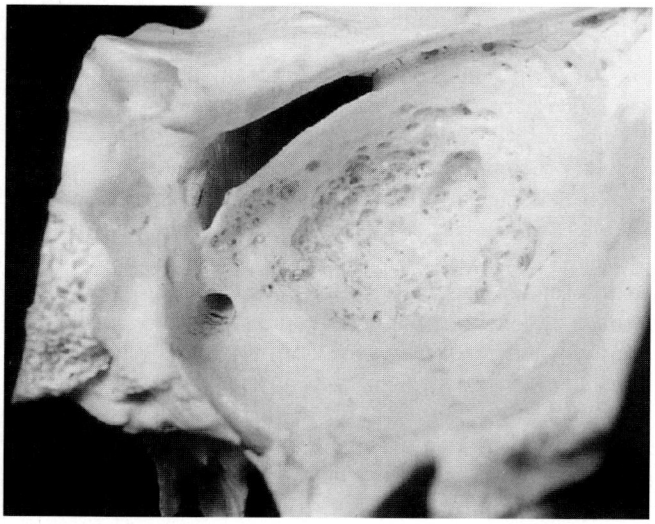

FIG 7-3
Photograph of disarticulated right sphenoid bone, as viewed from an intracranial perspective, showing extensive "pitting" of the cranial base. These arachnoid pits are sometimes associated with developing CSF fistulas (see text). (Superior orbital fissure is seen across the top of the photo; foramen rotundum is at bottom left.)

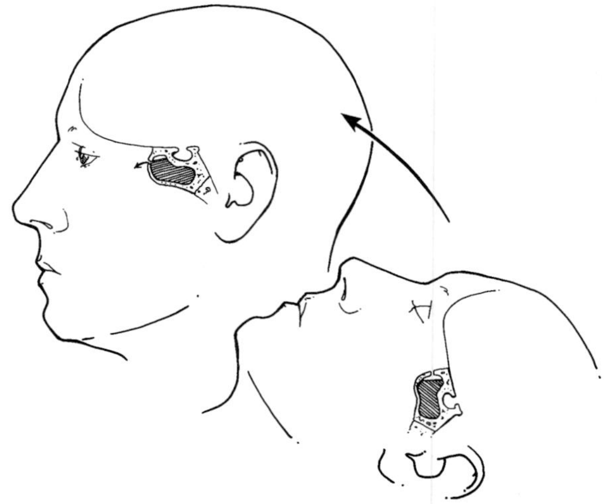

FIG 7-4
Diagram demonstrating the "reservoir sign." CSF accumulates in sphenoid sinus when patient is recumbent, and is suddenly discharged when head is leaned forward. (From Nuss, DW: Diagnosis and Management of Cerebrospinal Fistulas. In *Advances in Otolaryngology—HNS,* vol. 8, 1994.)

does not justify a wait-and-see approach to therapy, however, since even on bout of meningitis can have dire consequences.) Headache is a prominent clinical feature and is often flow-related. Typically patients will report headache that begins at low severity and intensifies over a few days, until a sharp increase in rhinorrhea suddenly occurs. Once CSF flow commences, headache is relieved until the cycle begins again some time later. Nontraumatic leaks are more common in adults who are over 30 years of age and twice as common in females as in males. (Traumatic leaks show no special age or gender predilections.) In our experience, nontraumatic leaks seldom resolve without surgical intervention, and the recurrence rates after treatment are higher than those with traumatic leaks. This latter finding is undoubtedly related to the more complex and diverse etiologic factors that are involved in the genesis of nontraumatic fistulas.

DIAGNOSIS OF CSF LEAKS

Clinical Diagnosis

The task of diagnosing CSF leakage is sometimes quite simple and at other times exceedingly difficult. Regardless of the clinical circumstances, the diagnostic process must begin with a thorough history, since there are several classic symptoms and clinical presentations that are highly suggestive of CSF leakage. The majority of patients with CSF fistulas will give convincing and reliable evidence of the leakage if the proper inquiries are made by the physician. Any patient with a complaint of clear, watery drainage from the nose or ear must be considered to have a CSF leak until proved otherwise, especially if that drainage is unilateral. As discussed above, the description of a headache that is relieved by the commencement of a liquorrhea from the nose or ear is suspicious as well. Sometimes patients will perceive a metallic, sweet, or salty taste associated with CSF in the throat. Symptoms such as anosmia, nasal obstruction (as in the case of meningoencephalocele), fullness in the ear, and conductive hearing loss may also be valuable clues. Obviously, the physician should inquire about prior surgery or injuries to the head or facial regions.

A particularly convincing detail in patients with CSF rhinorrhea is the so-called "reservoir sign." When a CSF fistula involving the frontal, ethmoid, or sphenoid sinus is present, CSF tends to accumulate in the sphenoid sinus (the reservoir) while the patient is recumbent.[39] When he or she resumes the erect position, the CSF remains in the dependent portion of the sinus until the head is leaned forward. At that moment the fluid leaks back out of the ostium of the sinus and appears as profuse rhinorrhea (Fig. 7-4). This reservoir sign was originally believed to be a sign specific for sphenoidal fistulas, but it may signify a leak anywhere along the anterior cranial base. Even though it is not anatomically specific, the sign when present is highly suggestive of CSF leakage, since there are few (if any) other sinonasal disorders that will give profuse intermittent drainage from the nose. Furthermore, it provides an opportunity for retrieval of a significant volume of fluid for confirmatory chemical testing; the patient is given a suitable container (such as a test tube) to take home and instructed to lean forward and collect any discharge as soon as he arises in the morning.

The physical examination should always include general head and neck evaluation as well as complete neurologic examination. Next, a thorough inspection of the ears, nasal cavity, and nasopharynx is performed. Careful visualization of the sinonasal tract, including the eustachian tube orifices, using a sinus endoscope is strongly recommended as a part of the initial examination. Otomicroscopic examination is also strongly recommended, since CSF leaks involving the temporal bone may be easily missed by routine inspection. Unless there is a perforation of the tympanic membrane, otorrhea will not be seen. In patients who have intact eardrums, CSF will either accumulate in the middle ear or will flow through the eustachian tube, presenting in the nose as so-called paradoxic rhinorrhea. With otomicroscopy, it is sometimes possible to see subtle air-fluid levels that suggest the presence of CSF in the tympanic cavity.

If no such signs of fluid are detected but the patient gives a history consistent with gross drainage, several provocative maneuvers may be attempted. The Valsalva maneuver (forced abdominal strain against a closed glottis) and Queckenstedt maneuver (bilateral digital jugular vein compression) both cause transient elevation of intracranial pressure, and may thereby accelerate CSF leakage when a fistula is present. Both of these maneuvers can be performed with the patient seated and leaning forward, which exaggerates the ICP even more.

If these investigations are done carefully, it is often possible to visually confirm that CSF is indeed leaking. This is no small accomplishment, since knowledge of the site (or even the general vicinity) of the fistula helps to streamline subsequent imaging studies and surgical planning.

The patient with unexplained meningitis. Occasionally a patient comes to the attention of the otolaryngologist without any specific complaints but with a history of unexplained meningitis. Typically, this will be an otherwise healthy person who suddenly developed meningitis but did not have acute sinusitis, otitis media, or any apparent source for the meningitis and also did not have any underlying illness that would predispose to it. Such a patient must be thoroughly questioned and examined for the kinds of details outlined above, because any episode of unexplained meningitis—especially if it is recurrent—must be presumed to be the result of an occult CSF fistula until proved otherwise. Even if thorough history and examination fail to confirm CSF leakage, these patients should undergo additional testing (outlined below) to rule out a CSF leak.

Biochemical confirmation of CSF leakage

In most patients with CSF leaks, history and physical examination are sufficient to establish beyond reasonable doubt that the leak is present. Before treatment is rendered, though, and prior to undertaking multiple invasive or expensive imaging studies, it is always prudent to confirm, if possible, the clinical impression with chemical tests. When the history and physical examination leave room for doubt, these confirmatory tests assume an even greater importance.

Retrieval of specimen for testing. When gross rhinorrhea or otorrhea is present, the fluid may be collected by simply allowing it to drip into an open container such as a test tube or cup. If drainage is scant or questionable, it is useful to place a Merocel sponge of appropriate size into the suspect area (nose or external ear canal). The sponge is left in place until it becomes moist. It may then be placed into the barrel of a syringe and compressed by the plunger of the syringe until all of the fluid is squeezed out and collected in a test tube. If the patient is suspected of having CSF in the middle ear but has an intact tympanic membrane, tympanocentesis is recommended.

Glucose testing. Normal nasal and aural secretions, including mucus and lacrimal fluid, are very low in glucose (less than 30mg/dL), while CSF glucose content is generally much higher (50 to 80mg/dL, or about two-thirds the content found in blood plasma). When trying to determine if a patient has true CSF leakage, glucose testing offers several definite advantages in that it is a universally available, simple, quick, and inexpensive test.

Unfortunately, problems with glucose testing arise in certain situations. First, glucose content will be increased if there has been recent trauma in which blood has been mixed in with the suspect fluid, leading to the possibility of a false positive result. This seriously limits its utility in trauma patients. Second, the most widely used methods of checking for glucose content—multireagent strips such as Dextrostix and Urostix—are so sensitive that they frequently give false positive readings occurring in 45% to 75% of cases.[30,36] Third, if a patient has meningitis at the time of the glucose test, a low glucose content will be found that could be wrongly interpreted as a negative test for CSF, since the glucose level in CSF falls dramatically in the presence of bacterial meningitis.

Besides glucose testing, assays for protein and chloride have been used to screen for the presence of CSF. Each of these has limitations that render them unreliable, so that we generally discourage their use.

Beta-2-Transferrin Testing. Because of the pitfalls of glucose testing in the diagnosis of CSF leakage, the beta-2-transferrin (B2T) assay is emerging as the most reliable way to determine whether CSF is present in a specimen or not.[11,25,26] The protein transferrin is ubiquitous in the human body, but in the central nervous system (CNS) it is converted (by the neuraminidase enzyme) to a slightly changed version of itself that has a different electrophoretic profile. This converted transferrin molecule exhibits a separately identifiable protein band (the beta-2 or *tau* fraction) when subjected to electrophoresis. Only the beta-1 fraction is normally found in tears, saliva, mucus, and serum, so the test provides a very sensitive and specific method of distinguishing these types of fluids from CSF.

Other than CSF, only the vitreous humor of the eye and perilymph of the inner ear are known to contain B2T. (This finding is very understandable when one considers that these special sense organs are really just specialized extensions of the CNS.) Neither of these fluids would be likely to confound the test interpretation because vitreous leakage portance if the CT leaves unanswered questions about the neuroanatomy, as in the case of a small intracranial lesion that may represent either tumor or herniated brain, for example (Fig. 7-7). The CT-cisternogram becomes necessary if the plain CT leaves doubt about the site of leakage, or if there are several abnormal areas on the CT that could each potentially be responsible for leakage. CT-cisternography is most productive in patients who have clinically evident leakage. If the patient is not experiencing drainage on the day of the test, the scan will likely be negative.

Perhaps the most difficult circumstance is that of the patient who, on clinical grounds, is either known to have or very strongly suspected of having a CSF leak, but the leakage is sparse and intermittent. For that reason, the CT and even the CT-cisternogram may fail to localize the fistula site. Often these patients have already experienced one or more bouts of meningitis, accentuating the urgency of intervention. In these patients, several options may be considered. Arrangements may be made with a radiology department for such patients to have "on-call" cisternograms—to be ready to perform the study on any day that the patient experiences definite drainage. Nuclear radioisotope scans may be conducted over several days, as described above, to try to identify the "slow leak." Pressure-infusion cisternograms may be performed in which the contrast is infused into the subarachnoid space under controlled but supraphysiologic pressure, thus encouraging leakage. Obviously such a study would be conducted only with the support of the neurosurgical consultant.

In rare circumstances, all of the above studies may be inconclusive. When faced with such a situation, the patient must be counseled accordingly. The alternatives then include close observation and periodic reimaging or "exploratory" surgical intervention without knowing exactly where the fistula is.

TREATMENT OF CSF LEAKS

As stated earlier, because of the likelihood of meningitis and other intracranial complications, optimal treatment for any patient who has a CSF leak is to have the leak closed. Closure of a CSF fistula may be accomplished by either operative or nonoperative means, but in the majority of cases surgical intervention is necessary. Surgical approaches to the repair of CSF fistulas can be divided into intracranial and extracranial approaches.

Intracranial approaches

Intracranial surgery for closure of CSF leaks has been practiced for many decades. The exact operation depends upon the location (or presumed location) of the fistula. For leaks emanating from the anterior cranial fossa, frontal craniotomy is done. For those involving the middle fossa, temporal craniotomy or combined fronto-temporal craniotomy is needed. For leaks that originate in the posterior fossa, occipital craniotomy is chosen.

Once inside the cranium, the neurosurgical approach to the fistula may be either intradural or extradural. In the former, the dural envelope is incised at a site remote from the fistula, and the fistula site is located and repaired "from above."[34] This kind of repair typically is carried out using grafts of fascia, muscle, pericranium, or homologous dura, which are inserted between the brain and the dura. In the anterior fossa, it is also possible to develop pedicled flaps from the nearby falx cerebri that can be rotated into position to cover the fistula site.

In the extradural method, the same principles apply, the

A

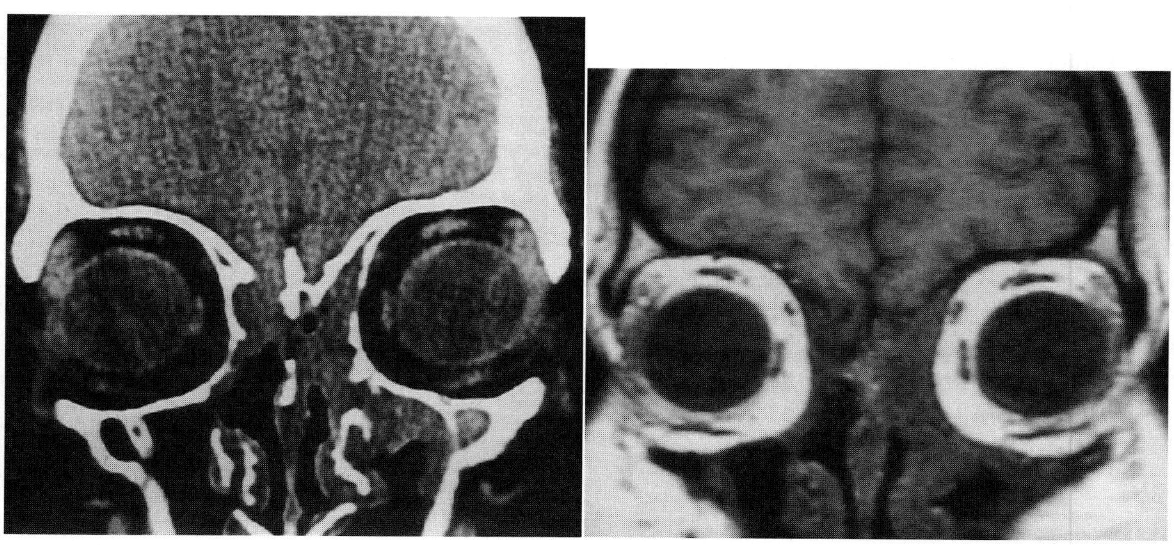

B

FIG 7-7
A, Coronal CT scan of patient with history of unexplained meningitis, showing defect in cranial base with associated soft tissue abnormality. On this CT, it is not possible to tell whether the soft tissue represents sinus mucosal disease or encephalocele. **B,** Coronal MR scan of same patient, demonstrating a small encephalocele herniating into right ethmoid sinus.

main difference being that the dural defect is approached without actually entering the meningeal envelope.[35] In this approach, the plane of dissection is between the dura and the bony cranial base. Thus, the graft or flap that is used to obliterate the fistula site is placed extradurally. Whenever possible, the dural rent is also repaired directly, using sutures prior to placement of the graft or flap along the cranial base. With an extradural approach, it is possible to employ pedicled flaps of pericranium, galea, fascia, or temporalis muscle in the repair.

The intracranial approaches (intradural and extradural) offer one very significant advantage compared with the extracranial approaches for repairing CSF leaks: they permit direct access to the fistula site and adjacent intracranial structures at the same time. In cases of leaks that occur as a result of intracranial tumors or complicated head trauma, for example, this simplifies management because the CSF leak and the intracranial pathology or injury can be fixed simultaneously.

Unfortunately, intracranial approaches also carry several disadvantages that limit their usefulness for repair of many CSF leaks. First, whenever the cranial base is approached via standard craniotomy (i.e., traditional neurosurgical craniotomy not employing any special cranial base exposure), it is necessary to displace the brain by some form of retraction. Brain retraction can have both immediate and delayed consequences. Because brain tissue is relatively inelastic, retraction provokes an inflammatory response that leads to cerebral edema, which can cause serious neurologic complications in the postoperative period. Retraction and displacement of brain also creates the opportunity for postoperative hemorrhage in the epidural and subdural spaces as well as in the substance of the brain itself, again with significant neurologic compromise.

Brain retraction can also lead to delayed complications, which are usually not as dramatic but are nonetheless serious. Retraction-related injury of cerebral cortex is well recognized as a cause of seizures, especially if the temporal lobe has been manipulated. Seizures are usually not life threatening but they make it extremely difficult for patients to return to work, to resume driving automobiles, and to obtain health insurance, not to mention the inconvenience, expense, and potential risks of having to take anticonvulsant medication. Besides seizures, retraction is also known to cause encephalomalacia of the retracted cortex, which can often be seen on postoperative MRI studies.[4] Encephalomalacia, depending on the site, can produce permanent cognitive and intellectual deficits as well as changes in emotional behavior.

Another potential problem that accompanies intracranial approaches concerns the olfactory apparatus. Since most CSF leaks occur in the anterior fossa, the olfactory nerves present an obstacle because they essentially "tether" the frontal lobes at the cribriform area. This tethering limits surgical access to the fistula site, which is commonly situated in either the cribriform area itself or the adjacent fovea ethmoidalis. In most cases, it is therefore necessary to either stretch or divide these nerves, and the patient is rendered anosmic as a result.

Intracranial approaches can be especially troublesome for CSF leaks originating from the sphenoid sinus. Because of the unique location of the sphenoid sinus at the "center of the head," surgical exposure via craniotomy is very difficult, requiring extensive retraction of the frontal lobes and sometimes also the temporal lobes as well. Access to the sinus is limited even further by the presence of the cavernous sinuses and associated neurovascular structures on either side.

Extracranial approaches

Because of the considerable potential for problems with intracranial surgery for repair of CSF leaks, extracranial approaches have been increasingly used clinically. The first successful extracranial repair of a CSF leak was reported in 1948 by Dohlman,[6] who was able to close a nontraumatic fistula involving the ethmoid fovea via an external ethmoidectomy approach. Since that time, a number of clinicians, including Hirsch, Montgomery, Calcaterra, Papay, Mattox, and others,[1,3,8,10,16,19,32,33] have contributed technical refinements that have made extracranial repair a safe and effective alternative to intracranial operations for CSF leakage in many cases. In fact, extracranial repair is now gaining acceptance as the preferred method for initial treatment of CSF leakage in many institutions, because the success rates are actually better than with intracranial repair in properly selected cases and the morbidity is lower.[9,18]

Certainly, the fairly recent appearance of multidisciplinary cranial base surgery "teams" in tertiary health care centers has been a key factor in the increasing appreciation for the value of extracranial approaches. Because these kinds of teams integrate the techniques and treatment philosophies of neurosurgeons and otolaryngologists working together, the range of options for management of patients with CSF leaks has become both broader and better defined.

Obviously, not every patient with a CSF fistula will be a candidate for an extracranial operation. Examples previously mentioned, such as a patient with CSF leakage due to an intracranial tumor or due to extensive transcranial injury, illustrate that there will always be a role for purely intracranial surgery in treating CSF leaks. Identification of such patients is usually straightforward using information from the CT and/or MR scans. Most CSF leaks, however, are not associated with extensive intracranial pathology, and the otolaryngologist has much to offer in these cases.

Anterior, middle, and posterior cranial base access. CSF fistulas may arise from any of the three cranial fossae: anterior, middle, or posterior. Extracranial approaches to all of these regions of the cranial base are familiar to all otolaryngologists by virtue of their training in surgery of the nose, paranasal sinuses, and temporal bone. Therefore, the various surgical routes of access for exposure of CSF fistulas will be reviewed here only briefly. (For must recognize that a CSF fistula always consists of defects at two different levels: (1) a rent in the dura and (2) a hole in the bony cranial base. When possible, closure of both defects is desirable. Principles of definitive repair can be condensed to the following steps: (1) getting enough room to work, (2) defining the bony margins of the cranial base defect, (3) locating and closing the dural defect if possible, (4) closing the cranial base defect.

Getting enough room to work.—The ability to fix both the rent in the dura and the hole in the cranial base depends upon the adequacy of surgical exposure; i.e., one must be able to see the fistula well in order to repair it well. Exposure is related to the choice of the surgical approach, as already discussed. After the initial approach is made, one of the most important tasks in getting room to work is to precisely clear out any surrounding scar tissue, excess mucosa, and other obstructions from around the fistula site. Microsurgical dissectors are extremely helpful in this regard. The Fisch "hockey stick" raspatory, the Rhoton microneurosurgical dissectors, and a variety of middle ear dissecting tools, including the Tabb elevator, are all excellent tools for this work. They are equally valuable for CSF leaks involving the sinuses as well as the middle ear. In addition to clearing the immediate area, it is sometimes necessary to correct any gross anatomic deformities that limit the access, such as a deviated septum or large concha bullosa.

Defining the bony margins of the cranial base defect.—Once the area around the fistula has been cleared of obstructions, margins of the bony defect are defined by carefully palpating the cranial base along the entire perimeter surrounding the fistula. This confirms the precise shape and dimensions of the defect and therefore facilitates accurate repair. Again, the microsurgical dissectors are very useful for this maneuver.

Locating and closing the dural defect.—If the bony defect is large enough, the dura will be visible in its midst. In some instances, it will be possible to see the dural rent directly. In others, the dural rent will be remote from the site of the bony defect. If the actual dural rent is visible, an attempt is made to directly repair it. Occasionally it may be possible to place fine sutures that coapt the dural edges. More often the best solution is to bridge the dural gap with a tissue graft, usually of fascia (using fascia temporalis or fascia lata).

If the dural rent is not directly visible, it is often because the bony defect is very small. In this situation, the surgeon has two options. One of these is to simply cover the area with an extracranial graft (or flap). This method obviously foregoes the possibility of directly repairing the dura and relies on repair of the cranial base alone to obliterate the fistula. The other option is to enlarge the bony defect enough so the dura can be directly patched. After the dural patch is placed, repair of the cranial base as a second layer would follow. Either of these methods can be successful.

In our experience, a dural patch has a better chance of stopping a CSF leak if the fascia graft is "oversized" slightly larger than the actual size of the cranial base defect. The graft is placed directly against the dura, with its edges "tucked in" above the perimeter of the bony defect (i.e., intracranial graft placement) (Fig. 7-8). Other authors have reported success with techniques that simply place fascia against the outside edges of the bony defect (extracranial graft placement). Intracranial graft placement seems to be more appealing because the graft is mechanically held in place, "sandwiched" between the brain above and the bony margins below.

Closing the cranial base defect.—After the dural defect has been patched, it is advisable to bolster that closure with a second layer that obturates the cranial base defect, as sort of a "belt and suspenders" strategy. The question of whether to reconstruct the bone at the cranial base is often asked. Generally, this is only necessary if the defect is so large that herniation of intracranial contents is considered likely in the absence of such bony repair. Practically speaking, herniation is not likely unless a defect is on the order of one centimeter in diameter or greater. Donor site options for bone replacement include the middle turbinate, septum, anterior wall of the maxilla, or, in case of very large defects, split cranial bone grafts. In the majority of cases, though, bony reconstruction is not necessary; what is more important is to close the cranial base in such a way as to promote rapid healing that will lead to permanent wound repair. This second layer of closure is naturally dictated by the location of the fistula. Options in the nasal cavity include septal mucosal flaps, middle turbinate mucosal flaps, or free mucosal grafts. In the frontal and sphenoid sinuses, this second layer usually consists of a fat graft that obliterates the sinus cavity. In the temporal bone, it may be either a fat graft, temporalis muscle flap or graft, or temporalis fascial flap.

Other technical considerations. Other technical considerations also have an impact on the success of the repair. *Magnification and illumination* by microscope or telescope are indispensable items. *Fibrin glue* is very helpful for stabilizing the fascial and mucosal grafts and/or flaps, (Our recipe for obtaining reliable autologous fibrin glue is shown in Fig. 7-9). The glue is used only sparingly, however, because of the concern that excessive collections of fibrin may interfere with wound healing. To further promote wound healing, it is preferable to use *autologous tissues* in the repair whenever possible. Thus, the fascia and other tissue grafts used in this work are nearly always taken from the patient rather than using stored, processed, radiated, or otherwise commercially prepared tissues. Also, in the interest of promoting rapid wound healing, use of *vascularized tissues* is recommended when feasible. Examples would include the previously mentioned septal and middle turbinate mucosal flaps, pericranial flaps, and pedicled temporalis fascial flaps.

In the rare circumstances when autologous tissues or vascularized flaps are judged to be inadequate, perhaps because of prior surgery or trauma to the area, a variety of *biomaterials* have been used to obliterate the fistula site. Methylmethacrylate in particular has been employed in the past

A

FIBRIN GLUE FOR USE IN REPAIR OF CSF FISTULAE

Ingredients:

1. Thrombin (1000 u/ml)
2. Amicar (5gm/20ml)
3. Cryoprecipitate (the fibrin-rich component)
   May be either autologous (must be arranged in advance) or homologous (single-donor blood component from blood bank). Both are available in aliquots of 2-5 ml each. One aliquot is nearly always sufficient.
4. Two 3-ml syringes
5. Two sterile medicine cups
6. Two spinal needles, any gauge

Directions:

1. Reconstitute thrombin by adding 10 ml saline to make 100 u/ml concentration.
2. Mix 1 ml of reconstituted thrombin with 2 ml of amicar in the first medicine cup. NOTE: The thrombin-amicar solution is now ready for use and should be used within about 30 minutes.
3. Place the cryoprecipitate (fibrin) in the second medicine cup. If the fibrin has been frozen, allow sufficient time for thawing before use.
4. Draw up the desired amount (usually 3 ml) of fibrin in one syringe and an equal volume of the thrombin-amicar solution in the other syringe.
5. The fibrin is activated immediately on contact with the thrombin-amicar solution. It is therefore desirable to apply the two components to the operative site simultaneously. To do so, apply a spinal needle to each syringe, and then fasten the syringes together in parallel side-by-side fashion (using steri-strips) so that both plungers can be depressed simultaneously. The ends of the needles are then bent so that they converge, allowing direct mixing of the two components at the wound surface. (Alternatively, a double-barrel syringe kit is available from Micromedics Corporation). Apply the "glue" evenly to the operative site. Best results are obtained when the field is as dry as possible.

B

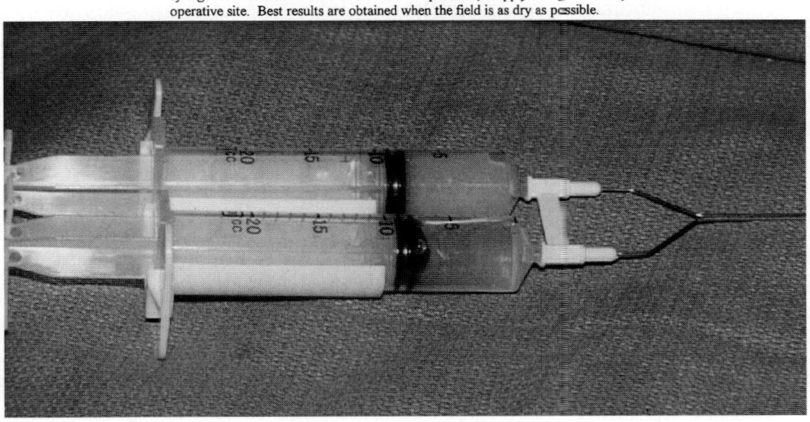

FIG 7-9
A, Recipe for mixing fibrin glue from cryoprecipitate and other components. **B,** Photograph of dual syringes with converging needles for application of fibrin glue directly to operative site.

for repair of CSF fistulas, especially in the frontal sinus and anterior cranial base. Both of the authors have had the unpleasant experience of having to remove methylmethacrylate from patients whose operations were initially successful only to later become infected, leading to resurgence of the CSF leakage. Methylmethacrylate is therefore mentioned only to illustrate the following point: it does not perform well when placed in contact with the nose, paranasal sinuses, or pneumatized portions of the temporal bone.

One biomaterial that appears to be very promising for dealing with difficult CSF fistulas is hydroxyapatite (HA).[5] Previously, HA was only available in its hard crystalline form, either as large blocks that had to be carefully sculpted or as minute granules. Neither of these configurations was practical for repairing CSF leaks. Recent development of the substance in a "cement" form, however, makes it very appealing for use in repairing fistulas because it can be applied directly into the cranial base defect, in much the same way as spackling paste is applied to seal a crack in a wall. The ingredients for the cement are mixed to form a paste at the time that they are needed and are placed into the fistula site. The cement gradually hardens, over several hours until it is comparable in density to the bone of the cranial base.

Unlike methylmethacrylate and other materials, HA is osteoconductive, allowing it to serve as a matrix for ingrowth of living osteocytes until it is eventually replaced to a large extent with new bone.[7] Use of the new HA cement on an investigational basis in several difficult cases of CSF leakage has been successful. Long-term outcomes are under study and the U.S. Food and Drug Administration (FDA) approval of the cement form of HA is pending.

Intraoperative adjunctive measures

In the process of repairing a CSF fistula, the volume of CSF draining through the site may sometimes be considerable, interfering with the placement of grafts and positioning of flaps. (An analogy can be made to fixing a leaking pipe in a plumbing system; once the leak has been located, it is helpful to shut off the flow while the repair is in progress.) Temporary measures to reduce or eliminate the flow are therefore helpful. All of these measures exert their influence on CSF egress by reducing intracranial pressure

(ICP). *Positioning of the patient with the head elevated* is the simplest of these measures but is quite effective. *Administration of diuretics* such as furosemide or mannitol reduces intravascular volume, which in turn reduces intracranial volume (since blood accounts for a significant proportion of the brain's volume), reducing CSF pressure further. *Administration of steroids* is occasionally helpful, but in general steroids do not reduce ICP except when there is preexisting inflammation or brain edema. Controlled *hyperventilation* can also reduce ICP, since hypocapnea induces a reflex reduction in cerebral blood flow. The patient is monitored by capnography, with the target $P\ CO_2$ in the range of 28 to 33 mm Hg.

Preoperative placement of an indwelling lumbar spinal drain is the most direct way to control intraoperative CSF flow. A spinal catheter is inserted into the subarachnoid space, usually at the interspace between the second and third lumbar vertebrae. The catheter is connected to a sterile drainage system with a control valve interposed so that flow can be regulated. Initially the valve is closed, because it may be difficult to locate the fistula if too much CSF is drained preoperatively. Once the fistula has been located, however, the valve may be opened to allow CSF drainage to commence. This diverts CSF flow away from the fistula site, making repair easier. Typically, the flow of CSF through the fistula is eliminated or substantially reduced after 50 to 75 ml has been evacuated through the drain.

The spinal drain's utility is not limited to intraoperative decompression of the subarachnoid space. As previously mentioned, it can also be used to help locate the precise site of a fistula during surgery. This is accomplished by injecting fluorescein into the catheter and, after allowing time for it to circulate in the CSF, observing for its appearance in the nasal cavity (in cases of rhinorrhea) or temporal bone (in cases of otorrhea). Because of potential neurotoxicity, specific recommendations for its concentration, volume, and method of injection must be carefully followed.[28,37] The spinal drain is also valuable postoperatively (discussed below).

Postoperative adjunctive measures

Even the most technically perfect repair of a CSF fistula may be unsuccessful if the patient is not properly managed in the postoperative period. Especially in the first postoperative week, it is crucial to keep the patient's intracranial pressure from becoming elevated because even a transient rise in ICP can disrupt the repair and result in failure. With this in mind, we recommend a number of simple precautions.

The patient is generally kept at rest with his or her *head elevated.* Regardless of whether the fistula involved the nose, sinuses, or temporal bone, the patient is *restricted from nose-blowing,* since this activity generates positive pressure that can insufflate air intracranially through the fresh operative site. Although sneezing is not preventable, the patient is instructed to *sneeze if necessary with the mouth open,* so the force of the sneeze is not directed through the nasal cavity. *No bending, lifting, or straining* of any kind is allowed during the first week. *Antitussives, antiemetics, and laxatives* are administered as needed to reduce coughing, retching, or abdominal straining that can increase ICP.

If a *spinal drain* is used intraoperatively, it is usually left in place for several days (most commonly 3 to 5 days) to continue postoperative decompression of the subarachnoid space. The rate of CSF drainage is regulated by the position of the drainage collection bag relative to the patient, and flow can be interrupted when necessary by closing the control valve. Generally, about 25 to 50 ml of CSF is allowed to drain every eight hours (for adults). This amount is usually sufficient to keep ICP down without causing problems. More vigorous drainage is certainly possible and sometimes necessary, but the incidence of complications is higher when drainage is too aggressive.

Any patient who has a spinal drain must be cautiously monitored and the volume and rate of drainage carefully controlled. Overdrainage can lead to severe ex vacuo headache ("spinal headache") and nausea or vomiting. More seriously, it can also lead to the so-called siphon effect, in which a too rapid egress of CSF through the drain creates a relatively low intracranial pressure and air is then sucked intracranially through the newly repaired but still fresh fistula site. The resulting intracranial air may become a life-threatening tension pneumocephalus[14] or may insufflate nasal microbes intracranially resulting in meningitis. Thus, the use of an indwelling spinal drain is not to be considered lightly. Such patients should be cared for in units where nursing personnel are experienced in monitoring and managing neurosurgical problems.

Nonoperative management of CSF leaks

Although the majority of CSF leaks do require surgical intervention, there are a few situations in which a nonoperative approach can be successful. Generally speaking, nonoperative management can be expected to work only in patients who have relatively small dural fistulas, who do not have elevated intracranial pressure, and who do not have impaired potential for wound healing. Therefore, a nonoperative approach is most appropriate when the CSF leak: (1) is of recent onset, (2) is low in volume, (3) occurs early in the postoperative period, (4) is the result of an injury that would not otherwise require surgical intervention (as in some cases of closed head trauma), (5) occurs as a result of a facial fracture without neurologic injury (early reduction of the fracture in such cases frequently solve the problem of CSF leakage without direct repair of the fistula), and, (6) occurs in a patient who is unwilling or not able to undergo anesthesia or surgery.

Nonoperative management essentially consists of the same measures described above in the section on postoperative adjunctive measures. In most patients managed nonoperatively, all of those measures are instituted immediately except for the placement of the spinal drain. (This scenario is sometimes referred to as "conservative management.") If liquorrhea does not stop within a day or so, the spinal drain is placed and drainage is implemented, as previously outlined. The length of time considered to constitute an adequate trial of nonoperative management is variable. In our experience, if CSF leakage persists beyond 5-7 days, nonoperative management is not likely to solve the problem.

CSF leaks and endoscopic sinus surgery

As the techniques of endoscopic sinus surgery (ESS) have become widely practiced, the incidence of iatrogenic CSF rhinorrhea has risen. A number of factors contribute to this problem, including the delicate, thin quality of bone at the ethmoid roof, the fragility of the adjacent cribriform plate, and the potential for fracture of these areas when removing disease from within the ethmoid sinus. Because the dura over these areas is quite thin and subject to tearing easily, CSF leakage may occasionally result after ethmoidectomy, even when the surgery has been carefully performed.

Stankiewicz[38] has reviewed this topic in detail and has reported an incidence of less than 1% in his large series of ESS patients treated in a major referral center. Although the true incidence in other circumstances is difficult to establish, it is safe to assume that it is significantly higher when patients are treated by less experienced surgeons or in training programs.

According to Stankiewicz, patients operated upon under general anesthesia were at significantly higher risk for CSF leakage than those operated upon using local anesthesia. This is explained by inability of the use of local anesthesia alone, to effectively anesthetize the dura. Thus, the patients's complaint of pain would alert the surgeon to the possibility that the cranial base is being manipulated and further transgression would be obviated. With general anesthesia, this "early warning system" is not possible. As a result, Stankiewicz recommends avoiding general anesthesia for ESS whenever possible.

Treatment of CSF leakage that occurs during or after ESS is usually straightforward since the site of the fistula is usually readily apparent and the etiology is as well. If CSF is observed to be leaking during ESS, the leak is repaired according to the techniques previously outlined. Most often, a fascia graft and/or mucosal flap will solve the problem. If the leak is not recognized (or does not develop) until some time in the postoperative period, the patient may be treated operatively or nonoperatively, depending on the timing and the volume of leakage. Minute amounts of CSF drainage that occur early in the postoperative period will usually resolve with conservative measures, whereas high-volume leaks or those that develop more than a week postoperatively are likely to require surgical intervention. Successful repair in these cases can almost always be achieved by extracranial methods and should seldom require craniotomy.

The role of antibiotics in patients with CSF leaks

As mentioned in the earlier discussion of the clinical importance of CSF leaks, prophylactic antibiotics are controversial in the management of patients who have CSF fistulas. Indeed, there is little evidence to support either the routine use or the withholding of antibiotics in these patients, since the only properly conducted trials have not demonstrated any significant difference between those who received antibiotics and those who did not. The risk of selecting for resistant organisms that can cause meningitis, however, is very real with prolonged prophylactic antibiotic use, and such cases of meningitis can be lethal or neurologically devastating.[13] Therefore, we do not recommend long-term use of antibiotics for the purpose of preventing meningitis in patients with CSF leaks. Whether short-term antibiotic prophylaxis—such as a brief course of therapy during an upper respiratory infection, for example—offers any benefit for patients with CSF leaks is by no means certain.

Beyond the question of *prophylactic* antibiotic use, the indications become clearer. Certainly, *perioperative* antibiotics are indicated and have been shown to be beneficial in reducing the incidence of meningitis in patients undergoing all kinds of cranial base procedures. Perioperative antibiotic use is therefore strongly recommended whenever repair of a CSF leak is undertaken. Antibiotics that achieve therapeutic levels in the CSF and have a broad spectrum of antimicrobial coverage, such as ceftriaxone or related cephalosporins, are favorable in this setting. The first dose is given just before surgery, and repeat doses are given every 12 hours for a total of 48 hours. If the patient has intranasal packing or an indwelling spinal drain, the antibiotics are continued until the packing is removed and/or the spinal drain is withdrawn.

Long-term management of intracranial pressure

Of all the factors that influence the outcome in treating patients with CSF leaks, intracranial pressure is certainly the most consequential. ICP necessarily becomes a recurring theme in the management of these patients, because it can play a role in the genesis as well as the recurrence of the problem. Many, if not most, patients who have had CSF fistulas repaired continue to have abnormal CSF reabsorption long after the leak has been fixed. The disturbed CSF dynamics in these individuals are the predictable result of previous episodes of meningitis, trauma, or surgery. If intracranial hypertension persists, however, the likelihood of recurrent CSF leakage is high. Therefore, long-term control of ICP is of the utmost importance.

Diagnosis and management of intracranial hypertension involve complex issues, the details of which are beyond the scope of this discussion. It is absolutely essential, however, that the otolaryngologist who treats patients with CSF leaks be acutely aware of the need for careful monitoring of ICP during long-term follow-up. Clinically, the presence of headaches or early optic disc changes may be early warning signs of elevated ICP. In follow-up CT scans, the size of the ventricles should be noted, since the ventricular system will dilate in some cases of intracranial hypertension. Any of these findings should alert the clinician, and evaluation by a neurosurgeon should be requested. Long-term treatment options depend on the severity of the hypertension. If mild, the patient can sometimes be managed with acetazolamide (Diamox) to decrease CSF production. If ICP is grossly elevated, then a CSF shunt (ventriculo-peritoneal or lumbar peritoneal) is usually needed.

From this and all of the above discussion, it should be clear that the otolaryngologist who engages in treatment of patients with CSF leaks must maintain a close working relationship with a colleague who is a neurosurgeon. CSF leakage, like all other cranial base disorders, is a complex problem, the complications of which are often brain related. Therefore these patients deserve the expertise of both specialists, who together can cooperate to deliver the most sophisticated care.

SUMMARY

Cerebrospinal fluid leaks are problematic because they predispose patients to meningitis and other central nervous system complications. Antibiotics do not reliably prevent these risks, and therefore surgical intervention is usually necessary. Otolaryngologists play an increasingly important role in the management of patients with CSF leaks because many fistulas can be repaired using surgical approaches through the nose, paranasal sinuses, and temporal bones.

CSF leaks may be either traumatic or nontraumatic in origin, a distinction that is significant because the clinical features, treatment strategies, and prognoses are somewhat different for each. Abnormalities of CSF circulation and reabsorption contribute to the development and/or persistence of leakage in some instances, and these must be recognized before successful treatment can commence.

Diagnosis of CSF fistulas can most often be made on clinical grounds but should be confirmed by biochemical testing and imaging procedures to facilitate treatment planning. After a leak is localized, treatment generally consists of surgical repair, which may be carried out by intracranial or extracranial means, depending on individual circumstances and pathology present. In selected patients, nonoperative treatment may also give satisfactory results. Adjunctive treatment consists mainly of measures to control intracranial pressure, which may sometimes be abnormally high in patients who have had CSF leakage.

The modern approach to diagnosis and treatment of CSF leaks is embodied in the concept of the "cranial base team," which incorporates the treatment philosophies and technical expertise of otolaryngologists and neurosurgeons, working together to arrive at the optimal solution in each case.

REFERENCES

1. Briant TDR, Snell E: Diagnosis of cerebrospinal rhinorrhea and the rhinologic approach to its repair. *Laryngoscope* 77:1390-1409, 1976.
2. Brisman R, Hughes JEO, Mount LA: Cerebrospinal fluid rhinorrhea. *Arch Neurol* 22:245-252, 1970.
3. Calcaterra TC: Extracranial surgical repair of cerebrospinal and rhinorrhea. *Ann Otol* 89:108-116, 1980.
4. Carrau RL, Weissman JL, Janecka IP, et al: Computerized tomography and magnetic resonance imaging following cranial base surgery. *Laryngoscope* 101:951-959, 1991.
5. Costantino PD, Friedman CD, Jones K, et al: Hydroxyapatite cement: I. Basic chemistry and histologic properties. *Arch Otolaryngol Head Neck Surg* 117:379-384, 1991.
6. Dohlman G: Spontaneous cerebrospinal rhinorrhea. *Acta Otolaryngol (Stockh)* 67(Suppl):20-23, 1948.
7. Friedman CD, Costantino PD, Jones K, et al: Hydroxyapatite cement: II. Obliteration and reconstruction of the cat frontal sinus. *Arch Otolaryngol* 117:385, 1991.
8. Hirsch O: Successful closure of cerebrospinal fluid rhinorrhea by endonasal surgery. *Arch Otol* 56:112, 1952.
9. Hubbard JL, McDonald TJ, Pearson BW, et al: Spontaneous cerebrospinal fluid rhinorrhea: Evolving concepts in diagnosis and surgical management based on the Mayo Clinic experience from 1970 through 1981. *Neurosurgery* 16:314-321, 1985.
10. Hudson WR, Hughes LA: Cerebrospinal rhinorrhea: Diagnosis and management. *South Med J* 68:1520-1523, 1975.
11. Irjala K, Suonpaa J, Laurent B: Identification of CSF leakage by immunofixation. *Arch Otolaryngol* 105:447-448, 1979.
12. Kaufman B, Nulsen FE, Martin HW, et al: Acquired spontaneous, nontraumatic normal-pressure cerebrospinal fluid fistulas originating from the middle fossa. *Radiology* 122:379-387, 1977.
13. Klastersky J, Sadeghi M, Brihaye J: Antimicrobial prophylaxis in patients with rhinorrhea or otorrhea: A double-blind study. *Surg Neurol* 6:111-114, 1976.
14. Komisar A, Weitz S, Ruben RJ: Cerebrospinal fluid dynamics and rhinorrhea: The role of shunting in repair. *Otolaryngol Head Neck Surg* 91:399-403, 1983.
15. MacGee EE, Cauthren JC, Brackett CE: Meningitis following acute traumatic cerebrospinal fluid fistula. *J Neurosurg* 33:312-316, 1970.
16. Mattox DE, Kennedy DW: Endoscopic management of cerebrospinal fluid leaks and cephaloceles. *Laryngoscope* 100:857-862, 1990.
17. McCabe BF: The osteo-mucoperiosteal flap in repair of cerebrospinal fluid rhinorrhea. *Laryngoscope* 86:537-539, 1976.
18. McCormack B, Cooper PR, Persky M, et al: Extracranial repair of cerebrospinal fluid fistulas: Technique and results in 37 patients. *Neurosurgery* 27:412-417, 1990.
19. Montgomery WW: Surgery of cerebrospinal fluid rhinorrhea and otorrhea. *Arch Otolaryngol* 84:92-104, 1966.
20. Nabawi P, Mafee M, Phillips J, et al: The success rate of metrizamide CT cisternography in the evaluation of cerebrospinal fluid (CSF) rhinorrhea. *Comput Radiol* 6:343-354, 1982.
21. Naldich TP, Moran CJ: Precise anatomic localization of atraumatic sphenoethmoidal cerebrospinal fluid rhinorrhea by metrizamide CT cisternography. *J. Neurosurg* 53:222-228, 1980.
22. Narayan RK: Head injury, in Grassman RG, Hamilton WJ, editors: *Principles of Neurosurgery,* New York, 1991, Raven Press.
23. Nicklaus P, Ducher PO, Hengerer AS, et al: New imaging techniques in diagnosis of cerebrospinal fluid fistula. *Laryngoscope* 98:1065-1068, 1988.
24. Nuss DW, Janecka IP: Cerebrospinal fluid rhinorrhea and the extensively pneumatized cranial base: A new method for repair. *Transactions of the American Laryngologic, Rhinologic, Otologic Society,* 1991, (Abstr.)
25. Oberascher G: A Modern concept of cerebrospinal fluid diagnosis in oto- and rhinorrhea. *Rhinology* 26:89-103, 1988.

26. Oberascher G: Cerebrospinal fluid otorrhea—new trends in diagnosis. *Am J Otol* 9:102-108, 1988.
27. Oberascher G: Personal communication.
28. Oberascher G, Arrer E: A new method for using fluorescein to demonstrate oto- and rhinoliquorrhea. *Arch Otorhinolaryngol* 243:117-120, 1986.
29. Oberascher G, Arrer E: Efficiency of various methods of identifying cerebrospinal fluid in oto- and rhinorrhea. *ORL J Otorhinorlaryngol Relat Spec* 48:320-325, 1986.
30. Ommaya AK: Cerebrospinal fluid fistula, in Wilkins RH, Rengacharry SS, editors: *Neurosurgery,* vol 1, New York, 1985, McGraw-Hill.
31. Ommaya AK, DiChiro G, Baldwin M, et al: Non-traumatic cerebrospinal fluid rhinorrhoea. *J Neurol Neurosurg Psychiatry* 31:214-225, 1968.
32. Papay FA, Benninger MS, Levine HL, et al: Transnasal transseptal endoscopic repair of sphenoidal cerebral spinal fluid fistula. *Otol Head Neck Surg* 101:595-597, 1989.
33. Papay FA, Maggiano H, Dominquez S, et al: Rigid endoscopic repair of paranasal sinus cerebrospinal fluid fistulas. *Laryngoscope* 99:1195-1201, 1989.
34. Ray BS, Bergland RM: Cerebrospinal fluid fistula: Clinical aspects, techniques of localization and methods of closure. *J Neurosurg* 30:399-405, 1969.
35. Samii M, Draf W: Surgery of traumatic lesions of the anterior skull base. In Samii M, Draf W, editors: *Surgery of the Skull Base.* Berlin, 1990, Springer-Verlag.
36. Spetzler RF Zabramski JM: Cerebrospinal fluid fistulae: Their management and repair. In Youmans JR, editor: *Neurological Surgery.* Philadelphia, 1990, WB Saunders.
37. Stammberger H: Special problems: Detection and treatment of cerebrospinal fluid leaks. In Stammberger H, editor: *Functional Endoscopic Sinus Surgery.* Philadelphia, 1991, BC Decker.
38. Stankiewicz JA: Cerebrospinal fluid fistula and endoscopic sinus surgery. *Laryngoscope* 101:250-256, 1991.
39. Tamakawa Y, Hanafee WN: Cerebrospinal fluid rhinorrhea: The significance of an air- fluid level in the sphenoid sinus. *Radiology* 135:101-103 1980.
40. Tourtellotte WW, Shorr RJ: Cerebrospinal fluid. In Youmans JR, editor: *Neurological Surgery.* Philadelphia, 1990, WB Saunders.

8

OSHA and the Otolaryngology Office

J. David Osguthorpe, M.D. and William J. Dichtel, Jr., M.D.

In the United States, approximately one and a half million harbor the Human Immunodeficiency Virus (HIV) and most are unaware of their predicament.[12] As their disease passes a long quiescent phase, averaging a decade, into the clinical manifestations of immunodeficiency, affected individuals seek physician attention for any one of a number of diseases. In 40%, the first manifestations of immunodeficiency are in the head and neck region, and at least 75% will develop a head and neck disease in the last year of life.[11,12] Common manifestations include recurrent or refractory infections of the middle ears or sinuses, oral herpes or candidiasis, oral leukoplakia, cervical adenopathy, salivary gland hypertrophy, and Kaposi's sarcoma. Though surgeons are still most likely to occupationally acquire an HIV infection in the operating room, such as from a contaminated needle stick, the preponderance of health care workers (HCW) are at risk in other settings such as physician's offices and hospital, ambulatory and home health care facilities.[3,10]

The Occupational Safety and Health Administration (OSHA) was created by the United States Congress in 1970 and is responsible for the promulgation and enforcement of safety regulations for the workplace. With recognition of the HIV epidemic in the later 1980s and the long-standing Hepatitis B virus (HBV) transmission problem for HCWs, a "Bloodborne Pathogen Standards" was added to OSHA responsibilities by Congress in 1991, with a phase-in of provisions to July of 1992 to cover the 5.6 million in health care and public safety occupations.[4,5,9] The standards contain instructions for the employers of workers who may reasonably be anticipated to have "skin, eye, mucous membrane, or parenteral contact with blood or other potentially infectious materials" during work tasks. The aforementioned applies to otolaryngologists in private office settings, as part owners of ambulatory care centers and the like. Though the inspections of physician's offices by OSHA have been infrequent, less than 300 in 1992, and usually prompted by a written complaint from an employee or patient, inspections will likely increase as an unofficial "grace" period wanes. OSHA inspections can occur without prior notice and in most states are accomplished by the states' own health services. The penalties for most infractions are $7,000 but are reduced by 60% for employers with 25 or fewer workers. Though further reductions in penalties are common for demonstrated "good faith efforts" to meet safety standards, willful or repeated violations can draw penalties to $70,000. The most commonly cited violations for physician employers to date are, in order of frequency, failure to have a hazard communication and/or exposure control plan, failure to maintain an employee illness and injury log, failure to meet employee training requirements, and inadequate housekeeping and/or waste disposal.

BLOODBORNE PATHOGENS STANDARDS

The Bloodborne Pathogens Standards codify the practice of "Universal Precautions," a concept first introduced by the Centers for Disease Control in 1987 and which states the "need for the HCW to consider all patients potentially infected with HIV and/or other bloodborne pathogens and to adhere rigorously to infection control precautions for minimizing the risks of exposure to blood and body fluids of all patients."[7] Personal barrier protection, environmental disinfection/sterilization, and engineering and workplace improvements to minimize HCW exposures comprise the universal precautions "triad." Though the original guidelines applied to all body fluids, in the head and neck region universal precautions no longer apply to nasal secretions,

Reprint Requests: J. David Osguthorpe, MD Department of Otolaryngology & Communicative Sciences 171 Ashley Avenue Charleston, S.C. 29425

Exposure Control Plan*

Exposure Determinations for Employee Duties
Employee Training in Universal Precautions and Workplace Engineering Controls
Identification and Communication of Hazards in the Workplace
Ready Availability of Personal Protective Clothing and Equipment
Hepatitis Vaccinations for Employees
Hepatitis B Vaccinations for Employees
Postexposure Protocol
Recordkeeping for Training and Exposures

*Mandated by OSHA 29 CFR 1910.1030 (1991).

TABLE 8-1
Employee "exposure determination" categories

Categories	Definition	Examples
I	All may come in contact with blood and other potentially infectious materials	Physicians, nurses
II	Some may come in contact with blood or other potentially infectious materials	Audiologists, housekeeping staff
III	All do not routinely have involvement with or exposure to blood or other potentially infectious materials	Receptionists and clerical workers

sputum, saliva, sweat, tears or vomitus unless such are obviously or likely to be contaminated by blood (such as nasal secretions in a patient with epistaxis or saliva after an oral biopsy). Blood is the predominant transmission vehicle for HIV and HBV, and no transmission of HIV in a medical setting by other than blood or blood contaminated material has been reported.

With universal precautions as the desired goal, OSHA requires employers of HCWs to have a written "Exposure Control Plan" which is available to all employees and is updated at least annually, more frequently when new work tasks or procedures are instituted or old ones modified (box above).[4,9] The plan must include exposure risk determinations for all employee positions, documentation of employee training in universal precautions and exposure control measures relevant to their job positions, procedures for handling blood and other potentially infectious materials (OPIM), records of Hepatitis B vaccinations for employees, a protocol for inadvertent exposures to blood or OPIM, the identification by label and oral communication of hazards in the workplace, the provision of personal protective clothing and equipment (PPCE) appropriate to work tasks, and record keeping for all of the aforementioned.

Exposure determination

"Exposure Determination" requires the employer to list all workplace tasks and procedures which might be associated with exposure to blood or OPIM and the job classifications for which some or all employees may have such exposure. Exposure classifications are commonly divided into 3 categories (Table 8-1) as follows: Category I—all employees may come in contact with blood or OPIM; Category II—some may make contact with those materials; Category III—employees who do not routinely have involvement with or occupational exposure to potentially infected materials. For practical purposes, most treat Category I (e.g., physician, nurse) and Category II employees (housekeepers, audiologists) identically, reserving Category III for receptionists, billing clerks and the like who do not deliver patient care or handle housekeeping tasks in patient care areas. If Category II employees are treated differently from Category I, all tasks which risk blood or OPIM exposure for Category II employees must be listed, along with PPCE for each task, such as requiring gloves for cleaning patient care areas, plus a mask and gown when assisting in incision and drainage procedures, and the like.

Category I and II (many also advocate Category III) employees must be provided with specified information and training at no cost during regular working hours prior to job assignment and also be provided with "refresher" information at least once a year. The initial training must include the workplace exposure control plan, information on the epidemiology, symptoms, and transmission of bloodborne pathogens, workplace tasks with possible exposure to blood or OPIM, the appropriate use of PPCE, and work practice and engineering controls which minimize disease transmission. Discussion of how to handle an exposure incident and implement a postexposure protocol is mandatory. Hazards in the work place, such as sharps containers, noxious chemicals and the like, must be identified in a workplace orientation for the employees and also be designated with warning labels or signs.

Personal protective clothing and equipment

Personal protective clothing and equipment (PPCE) must be readily available and at no cost to employees in work areas where contact with blood or OPIM is anticipated (box on p. 99). Gear appropriate for an otolaryngology office might include gloves, gowns, or laboratory coats and face shields or other eye protection and masks. Hypoallergenic gloves are provided to employees who need them. The cleaning and/or disposal of the aforementioned PPCE equipment is the responsibility of the employer and is guided by both OSHA regulations and the local health

Personal Protective Clothing and Equipment*
Gloves (Both sterile and nonsterile, hypoallergenic if needed by employee)
Masks, face shields, or eye protection
Gowns
Foot wear and head wear
Mucosa- and secretion-isolated resuscitation gear
*Type of clothing/equipment required is dependent on employee task; must be readily available and provided at no charge to employee

codes. After the initial training session in proper use of the equipment, the employer remains responsible for continued employee compliance. In general, gloves are required when there is a "reasonable anticipation" of hand contact with blood or OPIM and are discarded between patient contact with the HCWs hands washed immediately thereafter. Utility (housekeeping) gloves may be reused if intact and appropriately decontaminated. What constitutes "reasonable anticipation" is unclear and only general guidelines are available. The American Academy of Otolaryngology-Head and Neck Surgery has contacted OSHA regarding more specific information on procedures common to the specialty and will make this available when received.

Face and/or eye protection is required when potentially infectious materials are likely to be splashed or sprayed. Gowns, aprons, or the like are used when appropriate (e.g., nasal packing for epistaxis) and caps and shoe covers when substantial contamination is possible. Resuscitation equipment must isolate employees from patient secretions and mucosal contact, such as with a face mask and ambu bag combination rather than a mouth-to-mouth resuscitation.

Engineering and work practice controls

The OSHA Bloodborne pathogen standards also mandate "engineering and work practice controls." These are procedures, techniques, and mechanical systems to be installed in the office to limit physician and employee exposure to bloodborne pathogens. Engineering and work practice controls must be instituted and reviewed on at least an annual basis in the practice to decrease the risk of employee exposure to blood and body fluids. These include but are not limited to the following[5]:

Handwashing facilities. Handwashing stations must be readily available to the professional staff. Employees must wash hands after each patient contact, after removing gloves or after contact with contaminated surgical instruments or work surfaces. Antiseptic hand cleaner and paper towels must be available at each of the wash stations. Mucous membrane surfaces that become contaminated must be washed promptly after exposure occurs.

Eyewash facilities. An eyewash station must be available for employee use. Copious eye irrigation is warranted in the case of eye exposure to blood or body fluid aerosols or office chemicals.

Sharps disposal. Containers for disposal of sharps must be rigid and water-tight. They must be readily available at the site where they are used and must not, in themselves, present a source of danger to employees or the public. Sharps containers must be replaced before the filling to the point where the health care worker could come in contact with needles or syringes that have already been placed in the container. Needles should not be recapped except in the unusual circumstance in which the procedure necessitates such technique. The one most likely circumstance for need to recap needles in the otolaryngology office would be during needle aspiration of lymph nodes, salivary gland, or thyroid masses when cytologic specimens must be plated on glass slides. In such circumstances, a "one handed" recapping technique such as placing the cap on a counter top and not holding it with the unused hand or using a hemostat to grasp the hub of the needle to remove and replace it should be routinely adopted to decrease the likelihood of needlestick injury.

Employees must be taught the technique of removing scalpel blades from handles safely, or disposable scalpels should be used. Wires removed from arch bars or dental appliances must be treated as sharps. Suture needles should be disposed of in a sharps container immediately as the procedure is completed. Glass microscope slides should be treated as sharps and should be placed in cardboard carrying containers made for them and disposed of in sharps containers if no longer needed.

Soiled linens. Soiled linen must be gathered in a clearly marked (usually orange, red, or yellow) impermeable bag. Care must be taken to assure that sharps, including skin staples, have been removed from drapes to avoid potential exposure of laundry personnel. Potentially infectious linens must be clearly marked for the laundry. Most otolaryngology offices will contract with a commercial laundry to clean linens in a prescribed manner to ensure decontamination. It is advisable to receive written confirmation from the laundry that proper techniques and handling procedures are being followed. In some cases, having laundry facilities on site in the office or clinic may be appropriate. In such cases, the practice must follow prescribed guidelines such as ensuring handling of potentially contaminated linens with gloves and appropriately hot water to ensure sterilization. Employees cannot be allowed to take potentially infected linens (e.g., laboratory coats) home for washing in home facilities.

Nondisposable sharps (sinus trocars, otologic picks, etc.) must be kept separate from other surgical instruments. Such sharps will be rinsed with water and placed in a container of glutaraldehyde or other disinfectant and be allowed to soak for the prescribed interval before they are further cleaned and autoclaved.

Spilled blood. Cleaning of spilled blood or other potentially infectious materials must also be done in a prescribed manner. Office infection control policies must document and employees must be trained in these techniques. Spilled infectious materials are mopped up or wiped clear by an employee using gloves and other appropriate personal protective equipment. Counter tops and other work surfaces are wiped with a one to ten dilution of household bleach or other surface decontaminant which is bacteriocidal, mycobacteriocidal, virucidal, and fungicidal. Larger quantities of blood should be congealed with commercially available encapsulating powders. Solutions should be disposed of in a sanitary sewer system.

Surgical instruments. Cleaning of surgical instruments must be done by personnel wearing gloves, goggles, if splashing may occur, and other appropriate personal protective equipment. Grossly soiled materials should be washed off with detergent and water, and the equipment should be steam autoclaved or treated with gluteraldehyde or other sterilizing solutions for an appropriate period of time. Atomizers used for applying aerosolized medications to the nasal or oral mucosa or other surfaces must be shielded or cleaned with disinfectant solutions after each use. Any equipment that may leave the office for use or servicing elsewhere such as endoscopes or surgical instruments are decontaminated, disinfected, or sterilized prior to leaving the office.

Endoscopes. Fiberoptic laryngoscopes are used frequently in otolaryngology offices and must be cleaned between each use. Disinfection of fiberoptic scopes can be performed in two ways: (1) utilizing gluteraldehyde or similar disinfecting solutions or (2) using sheathing materials and subsequently removing the sheath after each use. Sheathing the scopes is generally more expensive, but it offers the advantage of faster turnaround time. For some practices, the purchase of multiple scopes to allow the necessary turnaround time for disinfection would be the best option. In others, sheathing the scopes will prove more time effective. Recently, more-concentrated solutions of gluteraldehyde have become commercially available that shorten the time required to sterilize endoscopes and other equipment to ten minutes. These solutions are potentially more damaging to the scopes when used over protracted periods. Telescopes should not be left in solutions to soak overnight.

If soaking the scopes in glutaraldehyde is the selected method of disinfection, the following steps should be adhered to:

1. The scope is thoroughly cleaned with a soap and water solution to remove all debris, crusts, or other materials.
2. The scope is immersed in the disinfecting solution. Disinfection with lower concentration glutaraldehyde solutions occurs within several minutes for HIV, ten minutes for hepatitis B virus, and twenty minutes for *Mycobacterium* species. Thus, twenty-minute soak times are recommended. An adequate reservoir of the disinfecting solution must be used to immerse the fiber portion of the scope. Covered scope disinfecting basins are available for this step.
3. Scopes should be thoroughly rinsed clean and wiped clean.
4. Some scopes (Pentax and others) have inflation devices to check the integrity of the rubber sheath of the fiber bundles.
5. Lenses and eyepieces should be checked for clarity and cleaned as indicated.
6. The scope should be returned to its case or caddie for safe storage.

Rigid telescopes such as the "Hopkins Rod" laryngoscope, sinus endoscopes, or otologic endoscopes also can be sterilized by immersion in appropriate solutions for the prescribed period of time.

No two otolaryngology offices are exactly alike, and the requirements to afford protection to employees and to comply with the OSHA bloodborne pathogen standards may vary. It is strongly recommended that otolaryngologists fully familiarize themselves with protective techniques for the benefit of themselves, co-workers, and employees. They should then document a "customized" infection control plan to apply to their clinical requirements and personnel.

Handling of laboratory specimens. All blood and tissue specimens must be handled in ways to reduce contamination by splashing, spraying, splattering, or generation of droplets. Biopsies are sent with bottles tightly capped in plastic bags supplied. Microscope slides sent from needle aspirate specimens are sprayed with fixative and placed in cardboard microscope slide carriers.

Smoking, food, cosmetics. Smoking should be prohibited in the office and no eating and drinking should take place in the laboratory, allergy treatment area, patient examining rooms, nurses' stations, or audiology areas. Hands must be washed after each patient contact and before eating. Applying cosmetics and handling contact lenses should not be performed in any patient care areas. Food must not be stored in refrigerators or freezers used for medicines, allergy solutions or clinical specimens.

TUBERCULOSIS REGULATIONS

Tuberculosis remains a major pathogen in the United States. Despite efforts to eradicate the disease, there has been an 18% increase in the number of cases of TB reported to the Centers for Disease Control. In 1990, there were 25,500 new cases of TB reported in the United States, with 3700 new cases in New York City alone. This rise in incidence of TB is felt to be due to several factors, including increased population at risk because of concurrent AIDS and because of the emergence of multiple drug resistant strains of TB.[2]

Between 1988 and 1993, sixteen HCWs have been reported to develop active TB with multidrug-resistant strains (MDR-TB). Five HCWs died of the disease during that period. These facts prompted OSHA to examine this data and to begin development of regulations to protect health care workers from this additional threatening pathogen acquired in the workplace. *Mycobacterium tuberculosis* is a bacteria spread primarily in 1 to 5 micron infectious droplets aerosolized when an infected individual coughs or expectorates. Medical procedures that increase the likelihood that a patient would exhibit such behavior in close proximity to a HCW could increase the likelihood of the health care worker contracting TB.[2]

In December 1990, the CDC published "Guidelines for preventing the Transmission of Tuberculosis in Health-Care Settings, with Special Focus on HIV Related Issues."[6] In that report, the authors noted that TB was particularly likely to be spread from patients who have unrecognized laryngeal and pulmonary TB. In addition, they cited cough-inducing procedures such as bronchoscopy, laryngoscopy, sputum induction, and administration of aerosolized medications as potential means of spread of the TB bacillus.

The guidelines developed by the CDC to control the spread of TB in health care facilities include the following principal points:

- Early identification, isolation and treatment of patients with TB infection
- Prevention of generation of infectious droplet nuclei
- Reducing microbial contamination of air
- Decontamination of medical equipment and surfaces in patient care areas
- Conducting surveillance for TB transmission to HCWs

From these general guidelines, the CDC went on to make specific recommendations to be followed by health care facilities including the following points:

- Patients at risk for TB should be screened with Mantoux tuberculin skin tests. Those with positive skin tests are evaluated for possible preventive antimycobacterial therapy.
- Vigorous efforts should be made to identify and treat patients who may have active tuberculosis. Patients with active pulmonary symptoms such as frequent and productive cough persisting at least three weeks, dyspnea, weight loss, fever, anorexia or fatigue should have TB included in their differential diagnosis and should be tested accordingly. For patients with other diagnoses that explain their pulmonary symptoms, the possibility of concurrent TB infection should be considered.
- Isolation precautions should be taken in those cases where active TB is suspected or proven to exist. Patients with suspected TB should not be returned to busy common waiting rooms.
- In facilities serving populations with a high incidence of TB or in those facilities frequently treating patients for symptoms common with active TB, attention must be paid to ventilation to decrease risk of transmission of the bacillus, and
- When specific procedures are performed that generate expectorated aerosols or droplets, procedure-specific precautions should be taken.

As of this time, most of the attention on the part of the CDC and OSHA in this area has been directed toward hospitals and other inpatient facilities. However, under the "General Duty Clause" of the OSHA regulations, if an employer knows of an increased risk to which he may be subjecting his employees, he can be held accountable even though specific regulations and guidelines may not have been violated.[13] It would be wise for any physician practicing in an area where there is a high incidence of TB or where the incidence of TB is increasing to take precautions to prevent infection from being spread within his or her practice.

At this point, it is recommended that otolaryngologist conduct Mantoux PPD tests on all of their personnel who have not previously tested positively. Testing should be performed on an annual basis in those employees who have not developed a positive test. Such testing may be indicated as frequently as every six months in clinical situations with particularly high risk of exposure. Employees not desiring to undergo testing and unable to document prior positive PPD testing should sign a waiver and may need to avoid contact with immunosuppressed or other susceptible patients.

Otolaryngologists should be on the lookout for patients with active pulmonary or laryngeal TB. A thorough history should be taken looking for evidence of active TB in patients who have had symptoms suggestive of the diagnosis or in patients who are immunosuppressed. A history of prior TB testing should be elicited, and in those patients without documentation of prior positive testing Mantoux TB tests should be applied. Otolaryngologist should examine the larynx for signs of active laryngeal TB, and, if findings suggest that diagnosis, infectious disease consultation and hospitalization, isolation, and treatment should be instituted as expeditiously as possible. Chest x-rays are appropriate for patients with suspected active TB.

By virtue of performing frequent office examinations of the upper aerodigestive tract, otolaryngologists frequently may induce the production of droplet nuclei that may spread the TB bacillus from a patient with known active TB. This can occur in oral, pharyngeal, or laryngeal examinations with tongue blades or mirrors or with laryngoscopic examinations with fiberoptic or rigid telescopes. In such situations, when the otolaryngologist is examining patients suspected of having active TB, additional steps to control risk of infection to the physician and coworkers should be instituted.[2,6] Steps to be followed include:

- Having unnecessary personnel clear the examining area.
- Those workers present should wear particulate respirators. These are masks capable of filtering out droplet nuclei of one to five microns in diameter. Typical surgical masks are not particulate respirators because they do not filter out small particles capable of spreading the TB bacillus because the filter size of the mask is too large and the masks do not fit tightly enough around the face to prevent ingress or egress of small particles.
- Working in rooms with ventilating systems capable of cleansing the air or otherwise decreasing the concentration of small, potentially infectious droplet nuclei.
- Sterilizing all instruments and equipment adequately to ensure destruction of all *Mycobacterium tuberculosis*. Following the criteria outlined in Section II of this manual (Bloodborne Pathogen Standards) should eradicate the TB bacillus.

At this point, OSHA has not mandated the need for special ventilating systems in physicians offices or other outpatient clinics in which bronchoscopy is not performed, in which tracheal aspirates are not obtained, or aerosolized medications are not administered. It is anticipated that, particularly in areas with large HIV positive populations at particular risk to develop active TB or in areas where active TB is relatively common, such mandates may be forthcoming in the near future. Steps that can be taken include the following;

- Placing ventilation systems in one or two examining rooms that ventilate directly to the outside and have at least six air exchanges per hour.
- Placing ventilation systems in examining rooms that incorporate HEPA filters, ultraviolet radiation, or some other means of sterilizing the air. Air cleaned with HEPA filters should not be directed back into the general air circulation of the building.
- In addition, rooms in which patients with or suspected of having active TB are treated should have relatively negative air pressure (i.e., air is drawn into the room when the door is opened) to decrease dissemination of potentially infectious droplet nuclei into other areas of the office, clinic, or health care facility.[6]

For those otolaryngologist and administrators working in "endemic" areas for TB, consultation with a qualified ventilation engineer is advisable before new construction of patient care areas or before "retrofitting" older facilities to meet these recommendations.

HAZARDOUS SUBSTANCE CONTROL PLANS

OSHA regulations addressing potential exposure of workers to chemicals are not new: they were initially enacted in 1985.[8] Physicians, hospitals, clinics, and their staffs were relatively poorly informed and noncompliant of these regulations until the Bloodborne Pathogen Standards went into effect and physicians were "introduced" to OSHA and *vice versa*. OSHA estimates that as many as 30 million workers are exposed to hazardous chemicals in the workplace and that nearly 600,000 potentially hazardous chemicals may be found in the work environment. Initially, only manufacturers were covered by the hazardous chemical standards and regulations, but in 1990 the United States Supreme Court ruled that the regulations apply to all industry sectors including the health care industry.[1,8] Since October 1990, OSHA has had the authority to examine health care facilities for compliance with these standards.

The OSHA Hazard Communication Standard (29 CFR 1910.1200) mandates all of the following:

- Employers must have a written Hazard Control Plan on site and available to the employees.
- Employers must keep and up-to-date inventory of all potentially hazardous substances used by or accessible to employees.
- Potential hazards of each of the above chemicals and substances must be assessed. This is true for proper use of the chemicals as well as for inadvertent or emergent exposure to them.
- The substances must be properly labeled.
- Employees must be properly trained regarding the handling, dangers, and disposal of the chemicals. This training must be repeated at least annually.
- Material Safety Data Sheets (MSDS) must be kept up to date, complete, and readily available to employees.

To comply with the Hazard Communication Standards, an otolaryngologist must complete the following tasks:

- Appoint a practice or clinic "safety officer." The safety officer may be a physician, administrator, nurse, or other individual in the practice who will have the responsibility for making sure that all of the subsequent steps are carried out.
- Write a "Hazard Control Plan." The Hazard Control Plan, like the "Bloodborne Pathogen Standard" of Section II of this manual, relays the important concepts of control of hazardous chemicals to the employees and staff.
- Conduct an inventory of the practice, listing all of the chemicals and substances found and determining if they present any danger to employees either in their usual means of use or with emergent exposure.
- Make sure that all of the chemicals found are properly labeled.
- Collect Material Safety Data Sheets on each of the chemicals found.
- Direct educational programs for employees, at least annually, on hazardous chemicals in the practice.

- With each new chemical arriving in the practice, make sure that it is properly labeled, that the Material Safety Data Sheet is added to the catalog, and that employees are alerted to potentially dangerous chemicals in either proper use or with misuse.

An inventory of chemicals found in an otolaryngology practice or clinic can be surprisingly long. Included are preserving solutions such as formaldehyde, surgical soaps such as iodophors, disinfecting solutions such as glutaraldehyde, bleach, etc., cleaning solutions such as ammonia, soaps, and window washing solutions. In addition, local anesthetics, topical anesthetics, neosynephrine, and other vasoconstrictive solutions must be listed. Any gel, liquid, lotion, suspension, or nonsolid form of medication must be included in the log. Solid medications are exempted from inclusion. Office chemicals such as copy machine chemicals and lubricants are included.

Material Safety Data Sheets (MSDS) must be obtained for each chemical listed in the inventory.[1,8] Material Safety Data Sheets are completed and supplied by the manufacturer of the chemical. They must be supplied to the practice by the local distributor. These responsibilities of the manufacturer and distributor of the chemicals is also mandated by the OSHA Hazard.

Communication Standards and most are cooperative with requests for such data. MSDSs contain all of the following data;

- Chemical identity
- Hazardous ingredients—chemical and common names of potentially hazardous components
- Physical and chemical characteristics—physical chemical data such as vapor pressure, flash point, boiling point, color, appearance, etc.
- Fire and explosion hazard—potential for fire and/or explosion
- Reactivity data—other chemicals likely to react with this substance
- Health hazards—acute and chronic health problems with signs and symptoms that could develop with exposure
- Precautions for safe handling and use—general precautions and instructions for optimal use of the chemical
- Control measures—work policies, protective equipment, and engineering controls needed for safe use of the chemical.

A few chemicals potentially found in an otolaryngology office warrant special mention. Glutaraldehyde and formaldehyde are very aromatic, and even opening containers for a brief period can result in significant dangers to physicians or other employees of the practice. Formaldehyde and glutaraldehyde used in tissue preserving solutions should be opened only long enough to allow placement of a biopsy specimen into the container. Glutaraldehyde solution used for disinfecting should be kept closed as much as possible to minimize "outgassing" from the solutions. Special air-monitoring requirements have been mandated for these solutions.[1]

As mentioned above, liquid, gel, cream, lotion, or other nonsolid medications require Material Safety Data Sheets. This is true whether the drug was given to the physician or office to distribute as samples or whether they were purchased by the office: the hazard remains the same in either case. In such cases, pharmaceutical representatives should be asked for the MSDS for the drug, and, if not available, the samples should not be accepted into the office. Compressed gasses such as bottled oxygen or nitrous oxide present potential problems as well. Care must be taken that the bottles for such gasses are secure. They must be stabilized in a cart or stand and should be positioned in the office away from heavily trafficked areas where they could be knocked over.[13] One of the major concerns with such gasses is the potential for the valve to shoot off of the bottle under pressure, forming a potentially dangerous projectile.

Of all of the OSHA regulations, the Hazard Communication Standards present the greatest challenge for the office trying to remain current. It is prudent for the physicians and/or the practice safety control officer to repeat the inventory three or more times per year to make sure that additional protectively harmful chemicals have not "crept in" to the practice unnoticed.

FIRE SAFETY STANDARDS

Fire safety is another area of great concern to businesses and employees. In 1988, workplace fires resulted in 3.1 billion dollars damage in the United States. Potential loss of life in such fires is of even greater concern. Fire safety regulations in the workplace are mandated by the OSHA Emergency Planning Standard, 29 CFR 1910.38.

Fire is unlikely in the otolaryngology office, though a few potential points of fire danger must be considered: Any building is potentially a source of fire. This may emanate from a furnace, boiler or heating system, from electrical fire, from outside sources such as lightning or adjacent fire, etc. There are several sources of heat within an otolaryngology practice that could serve as a source of a fire. These include autoclaves, hot bead sterilizers, alcohol lamps or other mirror heating devices, light sources, etc.

OSHA standards require that employers provide properly maintained, marked, and functional exits, appropriate fire retardant or fire fighting equipment such as fire extinguishers and/or sprinkler systems, written and diagrammatic fire safety plans for response and evacuation, and employee training about implementing such plans in case of a fire emergency. All employees must be trained and know their responsibilities in the event of fire. Location of fire extinguishers, fire exits, and evacuation routes must be established for the employees. Their responsibilities in notifying the fire department and other authorities and in helping patients and other employees must be well understood.

A fire emergency response plan must be written and contain all of the specifics on how the employees should respond. Fire professionals frequently use the acronym "RACE" to remind employees of their responsibilities. The letters stand for the following responsibilities:

Rescue any person in immediate danger.
Alarm all other persons, whether employees or patients in the facility, and call the fire department
Confine the fire by closing windows or doors in the immediate area and,
Extinguish the fire if it is small and can reasonably be extinguished with available extinguishers and equipment and/or evacuate the building

A fire safety plan may reasonably define different categories of emergency, delineating a different set of responsibilities for a "minor fire" as opposed to a major one. A minor fire would be one limited to a small area or container and for which use of available fire extinguishers would in all likelihood control the problem. In such instances, the building may not need complete evacuation, but the patients in the immediate vicinity of the fire are moved. Flammable materials in the area such as volatile liquids, paper and other combustibles, and oxygen cylinders should be moved from the area. The area should be contained by closing doors, windows, etc., and the fire extinguishers should be used. The fire safety plan should list specific steps followed in using the particular type of fire extinguisher that is available in the office, and which type of extinguisher to use in what variety of fire (Table 8-2). The plan must also specify a fire safety officer (e.g., a physician or practice administrator) who is to be notified of the fire, who can report it to the proper authorities, and who can replenish the fire fighting equipment used. Ideally, the fire safety office should inspect the area and give approval before employees or patients are allowed to return to the area.

A separate section of the fire safety plan should delineate steps to be followed in the event of a major fire such as a fire of the building structure itself or of appliances or electrical equipment. In such cases, the fire safety plan should restate the RACE acronym, delineating responsibilities of employees but emphasizing "Evacuation" as opposed to "Extinguishing the fire" as the final "E." Plans should be constructed to promote patient and employee safety as opposed to extinguishing the fire source. Efforts must be made to determine that all patients and employees have been evacuated and the fire safety plan should delineate how this is accomplished. Ideally, the fire safety office or receptionist should be charged with the responsibility of taking a daily patient list or roster with him or her when evacuating the office.

TABLE 8-2
Fire extinguishers

Type of fire extinguisher	Type of fire
A	Wood and paper
B	Flammable liquids and gasoline
C	Electrical wiring and equipment
A B C	Combination fires
D	Combustible metals (e.g., Mg, Na)

Another major portion of fire safety plan must be evacuation planning. The plan should be specifically written for the office building, stating which doors, hallways, stairwells, and other routes are used in the evacuation. Elevators are avoided in the event of fire and the evacuation plan must take this into account. Employees must be instructed in these routes and, ideally, fire drills should be held on a periodic basis. Fire exits must be clearly marked with exit signs and other internal passages that do not lead to the outside or evacuation routes should be marked "Not an Exit" to help avoid confusion. Restrooms or storerooms should be clearly marked to avoid confusion. Maps of the office layout with fire evacuation routes clearly marked should be posted prominently in the office. Locations of fire extinguishers and alarm boxes should be marked on the diagram as well.

The fire safety plan must clearly state who the fire safety office for the practice is. It must state how the contact the local authorities (whether by dialing 911, or via another number). It should remind the employee contacting the authorities to relay:

- The exact location of the fire (e.g., address, suite, room)
- The type of fire
- Whether the building has been evacuated
- Patient or employee injuries
- Any other information requested

The fire safety plan must delineate the fire extinguishers present in the practice. It must relay the type of extinguisher (i.e., "A," "B," and/or "C," or "D")(Table 8-2). In addition, it must relay requirements and responsibilities for maintenance and recharging, and in employee instruction in the use of the extinguishers. Sprinkler systems in buildings do not obviate the need for fire extinguishers.

Fire prevention should be an important part of the fire safety plan as well. Volatile chemicals must be stored safely away from sources of spark or heat with adequate ventilation. Electrical guidelines should be listed, including avoidance of use of "cheater cords" to bypass grounded electrical outlets and overloading of circuits with electrical appliances. Periodic inspection of electrical equipment and cords must be specified in the plan.

Most municipalities will have very specific fire codes for new and old buildings. In addition, many will have specific requirements that must be adhered to in the fire safety plan. The local fire marshall should be consulted if assistance is required in developing the plan.

EMPLOYEE TRAINING

Employee training in the OSHA standards and the means taken by the office to comply with them is vital. Employees should be informed of what OSHA is, why they have developed the standards, of the fact that the standards are promulgated for employee safety, and of the fact that employees have avenues to pursue grievances through OSHA if employer compliance is not forthcoming. The OSHA standards require that a poster be posted prominently in the workplace to make sure that employees have been informed of their rights under these standards.[5,13]

The OSHA Bloodborne Pathogen Standard states that employees must undergo training in compliance with the practices' exposure control plan before beginning work with possible exposure and at least annually thereafter. Employees must have training in the fire safety and the fire safety plan of the practice and with potential hazardous chemical exposures in the practice as well. In particular, each of the following topics must be addressed:

- Potential sources of exposure to infectious waste and materials
- Work practice controls used to limit exposure
- Engineering controls
- Personal protective equipment
- Housekeeping, waste disposal and laundry
- Hepatitis vaccine: Potential benefits and indications
- Postexposure evaluation and follow-up
- Record keeping to comply with OSHA regulation
- Hazardous chemicals used in the practice
- Fire safety

Training should be both in general terms (i.e., as would apply to any medical or surgical practice) and in practice-specific terms (i.e., the measures mandated by the exposure control plan, fire safety plan or hazard communication plan of the individual practice). Date, topics discussed, which employees were in attendance, and who was the instructor should be documented with a sign-in sheet and attached to the practices OSHA compliance records.

DOCUMENTATION

Along with the other requirements, the OSHA regulations require documentation that all of the steps have been followed.[1,5] Documentation required includes:

- Written exposure control plan
- Written hazard communication plan
- List of potentially hazardous chemicals
- Material Safety Data Sheets for above chemicals
- Written fire safety plan
- Documentation of employee training
- Postexposure documentation
- Hepatitis vaccine documentation
- OSHA 200 log for exposure incidents

The OSHA standards mandating record keeping requirements are found in 29 CFR 1910.20. OSHA has produced a publication entitled *Record Keeping Guideline for Occupational Injuries and Illnesses,* 29 CFR 1904, O.M.B. No. 1220-0029 which is available without charge through your OSHA office.

This following is a brief review of some of the more important steps that must be followed to document compliance with OSHA Regulations:

OSHA 200 Log: Postexposure documentation

The OSHA 200 log is a vehicle to document occupational accidents, injuries, or illnesses. OSHA requires that an OSHA 200 Log be kept by all businesses with at least 10 employees, but it is advisable that smaller offices go "beyond compliance" and maintain such a log as well.[5,13] In addition, even employers with less than 10 employees are required to report on any employee who has suffered a fatality, multiple hospitalizations, or accidents.

For each employee work-related injury or illness, employers are required to document within six working days of the accident, injury, or exposure the following information:

- Date and time of the incident
- Date and time that the form was completed
- Name of the individual exposed
- Source of the exposure
- Description of employee's duties at the time of the exposure
- How the incident occurred
- Specific route of exposure
- Material to which employee was exposed.

In addition, the employer or his/her safety officer must assess specifically whether universal precautions, engineering controls, workplace controls, personal protective equipment, and other precautions were available to the worker and adhered to.

Employee medical record

OSHA regulations require that the employer maintain a medical record for all employees who have exposure incidents or who suffer work-related injuries of illnesses. Under the bloodborne pathogen standards 29 CFR 1910.1030 and the OSHA record-keeping requirements 29 CFR 1910.20, employers must keep medical records on exposed employees that include all of the following information:

- Name and social security number of the employee
- Documentation of the employee's hepatitis B vaccination status
- Any medical records relevant to whether or not the employee can receive the hepatitis B vaccine
- Copies of medical examinations, medical testing, and follow-up relevant to the incident
- Copies of information sent with the employee to the examining physician after the incident

All of the above medical records must be handled with the strictest confidentiality. They may only be released with the employee's written permission with the exception that OSHA or the National Institute of Safety and Health may examine the records without the employee's or employer's permission. Such medical records must be maintained by the employer for a period of thirty years after the incident or exposure. Provisions are made in the codes for transfer of those records to OSHA if the employer closes business or is otherwise not available to maintain those records.[5]

When referring the employee to an examining physician after the exposure (at the expense of the employer), the employer should supply the following information confidentially to that physician:

- Name of the employee
- Job description
- Date of the exposure
- Type of exposure
- Details of how the exposure occurred
- Employee's hepatitis B vaccination status
- If the exposure is to a bloodborne pathogen, the HIV and HBV status of the patient, if available or as it becomes available (name of patient should not be stated)
- Signature of employer or his or her representative and date completed
- Person to contact or relay record of examination and recommendations to on behalf of the employer

In addition, the employer must make it clear to the examining physician that the purpose of the examination is for appropriate diagnosis and care for the exposure incident and that all appropriate steps must be taken. Billing for such services is to the employer.

In turn, the examining physician must relay the following information back to the employer to keep on file in the employee's confidential medical record:

- Employee name
- Date of the examination
- A written opinion limited to whether hepatitis B vaccination is indicated for the employee and whether or not such a vaccination was administered to the patient
- A statement confirming that the patient was appropriately counseled regarding possible subsequent development of medical conditions related to the exposure

Other medical information should *not* be relayed back to the employer. The employee's medical record is otherwise confidential.

Hepatitis B vaccination documentation

Under the requirements of the Bloodborne Pathogens Standards, employees who have not previously been vaccinated and who do not have other contraindications must be give the opportunity to undergo hepatitis B vaccination at the expense of the employer. The employer must maintain confidential records of the dates of hepatitis B vaccinations or any records relevant to the employee not being a candidate for not being vaccinated. If the employee *elects* not to be vaccinated, he or she must sign a release form stating that he or she declines the opportunity to be vaccinated. An example of wording for such a form is as follows:

> *I, (*typed or printed name*), understand that because of my occupation and employment with (*name of otolaryngology practice*), I may become exposed to blood or other potentially infectious materials that present risk of my acquiring hepatitis B virus (HBV) infection. I understand that infection with hepatitis B virus may lead to serious and, at times, life-threatening illness. I have been given the opportunity to be vaccinated with hepatitis B vaccine, with provision of the vaccine and its administration paid for by (*name of practice*). This would be provided without personal expense on my part. I understand that by declining to be vaccinated, I will remain at risk of acquiring hepatitis B. I realize that if I elect to change my mind in the future while employed by (*name of practice*), I will be provided the vaccine at no expense to me unless its administration is contraindicated for other medical reasons at that time.*
>
> *Signed:* (employee signature) *Date:* ________
>
> *Witness:* (witness signature) *Date:* ________

If the employee elects to receive the vaccine, a confidential vaccination record is kept and includes:

- Employee name
- Date of birth
- Social security number
- HBV antibody screening results and date (if performed)
- Dates of administration of vaccination dosages 1, 2, and 3
- Date of administration of HBV booster (if given)

- Repeat antibody screening results and dates (if performed)
- Any additional relevant notes

Training records

As noted in the above sections, employers are under mandate to provide training regarding the Bloodborne Pathogen Standards, the practice's Exposure Control Plan, the Fire Safety Plan, and the Hazard Communication Standards. All formal training sessions for employees should be documented with a statement signed by all employees in attendance, the instructor, and the employer or his or her representative. This statement should include all of the following information.

- Date of the session
- Material covered during the session (e.g., purpose of the OSHA regulations, bloodborne pathogens, exposure control plan)
- Instructor and his or her qualifications
- Names and job titles of all in attendance
- Signatures of all involved

Records of all training sessions are kept for at least three years.

CONTACTING OSHA

There are several methods of contacting OSHA representatives for assistance in meeting OSHA regulations, including all of the following:

Approved sources of OSHA-funded consultation

Business owners may request free on-site consultation through the 7(c)(1) Onsite Consultation Program. Through this program, consultants, funded by OSHA, will inspect the business or medical practice looking for any areas which would place employees at risk or would appear to violate OSHA standards. They will not write citations for infractions found. However, if any conditions or situations are noted that would place employees in "imminent danger" and if the business does not take steps to immediately correct the situation, the consultant is required to notify OSHA so that enforcement steps can be taken. Other "serious" hazards, if identified, must be corrected on a timetable set by the consultant and the business together. If the corrective actions are not taken within the prescribed timetable, OSHA officials would intervene. Thus, only deliberate inaction on the part of the business following such an inspection could result in citations.

Contacting OSHA offices

Your local office is source of information, publications or assistance in understanding the OSHA requirements and standards. Contacting OSHA will not trigger an inspection, but if you request an inspection from the OSHA Office, they may issue citations for infractions.

State-operated compliance programs

OSHA encourages each state to assume responsibility for administration and enforcement of OSHA regulations and standards within that state. States are invited to assert jurisdiction over additional areas of occupational safety whether covered or not by federal laws. The state must first submit a plan for approval by the OSHA.

Some states are now operating under approved state plans. These states may have adopted the existing federal standards or may have developed their own standards. You need to know whether you are covered by state plan operation or are subject to the federal program in order to determine which set of standards and regulations (federal or state) apply to you. The easiest way to determine this is to call the nearest OSHA Area Office.

The following states were operating under OSHA-approved state plans in 1994.

Alaska	Michigan	Tennessee
Arizona	Minnesota	Utah
California	Nevada	Vermont
Hawaii	New Mexico	Virginia
Indiana	North Carolina	Virgin Islands
Iowa	Oregon	Washington
Kentucky	Puerto Rico	Wyoming
Maryland	South Carolina	

Connecticut and **New York** have programs which cover only state and local government operations.

SUMMARY

The regulations promulgated by the Occupational Health and Safety Administration were largely unknown by the medical community until the Bloodborne Pathogen Standards went into affect in 1992. The Bloodborne Pathogen Standards codify steps that must be taken within physicians offices, hospitals, and other workplaces where employees may be exposed to blood or other potentially infectious diseases. These standards promote the adoption of "Universal Precautions" and require the provision and use of "personal protective clothing and equipment," the design and incorporation of "workplace engineering controls," and the delineation and compliance with "work practice controls." Each practice must design and adopt a practice specific "infection control plan." "At risk" employees must be offered and supplied the hepatitis B vaccination series. The Bloodborne Pathogen Standards also mandate employee training requirements and record keeping requirements.

Tuberculosis in the medical workplace represents a re-emerging hazard in the 1990s. New standards have been directed at hospitals, but it is anticipated that requirements may be directed at physicians' offices as well. Procedures mandated include TB testing of employees, early identification of patients with TB, HEPA filters and masks, and appropriate ventilation and air exchange in selected patient care areas.

Older regulations, the Hazard Communication Standards, require that all chemicals used in the workplace be cataloged and that Material Safety Data Sheets be collected on them. All chemicals in the workplace must be labeled appropriately. Fire safety standards for the workplace are also codified in the OSHA regulations.

Compliance with the OSHA regulations promotes a high level of health care worker safety and reduces physician and employer liability. Failure to comply may result in stiff punitive measures.

REFERENCES AND OTHER SOURCES OF INFORMATION

Cited Literature

1. *Access to Medical and Exposure Records,* OSHA 3110
2. American Hospital Association and the American Society for Hospital Engineering: Hospital controls for tuberculosis: OSHA's role, American Hospital Association, 1994.
3. Bell DM: Human immunodeficiency virus transmission in health care settings: risk and risk reduction. *Am J Med* 91(suppl 3B):294, 1991.
4. *Bloodborne Facts: (information sheets)* OSHA Publication Office
   Hepatitis B vaccination--Protection for you
   Holding the line on contamination
   Personal protective equipment cuts risk
   Protecting yourself when handling sharps
   Reporting exposure incidents
5. Bloodborne Pathogen Standards. *Federal Register* 56:64175, 1991.
6. Centers for Disease Control: Guidelines for preventing the transmission of tuberculosis in health-care settings, with special focus on HIV-related issues. *MMWR* 39:1-29, 1990.
7. Centers for Disease Control: Guidelines for prevention of HIV transmission in health care settings. *MMWR* 36(Suppl 2s), 1987.
8. *Chemical Hazard Communication Guidelines:* OSHA 3111.
9. Occupational Safety and Health Administration: General Industry Standards for Bloodborne Pathogens. *Federal Register* 56:64175, 1991.
10. Osguthorpe JD: Occupational human immunodeficiency virus exposure: risks to the health care worker. Otolaryngol Clin North Am 25:1341,1992.
11. Smith RV, Eisele DW: Human immunodeficiency virus: transmission concerns in clinical practice. *Ear Nose Throat J* 70:271, 1991.
12. Tami T, editor: Otolaryngologic manifestations of acquired immunodeficiency syndrome, *Otolaryngol Clin North Am,* 25:6, 1992.
13. Williams-Steiger Occupational Safety and Health Act of 1970, Code of Federal Regulations: Title 29, Parts 1910 (1910.1000 to end) S/N 869-017-00110-4.

OSHA Publications

OSHA publications may be obtained by one of the following routes:

1. Call your state OSHA office

2. Write or call the OSHA Publication Office c/o
   OSHA Publication Office
   Room N-3101
   200 Constitution Avenue, N.W.
   Washington, D.C. 20210
   (Please send a self-addressed label)

3. Write or call the US Government Printing Office, c/o
   Superintendent of Documents
   Government Printing Office
   Washington, D.C. 20402
   (or call (202) 783-3238)

Currently available OSHA publications include

All About OSHA: OSHA 2056

Bloodborne Pathogens and Acute Health Care Workers: OSHA 3128

Bloodborne Pathogens and Dental Workers: OSHA 3129

Bloodborne Pathogens and Emergency Responders: OSHA 3130

Bloodborne Pathogens and Long-Term Health Care Workers: OSHA 3131

Consultation Services for the Employer: OSHA 3047

Employer Rights and Responsibilities and Courses of Action Following an OSHA Inspection: OSHA 3000

Materials Handling and Storing: OSHA 2236, GPO order #029-016-00138-7 ($2.00)

Occupational Exposure to Bloodborne Pathogens: OSHA 3127

Occupational Exposure to Bloodborne Pathogens, Federal Register 56(235):64004-64182, December 6, 1991. GPO order #069-001-00040-8 ($2.00)

OSHA Publications and Audiovisual Programs: OSHA 2019

OSHA Handbook for Small Businesses: OSHA 2209

Personal Protective Equipment: OSHA 3077

Other United States Government Publications

Centers for Disease Control, Atlanta, GA, 30333 (or call 404-639-1547) for the most current information on universal precautions, post-exposure prophylaxis and the like.

Centers for Disease Control: Advisory Committee for the Elimination of Tuberculosis: A strategic plan for the elimination of tuberculosis in the United States, *MMWR* 38(suppl S-3), 1989.

Centers for Disease Control: AIDS and HIV update: Acquired immunodeficiency syndrome and human immunodeficiency virus infection among health-care workers, *MMWR* 37:229-34, 1988.

Centers for Disease Control: Core Curriculum on Tuberculosis. Printed by the American Lung Association, 1991.

Centers for Disease Control: Guidelines for prevention of transmission of human immunodeficiency virus and hepatitis B virus to health care and public safety workers, *MMWR* 38(suppl. S-6):1-37, 1989.

Centers for Disease Control: Infection-control practice for dentistry, 1993, *MMWR* 42:1-12, 1993.

Centers for Disease Control: Investigations of patients who have been treated by HIV-infected health care workers, *MMWR* 41:344-6, 1992.

Centers for Disease Control: Protection against viral hepatitis: Recommendations of the immunization practices advisory committee (ACIP), *MMWR* 39 (no. RR-2):1, 1990.

Centers for Disease Control: Recommendations for preventing transmission of human immunodeficiency virus and hepatitis B virus to patients during exposure-prone invasive procedures, *MMWR* 40:1-9, 1991.

Centers for Disease Control: Recommended infection-control practices for dentistry, *MMWR* 35:237-42, 1986.

Centers for Disease Control: Statement on management of occupational exposure to human immunodeficiency virus, including considerations regarding Zidovudine post-exposure use, *MMWR* 39:1-14, 1990.

Centers for Disease Control: Update: Universal precautions for prevention of transmission of human immunodeficiency virus, hepatitis B virus, and other bloodborne pathogens in health-care settings, *MMWR* 260:462-5, 1988.

Other References and Sources of Information

American Medical Association. 515 N. State St., Chicago, IL 60610 (or call 800-262-3211); request (for $150) "For Your Protection: The OSHA Regulations on Bloodborne Pathogens", a package of bloodborne pathogen training manuals (different ones for physicians and employees), a videotape, and a "model" exposure control plan.

American Society for Hospital Engineering Technical Document: TB control in the hospital environment: American Hospital Association, 1993.

Benninger MS, Gupta N, Gilmore K: Intraoperative infectious disease exposure to otolaryngology operating room personnel. *Laryngoscope* 101:1276-9,1991.

Chamberlain ME, Conley LJ, Bush TJ, et al: Health Care Workers with AIDS: National Surveillance Update. *JAMA* 226:3459-62, 1991.

Davidson TM, Stabile B: Acquired immunodeficiency syndrome precautions for otolaryngology-head and neck surgery. *Arch Otolaryngol Head Neck Surg* 117:1343-4, 1991.

Endres A, Alun-Jones T, et al: The effectiveness of double-gloving in otolaryngology. *Clin Otolaryngol* 15:535-536, 1990.

Fry DE: Blood exposure in the operating room: reducing the risk. *Am Coll Surgeons Bulletin* 76:16-21, 1991.

Gerberding JL, Littell C, Tarkington A, et al: Risk of exposure of surgical personnel to patients' blood during surgery at San Francisco General Hospital. *N Engl J Med* 322:1788-93, 1990.

Godin MS, Lavernia CJ, Harris JP: Occult surgical glove perforations in otolaryngology-head and neck surgery. *Arch Otolaryngol Head Neck Surg* 117:910, 1991.

Henderson DK: Postexposure chemoprophylaxis for occupational exposure to human immunodeficiency virus. *Am J Med* 91(suppl 3B):312, 1991.

Jagger J, Hunt EH, Brand-Elnaggar J, Pearson RD: Rates of needle-stick injury caused by various devices in a university hospital. *N Engl J Med* 319:284-288, 1988.

Kelly KE, Lee KC, Tami TA: Prevention of surgical glove perforations with cut-resistant gloves. *Otolaryngol Head Neck Surg* 104:291, 1991.

Klein RS, Phelan JA, Freeman K, et al: Low occupational risk of human immunodeficiency virus infections among dental professionals. *N Engl J Med* 318:86-90, 1988.

Kriebel D, Sama SR, Cocanour B: Reversible pulmonary responses to formaldehyde. A study of clinical anatomy students. *Am Rev Respir Dis* 148:1509-15, 1993.

Mandelbrot DA, Smythe WR, Norman SA, et al: A survey of exposures, practices and recommendations of surgeons in the care of patients with human immunodeficiency virus. *SGO* 171:99-106, 1990.

Marcusen DC and Sooy CD: Otolaryngologic and head and neck manifestations of the acquired immunodeficiency syndrome (AIDS). *Laryngoscope* 95:401-405, 1985.

Medical College of Pennsylvania and Legal Economic Guidelines: Bloodborne pathogens: Exposure and risk reduction based on 1992 OSHA standards. Medical College of Pennsylvania. Continuing Medical Education, 3200 Henry Avenue, Philadelphia, Pennsylvania, 19129, 1992.

Panlilio AL, Foy DR, Edwards JR, et al: Blood contacts during surgical procedures. *JAMA* 265:1533-7, 1991.

Popejoy SL, Fry DE: Blood contact and exposure in the operating room, *SGO* 172:480-483, 1991.

Pugliese G: TB respirators: What's required and what isn't. *Materials Management* 38-42, April 1994.

Reider HL, Cauthen GM, Kelly GD, et al: Tuberculosis in the United States, *JAMA* 262:385-389, 1989.

Smith JW, Nichols RL: Barrier efficiency of surgical gowns: Are we really protected from our patients' pathogens? *Arch Surg* 126:756-763, 1991.

Sooy CD, Gerberding JL, Kaplan MJ: The risk for otolaryngologists who treat patients with AIDS and AIDS virus infection: report of an in-progress study. *Laryngoscope* 97:1-4, 1987.

Tokars JI, Bell DM, Culver DH, et al: Percutaneous injuries during surgical procedures, *JAMA* 267:2899-2904, 1992.

Weaver VM, McDiarmid MA, Guidera JA, et al: Occupational chemical exposures in an academic medical center. *J Occup Med* 35:701-706, 1993.

Wright JG, McGeer AJ, Chyatte D, Ransohoff DF: Mechanisms of glove tears and sharp injuries among surgical personnel. *JAMA* 266:1668-1671, 1991.

Zuger A, Miles SH: Physicians, AIDS, and occupational risk: historic traditions and ethical obligations, *JAMA* 258:1924-1928, 1987.

9

Practical TMJ Management for Otolaryngologists

Cedric A. Quick, M.D., M.B.A., and Philip J. Smith, D.D.S.

Temporomandibular joint disorders (TMJ) or more currently termed temporomandibular disorders (TMDs) are defined as a collection of mandibular joint and craniofacial muscle problems embracing many different clinical entities.[4,17,18,21] They are considered a subclassification of musculoskeletal and rheumatic disorders, and current research supports the view that TMD is a cluster of related disorders in the masticatory system with many common clinical features.[7] The most common initial symptom is pain, usually localized in the muscles of mastication in the periauricular area or the temporomandibular joint.[14] The pain is usually aggravated by chewing or other jaw functions. Other common symptoms include: earache, jawache, headache, facial pain, tinnitus, and "fullness" in the ear. Associated features may involve limitation in range of motion of the jaw and various joint sounds described by the patient as clicking, popping, grating, or crepitus. Pain or dysfunction caused by nonmusculoskeletal causes (neurologic, vascular, neoplastic, or infectious disease) in the oral facial region must be distinguished from primary TMD.

The progression or resolution of TMD cannot be predicted accurately at the initial consultation or any single point in time. Previous signs, symptoms, and diagnoses are often unreliable. Also several indeterminable factors may influence the forward course of the problem. Fortunately, most of TMDs are self-limiting or are limited to mild and transient symptoms. There is, however, a patient population that has chronically recurrent or persistent TMDs with a variety of symptoms. Demographic studies in the U.S. show that at any time approximately 5% of the population is in need of treatment and that approximately 5% of the U.S. population is in treatment.[5] Unfortunately, these two groups do not always match. In the treatment of TMD, goals must be established that will give a reasonable expectation to both the patient and the clinician regarding the outcome of treatment. Ideally these should include reduction of pain, restoration of normal jaw function, reduction of the need for future treatment, and the restoration of a normal life style. The objective of this paper is to show how most of the patients we see can be treated conservatively and cost effectively without the risk of irreversible changes or the necessity for invasive procedures.

CLINICAL FEATURES

When discussing the temporomandibular joint complex, the terms loading and unloading of the joint are commonly used. The joint is unloaded when the mouth is empty and at rest. However, during the actual chewing, the working side (the side chewing the food) has the joint distracted and that joint will be unloaded. The balancing side, the side opposite the working side during chewing, is the loaded joint and experiences increased intra-articular pressure. Later in our discussion we will introduce the idea of splint therapy in order to unload the joint and to place it at rest.

Pain

When first appearing for treatment, the patient will usually give a history of pain, either chronic or acute, and previous treatment for presumed sinusitis, ear infections, or dental disorders. The pain may be muscular, involving either a dull ache over a diffused area, or described as a feeling of tenseness or tightness in the face or jaw. In the area of the temporomandibular joint, the pain may be dull or sharp and more localized, seeming to the patient that a single point is the origin of the pain. Patients often describe a pulling sensation and the inability to open the mouth fully. In instances in which there is a description of pain that defies biological reason, a psychogenic origin of the pain has to be suspected. These patients may often exhibit an abnormal pain reaction. Neurologic pain is usually described as sharp and/or shooting, burning, or numbing and has a constant response to stimulation. It will follow the neural path-

should be worn at all times, including meals. The patient must remove the splint to clean their teeth and the appliance following each meal. They should wear this appliance both day and night in order to obtain maximum benefit. After a period of two to eight weeks, if improvement is seen, the patient may then be allowed to stop wearing the appliance during the day and wear it only at night or in times of intense activity. In the group of patients classified as bruxers or clenchers, it might be necessary for them to wear a night splint for prolonged periods of time. Additionally, analgesic blocking of the involved muscles might help in overcoming acute symptoms or recalcitrant painful spasm. Slow stretching of the muscles and exercises to increase the patient's range of motion should be initiated when spasm subsides, and the patient should be instructed to continue these exercises well beyond the period of spasm. Patients who exhibit signs and symptoms of psychological or behavioral problems should be referred for appropriate counseling and behavior modification.

For patients that have clicking problems due to displaced disc or blockage of motion caused by the disc, a hard acrylic splint has been advocated to reduce the pain and recapture the disc. Historically, many clinicians held the belief that the displaced disc could be "recaptured" by splint therapy. Using MRI images, it has now been demonstrated that the disc becomes remodeled and adapts to the new position.[13]

In cases in which there is persistent inability to open the mouth or an extreme limitation of motion, and the above conservative measures have failed repeatedly, surgery may be considered.

SURGERY

If conservative, nonsurgical treatment fails to resolve the symptoms, then surgical treatment of the internal derangements may be indicated. Surgical arthroscopy is used in the treatment of displaced discs, closed locks, hypermobility, and arthritides. Among the typical findings with arthroscopy are: adhesions, fibrillations, perforations, synovitis, and hyperemia. Arthroscopic treatments include lysis and lavage, suturing of the disc, laser surgery, and injection of sclerosing agents or steroids.[11,12,15,16,19,20] Procedures that are used in open TMJ surgery include: discoplasty-repair of perforations, reattachment of the disc, or excision of the disc combined with autogenous replacement.[6,10]

ALTERNATIVE TREATMENTS

Although there are many other modalities of treatment for TMD which are recommended by various authors, many do not stand the scrutiny of well-researched clinical and scientific appraisal. Some of these controversial methods include: the use of electromyography for stabilizing the patient's occlusion, grinding of one or more teeth in order to obtain a "more ideal" occlusion, and the construction of various exotic splints which can cause teeth to supererupt and change permanently the patient's occlusal relationships.

SUMMARY

Patients that present with the signs and symptoms of TMD should be examined and evaluated in a logical manner. Pain, joint sounds, and deviation or limitation in jaw motion are the common initial complaints. Diagnostic tests should include screening radiographs, psychological testing when indicated, and local anesthesia to localize and differentiate the source of pain. Initial management should be conservative, progressing to more aggressive modalities as indicated by patient response. Placing the patient on a soft to liquid diet, NSAID, and warm moist soaks will alleviate symptoms in 80% of TMD patients. Bite splints and stress management are the next level of therapy. Surgical treatment must be reserved for those patients that do not respond to conservative therapy and have positive indicators for the surgery.

REFERENCES

1. Anonymous: Assessment. In McNeill C, editor: *Temporomandibular disorders.* Chicago, 1993, Quintessence Publishing Co., Inc.
2. Anonymous: Epidemiology, In McNeill C, editor: *Temporomandibular disorders.* Chicago, 1993, Quintessence Publishing Co., Inc.
3. Anonymous: Etiology. In McNeill, C, editor: *Temporomandibular disorders.* Chicago, 1993, Quintessence Publishing Co., Inc.
4. Anonymous Panel Discussion: Definition of Terms. In McNeill C, editor: *Current controversies in temporomandibular disorders.* Chicago, 1992, Quintessence Publishing Co., Inc.
5. Anonymous: Panel Discussion: TMD Epidemiology. In McNeill C, editor: *Current controversies in temporomandibular disorders.* Chicago, 1992, Quintessence Publishing Co., Inc.
6. Chuong R, Piper MA: Avascular necrosis of the mandibular condyle-pathogenesis and concepts of management. Oral Surg Oral Med Oral Pathol 75:428-432, 1993. (Review.)
7. Clark GT: Etiologic theory and the prevention of temporomandibular disorders. Adv Dent Res 5:60-66, 1991. (Review.)
8. Clark GT, Merrill RL: Diagnosis and nonsurgical treatment of internal derangements. In Sarnat BG. Laskin DM, editors: *The Temporomandibular joint: a biological basis for clinical practice.* ed., 4 Philadelphia, 1992, W.B. Saunders Co.
9. Dworkin SF, LeResche L, Von Korff MR: Diagnostic studies of temporomandibular disorders: challenges from an epidemiologic perspective. Anesth Prog 37:147-54, 1990.
10. Gundlach KK: Long-term results following surgical treatment of internal derangement of the temporomandibular joint J. Craniomaxillofac Surg 18:206-209, 1990. (Review.)
11. Heffez L.B. Arthroscopy broadens TMJ treatments. J. Am Dent Associates, 123:107-108; 111-112, 1992. (Review.)
12. Holmlund A., Hellsing G., Axelsson S: The temporomandibular joint; a comparison of clinical and arthroscopic findings. J. Prosthet Dent 61:61-5, 1989.
13. Kirk WS, Jr: Magnetic resonance imaging and tomographic evaluation of occlusal appliance treatment for advanced internal derangement of the temporomandibular joint. J. Oral Maxillofac Surg, 49:9-12, 1991.
14. Laskin DM, Greene CS: Diagnostic methods for temporomandibular disorders: what we have learned in two decades. Anesth Prog 37:66-71, 1990. (Review.)
15. McCain JP, Podrasky, AE, Zabiegalski NA: Arthroscopic disc repositioning and suturing: a preliminary report. J. Oral Maxillofac Surg 50:568-579, 1992.
16. McCain JP, Sanders B, Koslin MG, et al: Temporomandibular joint arthroscopy: a 6-year multicenter retrospective study of 4,831 joints.

J. Oral Maxillofac Surg 50:926-30, 1992. (Published erratum appears in J. Oral Maxillofac Surg: 50:1349, 1992.)
17. Mohl ND: Reliability and validity of diagnostic modalities for temporomandibular disorders. Adv Dent Res, 7:113-9, 1993. (Review.)
18. Murakami K, Clark GT: Diagnosis of intracapsular pathology associated with temporomandibular joint disorders. Adv Dent Res, 7:113-9, 1993. (Review.)
19. Nitzan DW, Dolwick MF, Martinez GA: Temporomandibular joint arthrocentesis: a simplified treatment for severe, limited mouth opening. J. Oral Maxillofac Surg 49:1163-1167, 1991.
20. Sanders B., Murakami K., Clark GT: *Diagnostic surgical arthroscopy of the temporomandibular joint*. Philadelphia, 1989, WB Saunders Co.
21. Talley RL, Murphy GJ, Smith SD, et al: Standards for the history, examination, diagnosis, and treatment of temporomandibular disorders (TMD): a position paper. Cranio. 8:60-77, 1990. (Review.)
22. Westesson PL: Reliability and validity of imaging diagnosis of temporomandibular joint disorder. Adv Dent Rse 7:137-51, 1993. (Review.)
23. Wilkinson TM: Equilibration and restorative dentistry. In McNeill C, editor: *Current controversies in temporomandibular disorders*. Chicago, 1992, Quintessence Publishing Co., Inc.
24. Wink CS, St. Onge M., Zimny ML: Neural elements in the human temporomandibular articular disc. J Oral Maxillofac Surg 50:334-337, 1992.

SELECTED TMJ BIBLIOGRAPHY AND ADDITIONAL READINGS

Myofacial pain and dysfunction: the trigger manual
Travell and Simons
Williams and Wilkins, 1983.

Temporomandibular disorders: classification, diagnosis, and management, edition 3
Bell
Yearbook Medical Publishers, Inc.

Orofacial pains Classification, Diagnosis, Management, ed 4
Bell
Yearbook Medical Publishes, Inc.

TMJ internal derangement and arthrosis: surgical Atlas
Dolwick and Saunders
Mosby, 1985.

Diagnostic and surgical arthroscopy of the temporomandibular joint
Sanders, Murakami, and Clark
W.B. Saunders, 1989.

Management of facial, head, and neck pain
Cooper and Lucente
W.B. Saunders, 1989.

Wolff's headache and other head pain
Wolff
Oxford Press, 1980.

10

Reading Between the Lines in Medical Journals

Richard M. Rosenfeld, M.D., M.P.H.

This chapter will help make you an informed consumer of medical journals. If you read, write, or review articles, you will benefit from learning how to read between the lines. But shouldn't that mystical process called "peer review" assure you of high quality in published articles? Unfortunately manuscript assessment, like even the most sophisticated diagnostic tests, has a certain sensitivity and specificity[12]; reviewers may be biased, unqualified, or possess widely discrepant opinions about a study. Even when the research is sound, the author's conclusions may not be supported by data or generalizable to your particular situation. The bottom line? Caveat lector; beware of what you read even in excellent journals!

A first-rate journal article is hard to refute. The authors state their focused problem of study, present evidence, assess its validity, and form persuasive conclusions after considering supportive and conflicting evidence. But not all articles are first rate. You can, however, spot the clinkers by knowing ahead of time what constitutes a great article and then methodically checking for flaws, distortions, and omissions. An expert clinician considers something abnormal until they examine it and prove otherwise; reading between the lines means treating a journal article the same way.

When learning to read between the lines, two feared disciplines become unavoidable: epidemiology and statistics. Epidemiology deals with the patterns of disease and the factors that influence these patterns.[16] If you thought you left it behind in medical school, think again; epidemiology permeates nearly every aspect of medicine. Statistics is the art and science of collecting, summarizing, and analyzing data that are subject to random variation.[13] Because *all* research data and clinical observations are subject to random variation, statistics must be used to separate chance occurrences from true associations.

FIVE TYPES OF JOURNAL ARTICLES

The first step in reading between the lines is to determine the type of study with which you are dealing. The classification that follows lists publication types in order of increasing ability to establish causal associations. Key features pertinent to study design are summarized in Table 10-1.

Review articles

Review articles attempt to identify general trends unlikely to emerge in any single study, by synthesizing previous research through qualitative (narrative) and quantitative (numerical) techniques. The underlying philosophy is that science is a cumulative process, and that a single study, no matter how elegant or well-designed, is rarely decisive.

Narrative reviews emphasize qualitative techniques. Because they are often subjective and unsystematic, narrative reviews have been criticized as being an inefficient and scientifically unsound way of extracting useful information from a large body of evidence.[15]

Meta-analyses emphasize quantitative techniques. They permit systematic, organized, and structured evaluation of a problem of interest, using statistical tables or other data from a number of independent studies. Meta-analyses are frequently used to pool results from a number of small randomized trials, none in itself large enough to demonstrate statistically significant differences, but in aggregate capable of so doing. In contrast to the traditional subjective literature review, meta-analyses use a hypothesis-driven protocol to synthesize objectively selected studies of known quality and combinability.

Case reports

Case reports are case history studies. Though no longer as popular as in earlier years, the "case report with review of the literature" still merits publication if it describes[11]:

TABLE 10-1
Types of journal articles

Study design	What it can do	What it cannot do	What to beware of
Case report	Share experience; generate hypotheses	Test hypotheses	Don't blink; you may never see the case again
Retrospective	Study rare events; assess safety, feasibility, and prevalence	Test hypotheses, unless a control group is present	Difficulties in choosing controls; data not initially collected for research
Prospective	Study multiple outcomes; assess safety, feasibility, and incidence	Test hypotheses, unless a control group is present	Dropouts and limited follow-up of participants
Randomized clinical trial	Determine efficacy; control selection bias and unknown confounders	Determine effectiveness under real world circumstances	Overly restrictive entry criteria; definitions of disease and outcomes
Review article	Share expert opinion and narrative insights	Provide new data	Reviewer bias; selective exclusion of articles
Meta-analysis	Provide new integrative data; assess consistency and publication bias	Substitute for well-designed large scale studies	Lack of a priori protocol and hypothesis; mixing apples and oranges

- A previously undocumented syndrome or disease
- An unexpected association of two or more diseases or disorders that may represent a previously unsuspected causal relation
- A new and important variation from an expected pattern: the "outlier" case
- An unexpected event that suggests a therapeutic or adverse drug effect
- Good case reports are short, concise, focused, and unique.

Retrospective study

Retrospective studies begin *after* subjects have developed or have failed to develop the disease or outcome of interest.

Case series typically consist of a series of short case reports followed by generalizations drawn from the cases and a brief literature review. There is often a tabular presentation of data which includes the author's cases, treating them as if they had already been published. Although case series are generally descriptive, an analytic tone occasionally prevails. Specific hypotheses are posed, cases are defined precisely, comparison case data are sought, and data are tested statistically.

Cross-sectional studies are controlled studies that examine the relationship between diseases and other variables of interest as they exist in a defined population at one particular time. Examples are surveys, prevalence studies (diagnosis and staging), and evaluations of diagnostic tests.

Case control studies are controlled studies that examine the relationship between *current* presence or absence of disease and *prior* exposures or conditions. They provide stronger evidence for causality than cross-sectional studies. Unlike analytic case series, which are primarily descriptive, case control studies seek to explain phenomena by evaluating previous events.

Prospective study

Prospective studies begin *before* subjects have developed or have failed to develop the disease or outcome of interest.

Cohort studies identify subsets of a defined population who are, have been, or in the future may be exposed or not exposed to some factor of interest (e.g., a surgical procedure) and then observe the population sufficiently long to determine outcome. Cohort studies are also called concurrent, incidence, longitudinal, and natural history studies.

Historic cohort studies use existing records about the health or other relevant aspects of a population as it was at some time in the past and determine the current status of members of this population with respect to the condition of interest. Unlike case series, which contain only cases, a historic cohort study contains controls or a group of unexposed subjects.

Randomized clinical trial (RCT)

Also called a randomized controlled trial, this is an *experimental* study in which each subject has a known probability of being assigned to a treatment or control group. In contrast, retrospective and prospective studies are *observational;* the probability of ultimate assignment is unknown. Randomization provides two critical advantages. First, selection bias is eliminated in deciding whether a particular subject will enter the control or treatment group. Second, known and unknown factors which may influence the outcome of interest are balanced among groups, thereby reduc-

TABLE 10-2
Flaws in study design

The flaw	What it is	What it implies
Hypothetical hypotheses	Investigators do not pose a clear, a priori hypothesis	Results of statistical tests may be invalid
Schizophrenic study type	Limitations of study type (Table 10-1) are ignored	Conclusions are unsupported by data
Sampling by prestidigitation	Study sample magically appears without mention of sampling scheme (Table 10- 3)	Results may not be applicable outside the study
Clandestine controls	Statements are made about causality, associations, or efficacy without control groups	Inferences are unsupported by data
Confounded outcomes	Authors fail to consider all possible explanations for study results	Bias, chance, or confounding may be responsible for the observed results

ing their ability to distort the treatment effect of interest. RCTs are considered the most scientifically rigorous method of hypothesis testing available in epidemiology.

Study design in otolaryngology

Nearly 80% of articles published in otolaryngology journals are clinical research.[21] The distribution of study types in 1989 was 2.5% review articles (no meta-analyses), 57% case report or case series, 20% cross-sectional studies, 10% case control studies, 4% prospective studies, and 6.5% RCTs. Over the past two decades, the quantity and quality of clinical research in otolaryngology journals have steadily increased. In general, reviews and case series are decreasing, analytic studies are increasing, and meta-analyses and outcomes research are gaining in popularity.

FIVE FLAWS IN STUDY DESIGN

Although study type generally correlates with credibility, a well-designed case series can be more meaningful than a poorly designed RCT. The arch enemy of credibility is *bias:* any trend in the collection, analysis, interpretation, publication, or review of data leading to conclusions that systematically differ from the truth. Because a common technique for dealing with bias is to ignore it, you have to read between the lines. Suspect bias if you encounter any of the five flaws in study design described below and summarized in Table 10-2.

Hypothetical hypotheses

Every article should begin with a clear, concise, and plausible statement of purpose. The purpose may be either descriptive (hypothesis-generating) or analytic (hypothesis-driven). Beware of studies that leave it to the reader to guess the purpose of the study, present more than a few hypotheses, or formulate hypotheses *after* collecting the data (post hoc) yet treat them the same as hypotheses formulated before the study (a priori).

Studies that use statistical tests (e.g., generate p values) must state their hypotheses. A hypothesis is any conjecture cast in a form that will allow it to be *tested* and *refuted.* The last two words are critical; they distinguish dogma from hypotheses. Hypotheses are often stated in the null, meaning that the results observed in a study, experiment, or test are no different from what might have occurred as a result of the operation of chance alone.

Depending on whether the hypothesis concerns any difference between groups, or a difference in a certain direction (for better or for worse), a two- or a one-tailed statistical test will be used. Why should you care what type is used? Because it's easier to produce small p values with a one-tailed test; about half as many subjects are required to achieve statistical significance. However, results are invalid if the researchers began with a two-tailed hypothesis and switched to a one-tailed hypothesis after examining the data.

Schizophrenic study type

This occurs when an author selects a particular study type (as defined above) but ignores the consequences and limitations which necessarily follow. Here are the most common types.

Schizophrenic review articles think they are prospective studies. A single-authored review, lacking specific criteria for article selection and quality assessment, is a prime candidate for "garbage in, gospel out." Meta-analysis overcomes this problem to some extent but is still limited by the quality and combinability of papers studied. A good review or meta-analysis is a necessary bridge between past and future research but can never substitute for a large, well-designed, prospective study.

Schizophrenic case reports think they are case series or review articles. Based on one or two cases, sweeping conclusions are presented about the population at large, and practitioners are urged to awaken each morning with a "high index of suspicion" for the disorder in question. The salient case features are then buried in a "review of the world literature" followed by a long reference list. Because these reviews are generally unsystematic and poorly documented, biased conclusions may arise.

TABLE 10-3
Methods for sampling a population

The method	How it is performed	Comments
Brute force sample	Includes all units of study (charts, patients, laboratory animals, or journal articles) accessible to the researchers	Time consuming and unsophisticated; bias prone because missing units are seldom randomly distributed
Convenience (grab) sample	Units are selected on the basis of accessibility, convenience, or subjective judgments about eligibility	Assume this method when none is specified; study results cannot be generalized because of selection bias
Consecutive sample	Every unit is included over a specified time interval or until a specified number is reached	Excellent method when intake period is long enough to adequately represent seasonal and other temporal factors
Systematic sample	Units are selected using some simple systematic rule, such as first letter of last name, date of birth, or day of week	Less biased than a grab sample, but problems may still occur because of unequal selection probabilities
Random sample	Units are assigned numbers then selected at random until a desired sample size is attained	Best method; bias is minimized because all units have a known (and equal) probability of selection

Schizophrenic retrospective studies are most often case series (often surgical) that discuss treatment efficacy without mentioning either natural history or the placebo effect. Many acute and chronic problems resolve on their own, an effect which is difficult to estimate without a concurrent untreated control group. Further, patients with chronic conditions typically have fluctuating symptoms and seek medical care (and enroll in research studies) when symptoms are at their worst. Thus, the next change is likely to be an improvement (independent of therapy), a phenomenon called regression to the mean.

Recent studies have shown that the *placebo effect* may account for on average 70% of good to excellent outcomes seen in medical and surgical case series.[20] This contrasts with initial reports in the 1950s suggesting a much lower impact of approximately 33%. Components of the placebo effect include physician attention, interest, and concern in a healing setting; patient and physician expectations of treatment effects; the reputation, expense, and impressiveness of the treatment; and characteristics of the setting that influence patients to report improvement.[25]

Schizophrenic prospective studies equate themselves with RCTs. However, only random assignment to study groups eliminates the numerous biases introduced by permitting subjects or investigators to decide which treatment (or lack of treatment) will be administered to any given participant. Outcomes research is a special form of prospective study in which special techniques are employed to adjust for variations in disease among participants.

Schizophrenic RCTs are victims of their own experimental design. By using rigid eligibility criteria, assuring compliance with treatment, and measuring disease and outcomes with sophisticated tools, the researchers create an environment very different from usual clinical conditions. The *efficacy* measured under ideal circumstances, however, often exceeds the *effectiveness* in a clinic, hospital, or private office. Therefore, beware when the conditions under which the RCT was performed differ dramatically from the conditions to which you intend to apply the results.

Sampling by prestidigitation

At the heart of every article lies a *sample* of patients, laboratory animals, medical records, or journal articles that the investigators selected for study from the larger *population* of all possible choices. A wondrous aspect of many studies is how the sample magically appears. This poses no problems provided any conclusions drawn are limited only to the sample studied; however, bias can run rampant when attempts are made to generalize results beyond the sample, unless the sample is representative of the intended population. Unfortunately, magical samples are rarely representative.

Every article (including reviews) should provide *eligibility criteria* —the specific temporal, geographic, and demographic characteristics required for inclusion in, or exclusion from, the study. The authors must then specify the *sampling frame* —where they looked to find subjects. How this frame was compiled—manual search of clinic charts, computerized medical records search, access of on-line databases for review articles—has important implications when generalizing results. Finally, the *sampling method* is defined. Researchers rarely study the entire sampling frame, but instead select a more manageable sample to examine in detail. Common sampling methods are listed in Table 10- 3.

Clandestine controls

There is nothing wrong with an uncontrolled study; however, once the authors attempt to assess causality or efficacy (see "Schizophrenic retrospective studies" above) credibility vanishes and clandestine controls appear—controls the authors wish they had but really do not. Also beware when controls are borrowed from other researchers or previously published work (historic controls); there is a much greater potential for bias with these *nonconcurrent* controls than for *concurrent* controls (parallel groups; crossover groups; paired organs). Control groups are relatively uncommon in otolaryngology journals, found in less than 20% of clinical research studies.[21]

Why are controls so important? If 80% of subjects with disease X possess gene Y should we get excited? Only if another group of subjects without disease X turns out to have a prevalence of gene Y that differs significantly from 80%. A similar phenomenon occurs in treatment studies because of the omnipresent placebo effect, underlying up to 70% of all medical interventions. Without a comparison group, it is impossible to distinguish placebo effects from treatment effects (absolute efficacy) or to determine the relative value of different interventions (comparative efficacy). Patient surveys are particularly prone to bias from clandestine controls. On any given survey of patient satisfaction, approximately 80% of respondents will report "satisfaction" or "willingness to undergo the intervention again," even for procedures of dubious benefit. Only with a comparison or control group do such skewed responses become interpretable.

Here is a final note on control groups. An *uncontrolled* prospective study can define natural history and prognosis but cannot determine risk factors or causation. A partial solution is to compare subjects in the cohort who eventually develop the outcome of interest with those who do not. This creates a "nested case control study" within the cohort study, which is equivalent to the classic case control study, except that the data have been collected in a planned fashion.

Confounded outcomes

Most studies record and analyze some outcome or endpoint of interest and then draw conclusions based on results. Conclusions are valid, however, only when the study has been conducted in such a fashion as to control for the effects of bias, chance, and confounding.[1]

Bias can be introduced during any stage of research: reading-up on the field, specifying and selecting the study sample, executing the study, measuring exposures and outcomes, and analyzing the data.[24] A few common types of bias to check for are:

- *Detection bias.* A systematic error in the ascertainment, diagnosis, or verification of cases in a case series or case control study.
- *Selection bias.* A systematic difference between a study sample and the larger population they are supposed to represent or from a second group of subjects with whom they are supposedly comparable. For example, volunteers are rarely representative of a target population (volunteer bias), and subjects drawn from hospitals or clinic registries tend to have distorted relationships between exposure and disease (Berkson bias).
- *Response bias.* A systematic error that results when subjects respond inaccurately—whether deliberately or unintentionally—to a questionnaire or interview.
- *Attention bias.* An apparent response to medical or surgical therapy which in fact was caused by the extra attention given to patients in a case series or in a specific treatment arm of a clinical trial. Attention bias is a component of the placebo effect.
- *Hawthorne effect.* The epidemiologic equivalent of the uncertainty principle in physics: the act of observing a phenomenon changes the phenomenon itself. Particularly troublesome in satisfaction surveys, where people may change behavior just because they know they are being studied.
- *Observer bias.* Observers may systematically err in measuring and recording observations so that they concur with prior expectations. Further inaccuracies may be introduced by interobserver and intraobserver variation.

Chance may explain an apparent trend in any uncontrolled study or in controlled studies that provide only descriptive analysis (e.g., omit p values). The difference between 60% and 80% successful outcomes in two groups may seem intuitively "significant," but may fall well within random error (chance variation) if each group contains a relatively small number of subjects. Investigators should present a *p value* to assist you in analyzing the potential impact of chance. Stating "$p < 0.05$" means there is less than a 5% probability that observed differences represent random error, suggesting the finding is truly nonfortuitous.

Confounding [from the Latin confundere, to mix together] refers to an apparent association between two variables when none really exists. It is caused by a confounding variable (e.g., age, sex, social class) that is associated with the outcome under study but itself has not been controlled for during analysis. A confounder must satisfy both of the following conditions: (1) it is associated with the disease or outcome of interest, and (2) it is associated with the intervention or exposure factor under study.

The time to address the issue of confounding is *before* the study starts, not during statistical analysis. For example, cure rates in a therapeutic trial for otitis media could be influenced by the age, sex, and race of the child; bottle feeding; passive smoke exposure; day care attendance; prior history of otitis media; recent antibiotic use; coexisting acute infections; underlying susceptibility (cleft palate, syndromes), etc. A thoughtful author measures these variables at the start of the study and considers them guilty as confounders until proven otherwise. Confounding is a particu-

TABLE 10-4
Popular statistical tests in otolaryngology journals

Hypothesis test	What it can do	What it cannot do
t-test	Compare the means of *two* groups of continuous data	Compare three or more groups; analyze sparse or skewed data
Analysis of variance (ANOVA)	Compare the means of *three or more* groups of continuous data	Analyze sparse or skewed data
Contingency table (chi-square)	Test for an association among two groups of categorical data	Analyze sparse data
Survival analysis	Estimate the time-related probability of an event; adjust for dropouts or censored data	Compensate for inadequate periods of follow-up
Multivariate analysis	Examine the simultaneous effect of multiple variables on an outcome of interest	Make valid predictions unless the fit of the model to the data is thoroughly assessed
Nonparametric analysis	Analyze small data sets without a normal distribution	Analyze very sparse data

lar problem in chart reviews because of variations in completeness. When reading a study, ask yourself: "What are the possible confounding variables?" Then seek them out. If the author does not satisfactorily address them, beware of the results.

Once identified, confounders can be controlled for in either the design phase or analysis phase of the study. Two design stage strategies are matching (typically in case control studies) and restriction (limiting participants to those with a comparable level of the potential confounder). In the analysis stage, stratified analysis and multivariate modeling are most commonly used to identify independent effects of variables.[4]

SIX POPULAR STATISTICAL TESTS IN OTOLARYNGOLOGY JOURNALS

The creatures below dwell in the Results section of a study; they have an uncanny ability to make the reader jump directly to the Discussion section to avoid looking them in the eye. However, the ultimate credibility of a well-crafted, unbiased study depends on the suitability and validity of the statistical analysis performed.

Despite the bewildering variety of statistical tests, there are many similarities.[23] They all test hypotheses, determine the probability that the null hypothesis is true (p value), and are valid *only* when fundamental assumptions about the data are satisfied. Therefore, authors must convince you that these assumptions (discussed below) have indeed been satisfied before expecting you to believe their results. Also, remember that even the most elegant statistics cannot substitute for faulty study design, cannot eliminate bias introduced during data collection, cannot assess causality, and cannot measure clinical significance.

Over the past 20 years, the prevalence of inferential statistics in otolaryngology journals has quadrupled[22]; approximately 30% of clinical research articles now contain at least one p value. Familiarity with only six statistical techniques, however, will provide access to over 90% of published articles. Salient features of the most popular tests in otolaryngology journals are listed below and summarized in Table 10-4.

t-tests

Description. These test whether the means of *two* independent or paired groups of continuous data differ significantly. T-tests are found in nearly 30% of analytic clinical research articles in otolaryngology journals.[22]

Interpretation. A significant p value implies a low probability that the mean values for the two groups are equal. Because valid results depend on relatively equal variances (standard deviation) within each group, a statistical test is required to verify this assumption (F test).

Precautions. t-Tests will produce an artificially low p value if the groups contain small samples with skewed data (not normally distributed) or unequal variance (F test is significant); instead, a nonparametric test (Mann-Whitney U or Wilcoxon signed-ranks) should be used. t-Tests should *never* be used to compare more than two groups; ANOVA is required.[8] When the outcome of interest is time related (e.g., cancer survival, duration of hospital stay, disease recurrence), survival analysis (see below) is more appropriate than a t-test.

Analysis of variance (ANOVA)

Description. ANOVA tests whether the means of *three or more* independent groups of continuous data differ significantly with regard to a single factor (one-way ANOVA) or two factors (two-way ANOVA). ANOVA is found in only 9% of analytic clinical research articles in otolaryngology journals[22] but is more common in basic research.

Interpretation. A significant p value implies a low probability that the mean values for all groups are equal. From a statistical standpoint, we say that the variance *between* groups is larger than the variance *within* each group.

Because valid results depend on relatively equal variances within each group, a statistical test is required to verify this assumption (F test). Note that ANOVA provides no information on whether *individual* pairs of groups differ significantly; it tests only for an overall global difference. For example, when comparing four groups of data (A, B, C, and D), the finding "p <0.05, ANOVA" means there is less than a 5% chance that the statement "A = B = C = D" is true; however, it says nothing about whether A ≠ B or C ≠ D or D ≠ A, etc. Once the investigators demonstrate a significant global difference, they can use *multiple comparison* procedures (Bonferroni, Tukey, Newman-Keuls, Scheffe, Dunnett) for individual group comparisons.

Precautions. ANOVA will produce an artificially low p value if the groups contain small samples with skewed data or unequal variance; instead, a nonparametric test (Kruskal-Wallis) should be used. Multiple pairwise t-tests cannot substitute for ANOVA; the effect is to greatly increase the odds of a false positive result (type I statistical error).

Contingency tables

Description. These test for an association between two dichotomous variables (data which can take on only one of two values, such as male vs. female) or categorical variables (data can take on only one of three or more values, such as tumor stage) by using the chi-square statistic. A modification, called the McNemar test, can be used for two groups of paired data. Contingency tables are found in 20% of analytic clinical research articles in otolaryngology journals.[22]

Interpretation. The chi-square test works by comparing the *observed* frequencies for each row-column combination (cell) in the contingency table with the *expected* frequencies assuming rows and columns are unassociated. A significant p value implies a probable association between rows and columns.

Precautions. As with t-tests and ANOVA, small samples can produce an artificially small p value. If the *expected* frequency for any single cell is less than 2, or if more than half the expected frequencies for all cells are less than 5, an exact test must be used (e.g., Fisher's exact test). Beware of authors who overinterpret a "significant" chi-square result. As with ANOVA, when p <0.05 we claim a *global* association between variables; we cannot specify which particular subgroups of rows and columns are or are not associated.

Survival analysis

Description. Survival analysis estimates the probability of an event (typically, but not necessarily, survival) based on the total period of observation and tests for associations with other variables of interest. Survival analysis permits maximum use of data from *censored* observations, which occur when a subject is lost to follow-up or if the study ends before the outcome of interest has occurred.

Interpretation. There are two main ways of analyzing survival data: the life table method divides the time into intervals and calculates survival at each interval; the Kaplan-Meier method calculates survival each time an event occurs. Both methods produce a graph (survival curve) showing the cumulative probability of the event vs. total period of observation. Authors sometimes eliminate the curve, and instead give event rates only for specific time periods (e.g. 1-year, 3-year, 10-year, etc). When two or more survival curves are compared, and the p value is low, a probable association exists between time to event and the factor used to stratify the curves.

Precautions. When you see a "survival cure," be sure that it has been calculated using survival analysis (life table or Kaplan-Meier), *not* by simply dividing cumulative events at a given time by the total subjects still around at that time. The latter method mistreats censored observations, yielding artificially low estimates. Nor is it desirable to simply exclude from analysis all subjects not meeting some arbitrary cut-off for observation time; resulting rates may be artificially high. When sample size is small the life table method can be biased, and Kaplan-Meier analysis is more suitable.

Multivariate procedures

Description. These procedures examine the *simultaneous* effect of multiple variables (generally three or more) on an outcome of interest. In contrast, t-tests, one-way ANOVA, chi-square, and survival analysis examine the *univariate* effect of variables on an outcome one at a time. Different multivariate procedures are used depending on the type of outcome studied. A continuous outcome is studied with multiple regression, a dichotomous outcome with logistic regression, a categorical outcome with discriminant analysis, and a censored outcome (survival) with Cox regression.

Interpretation. Multivariate analysis produces a statistical model which predicts outcomes based on combinations of individual variables. p Values are presented for both the model as a whole and for the *coefficients* of each variable in the model. The magnitude of the coefficient represents the relative effect of a particular variable on outcome when controlled for all the other variables in the model. A positive coefficient implies a positive association; a negative coefficient implies a negative association.

Precautions. Biased results may occur if the variables in the model are highly correlated with each other. Although a model may precisely fit the investigator's data, there is no guarantee that it will predict outcomes for subjects outside the study with equal precision. As with any statistical test, the result is garbage in—garbage out. No degree of multivariate analysis can adjust for confounding variables that were not recorded at the start of the study.

TABLE 10-5
Statistical deceptions used in journal articles

The deception	The problem	The solution
Standard error is used to describe the range of data	Range is artificially low, making data look better than they are	Always use standard deviation when summarizing data
Small sample study results are taken at face value	Results are imprecise and would likely vary if study were repeated	Determine the range of results consistent with data by using a 95% confidence interval
Extremely small p values are elevated to a god-like status	Trivial differences may be statistically significant if a large enough sample is used	Always examine the size of the clinical effect, not just its statistical significance
Some results are "significant" but there are too many p values to count in a single lifetime	"Significant" results may be false positives because each p value has a 5% error rate*	Reduce the number of p values through multivariate analysis or analysis of variance
Subgroups are compared until statistically significant results are found	If you torture the data sufficiently, they will eventually confess to something	Subgroup comparisons are valid only when all groups as a whole are significantly different
No significant difference is found between groups in a small sample study	A significant difference may have been missed because of inadequate sample size	Be sure the authors discuss power and sample size before believing study results
Significant p values are crafted through improper use of hypothesis tests	Small studies with skewed data require special methods of analysis	Do not believe results unless a nonparametric or exact statistical test was used

*Assuming that 0.05 is selected as the level of statistical significance.

Nonparametric tests

Description. Nonparametric tests test hypotheses *without* requiring that the data have a normal distribution. The nonparametric equivalents of the t-test, paired t-test, and one-way ANOVA are the Mann-Whitney U, Wilcoxon signed-ranks, and Kruskal-Wallis tests, respectively.

Interpretation. When an author uses a *parametric* test (e.g., t-test or ANOVA), the data must be either normally distributed or come from a large enough sample (about 30 or more subjects) that this assumption may be relaxed. Nonparametric tests avoid this requirement by ranking the data in each group and then comparing rank sums instead of the actual values of individual observations. Whereas the parametric tests discussed above make inferences about *means*, nonparametric tests make inferences about *medians*.

Precautions. Very sparse data sets are suitable neither for parametric nor nonparametric analysis; more sophisticated *exact* significance tests must be used. Fisher's exact test is a well-known exact procedure for 2 × 2 contingency tables. Exact tests for other situations require special computer software.[17]

SEVEN WAYS TO DECEIVE WITH STATISTICS

Over a century ago, Benjamin Disraeli noted: "There are three kinds of lies: lies, damn lies and statistics." Although such consummate skepticism is rarely justified, statistics can undoubtedly be misused—either by intent or through ignorance or carelessness—to produce incorrect conclusions. Because most physicians are either amateur statisticians or have no recollection of statistics beyond bad memories in medical school, misuse in the literature is common. Reviews of clinical research indicate that about 50% of published articles contain statistical flaws serious enough to question the validity of the conclusions (Table 10-5).

How does statistical misuse slip by editors, peer reviewers, and journal readers? This happens because of the "dazzle" phenomenon observed by Darrell Huff, author of *How to Lie with Statistics:* "If you cannot prove what you want to prove, demonstrate something else and pretend that they are the same thing. In the daze that follows the collision of statistics with the human mind, hardly anybody will notice the difference."[9] Be particularly wary of the following dazzling phenomena:

Standard error switcheroo

When you see results reported as "X ± Y" don't assume that Y is the standard deviation (SD) unless specifically stated. Sometimes Y is actually the standard error (SE), a number which is *always* smaller than the SD. Actually, SD and SE are very different; so understanding why many authors report the latter is difficult, unless they are enamored by the smaller value. When describing a set of data, SD is always preferred[2]; it summarizes how widely dispersed the observations are about the mean value. If the data are symmetric (normally distributed), the mean ± 2 SD will encompass about 95% of observations. If the SD is actually larger than the mean, the data is skewed and would be better described by the range or by percentiles. In contrast, the

SE is an inferential, not a descriptive, statistic; it permits inferences to be made about some population of interest based on data derived from a smaller sample.

Consider a study of 25 children undergoing tonsillectomy that reports a mean blood loss of 150 ± 30 cc where 30 is the SD. We now know that 95% of subjects had a blood loss of 150 ± 60 cc (assuming the data are normally distributed). To obtain the SE, we divide the SD by the square root of the sample size. In this example the square root is five, giving an SE five times smaller than the SD. The mean blood loss now is written as 150 ± 6 cc, where 6 is the SE. Obviously this looks "better" than the SD, but what exactly does this mean? It means "based on our results, if we extrapolate to the population of children outside our study undergoing tonsillectomy, we estimate with 95% confidence that the mean blood loss will be 150 ± 12 cc." This statement no longer describes the study data but makes an inference about some hypothetical population. Unless the authors clearly state that this is their intent, the SD should have been used.

Small sample whitewash

Because medical research is costly and time consuming, we rarely have the luxury of studying large samples. Fortunately, we can derive meaningful conclusions from small samples through the magic of statistics. Remember—statistics is the art and science of dealing with uncertain data; the smaller the sample, the greater the uncertainty. Beware when the authors claim their sample is "too small for statistical analysis"; that's when they need it most.

We define uncertainty in research by specifying the *precision* of a result, most often with a 95% *confidence interval* (CI). The CI tells you the *range of results consistent with the data*. Repeat this last statement five times aloud; it is a critical concept. Whereas descriptive studies rarely need p values, they nearly always benefit from a CI.

For example, while perusing the *Journal of Low Budget Research* an article on an innovative new surgical procedure captures your attention. The authors successfully perform the procedure on 4/4 elephants (100% success rate) and conclude that "testing in humans is indicated based on these wonderful results." Do you agree? Intuitively you wonder if a study on only four animals is really "meaningful." Actually, it is the precision of the result that is in question. The range of results (95% CI) consistent with this single experiment on four elephants is actually between 47% to 100%[17]! Knowing that the "true" success rate may be as low as 47%, you may now disagree with the need for human testing. What is really needed is a larger animal study with increased precision. Had the investigators successfully operated on 40/40 elephants the 95% CI would be 93% to 100%. Clearly these results have different impact than the former.

Because most authors don't bother to estimate precision, you may need to calculate the 95% CI yourself. For large studies, simple formulae are available.[7] When the data are skimpy (less than 20 observations), a computer program is necessary for an exact calculation.[17]

p value prowess

When you have to take off your shoes to count the number of zeros following the decimal point of a p value, you know you've encountered a very, very, very important result! Wrong! p Values tell you one thing and one thing only: the probability that the null hypothesis is true. When we wish to compare cure rates achieved by two treatments, we initially pose a null hypothesis of no difference between them. A p value of 0.01 tells us there is only a 1% chance that the results are explainable by the null hypothesis, so we concoct some alternative way to explain the findings (usually that one treatment is more effective than the other). A p value of 0.0000001 reduces the credibility of the null hypothesis to only 0.00001% but tells us nothing about the *clinical significance* of the findings.

A critical limitation of p values is that they offer no information on the *magnitude* or clinical significance. A treatment that is 5% better than a control ($p = 0.0000001$) would be less meaningful from a clinical standpoint than one that is 20% more effective but has a larger p value ($p = 0.01$). Therefore, look not at the p value alone but at the magnitude of the clinical effect observed.[14] Magnitude is commonly presented in relative terms (odds ratio, relative risk ratio) or absolute terms (rate difference, difference between groups); a 95% CI aids in interpretation.

Multiple p value phenomenon

p Values have a momentum of their own; once you start churning them out, it's hard to stop (especially if you have a nifty computer program that churns them out for you . . .). When you see a Results section or a data table chock full of p values, realize that some "significant" p values ($p < 0.05$) are likely to occur by chance alone.[3] If a researcher performs 20 individual hypothesis tests (e.g., calculates 20 p values) and we assume that the subjects studied do not differ beyond random variation, there is only a 36% chance that *none* of the p values will be significant! Further, the chance of getting 1, 2, or 3, significant p values is 38%, 19%, and 6%, respectively.

What accounts for the multiple p value phenomenon? The problem arises because each individual hypothesis test is based on a cut-off of $p < 0.05$ as a measure of significance; the effect of performing multiple tests is to inflate this 5% error level for the study as a whole. The probability of getting at least one spurious result is: $1\text{-}(1\text{-alpha})^n$, where alpha is the level of significance for each individual test (generally 0.05) and n is number of tests performed. Multiple p values are eliminated by multivariate analysis (see above). ANOVA is a special way of controlling for multiple p values when three or more groups of continuous data are compared.

Selective analysis of results

Check for this in every study that compares three or more groups of subjects, including animal research. Authors may pluck out a few groups for pairwise comparisons and then pontificate on the "statistically significant" findings they discover. Unfortunately, this violates a basic tenet of statistics—you *cannot* compare subgroups of your data *unless* you first check for statistically significant differences between *all* groups considered simultaneously. For categorical data, a chi-square is first calculated for the entire contingency table; if $P < 0.05$, the authors can then extract subsets of the table for selective analysis *provided* they adjust for multiple comparisons. For continuous data, ANOVA should be used (not multiple pairwise t-tests) as described previously.

Powerless equalities

Some authors would like to convince you that a new treatment or diagnostic test is *equivalent* to an established standard. In particular, support for the use of new antibiotics often arises from an RCT claiming "no significant difference ($p > 0.05$)" from another drug. When interpreting these results, look not at the p value but at the statistical *power;* the size of the p value is pertinent only when a statistically significant result is given. Power tells you the probability that the investigators would have detected a true difference, given that one really existed. With small samples, power is usually inadequate (<80%) to state confidently that the investigators didn't miss a real difference. Because very few articles calculate power you may need to calculate it yourself.[18] As with CI's, formulae are available to calculate power.[5,27]

Nonparametric nihilism

When sample sizes are modest—less than 30 observations per group—a nonparametric hypothesis test should be used *unless* the authors specifically examine the data and determine that it is normally distributed. However, despite the small and skewed samples common in clinical research, only 7% of articles from 1989 in otolaryngology journals contained nonparametric methods.[22] Using a garden variety t-test for small, skewed samples can produce deceptive results through artificially low p values. Even a single outlier (data that differs markedly from the rest of the values) can invalidate a parametric test result. In general, beware of conclusions drawn from small data sets analyzed with conventional parametric tests. Although nonparametric tests provide more meaningful results under these circumstances, very sparse data require more complicated exact techniques for analysis.[17]

FIVE CRITERIA FOR EVALUATING A STUDY

Scientific papers are built on the principles of *critical argument;* they must argue you into believing what they conclude.[11] Therefore, a credible paper must address the five criteria summarized in Table 10-6. The first two criteria are addressed in the article's Introduction, Methods, and Results sections and have been covered earlier in this chapter. The last three criteria are of particular importance, because they constitute the Discussion section to which many eager readers immediately turn their attention. Let us now focus on these three essential components of the Discussion.

TABLE 10-6
Five criteria for evaluating a study*

Criteria	Comment
1. Is the problem, question, or hypothesis adequately defined?	Meaningful results rarely occur by divine revelation; hypothesis generation must precede hypothesis testing.
2. Do the authors present clear and convincing evidence to support their conclusions?	This can occur only when a suitable study design is chosen (Table 10-1) and design flaws are avoided (Table 10-2).
3. Is the evidence valid?	The evidence is valid for the author's patients (internal validity) when statistical analysis is appropriate (Tables 10-4 and 10-5); it is valid for *your* patients (external validity) if sampling method is appropriate (Table 10-3).
4. Are you convinced of the author's conclusions after considering the evidence?	An initial answer or judgment on the validity of the hypothesis is based on study findings and supporting published studies.
5. Do you remain convinced of the author's conclusions after considering any counterevidence?	Final conclusions are made after considering limitations of study type, flaws in design, alternative explanations for associations, and conflicting published studies.

*A great study should have "yes" answers to all five questions.

Validity of the evidence

Validity is not an accident. It arises from attention to study design; avoidance of common flaws; sound sampling and subject selection; proper statistical analysis; and measures to control chance, bias, and confounding. In the Discussion section, authors should convince you of their study's internal and external validity.[10]

Internal validity is the degree to which the investigator's conclusions correctly describe what actually happened in the study. When the research has been conducted and analyzed in a sound fashion, we infer that the findings reported are credible, at least for the study sample.

External validity is the degree to which the investigator's conclusions are appropriate when applied to the universe outside the study. This universe has two components: (1) the accessible population from which the researchers obtained their sample, and (2) the target population about which they are ultimately interested. From the reader's point of view, the key question is "Can I apply the results of this study to the patients I see in my practice?" For the answer to be "yes," the sampling method must be sound and the demographic and disease characteristics must be comparable to the target population.

Implications of the evidence

Credible implications are *always* dependent on criterion no. 3 in Table 10-6: "Is the evidence valid?" They also depend on achieving a sense of perspective with the previously published body of similar literature. Indeed from a reviewer's standpoint, a new study, no matter how elegant or thought provoking, is only a single addition to the accumulated body of existing knowledge.[15] Particularly in the case of RCTs, there may already be a large number of previously published investigations (e.g., for acute otitis media there are over 200 RCTs). Unfortunately, many authors view their results as "the bottom line," warranting more attention and meaning than prior efforts. Do not take the author's assessment of "Implications of the Evidence" at face value unless a dedicated attempt has been made to compare, contrast, and reconcile the findings with prior literature.

Implications of the counterevidence

Once an author commits to a specific type of study, they are subject to certain inherent limitations. Beware of articles that fail to acknowledge the following potential problems:

- *Retrospective studies* are limited by the availability and completeness of the records from which subjects were identified, the accuracy of information in the records (remember, it was originally recorded for clinical care not for research), and the nonuniform lengths of follow-up of individual subjects. Case series without control groups cannot draw credible conclusions about treatment efficacy or causal associations.
- *Prospective studies* are limited by difficulties involved in maintaining follow-up of all participants; survival analysis should be used to control for censored subjects. If the study was conducted using volunteers, the findings may not be generalizable.
- *Randomized clinical trials* generally employ strict eligibility criteria and may not be applicable to less stringent situations. The efficacy demonstrated may exceed effectiveness in a general clinical setting where diagnostic certainty is lower, patient compliance may vary, and other uncontrolled factors impact on outcome. Further, the treatment end points used in the study may differ from those considered important by you and your patients.
- *Reviews and Meta-Analyses* are by definition retrospective research and are therefore subject to limitations in completeness, availability, and accuracy of source articles.

In the Discussion section the authors should acknowledge any potential flaws in study design (see Table 10-2). Pay particular attention to alternative explanations for associations (bias, chance, confounding, and the placebo effect) as described previously under "Confounded Outcomes." Finally, look for a comparison of conflicting studies with the present work and the impact of this evidence on the author's conclusions.

Special considerations for reviews and case reports

All scientific papers—including case reports and review articles and case reports—should present a critical argument as outlined above. In addition, the following considerations apply:

Case reports. Because these are often a budding academicians "first stab" at getting into print, be particularly wary of their content. A good case report contains these essential elements: [11]

1. A statement of why the case is worth reading about
2. An account of the case, with all relevant data
3. Discussion of evidence that the case is unique or unexpected
4. Possible alternative explanations for case features
5. Conclusion, with implications

Don't waste your time reading so-called "minor" case reports. Avoid the following varieties, unlikely to get published in first-rank journals:[11]

- The everyone-should-remember case
- The grand-rounds case
- The I-am-a-clever-chap case
- The variations-on-a-well-known-theme case
- The goodness!-book-of-medical-world-records case

Reviews or meta-analyses. Both should contain[19]:

1. A precise statement of hypothesis or purpose
2. Documentation of the literature search
3. Inclusion and exclusion criteria for articles discussed
4. Consideration of *publication bias,* a tendency for editors and authors to preferentially publish research with "significant" findings[6]

5. Narrative conclusions and recommendations
6. Unresolved issues and problems needing further study

Meta-analyses and quantitative reviews should also possess[26]:

1. Specific definitions of outcomes or treatment end points
2. Details of methods for combining studies and pooling data
3. A test for combinability (homogeneity) of studies pooled
4. Exploratory analysis for associations between outcomes and research design, treatment subgroups, or demographic factors
5. A sensitivity analysis to test the stability of results when analyzed using alternative methods

SUMMING UP

In this chapter I have emphasized a methodical approach to reading journal articles which incorporates fundamental concepts of statistics and epidemiology. Whereas a thorough application of the criteria in Table 10-6 to *every* article you read might lead to full-blown clinical depression, I do urge you to read between the lines of selected "important" articles. What constitutes an "important" article? Important articles are those that are newsworthy or contain results you are contemplating for use in your own research or clinical care. In addition, any manuscript or grant application you encounter as a peer reviewer should be read between the lines. Hopefully the information herein will help make the reading process a little more enjoyable.

REFERENCES

Abramson JH: *Making Sense of Data: A Self-Instructional Manual on the Interpretation of Epidemiologic Data.* New York, 1988, Oxford University Press.

Brown GW: Standard deviation, standard error: which 'standard' should we use? *AJDC* 136:937-41, 1982.

Brown GW: P values. *AJDC 144:493-5, 1990.*

Datta M: You cannot exclude the explanation you have not considered. *Lancet* 342:345-347, 1993.

Dawson-Saunders B, Trapp RG: *Basic and Clinical Biostatistics,* ed 2, Norwalk, Connecticut, 1994, Appleton & Lange.

Easterbrook PJ, Berlin JA, Gopalan R, et al: Publication bias in clinical research. *Lancet* 337:867-72, 1991.

Gardner MJ, Altman DG: Confidence intervals rather than p values: estimation rather than hypothesis testing. *Br Med J* 292:746-750, 1980.

Godfrey K: Comparing the means of several groups. *N Engl J Med* 313:1450-1456, 1985.

Huff D: *How to Lie with Statistics.* New York, 1954, WW Norton and Company.

Hulley SB, Cummings SR: *Designing Clinical Research: An Epidemiologic Approach.* Baltimore, 1988, Williams & Wilkins.

Huth EJ: *How to Write and Publish Papers in the Medical Sciences,* ed 2, Baltimore, 1990, Williams & Wilkins.

Kassirer JP, Campion EW: Peer review: crude and understudied, but indispensable. *JAMA* 272:96-97, 1994.

Last JM: *A Dictionary of Epidemiology.* ed 2, New York, 1988, Oxford University Press.

Laupacis A, Sackett DL, Roberts RS: An assessment of clinically useful measures of the consequences of treatment, *N Engl J Med* 318:1728-1733, 1988.

Light RJ, Pillemer DB: *Summing Up: The Science of Reviewing Research,* Cambridge, 1984, Harvard University Press.

Lilienfeld AM, Lilienfeld DE: *Foundations of Epidemiology.* ed 2, New York, 1980, Oxford University Press.

Mehta C, Patel N: *StatXact: Statistical Software for Exact Nonparametric Inference.* Cambridge, 1991, Cytel Software Corporation.

Moher D, Dulberg CS, Wells GA: Statistical power, sample size, and their reporting in randomized controlled trials. *JAMA* 272:122-124, 1994.

Neely JG: Literature review articles as a research form. *Otolaryngol Head Neck Surg* 108:743-748, 1993.

Roberts AH, Kewman DG, Mercier L, et al: The power of nonspecific effects in healing: implications for psychosocial and biological treatments. *Clin Psychol Rev* 13:375-391, 1993.

Rosenfeld RM: Clinical research in otolaryngology journals. *Arch Otolaryngol Head Neck Surg* 117:164-170, 1991.

Rosenfeld RM, Rockette HE: Biostatistics in otolaryngology journals. *Arch Otolaryngol Head Neck Surg* 117:1172-1176, 1991.

Rosenfeld RM: Taming the statistical shrew. In Johnson JT, Derkay CS, Mandell-Brown MK, Newman RK, editors: *Instructional Courses Volume 6.* St. Louis, 1993, Mosby–Year Book.

Sackett DL: Bias in analytic research. *J Chron Dis* 32:51-63, 1979.

Turner JA, Deyo RA, Loeser JD, et al: The importance of placebo effects in pain treatment and research. *JAMA* 271:1609-1614, 1994.

Wilson A, Henry DA: Assessing the quality of published meta-analyses. *Med J Austr* 156:173-187, 1992.

Young MJ, Bresnitz EA, Strom BL: Sample size nomograms for interpreting negative clinical studies. *Ann Int Med* 99:248-251, 1983.

11

Diagnosis, Testing, and Treatment of Olfactory Disorders

Michael H. Stevens, M.D.

Although the sense of smell in man is less crucial to survival than that in animals, the result may be equally catastrophic if one is unable to detect a gas leak or smoke from a fire. Olfactory dysfunction can also be a real disability by reducing the overall quality of life, not only because of the inability to detect pleasant odors but also because of the important enhancement that olfaction gives to the sense of taste.

It has been estimated that two million American adults suffer from disorders of taste and smell.[20] Since few physicians understand much about the evaluation and treatment of these disorders, a great deal of unnecessary impairment is present. Although a disability rating of 5% for total anosmia is suggested in the *1993 American Medical Association (AMA) Guides to the Evaluation of Permanent Impairment*,[1] this is certainly inadequate for those persons whose livelihoods depend on this sense, such as cooks, perfumers, and wine tasters.

A basic understanding of the anatomy and physiology is necessary for the clinician to understand some of the difficulties with diagnostic testing. The olfactory membrane occupies a position high in the nasal cavity on the superior aspect of the nasal septum and over the superior nasal turbinates. It occupies approximately 1 to 3 cc in area. Because of its location, it is out of the mainstream of airflow in normal, quiet breathing. A sniff, therefore, produces laminar flow of the incoming odor toward the olfactory recess. Since 30% to 50% of airway resistance in the respiratory tract is contributed by the nose, some of the incoming air may not reach the olfactory membrane because of turbinate hypertrophy from the nasal cycle. Odors must reach the olfactory membrane for them to be detected.

Histologically, the olfactory membrane is composed of bipolar neurons, which are the functional component of the system. It is also composed of sustentacular cells, basilar cells, and Bowman's glands. The bipolar neurons have 6 to 8 short processes known as the "olfactory rods." These rods extend to the surface as the olfactory vesicle. The vesicle has cilia which parallel the surface and are bathed in a blanket of mucous 20 to 50μ thick. The cilia are immotile, even though they have a normal relationship in the axoneme, since the dynein arms that are usually seen in motile cilia are absent.

The mucous that bathes the cilia is thought to come from Bowman's glands, since they are composed of an abundant amount of smooth endoplasmic reticulum. These are serous and located in the submucosa. This mucous may also come from the supporting cells and it gives the membrane a yellow-brown color grossly because of the pigment which is present. This pigment is a phospholipid and is speculated to play a role in the contact or adsorption of odors on the membrane's surface. The exact mechanism of action, however, is unknown.

Each bipolar neuron consists of peripheral receptors of first-order ganglion cells which project centrally to form the olfactory nerves. There are about twenty olfactory nerves on each side which penetrate the cribriform plate. They are surrounded by dura. These synapse in the olfactory bulb with mitral cells which are the secondary neurons. Approximately 100 neurons may synapse with a single mitral cell. These synapses form spherical structures called glomeruli. The axons of these mitral cells form the lateral olfactory tract, located beneath the frontal lobe, which connects the bulb to many bilateral cortical centers. In the bulb are also located some small tufted cells which form the medial olfactory tract. One of the unique features of this system is that it can regenerate.[14] It is therefore different from other central nervous system neurons. This may be explained by its origin, which is felt not to be from the neural crest but to be epithelial.

The physiology of the olfactory system is also rather remarkable. A normally functioning individual can smell 9

after surgery and long-term topical steroids, but significant improvement occurred in only 50% of these patients. Jafek[22] has suggested improvement in olfaction following endoscopic sinus surgery, but no definitive study has yet been done. As such, it remains for future therapeutic modalities to be determined that can be helpful for patients with disabling disorders of olfaction.

REFERENCES

1. American Medical Association: *Guides to the Evaluation of Permanent Impairment,* ed 4, Chicago, 1993.
2. Amoore JE, Johnston JW, Rubin M: The Stereochemical Theory of Olfaction. *Scientific American* 210:42-49, 1964.
3. Bakey L: Olfactory Meningiomas. *JAMA* 251:53-55, 1984.
4. Brown HM, Storey G, Jackson FA: Beclomethasone Disproportionate Aerosol in Treatment of Perennial and Seasonal Rhinitis. *Br J Clin Pharmacol* 4:2838-2865, 1977.
5. Doty RL: Causes of Olfactory and Gustatory Disorders. In *Smell and Taste in Health and Disease.* Getchell TV, editor: New York, 1991, Raven Press.
6. Doty RL: A Review of Olfactory Dysfunctions In Man. *Am. J Otolaryngol* 1:57-78, 1979.
7. Doty RL: Shaman P, Kilman CP, et al: University of Pennsylvania Smell Identification Test *Laryngoscope* 94:176-178, 1984.
8. Douek E: *The Sense of Smell and its Abnormalities.* Edinborough, 1974, Churchill Livingstone.
9. Duncan RB, Briggs D: Treatment of Uncomplicated Anosmia by Vitamin A. *Arch Otolaryngol* 75:36-44, 1962.
10. Eccles R, Jarvad MSM, Morris S: Olfactory and Trigeminal Thresholds and Nasal Resistance of Airflow. *Acta Otolaryngol* 108:268-273.
11. Eichel BS: Improvement of Olfaction Following Pansinus Surgery. *ENT Journal* 73:248-253, 1994.
12. Foulkes MA: Design Issues in Chemosensory Trials *Arch Otolaryngol* 116:65-68, 1990.
13. Goodspeed RB, Goul JF, Catalaanotto FA, et al: Corticosteroids in Olfactory Dysfunction. In Meiselman HI, Rivolin RS, editors: *Clinical Measurement of Taste and Smell.* New York, 1986, MacMullam
14. Graziadei PPC, Graziadei AGM: Regeneration in the Olfactory System of Vertebrates. *Am J Otolaryngol,* 4:228-234, 1983.
15. Henkin PI: Disordered Smell. *Lancet* 1:901-902, 1988.
16. Henkin RI: Olfaction in Human Disease. In English GM editor: *Looseleaf Seris in Otolaryngology.* New York, 1982.
17. Henkin RI, Schecter PJ, Friedwald WT, et al: A Double Blind Study of Effects of Zinc Sulfate on Taste and Smell Dysfunction. *Am J Med Sci* 272:285-299, 1976.
18. Hotchkis WT: Influence of Prednisone on Nasal Polyposis with Anosmia *Arch Otolaryngol* 65:478-479, 1956.
19. Jafek BW: Ultrastructure of Human Nasal Mucosa. *Laryngoscope* 93:1577-1599, 1983.
20. Jafek BW, Hartmann D, Eller PM, et al: Post Viral Olfactory Dysfunction. *Am J Rhinol* 91-100, 1990.
21. Jafek BW, Moran OT, Ellen PM: Steroid-Dependent Anosmia. *Arch Otolaryngol* 113:547-549, 1987.
22. Jafek BW, Murrow B, Johnson WW: Olfaction and Endoscopic Sinus Surgery. *ENT Journal* 73:548-554, 1994.
23. Kaufman MD, Lasiter KR, Shensy BV: Paroxysmal Unilateral Dysosmia. *Am Neurol* 3:450-451, 1988.
24. Mings R, Friedman WH, Linford PA, et al: Five-year Follow-up of the Effects of Bilateral Intranasal Sphenoidectomy in Patients with Sinusitis and Asthma. *Am J Rhinol* 2:13-16, 1988.
25. Moran DT, Jafek BW, Rolling JC: Electromicroscopy of Olfactory Epithelia in Two Patients with Anosmia. *Arch Otolaryngol* 111:122-126, 1985.
26. Mozell MN, Hornung DE, Leapold DA: *Initial Mechanisms Basic to Olfactory Perception.* 4:238-246, 1990.
27. Scott A: Caution Urged in Treating "Steroid-Dependent Anosmia". *Arch Otolaryngol* 115:109, 1989.
28. Shiffman SS: Taste and Smell in Disease. *N Engl J Med* 308:1275-1279, 1983.
29. Stevens CN, Stevens MH: Quantitative Effects of Nasal Surgery On Olfaction. *Am J Otolaryngol* 6:264-267, 1985.
30. Stevens MH: Olfactory Disorders: Diagnosis. In Johnson JT editor: *Instructional Courses Vol I,* St. Louis, 1989, Mosby.
31. Tarlo SM, Cockcroft DW, Dolovich J, et al: Beclomethasone Disproportionate Aerosol in Perennial Rhinitis. *J. Allergy Clin Immunol* 59:232-236, 1977.
32. Taylor LRS: ACTH and Nasal Polyps. *J Laryngol Otol.* 87:103-5, 1973.
33. Zusho H: Post-traumatic Anosmia. *Arch Otolarygol* 108:90-92, 1982.

Part Three

Head and Neck

12

Genetics of Squamous Cell Carcinoma of the Head and Neck Region

Michael S. Benninger, M.D., Maria J. Worsham, Ph.D., and Daniel L. Van Dyke, Ph.D., F.A.C.M.G.

Cancer is second only to heart disease as the leading cause of death in the United States, accounting for greater than 20% of all deaths. Cancer of the head and neck, including skin, accounts for 10% of all malignancies and 5% of all cancer deaths.[32] Squamous cell carcinomas (SCC) account for the majority of the nonskin head and neck malignancies. The risk factors for SCC are well recognized, with most occurring in patients with histories of prolonged exposure to tobacco or alcohol.[3]

The treatment of SCC of the head and neck has been well standardized, with traditional therapies relying on surgery, radiation therapy, or combined surgery-radiation therapy treatments. Recent efforts in new treatment strategies have revolved around adjuvant or concomitant chemotherapy. Despite intensive investigation, however, only modest improvements in survival have been identified in the past two decades. More recent efforts have been in determining predictors of outcome, and the effects of such predictors employing differing therapeutic modalities.[9,30,32,60,63,70,85,89] These efforts have directed the investigation of cancer therapy from new modalities or new applications of old modalities to attempting to understand the underlying pathogenic factors and mechanisms.

There is strong evidence that head and neck SCC has a genetic basis. In the East and Far East, oral cavity and oropharyngeal cancers account for almost one-half of all cancers.[47] Nasopharyngeal carcinomas are 25 times more frequent in people from the Kwang Tung Province of China than in whites with certain HLA haplotypes and familial clustering being identified.[19] In Bombay, 50% of all cancers are in the buccal mucosa.[19] Although environmental factors play a critical role as evidenced by the association of buccal cancer related to chewing pan, genetic predispositions for the development of cancer are likely to also be critical. Chinese who emigrated from Kwang Tung retain a significantly higher risk of developing nasopharyngeal carcinoma. Genetic segregation analysis showed strong evidence favoring an autosomal dominant pattern of inheritance for predisposition to malignancy in families with smoking-related malignancies.[72]

Genetic changes in many cancers have been identified, and frequently these cancers develop similar genetic changes (e.g., loss of the TP53, RB1, and DCC genes) which might suggest common pathways in tumorigenesis. The development of remarkable tools for molecular and genetic analysis have resulted in an explosion of information which allows for the elucidation of the mechanisms of cancer promulgation and is beginning to lead to innovations in cancer treatment which will likely become the alternatives to standard surgery, radiation, and chemotherapeutic modalities. With the undertaking of the Human Genome Project, it is foreseeable that genes will be identified for many if not most human cancers. Such efforts will likely result in rapid changes in cancer prevention, assessment, and treatment. Unfortunately, the knowledge of the genetics of head and neck SCC is still in its infancy.

This chapter will familiarize the reader with the basis for the genetics of human cancer, discuss the successes in other human cancers, and describe the present state of information related to SCC. The chapter will close with a model pathway of genetic changes in SCC and will raise questions related to ethical and practical issues which must be considered as the cancer genetic code unfolds.

HISTORIC CANCER GENETICS AND MOLECULAR BIOLOGY

Traditional efforts to treat head and neck SCC have revolved around efforts to develop new or different combinations of treatment modalities and to identify epidemiologic information which can suggest susceptible individuals or behaviors. As mentioned earlier, these efforts were very successful in identifying the few obvious susceptible patient groups and in showing that environmental exposures such as tobacco, alcohol, chronic mucosal irritation, actinic or low-dose radiation, and some industrial chemicals and products increase the risk of developing SCC.[3,10] Efforts at behavioral modification and screening have been effective in decreasing rates of SCC development in some groups and the growing national concern for the cost in lives and money due to tobacco-related diseases should further decrease the incidences of SCC. Nutritional and immunologic factors have been identified which seem to effect both treatment results and complication rates. Histologic grading and evaluation of tumor thickness have been used to predict survival and to develop algorithms for further treatment.[60,70] It is beyond the scope of this chapter to describe the many efforts to evaluate other factors responsible for SCC or potential value in treatment of SCC.[10] Hematologic factors such as the human eosinophil have been evaluated to assess the relationships of the host-tumor interaction.[34] The retinols, beta-carotene, and free radical scavengers have shown some benefit in prevention of human cancers including SCC, may reverse early cellular changes and have shown promise in the treatment of established cancers in some sites.[36,41]

The diploid human genome has 46 chromosomes: 22 pairs of autosomes and one pair of sex chromosomes (the X and Y chromosomes). The term haploid means having one each of the chromosomes typically found in the somatic (diploid) cells. This is typical of the gametes whose union restores the diploid number. Tetraploid cells have exactly double the number of normal chromosomes; in cancer cells, an abnormal DNA content in the tetraploid range suggests that part of the tumor cell population has had a doubling of the number of chromosomes, and these tetraploid cells universally have many abnormalities of individual chromosome as well. The term aneuploid describes any deviation from an exact multiple of the haploid number of chromosomes, whether more or fewer. In DNA content studies aneuploidy usually refers to a content greater than diploid. Cellular DNA content and ploidy have been found to be related to the aggressiveness of head and neck SCC and responsiveness to some treatments. Abnormal DNA content has been thought to reflect altered proliferation capacity of tumor cells[89] and has been associated with adverse biologic and clinical behavior.[85] Because of this relationship and the aggressive clinical behavior of malignant tumors, there have been substantial efforts in evaluating the role of aneuploidy in tumor response and treatment. The advent of flow cytometry has allowed for improved ease of ploidy analysis and more predictable results.

Nuclear DNA content as a prognostic factor in head and neck SCC has been confirmed in many studies. Aneuploid tumors have been shown to be radioresistant when compared with diploid tumors in early glottic carcinomas.[85] Chemosensitivity of aneuploid tumors has also been found to be lower when evaluating well or moderately differentiated tumors, although chemosensitivity was increased in aneuploid poorly differentiated tumors.[63] By using a measure of DNA content, the adjusted DNA index (aDI), the occurrence and frequency of metastatic neck nodes and time to recurrence after treatment of advanced laryngeal cancers have been identified.[89] Although most studies suggest poorer prognosis and more aggressive behavior in aneuploid tumors, these findings are not universal. Some have found a better prognosis in aneuploid tumors in some sites[33,34] and improved response with advanced differentiation.[63] Furthermore, some have also noted increased frequency of DNA diploid tumors in associated lymph node metastases.[9] Although the evidence favors that a high percentage of SCCs are aneuploid, DNA aneuploidy does not define all malignancy. Ploidy analysis may potentially help predict good versus poor responders and may help to guide treatment, but it is not of great benefit clinically at this time. Further study will clarify the role of ploidy analysis in the evaluation and treatment of patients with head and neck SCC.

ONCOGENES AND TUMOR SUPPRESSOR GENES

Human malignancies develop in individuals in four different relationships between human genetics and environmental factors: spontaneous mutations in people who have no environmental or genetic predisposition, individuals with genetic predisposition with no environmental exposure, individuals with environmental exposures with no genetic predisposition, and individuals who have both a genetic predisposition and environmental exposure.[18] Although such relationships are not well defined in SCC of the head and neck, information gained from the investigation in other malignancies are of great value in the approach to ongoing investigation of SCC.

The control of the normal cell cycle depends on a complex relationship between positive and negative regulatory factors. Mutational events which change the normal regulatory mechanisms can lead to poorly regulated cell growth, while those that alter the normal positive growth factors can result in prolific cell growth.[73] Genes that have been identified with regulatory control of the cell cycle have been called tumor suppressor genes. A loss or alteration of these genes may result in cancer development. Conversely, genes that have been identified with the development of cancer have been called oncogenes. In general, oncogenes are felt to be normal cellular genes which are altered or activated which allows them to induce tumor growth. Although speculation of the role of oncogenes has been discussed for some time, it is becoming evident that the change or loss of tumor suppressor genes may be an even more important genetic change in the development of human cancers. In most cancers both oncogenes and loss of tumor suppressor genes occur. To date, in colon cancer, at least four oncogenes and three tumor suppressor genes have been found to be involved along with an eighth gene which has not been classified. The altered three tumor suppressor genes have been identified in over 70% of tumors, while three of the oncogenes have been found in less than 5% of tumors.[57]

Chromosomal evaluations of various cancers have led to identification of specific chromosomes or chromosomal segments in which genetic changes most frequently occur. Subsequently, individual genes have been isolated which seem to be related to these cancers. Consistent chromosomal translocations between chromosome 8 and one of chromosomes 14, 2, or 22 in Burkitt's lymphoma led to the identification that one breakpoint was always in or near the region of c-myc gene (oncogene) at chromosomal band q24.1 in chromosome 8 and the other was in or near an immunoglobulin gene on the other chromosome. The effect is to deregulate the c-myc with subsequent stimulation of cell division.[49] Many other oncogenes have been identified. However, oncogenes have not been found to have a significant role in SCC at this time.

One question that has long been asked is whether or not there is a relationship between hereditary and nonhereditary cancers? In normal diploid cells, two mutational events would need to occur in order for the inactivation of a negative regulatory element (tumor suppressor gene).[73] This has been called the "two hit" theory (Fig. 12-1)). If, however, an individual had a hereditarily altered gene then only one spontaneously or environmentally mediated mutation (one hit) would need to occur to result in loss or inactivation of the suppressor gene. This theory would therefore describe the increased likelihood of certain individuals to develop the neoplasm. It would also explain why two individuals with similar environmental exposures may have significantly different likelihoods of developing a cancer. Early speculation of the two-hit mechanism was raised in evaluating retinoblastomas in which there appeared to be both a hereditary and a nonhereditary form. Forty percent of retinoblastomas occur in a hereditary pattern, where the likelihood of developing the cancer is almost 50% and the tumors frequently occur bilaterally. Often there is no family history of these tumors but the offspring of the individual have a 50% likelihood of developing retinoblastoma. This led to the postulation that a new mutational event results in the increased susceptibility. The other 60% of retinoblastomas occur in a nonhereditary mechanism and are unilateral. It was postulated that in the hereditary group, an inherited mutation had occurred so that only one "hit" was necessary in the retinoblast cell, whereas two "hits" were required in the retinoblast in the nonhereditary group.[49] The identification of the RB1 gene, which was the first tumor suppressor gene identified, confirmed this hypothesis. The RB1 gene produces a protein which interacts with DNA to regulate the transcription of other genes. In the absence of a normal RB1 gene, cell division is not normally regulated. Insertion of a normal gene results in return to normal cell regulation.[49]

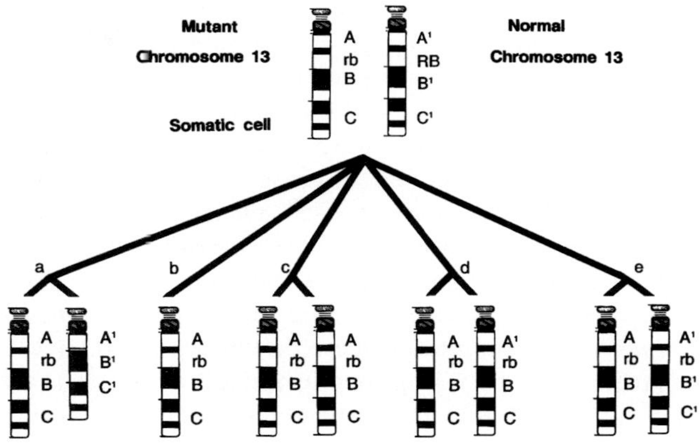

FIG 12-1
Genetic changes leading to loss of both copies (alleles) of a tumor suppressor gene can arise in the precursor cell to the tumor itself, or the first mutation can be inherited as a familial trait. When the first mutation is inherited, the liklihood of a second mutaton in a susceptible cell is much greater than the liklihood of a mutation in both alleles in the same cell. For this reason, familial tumors like retinoblastoma are often bilateral and have an earlier age of onset than do the typically unilateral sporadic tumors. In the example shown, one chromosome 13 in a retinoblast cell has an inherited or acquired mutation at the RB1 locus *(top left, "rb")* and has a normal RB1 gene on the other chromosome. The mechanisms that have been postulated[13] for acquiring the second hit in the remaining normal chromosome 13 include: (1) deletion of the RB1 locus, (2) loss of the entire chromosome, (3) loss of the entire normal chromosome and duplication of the abnormal chromosome, (4) recombination between the two 13's, resulting in both chromosomes being homozygous for the rb mutation and all genes distal to the RB1 locus, and (5) a new point mutation or possibly gene conversion at the RB1 locus on the normal chromosome.

A major cellular factor that occurs in all cancers is alteration in the control of the cell cycle with subsequent uncontrolled cell growth. The cell cycle regulatory gene that has attracted the most attention and interest in investigating human cancers, including SCC, is the TP53 gene, a tumor suppressor gene. Mutations in TP53 contribute to the development of 50% or more of all cancers.[58] The gene is located on the short arm of chromosome 17 and encodes for a protein which acts to control the cell cycle.[24,51,56,58] When cellular DNA is damaged, the p53 protein is produced, accumulates in the cell, and arrests cell replication in the G1 phase. The p53 protein binds with and blocks cyclin-dependent kinins which help to move cells through the cell cycle. This arrest in the cell cycle allows DNA repair to occur. In the absence of a normal p53 gene, cell cycle arrest and DNA repair fail to occur, resulting in increased numbers of chromosomal abnormalities.[24,49,59]

Loss of expression of p53 occurs with inactivation of either one or both copies of the gene. However, with the inactivation of one copy ("one hit") 50% of the normal suppressor protein is formed and no significant effect on cell cycle control occurs. With inactivation of both genes ("two-hit"), no suppressor protein is produced and the arrest in cell-cycle for DNA repair is lost.[24] Of interest is the significant interplay between tumor suppressors such as p53 and other tumor suppressor genes and oncogenes. As mentioned above, p53 interacts with cyclin-dependent kinases to control the cell cycle. If these cyclins are overproduced or produced at the wrong time in the cell cycle, then cell cycle control would again be lost. Cyclin D1 is a growth factor sensor which helps the cell to divide in the G1 phase. Once the cell is committed to DNA synthesis, then the entire cell cycle occurs.[59] Overexpression of D1 can lead to uncontrolled cell division and cancer development, and therefore these normal genes are potential oncogenes when uncontrolled.

Human papilloma viruses (HPV) have been implicated in the progenesis of human cancers and SCC. The DNA of HPV 16, 18, and 31 has been found in human genital cancers, and HPV 16 and 18 have been recognized in verrucous carcinomas of the larynx.[6,27] For cervical cancers in HPV-positive tumors, normal RB1 and p53 genes are found but appear to be deactivated by interaction with viral proteins. HPV-negative tumors demonstrate mutations in p53 and RB1.[49] HPVs produce proteins E6 and E7. E6 interacts with p53 and E7 interacts with the protein of RB1. In HPV 16 and 18, which are associated with cervical and laryngeal cancers, both E6 and E7 are interactive while only E7 is interactive for HPV 6 and 11, which have been found in association with benign laryngeal papillomas.[49] The lack of E6 would allow for normal cell cycle control via p53 and might account for the benign nature of these tumors.

THE IMPORTANCE OF UNDERSTANDING CANCER GENETICS

At the most basic cellular level, all cancers are genetic diseases. A clear understanding of genetic changes are important in cancer and can provide the basis for molecular strategies to control it. Knowledge of the clinically significant changes is central to characterization of genetic subgroups, prognostic applications, and treatment decisions. In squamous cell carcinoma (SCC), these goals are attainable and will benefit many people.

CHROMOSOME ABNORMALITIES, PROGNOSIS, AND TUMOR GENE LOCALIZATION

Many prognostically informative changes have been identified in preleukemia, leukemia, and lymphoma, and many therapeutic protocols now incorporate cytogenetic analysis or gene analysis of changes that were first identified by cytogenetics.[69] As with leukemia and lymphoma, evidence is emerging that some chromosomal defects in solid cancers are prognostically or diagnostically important.[26,69] For example, loss of 18q and 17p are common chromosome abnormalities in colorectal carcinoma.[61] A model fitting most colorectal carcinomas includes a cascade of gene mutations and losses, starting with 5q *(MCC/APC)* mutation in one copy of the gene (allele) and loss of the remaining normal allele to create an early adenoma. (Loss of one allele is often detectable by demonstrating loss of a highly polymorphic marker nearby on the chromosome. The marker locus, being highly polymorphic, is heterozygous in most people. Thus loss of heterozygosity (LOH) at the marker locus signifies probable loss of the nearby tumor suppressor gene from that chromosome.) Next, intermediate stages of carcinogenesis are marked with a variety of other genetic changes, many of which involve LOH and loss of tumor suppressor genes. Finally, the cascade culminates with 18q and 17p *(DCC* and *TP53 tumor suppressor loci)* mutations and LOH to create carcinoma.[84] Tumors with loss of 18q and 17p and those with multiple genetic losses comprise a poor prognostic group.

As prognostically important changes are identified in SCC, it will be possible to develop a molecular genetic basis for staging and classification analogous to that beginning to be applied to carcinomas of the colon and rectum, bladder, glia, and breast,[14,16,23,78] as well as presymptomatic testing in at-risk populations.[67,82]

Specific genetic changes have been described in many solid tumors, as technical problems with karyotyping have been overcome, including 3p deletion in bladder and small cell lung carcinoma,[1,87] deletion of 5q, 17p, and 18q in colon cancer, [61,74] loss of 9p and 6q in melanoma, [15,77] and mutations and deletions of 13q in retinoblastoma and osteogenic sarcoma.[30] Many investigators are scrutinizing these sites to determine the underlying genetic mechanisms. For example, Fountain et al.[28,29] localized 9p21 as the site of a tumor suppressor gene in malignant melanoma, the probable gene being *CDKN2/MTS1,* an inhibitor of cyclin-dependent kinase.[43]

The observation of consistent genetic losses in solid tumors has strengthened the concept (Knudson's hypothesis) that loss of a normal allele allows expression of a recessive mutation on the opposite homolog or loss of tumor suppression.[13,30] Sporadic and inherited retinoblastoma are associated with loss of both functional copies of the *RB1* gene at 13q14.[13,30] Using restriction fragment length polymorphism (RFLP) analysis and cytogenetics, our laboratory identified LOH for 13q loci in one endometrial carcinoma, and a breakpoint in the 13q11-q14 region in a second.[37,38] Subsequently, we found breakpoints and deletions of 13q11-14 in 25% of SCCHN.[81] These examples and others[2,4,11,22,44,64] underscore the fact that identification of nonrandom losses of genetic material in cancer is a powerful step to identify genes that are important in cell transformation and tumor progression.

Cytogenetics and prognosis in squamous cell carcinoma

Most cytogenetic studies of SCCHN have relied on analysis of later stage tumors and established cell lines. Heo et al[40] reported recurrent loss of 3p and trisomy 6 in HNSCC cell lines. Whang-Peng et al[88] evaluated primary explants and cell lines originating from esophageal SCCs. Chromosomes 1, 3, 9, and 11 were rearranged in most cases, usually resulting in deletions. Viegas-Pequignot et al[83] described recurrent loss of 3p, 5, 8p, 10p, 13, and the Y, and gain of 1q, 3q, and 7q in short-term cultures of seven lung SCCs. Mitelman and co-workers used short-term cultures to karyotype early and later stage SCC, and in tumors with only one principal clone, the recurrent chromosome changes were similar to those observed by others.[46] In most cases, these studies and our research on stage I-IV tumors show that the main effects of the cytogenetic changes in SCC are deletions that lead to loss of heterozygosity (LOH) at several specific sites. Loss of segments of chromosomes 3p, 5q, 8p, 9p, 10p, and 18q are among the most common.

Our initial interest in SCC was to identify nonrandom cytogenetic changes in this tumor type and to test for associations between anatomic site and specific chromosome rearrangements or specific aneuploidies.

We anticipated that the cytogenetic data would also serve as a guide for molecular studies aimed at locating genes involved in the initiation and progression of SCC. Another goal was to determine which consistent changes were involved in tumor progression and might therefore serve as prognostic biomarkers.

The recurrent genetic and cytogenetic changes in SCC

To determine the common chromosome abnormalities in SCC, we karyotyped 29 SCCHN, 7 SCC of the vulva (SCV), and one SCC each from uterine cervix, urinary bladder, and vagina.[7,12,39,90,92,93] The analysis included direct preparations and short-term cultures established from fresh tumors as well as established cell lines.

For each tumor and for the tumors as a group, we characterized the pattern of ploidy changes, recurrent rearrangements and rearrangement breakpoints, gains of segments, and losses of segments of the karyotype (Fig. 12-2 to 12-5).

FISH analysis of SCCHN

Because the karyotypes of some tumors are complex, it was not always possible to fully describe the gains and losses with complete confidence. The technique of fluorescence in situ hybridization (FISH) can be helpful in these situations (Fig. 12-6 and 12-7). FISH employs fluorescent-labelled DNA sequences to examine chromosomes and can be useful not only on metaphase cells but interphase cells as well, even in cells dissociated from or within histologic sections.[95,96]

We recently tested for in vivo tumor heterogeneity using centromeric FISH probes on interphase cells within delineated tumor and nontumor areas in histologic sections. This study demonstrated that the cytogenetic patterns observed in vitro do indeed reflect the chromosomal pattern of the original tumor.[94] We also showed that two synchronous primary tumors arising in the mouth and pyriform sinus had nearly identical genetic changes, suggesting that some apparently independent primary tumors have a common origin.[95]

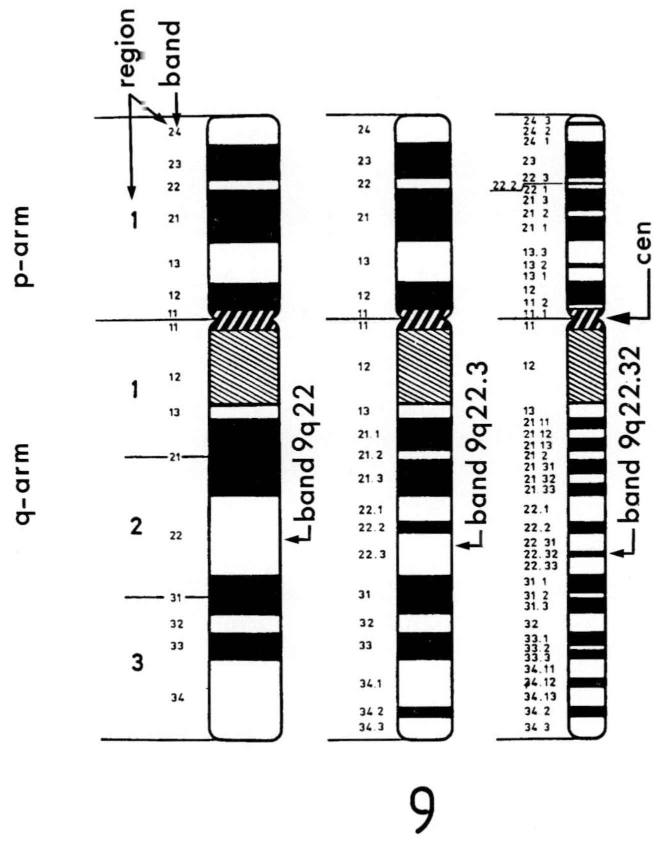

FIG 12-2
Cytogenetic nomenclature. Each chromosome is divided into two parts (arms) based on the position of the centromere. The smaller, or p, arm is placed at the top and the larger, or q, arm is placed at the bottom. Standard staining techniques, usually G-banding, produce a pattern of lighter and darker bands along the length of each chromosome, and each of the 22 autosomes and 2 sex chromosomes has a distinctive and constant pattern of bands. Based on an internationally accepted numbering system, presently ISCN(1985) and ISCN(1991), each chromosome arm is divided into numbered regions bounded by landmarks that include the centromere, major distinguishing bands, and the chromosome ends (telomeres). Each major band within a region is numbered, with region 1 and band 1 located nearest to the centromere. The centromere is termed cen, and the short and long arm telomere regions are pter and qter, respectively. Sub-bands that appear with increasing banding resolution are identified using a decimal point between the band and sub-band numbers. For example, 9q22.32 identifies chromosome 9, in the long arm, region 2, band 2, and sub-band 32.

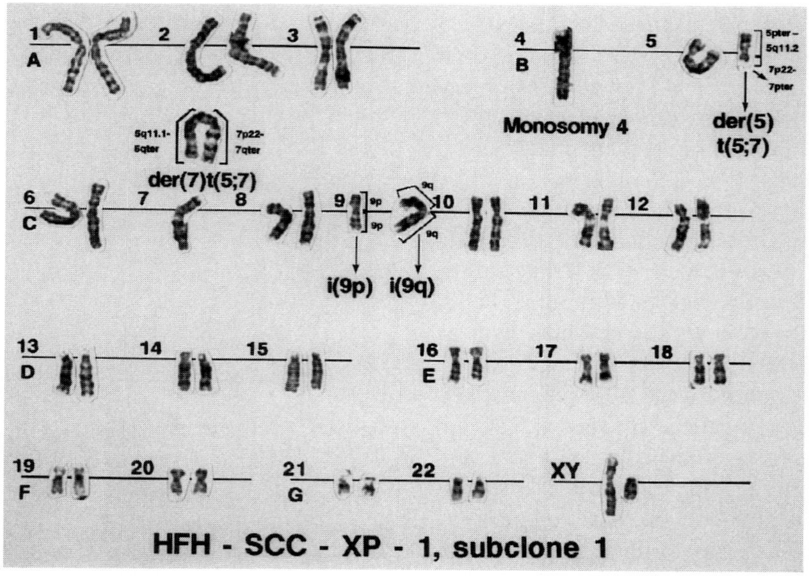

FIG 12-3

The karyotype of cultured cells from tumor HFH-SCC-XP-1, sub-clone 1, was 45,XY,−4,t(5;7)(q11.21;p22),i(9p),i(9q). This is a fairly simple karyotype for a solid tumor, with monosomy 4, a balanced translocation between chromosomes 5 and 7 and isochromosomes for the short and long arms of chromosome 9 as the only abnormalities. (From Worsham MJ, et al: Genes Chromosomes Cancer 7:158-164, 1993. Reprinted by permission of John Wiley & Sons Inc.)

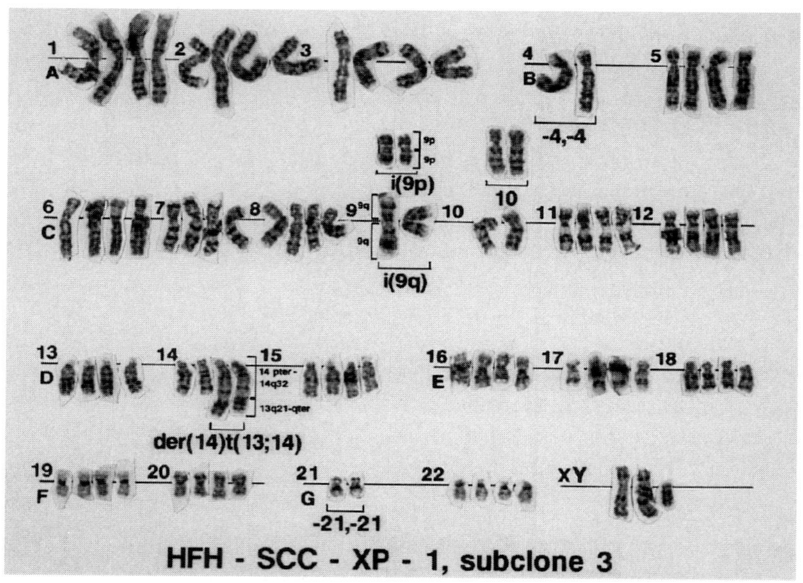

FIG 12-4

The karyotype of cultured cells from tumor HFH-SCC-XP-1, subclone 3, was hypotetraploid. The ISCN(1991) nomenclature is somewhat more complicated because the karyotype is near-tetraploid, but the changes are not much more complex than those shown for subclone 1 of this tumor (Fig. 12-3): 87,XXY,-Y,-4x2,i(9p)x2,i(9q)x2,der(14)t(13:14)(q21;q32)x2,-21x2. There are four copies of most chromosomes. The presence of only two copies of chromosome 4 and 21 suggests that the tetraploidization event occured after monosomy 4 and monosomy 21 developed in the near-diploid tumor cell population. Likewise, the presence of two copies of the unbalanced translocation between chromosomes 13 and 14 suggests that the translocation formed in the near-diploid cell population.

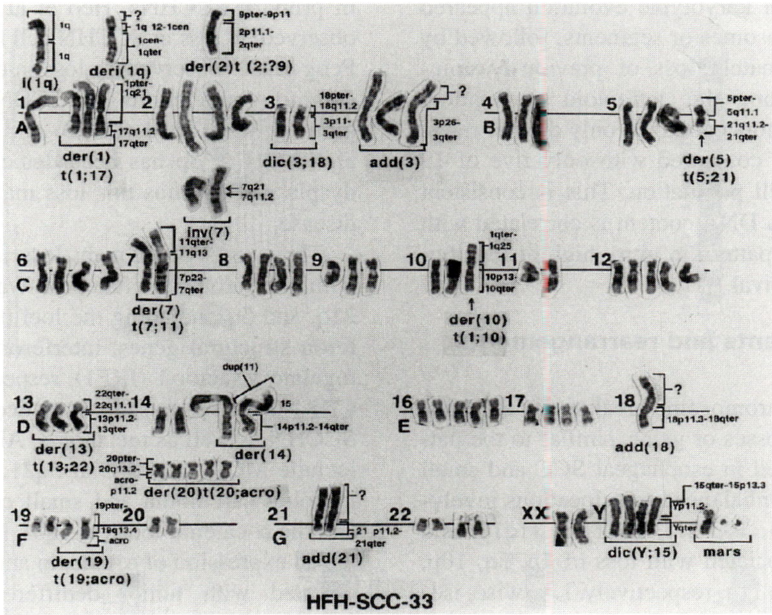

FIG 12-5
The karyotype of cells from tumor HFH-SCC-33 is hypotetraploid (88 to 92 chromosomes) and is complex, with numerous unbalanced translocations. In ISCN (1991) nomenclature, it is written as: 88-92,XX,dic(Y;15)(p13.3;p11.2)x4,der(1)t(1;17)(q21;q11.2)x3,+add(1)i(1q)(1qter-cen::cen-q12::?),+der(2)t(2;?9)(p11.1;p11),-3,add(3)(p26)x3,+dic(3;18)(p11;q11.2)x2,-4,der(5)t(5;21)(q11.1;q11.2),inv(7)(q11.2q21)x2,der(7)t(7;11)(p22;q13)x2,-9,-10,der(10)t(1;10)(q25;p13),-11x2,+12,-13,der(13)t(13;22)(p11.2;q11.1)x3,der(14)dup(11)(q13q23)t(11;14)(q23;p11.2)x2,+16,-18x3,add(18)(p11.3),der(19)t(19;acro)(q13.4;p11.2)x2,-20x2,+der(20)t(20;acro)(q13.2;p11.2)x4,-21x2,add(21)(p11.2)x2,+2-6mar[cp21]. As observed in the Fig. 12-4 karyotype, several of the rearrangements are present in two copies, suggesting that they arose before the tumor cell population became tetraploid.

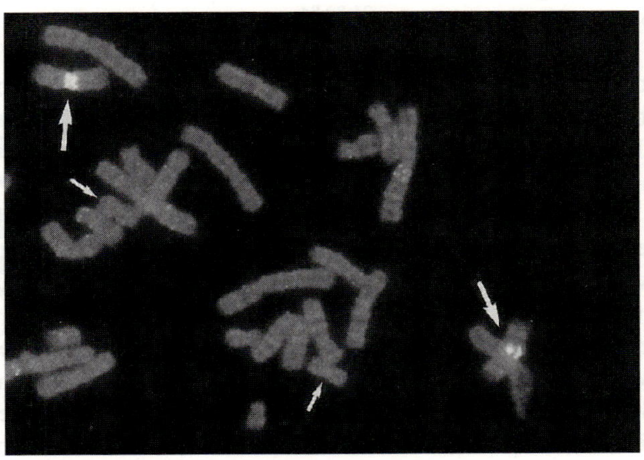

FIG 12-6
FISH of cells from tumor HFH-SCC-XP1 with a flourscent probe that is specific for the centromere of chromosome 9 (D9Z1) demonstrates 9 centromere signals on the isochromosome 9q only *(large arrows)*. The isochromosome 9p copies in this field *(small arrows)* did not give a hybridization signal with the 9cen probe. The G-banding of a similar cell from this tumor is shown in Fig. 12-3.

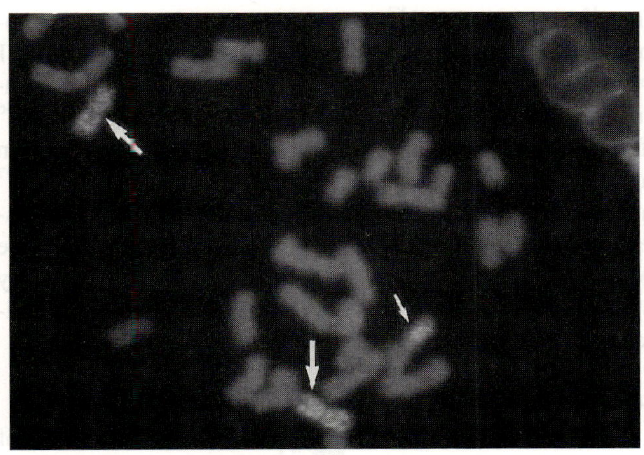

FIG 12-7
FISH of cells from tumor HFH-SCC-XP-1 with a cocktail of fluorescent probes derived from the entire length of chromosome 9, called chromosome paint because it colors all of the target chromosome. In this photo from a previously G-banded near-tetraploid metaphase, both copies of the isochromosome 9q *(large arrow)* and both of the isochromosome 9p *(small arrow)* are painted. This demonstrates that these chromosomes are all chromosome 9 derived, even though hybridization with the chromosome 9 centromere probe (Fig 12-6) was not evident on the short arm isochromosomes. The G-banding of a similar cell from this tumor is shown in Fig. 12-4.

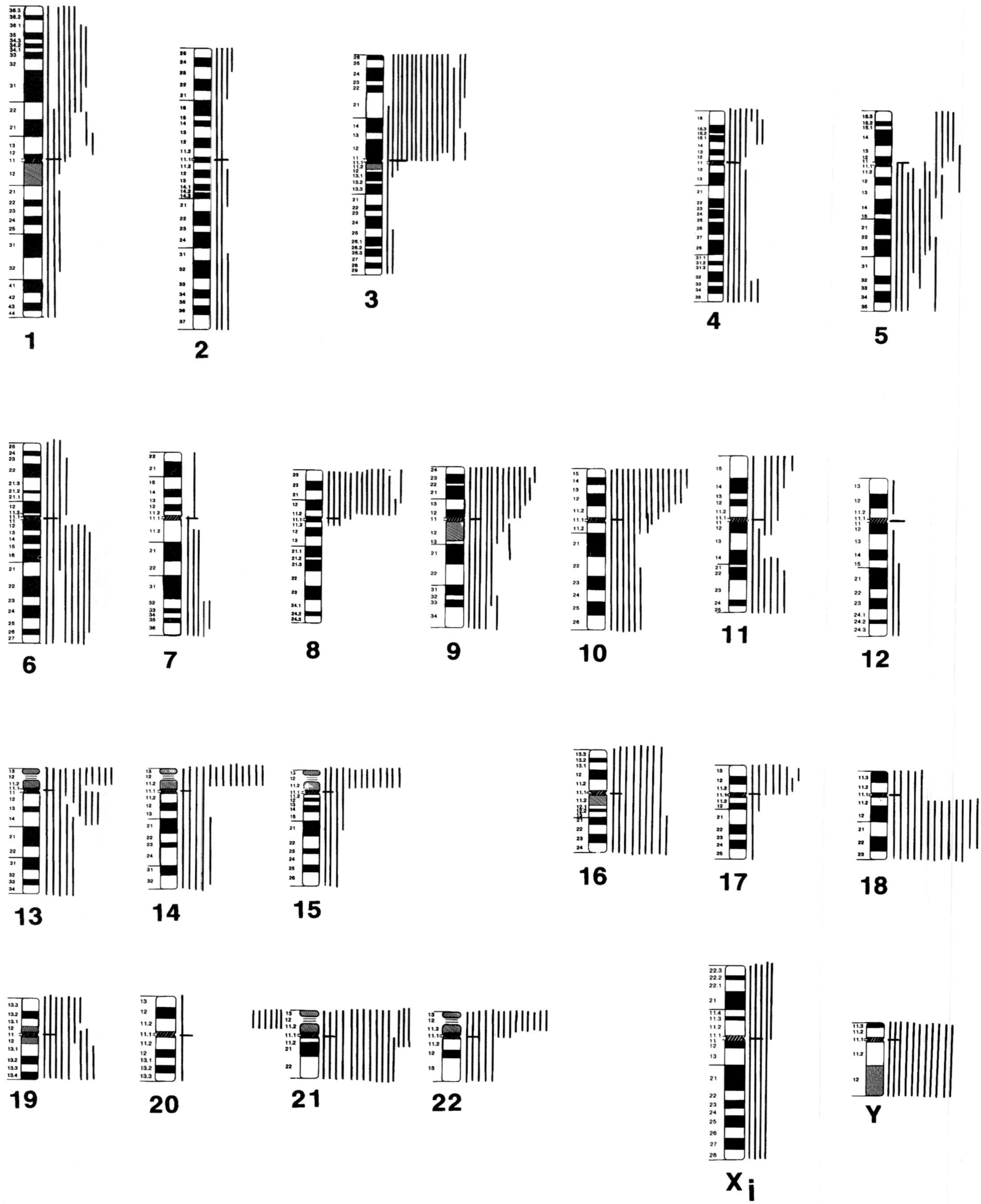

FIG 12-9

Losses of chromosomal segments in 29 SCCHN. Each vertical bar denotes loss of material in one of the tumors. The vertical lines to the right X chromosome indicate loss of the inactivated X. Loss of the genetically active X was never observed. Apparent loss of both copies of an autosomal segment was rare.

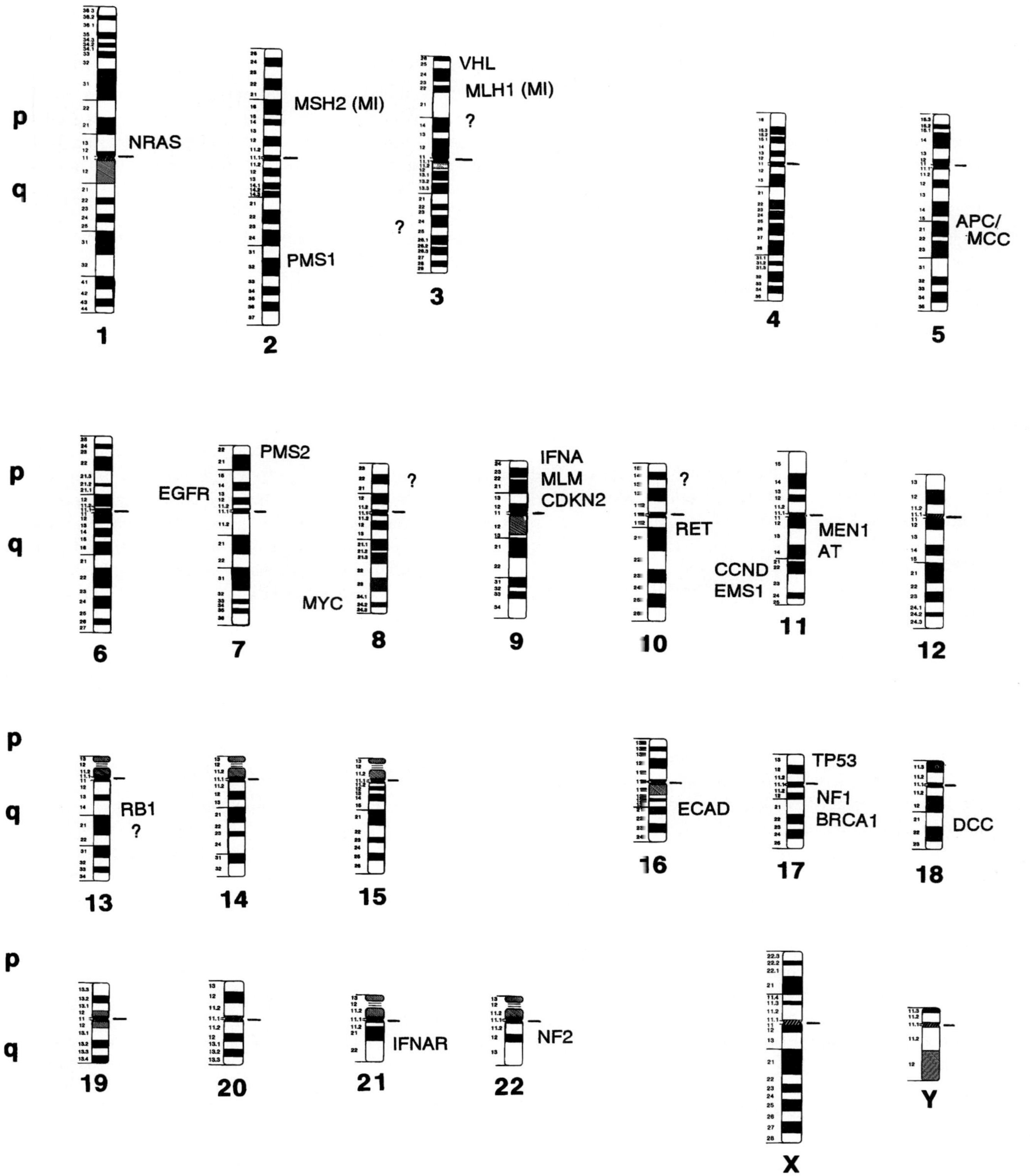

FIG 12-10
Some candidate genes that may be involved in SCCHN. Genes to the right of each chromosome are tumor suppressor genes, and to the left, oncogenes. Not all of these genes have been established as important in SCCHN, but they are shown here to indicate their location within regions that are commonly lost or gained in these tumors, thus their candidacy. Question marks in the figure, e.g., denote areas of the genome where genetic loss is common but where no candidate tumor suppressor gene has been mapped.

among the chromosome arms that were informative. (An arm is informative if the normal DNA was heterozygous for the marker locus. If 30 of 36 arms have a heterozygous marker in the patient's blood DNA, i.e., are informative, and 15 of the 30 informative arms demonstrate LOH in the tumor DNA, then the FAL = 0.50 for that tumor.) FAL also has prognostic significance in osteosarcoma[21] and non–small cell lung cancer.[79] Huang et al[42] described LOH involving four tumor suppressor loci (5q, 13q, 17p, and 18q) in esophageal carcinoma and postulated that loss at one locus either potentiates loss at other loci or that deletions are additive in their effect of conferring a growth advantage. Tsuchiya et al[79] emphasized the strong similarities in allelotype results between SCC and adenocarcinomas of the lung.

For our SCCHN series,[8] fractional segmental loss (FSL) and gain (FSG) were calculated as the proportion of losses observed among the autosomal arms that expressed recurrent loss. The risk ratio was elevated between FSL and survival, although a statistically significant relationship was not attained. Nevertheless, these results underscore the value of understanding the common genetic losses in SCC of the head and neck region.

Site specificity

For specific anatomic sites within the head and neck, there are clear differences in outcome based on stage at diagnosis, likelihood of recurrence, etc. However, no molecular data are available by site as yet; this requires a larger sample size and will be a target of the proposed studies.

Conversely, many of the recurring changes in SCC of the head and neck region have also been observed in SCC at other anatomic sites.[76,90] The overall similarities that do exist in the karyotypic patterns from these anatomic sites suggest that initiation, development, and progression of neoplasia in squamous epithelial cells are controlled by some of the same genetic pathways, irrespective of anatomic site. It also suggests that prognostically significant associations identified in SCCHN will be worth of investigation for their relevance in SCC at other anatomic sites, including esophagus and lung.

Moreover, many of the changes that are recurrent in SCCHN are found in diverse tumor types. For example, the demonstration that, in primary breast cancer, two distinct regions of 1p are frequently lost[5] is mirrored by our observations in SCCHN.

Histopathologic stage and karyotype

In our series of SCCHNs, earlier stage tumors tended to have simpler karyotypes. Within every pathologic stage there were also tumors that had more complex karyotypes. Most of the specific deletions were present in two or three of the seven early stage tumors.[8] This suggests that, if loss of individual regions has independent prognostic significance, they will find application as biomarkers of clinical outcome in early stage tumors.

Tobacco use

Lydiatt and Schantz presented data in August, 1994, that deletions of 9p were more common in tumors from eight patients who are nonsmokers than in tumors from 34 smokers.[54] Field et al[25] reported that nonsmokers' tumors had more MSRP loci expressing mitotic instability, but they did not find a difference in 9p LOH. These findings suggest that significant smoking-dependent differences exist in the evolution of SCCHN.

Summary

These preliminary data suggest that genetic losses are common at multiple specific sites in the genome in SCCHN tumors. Moreover, our data suggest that loss at specific anatomic sites is likely to be associated with tumor progression and patient survival. Fractional allelic loss is also likely to be associated with survival and other parameters and to reflect patterns of progressive genetic loss from SCC tumors as they evolve and become increasingly aggressive.

The available evidence suggests that some specific losses that arise early are implicated in tumor initiation and have little impact on survival, whereas other losses tend to occur later and are associated with a poor prognosis (Fig. 12-11).

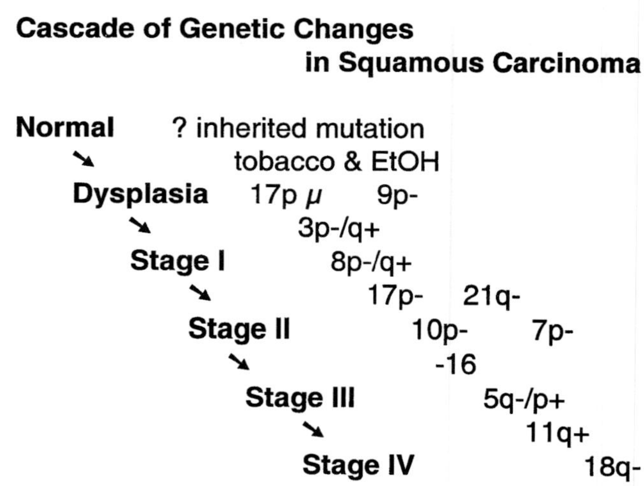

FIG 12-11
Cascade of genetic changes in squamous carcinoma of the head and neck region. Some chromosomal changes such as loss of the short arm of chromosome 3 (3p−) and gain of the long arm of chromosome 3 (3q+), appear to occur early in the progression of SCC and may have little impact on the progression to more aggressive stages. Conversely, changes that tend to appear at later stages may play a greater role in the invasiveness and the risk of recurrence and metastasis. This scheme does not imply that the abnormalities arise in the sequence shown. The appearance of each may be quite independent of the appearance of the others. However, it does seem likely that certain changes will be strongly associated with more advanced stages of the disease.

MICROSATELLITE REPEAT POLYMORPHISM (MSRP) ASSAY BY POLYMERASE CHAIN REACTION

MSRPs are di, tri-, and tetranucleotide repeat DNA sequences and short tandem repeat (STR) sequences that have gained attention because they are common and ubiquitous throughout the genome and are highly polymorphic,[53,86] as is the case with variable number of tandem repeat (VNTR) polymorphisms.[62] They commonly show levels of heterozygosity between 30% and 80%. Polymerase chain reaction (PCR) primers are designed for unique sequences flanking each MSRP, and tumor and normal DNA from each patient can be amplified (Fig. 12-12). After amplification, the PCR product is fractionated on denaturing 6% polyacrylimide gels. The alleles in the tumor lane can then be visualized on x-ray film and compared with those in the normal DNA lanes.

Microsatellite repeat polymorphism (MSRP) results

Loss of the short arm of chromosome 9 is a common and sometimes early cytogenetic change in SCCHN. This

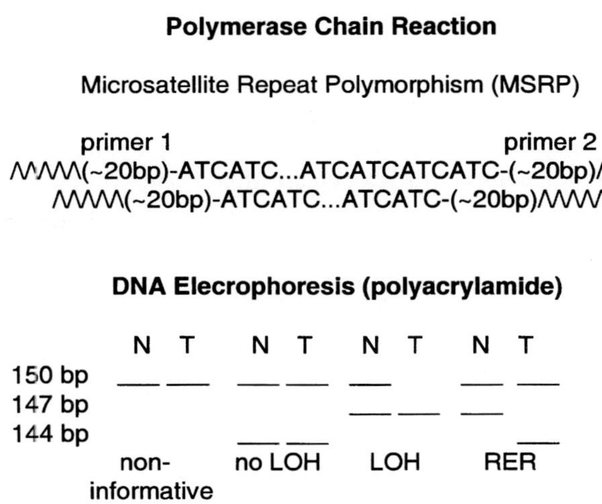

FIG 12-12
Polymerase chain reaction for microsatellite repeat polymorphisms. MSRPs are highly variable in length, so that most people are heterozygous at these loci. MSRPs that are located within a chromosomal region of interest are selected for analysis, and a primer on each side is employed in the PCR reaction to amplify the sequence in both tumor DNA and normal DNA from each subject. The DNA is electophoresed, and, in the example shown, if the subject is homozygous at this locus *(two far left lanes)* the probe is not informative with respect to the question of whether the tumor cells have lost one copy of this part of the genome. However, if the patient is heterozygous, retention of heterozygosity *(second pair of lanes)* indicates that no deletion occurred in the tumor or, alternatively, loss of heterozygosity is compelling evidence that one copy of the MSRP has been deleted. A change in the banding pattern, with retention of heterozygosity *(far right two lanes)*, indicates that an error (replication error, RER) has occurred within one of the MSRP alleles. The presence of RER at multiple loci appears to signify loss of replication accuracy in the tumor cell population.

loss was observed in three of seven stage I-II tumors,[81] and in one of these it was the sole autosomal abnormality.[92] For this reason, 9p was targeted using PCR typing of D9S199 and the closely linked IFNA and D9S126 MSRPs. D9S126 is the closest polymorphic target to MLM, the hypothesized malignant melanoma tumor suppressor[11,24] and is also lost in non–small cell lung carcinoma and other tumors.[65]

The experiments employed matched normal and tumor tissue DNA (and cell line DNA, when available). The results are consistent with our cytogenetic observations: of 29 patients who were heterozygous at this locus in their blood DNA, 12 (41%) exhibited LOH in tumor DNA. LOH was observed in seven of 14 (50%) informative patients who have died and in five of 15 (33%) informative patients who are still alive. Although the sample size is small, the trend is consistent with the predicted inverse association between LOH and survival.

For similar reasons, we targeted the ANK1 locus, a dinucleotide repeat polymorphism locus that resides proximal 8p. As with the chromosome 9 experiment, matched normal and tumor DNA were employed. Again, the results are consistent with the cytogenetic findings: there was LOH in the tumor DNA from three of 19 (16%) heterozygous patients, with no differences associated with survival.

In further studies that are continuing in our laboratory, we have thus far evaluated multiple MSRP loci from chromosomes 3, 5, 8, 9, 18, and 21 in 43 patients with SCCHN. The extent of LOH has approximated that expected based on the earlier cytogenetic studies. For example, loss of 9p was observed in 48% of tumors from the chromosome studies, and 52% of tumors expressed LOH for 9p loci. Although the data must be considered preliminary because relatively few loci have been evaluated and formal biostatistical analysis is pending, we observed more LOH in tumors of patients who have died than in tumors of patients who have survived more than two years since diagnosis. This is true for every MSRP tested. Similarly, replication errors at MSRP loci were observed in only 19% of patients who are still alive but in 53% of those who have died. These findings suggest that some combination of MSRPs may serve as useful biomarkers of prognosis in SCCHN patients.

ETHICAL ISSUES IN CANCER GENETIC RESEARCH

As cancer research progresses and the ability to identify cancer genes becomes more commonplace, a number of ethical issues will likely arise. Much of this is related to the new information and the effect of this information on genetic screening, therapy, and confidentiality. Such issues should be considered before genetic data is used widely in the care and prevention of cancer from any site, not just the head and neck. At the present time, with a few exceptions, head and neck cancer genetic research has revolved around the genetics of the tumors rather than the genetics of the individuals. However, using recent findings in other common cancers such as the familial predisposition identified in some individuals with breast cancer, it is not only conceivable but also likely that many head and neck cancers will be found to occur in patients with genetic predisposition to cancer. Three major potential ethical areas would seem to be present which need to be addressed: genetic therapy, genetic information, and genetic screening.

Two types of gene therapy are possible at this time: somatic and germ cell. In somatic gene therapy, a new gene is inserted into the cells of an individual to alter the course of a life-threatening disease or cancer, such as inserting a normal RB1 into patients with retinoblastoma. In germ line therapy, a new cell is implanted into a fertilized egg of an individual who carries a familial gene for a particular disorder, such as cystic fibrosis, thereby passing on a normal gene to subsequent generations.[35] Many questions arise when considering either of these interventions. There may be a substantial cost in screening for these individuals and subsequently applying the gene therapy. If so, who pays for this? If the cost is great enough to restrict some from receiving the treatment, who will decide how to ration? What at first may seem like a marvelous breakthrough in the prevention of a fatal disease may have substantial implications to subsequent generations. Many genetic changes occur to provide a selective advantage for the individuals who carry those genes. An obvious example is the sickle cell anemia gene. Homozygous individuals develop a severe and potentially fatal sickle disease, while heterozygous individuals develop minimal sequelae. It now seems apparent that this gene helps in protection against malaria and therefore may actually increase the survival rate of the population that carry the gene. A similar scenario may be present with cancer genes. Is there a selective advantage in the population to carry these genes, are those who die from the cancer doing so for the benefit of others, and might there be a more universal problem which might arise if these genes are eliminated by therapy? These are questions which cannot be answered until more information is accumulated, but such dilemmas need to be considered.

There are many implications to genetic screening. Many of these revolve around cost and limitations in resources. If there is a patient who has a hereditary predisposition to an environmentally mediated cancer such as smoking and alcohol in head and neck cancer, can identification of such people through genetic screening allow for early intervention with prevention and behavioral modification techniques. This, of course, is a considerable opportunity. However, screening may be able to identify only a few patients of the total population and the cost to screen the entire population may by excessive. In such cases, how are the resources allocated? Is there an opportunity for employers, the government, insurance companies, or other groups to use such information to restrict services, employment, or health care? What if consumer demand for screening surpasses the health care system's ability to provide such services? How will consents be obtained? Should screening be offered if no therapy is available? What are the potential economic and social discriminations which might ensue? Many more potential questions will arise and these will all need to be addressed.

The final, and perhaps most important, ethical area is related to the information itself. As implied above, this information has the potential to be used to discriminate against certain individuals or groups, which may affect their ability to receive health care, insurance, jobs, etc. Who owns the information once it is obtained? How do we as a society maintain the confidentiality of an individual's genetic fingerprint? What if such information has negative implications on the health of others? Does the family have the rights to such information and what happens to the information after death? Again, the potential questions that will be raised may be endless and these are just a few that have been presented to stimulate thoughtful consideration of such issues. As we make progress on the scientific efforts to identify the genetics of head and neck cancer, we must become aware of and plan for the significant social and economic ethical issues that will ensue.

SUMMARY

Physicians who treat patients with SCC, one of the most common human cancers, need better prognostic indicators. Recurrent genetic losses are clear prognostic indicators in other solid tumors. We hypothesize that recurrent genetic losses in SCCHN will have prognostic significance. Further research is desired because of the high probability that it will lead to the identification of discrete genetic events that commonly occur in squamous cancer cells and that are biologically important. Many of these events will probably be associated with disease progression, metastases, and poor survival. Identification of genetic biomarkers in SCC will provide important new parameters for clinical evaluation and will allow improved design of therapeutic protocols. Although ethical dilemmas as well as technical roadblocks certainly remain, such biomarkers will transfer readily to the general biomedical community and will be widely applicable.

REFERENCES

1. Babu VR et al: Tumor behavior in transitional cell carcinoma of the bladder in relation to chromosomal markers and histopathology. Cancer Res 47:6800-6805, 1987.
2. Benedict WF et al: Patient with 13 chromosome deletion: evidence that the retinoblastoma gene is a recessive cancer gene. Science 219:973-975, 1983.
3. Benninger MS: Presentation and evaluation of patients with epidermoid head and neck cancers. Henry Ford Hospital Med J 40:144-8, 1992.
4. Bigner SH et al: Chromosomal evolution in malignant human gliomas starts with specific and usually numerical deviations. Cancer Genet Cytogenet 22:121-135, 1986.
5. Blieche I et al: Two distinct regions involved in 1p deletion in human primary breast cancer. Cancer Res 53:1990-1994, 1993.

6. Bradford CR et al: Human papillomavirus DNA sequences in cell lines derived from head and neck squamous cell carcinomas. Otolaryngol Head Neck Surg 104:303-10, 1991.
7. Bradford CR et al: Chromosome 11p13 deletions and 11p breakpoints in squamous cell carcinoma: association with altered reactivity with the UM-E7 antibody. Genes Chromsomes Ca 3:272-282, 1991.
8. Buchagen DL et al: Hemizygosity on chromosome 3p correlates with cytogenetic losses in head and neck squamous cell carcinoma (SCC) cell lines. Fourth Res Workshop Biol Prevention Treatment Head Neck Cancer. Arlington, VA, September 8-11, 1994. Head Neck 16:475, 1994.
9. Burgio DL et al: DNA ploidy of primary and metastatic squamous cell head and neck cancers. Arch Otolaryngol Head Neck Surg 118:185-7, 1992.
10. Cann CI, Fried MP, Rothman KJ: Epidemiology of squamous cell cancer of the head and neck. Otolaryngol Clin 18:1-22, 1985.
11. Cannon-Albright LA et al: Assignment of a locus for familial melanoma, MLM, to chromosome 9p13-p22. Science 258:148-1152, 1992.
12. Carey TE et al: Characterization of laryngeal primary and metastatic squamous cell carcinoma cell lines UM-SCC-17A and UM-SCC-17B. Cancer Res 49:6098-6107, 1989.
13. Cavenee WK et al: Expression of recessive alleles by chromosomal mechanisms in retinoblastoma. Nature 305:779-784, 1983.
14. Collins VP, James CD: Gene and chromosomal alterations associated with the development of human gliomas. FASEB J 7:926-930, 1993.
15. Cowan JM, Halaban R, Francke U: Cytogenetic analysis of melanocytes from premalignant nevi and melanomas. J Natl Cancer Inst 80:1159-1164, 1988.
16. Dalbagni G et al: Genetic alterations in bladder cancer. Lancet 342:469-71, 1993.
17. D'Amico D et al: Polymorphic sites within the MCC and APC loci reveal very frequent loss of heterozygosity in human small cell lung cancer. Cancer Res 52:1996-1999, 1992.
18. Davidson BJ, Hsu TC, Schantz SP: The genetics of tobacco induced malignancy. Arch Otolaryngol Head Neck Surg 119:1198-205, 1993.
19. Decker J, Goldstein JR: Risk factors in head and neck cancer. N Engl J Med 306:1151-5, 1982.
20. Dolcetti R et al: p53 Overexpression is an early event in the development of human squamous-cell carcinoma of the larynx. Int J Cancer 52:178-182, 1992.
21. Emi M et al: Isolation and mapping of 88 new RFLP markers on human chromosome 8. Genomics 14:1261-6, 1992.
22. Fearon ER et al: Identification of a chromosome 18q gene that is altered in colorectal cancers. Science 247:49-56, 1990.
23. Fearon ER, Jones PA: Progressing toward a molecular description of colorectal cancer development. FASEB J 6:2783-2790, 1992.
24. Field JK et al: The role of p53 tumor suppressor gene in squamous cell carcinoma of the head and neck. Arch Otolaryngol Head Neck Surg 119:1118-22, 1993.
25. Field JK et al: Alelic imbalance and instability in squamous cell carcinoma of the head and neck. Head Neck 16:475, 1994.
26. Fletcher JA et al: Diagnostic relevance of clonal cytogenetic aberrations in malignant soft-tissue tumors. New Engl J Med 324:436-43, 1991.
27. Fliss DM et al: Laryngeal verrucous carcinoma: a clinicopathologic study and detection of human papillomavirus using polymerase chain reaction. Laryngoscope 104:146-50, 1994.
28. Fountain JW et al: Homozygous deletions within human chromosome band 9p21 in melanoma. PNAS 89:10557-10561, 1992.
29. Fountain JW et al: Genetic and physical map of the interferon region on chromosome 9p. Genomics 45:105-112, 1992.
30. Friend SH et al: A human DNA segment with properties of the gene that predisposes to retinoblastoma and osteosarcoma. Nature 323:643-646, 1986.
31. Furukawa Y et al: Structure, expression, and chromosome assignment of the human catenin (cadherin-associated protein) alpha 1 gene (CTNNA1). Cytogenet Cell Genet 64:74-78, 1994.
32. Gandour-Edwards RF et al: DNA content of head and neck squamous carcinoma by flow and image cytometry. Arch Otolaryngol Head Neck Surgery 120:294-7, 1994.
33. Goldsmith MM et al: Part I: DNA flow cytometry as prognostic indicator in head and neck cancer. Otolaryngol Head Neck Surg 96:307-18, 1987.
34. Goldsmith MM: The importance of the eosinophil in head and neck cancer. Otolaryngol Head Neck Surg 106:27-33, 1982.
35. Goldstein DA: Ethical dilemmas in molecular genetics. Arch Otolaryngol Head Neck Surg 119:1183-6, 1993.
36. Greenberg ER et al: A clinical trial of beta carotene to prevent basal cell and squamous cell cancers of the skin. N Engl J Med 323:789-95, 1990.
37. Grenman SE et al: UM-EC-1, a new hypodiploid human cell line derived from a poorly differentiated endometrial cancer. Cancer Res 48:1864-1869, 1988.
38. Grenman SE et al: Establishment and characterization of UM-EC-2, a tamoxifen-sensitive, estrogen receptor-negative human endometrial carcinoma cell line. Gynecol Oncol 37:188-199, 1990.
39. Grenman SE et al: Phenotypic characterization, karyotype analysis and in vitro tamoxifen sensitivity of new ER-negative vulvar carcinoma cell lines UM-SCV-1A and UM-SCV-1B. Int J Cancer 45:920-927, 1990.
40. Heo DS et al: Biology, cytogenetics, and sensitivity to immunological effector cells of new head and neck squamous cell carcinoma lines. Cancer Res 49:5167-5175, 1989.
41. Hong WK et al: Prevention of second primary tumors with isotretinoin in squamous cell carcinoma of the head and neck. N Engl J Med 323:795-801, 1990.
42. Huang Y et al: Loss of heterozygosity involves multiple tumor suppressor genes in human esophageal cancers. Cancer Res 52:6525-6530, 1992.
43. Hussussian CJ et al: Germ line p16 mutations in familial melanoma. Nature Genetics 8:15-21, 1994.
44. James CD et al: Chromosome 9 deletion mapping reveals interferon a and interferon B-1 gene deletions in human glial tumors. Cancer Res 51:1684-88, 1991.
45. Jiang W et al: Amplification and espression of the human cyclin D gene in esophageal cancer. Cancer Res 52:2980-2983, 1992.
46. Jin Y et al: Chromosome abnormalities in 83 head and neck squamous cell carcinomas: influence of culture conditions on karyotypic pattern. Cancer Res 53:2140-2146, 1993.
47. Johns ME Papel ID: Carcinoma of the oral cavity and pharynx. In Lee KJ, editor: Essential Otolaryngology, ed 4. New York, 1987, Medical Examination Publishing Company.
48. Kadowaki T et al: E-cadherin and α-catenin expression in human esophageal cancer. Cancer Res 54:291-296, 1994.
49. Knudson A: Genetics of tumors of the head and neck. Arch Otolaryngol Head Neck Surg 119:735-7, 1993.
50. Latif F et al: Chromosome 3p deletions in head and neck carcinomas: statistical ascertainment of allelic loss. Cancer Res 52:1451-1456, 1992.
51. Lee NK et al: p53, Retinoblastoma, and human papillomavirus in squamous cell carcinoma and adjacent normal mucosa of the upper aerodigestive tract. Arch Otolaryngol Head Neck Surg 119:1125-31, 1993.
52. Lindblom A et al: Deletions on chromosome 16 in patients with breast carcinoma are associated with development of distant metastases. Cancer Res 53:3707-3711, 1993.
53. Litt M, Luty JA: A hypervariable microsatellite revealed by in vitro amplification of a dinucleotide repeat within the cardiac muscle actin gene. Am J Hum Genet 44:397-401, 1989.

54. Lydiatt WM, Schantz SP: Loss of heterozygosity in head and neck tumors is more frequent in patients without a history of tobacco exposure. Head Neck 16:475, 1994.
55. Maestro R et al: Three discrete regions of deletion at 3p in head and neck cancers. Cancer Res 53:5775-5779, 1993.
56. Malkin P et al: Germline mutates of the -53 tumor-suppressor gene in children and young adults with second malignant neoplasms. N Engl J Med 326:1309-15, 1992.
57. Marx J: New colon cancer gene discovered. Science 260:751-2, 1993.
58. Marx J: How p53 suppresses cell growth. Science 262:1644-5, 1993.
59. Marx J: How cells cycle toward cancer. Science 264:319-21, 1994.
60. Mohit-Tabatabai M et al: Relation of thickness of floor of mouth Stage I and II cancers to regional metastases. Am J Surg 152:351-3, 1986.
61. Muleris M, Salmon RJ, Dutrillaux B: Cytogenetics of colorectal adenocarcinoma. Cancer Genet Cytogenet 46:143-156, 1990.
62. Nakamura Y et al: Science 235:1616-1622, 1987.
63. Nakashima T et al: Chemosensitivity and DNA ploidy in head and neck squamous cell carcinomas. Arch Otolaryngol Head Neck Surg 118:1031-6, 1992.
64. Nishisho I et al: Mutations of chromosome 5q21 in FAP and colorectal cancer patients. Science 253:665-669, 1991.
65. Olopade OI et al: Homozygous loss of the interferon genes defines the critical region on 9p that is deleted in lung cancers. Cancer Res 53:2410-2415, 1993.
66. Petty EM et al: Molecular definition of chromosome 9p21 germ line deletion in a woman with multiple melanoma. Am J Hum Genet 53:96-104, 1993.
67. Powell SM et al: Molecular diagnosis of familial adenomatous polyposis. N Engl J Med 329:1982-7, 1993.
68. Roa RA et al: DNA content of human squamous cell carcinoma cell lines. Arch Otolaryngol 111:563-575, 1985.
69. Rowley JD: The clinical applications of new DNA diagnostic technology on the management of cancer patients. JAMA 270:2331-2337, 1993.
70. Samedro A et al: Quantitative pathology of the intraepithelial laryngeal neoplasia. Otolaryngol Head Neck Surg 110:185-94, 1944.
71. Schipper JH et al: E-Cahederin expression in squamous cell carcinomas of the head and neck: inverse correlation with tumor dedifferentiation and lymph node metastasis. Cancer Res 51:6328-6337, 1991.
72. Sellers TA et al: Segregation analysis of smoking-associated malignancies: evidence for mendelian inheritance. Am J Med Genet 52:308-314, 1994.
73. Smith DI, Alonso M: Cloning of tumor suppressor genes involved in solid tumor development. Arch Otolaryngol Head Neck Surg 30:1210-1216, 1993.
74. Solomon E et al: Chromosome 5 allele loss in human colorectal carcinomas. Nature 328:616-619, 1987.
75. Sundaresan V et al: p53 and chromosome 3 abnormalities, characteristic of malignant lung tumors, are detectable in preinvasive lesions of the bronchus. Oncogene 7:1989-1997, 1992.
76. Testa JR, Siegfried JM: Chromosome abnormalities in human non–small cell lung cancer. Cancer Res 52:2702s-2706s, 1992.
77. Trent J et al: Identification of a recurring translocation site involving chromosome 6 in human malignant melanoma. Cancer Res 49:420-423, 1989.
78. Trent J et al: Clonal chromosome abnormalities in human breast carcinomas. II. Thirty-four cases with metastatic disease. Genes Chromo Cancer 7:194-203, 1993.
79. Tsuchiya E et al: Allelotype of non–small cell lung carcinoma—comparison between loss of heterozygosity in squamous cell carcinoma and adenocarcinoma. Cancer Res 52:2478-2481, 1992.
80. van der Bosch K et al: Deletions in the short arm of chromosome 8 are present in up to 90% of human colorectal cancer cell lines. Genes Chromo Cancer 5:91-95, 1992.
81. Van Dyke DL et al: Cytogenetic analysis of 29 squamous cell carcinomas of the head and neck. Genes Chrom Cancer 9:192-206, 1994.
82. Varesco L et al: A rapid screening method to detect nonsense and frameshift mutations: identification of disease-causing *APC* alleles. Cancer Res 53:5581-5584, 1993.
83. Viegas-Pequignot E et al: Recurrent chromosome aberrations in human lung squamous cell carcinomas. Cancer Genet Cytogenet 49:37-49, 1990.
84. Vogelstein B et al: Allelotype of colorectal carcinomas. Science 244:207-211, 1989.
85. Walter MA, Peters GE, Paiper SC: Predicting radioresistence in early glottic squamous cell carcinoma by DNA content. Ann Otol Rhinol Laryngol 100:523-6, 1991.
86. Weber JL, May PE: Abundant class of human DNA polymorphisms which can be typed using the polymerase chain reaction. Amer J Hum Genet 44:388-396, 1989.
87. Whang-Peng J et al: Specific chromosome defect associated with human small-cell lung cancer: deletion 3p(14-23). Science 215:181-183, 1981.
88. Whang-Peng J, Banks-Schlegel SP, Lee EC: Cytogenetic studies of esophageal carcinoma cell lines. Cancer Genet Cytogenet 45:101-120, 1990.
89. Wolf GT et al: DNA content and regional metastasis in patients with advanced laryngeal squamous carcinoma. Laryngoscope 104:479-83, 1994.
90. Worsham MJ et al: Consistent chromosome abnormalities in squamous carcinoma of the vulva. Genes Chromosomes Cancer 3:420-432, 1991.
91. Worsham MJ et al: Molecular and cytogenetic evidence for loss of DCC in squamous cell carcinoma. Am J Hum Genet 51:A74, 1992.
92. Worsham MJ et al: Deletion 9p22-pter and loss of Y as primary chromosome abnormalities in a squamous cell carcinoma of the vocal cord. Genes Chromosomes Cancer 6:58-60, 1993.
93. Worsham MJ et al: Clonal cytogenetic evolution in a squamous cell carcinoma of the skin from a Xeroderma Pigmentosum patient, HFH-SCC-XP-1. Genes Chrom Cancer 7:158-164, 1993.
94. Worsham MJ et al: Squamous carcinomas of the head and neck are monoclonal, cytogenetically stable, and exhibit minimal intratumor heterogeneity. Fifth International Workshop Chromo Solid Tumors, Tucson, January 10-12, 1993.
95. Worsham MJ et al: Common clonal origin of synchronous primary head and neck squamous cell carcinomas: analysis by tumor karyotypes and fluorescence in situ hybridization. Hum Path 26:251-261, 1995.
96. Worsham MJ et al: Karyotype aberrations identified in cultured squamous carcinomas arise in vivo: confirmation by fluorescence in situ hybridization. Head and Neck. Submitted, 1994.
97. Yin XY et al: Gene amplification and gene dosage in cell lines derived from squamous cell carcinoma of the head and neck. Genes Chromosomes Cancer 3:443-454, 1991.

13

Head and Neck Cancer Treatment Planning: Integrating Old and New Concepts

Sharon L. Collins, M.S., M.D., F.A.C.S.

This course was developed in response to a perceived need to educate otolaryngologists in the clinical and tumor biology principles underlying rational combination therapy available to the head and neck cancer (HNC) patient. (HNC refers to squamous cell carcinoma unless otherwise stated.) In the course of busy daily practice, treatment planning for the individual patient focuses on logistics and there is no time for interdisciplinary education; chemotherapists and radiotherapists do not have time to explain the principles underlying their modalities to surgeons, and surgeons do not have time to explain the variety of operations available. These constraints in the daily practice of head and neck oncology lead to the persistence of many misconceptions, i.e., the perception that surgery is "mutilating" whereas radiation and chemotherapy are not. It is hoped that presentation of the following information will provide the otolaryngologist/HNC surgeon with a data base to allow him/her to defend the role of surgery in multimodality treatment planning in a competent manner, and to be able to assess whether or not proposed regimens of multimodality treatment make sense, i.e., to transcend the role of a "technical consultant" and join the ranks of the "cognitive" specialists.

It is an unfortunate fact that surgeons have generally failed to become involved in planning clinical cancer protocols at the national level and such activity is dominated by chemotherapists and radiotherapists. The "cytoreductive" modalities (radiation therapy, chemotherapy) are gaining ascendancy as the preferred treatment for a variety of stages and sites of HNC because they seemingly lack the detriments on function and cosmesis pursuant to surgery. Surgeons have failed to provide viable surgical alternatives to "organ preserving" strategies using cytoreductive therapies (except for some sites of larynx cancer) by continuing to perform traditional procedures which are perceived as "mutilating." Consequently, surgeons are now at risk of seeing their modality relegated to the "salvage" context. Radiotherapists are competing successfully for "early" HNC, and treatments which combine chemotherapy and radiation sequentially or simultaneously are now considered by many practitioners to be "state of the art" for stage III and IV disease (and are gradually being extended to stage II disease as well). Where does this leave the surgeon in the initial management of a HNC patient? This perspective lends immediacy to the goals of this course.

This course reviews information from both the clinical and basic science arenas relating to the development, present status, and future directions of the treatment modalities used for head and neck cancer (HNC)—surgery, irradiation, chemotherapy. What has been learned in the past about the individual **clinical** treatment modalities and their present status and future use will be summarized, and a complementary discussion will describe clinically relevant tumor biology processes which influence tumor/host interactions and the impact of the various treatments upon them—both good and bad. This parallel information will be synthesized to present a different perspective on the pros and cons of single modality treatments and principles of combining the various treatment modalities for advanced cancers. Amalgamation of such information gives a broader perspective on **outcomes** in clinical oncology and the price paid to achieve such results—an area of emerging importance in the current medical-economic milieu.

Unanswered Questions in Head and Neck Oncology

- What are appropriate prognosis/treatment response predictors?
- How should the major treatment modalities be combined in previously untreated versus previously treated patients?
- Is surgery plus radiation better than either alone for HN/SCC?
- For cancers suitable for single modality therapy, is surgery or radiation better?
- For "advanced" lesions, how should multimodality therapy be combined to be most effective and least risky?
- Is chemotherapy part of the standard treatment for advanced HNC?
- Surgical oncology:
  - What historic principles and experience underlie the current practice of HNC surgical oncology?
  - What factors influence cancer regrowth in the head and neck?
  - What is the appropriate magnitude of resection in previously treated versus untreated patients?
  - What methods can be used intraoperatively to decrease the risk of implanting cancer cells?
  - What is the appropriate context for "conservation" versus "radical" surgery?
  - How can surgery be used in "organ preservation" strategies?
- Does achieving a wider anatomic margin on locoregional disease (e.g., skull base surgery) enhance locoregional control?
- What situations are suitable for reoperation?
- How big a radiation field is necessary? What are the best fractionation schemes? What is the role of adjuvant (hyperthermia, brachytherapy, sensitizers) modalities?
- Does chemotherapy benefit the patient with HN/SCC with respect to improving locoregional control, distant metastases, and/or survival?
- What chemotherapeutic agents should be used and how should they be interdigitated with other treatment modalities?
- What is the long-term fate of complete responders?
- Can the extent of surgery be reduced by upfront cytoreductive treatments?
- What is the proper treatment for microscopic residual disease—surgery and/or RT?
- Is MORE treatment necessarily BETTER?
- What are the best methods to palliate incurable patients?

This presentation should allow the reader to evaluate more critically some of the perennial, unanswered questions in head and neck oncology (box above). Some of the topics alluded to herein are discussed in more depth elsewhere by the same author.[13,14,127-129]

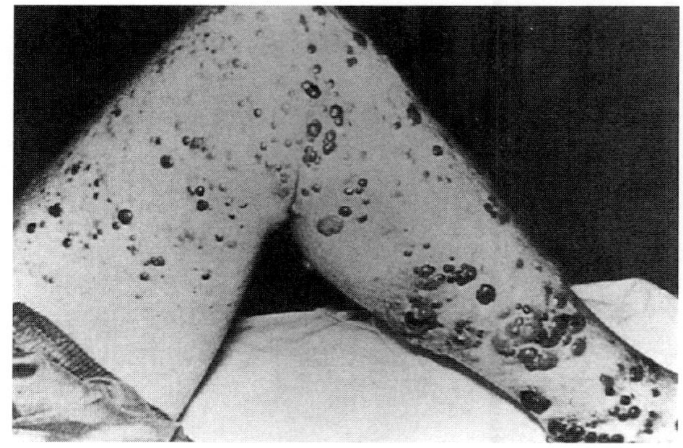

FIG 13-1
Example of tumor heterogeneity for pigmentation; melanoma metastases.

TUMOR BIOLOGY

Between the inadequacies of the clinical TNM staging system (inability of factors assessed—sex, age, performance status, site, T stage, histologic grade—to predict tumor recurrence or patient survival) and the complexities of cancer research at the cell and molecular level (largely incomprehensible to clinicians) are a variety of processes which relate to tumor/host interactions ("tumor biology") which are useful to consider when planning treatment for cancer patients. A description of some of these is presented, as well as a discussion of how the various treatment modalities impact on them in a positive or negative way.

Tumor heterogeneity

It is now known that cancer cells populating a primary neoplasm and metastatic deposits are not uniform but are biologically diverse with respect to a large number of phenotypic and genotypic characteristics, including morphologic features, cell-cycle-dependent phenomena, immunogenicity, tumorigenicity, ploidy, cell-surface receptors, enzyme markers, hormone receptors, growth rate, metabolic characteristics, pigment production (Fig. 13-1), **response to various treatment modalities,** and **metastatic potential.** Many metastasis researchers now believe that the successful establishment of metastases represents the selective emergence of pre-existing subpopulations of cells that are endowed with special properties which allow them to survive to complete the arduous and highly selective process of metastasis.[149,155,156,162]

The presence of multiple clonal subpopulations within neoplasms (intrinsic tumor heterogeneity/intraneoplastic diversity) is a universal adaptive mechanism that allows tumors to survive and adapt to adverse situations, analogous to genetic diversity in the evolution of organisms.[25,76] Multiple subpopulations arise during growth of a primary (or metastatic) neoplasm through processes of mutation, selection, and/or aberrant differentiation. Intratumoral heteroge-

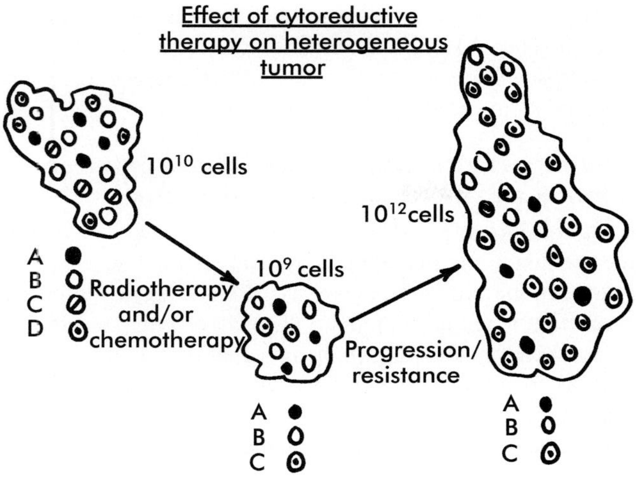

FIG 13-2
Effect of cytoreductive treatment on a heterogeneous tumor. Although tumor bulk may initially decrease and some subpopulations may be eliminated, altered relationships between the remaining tumor cell populations may lead to rapid tumor repopulation after chemotherapy and/or radiotherapy.

neity is a dynamic phenomenon with continual emergence of new variant subpopulations that can interact with each other to influence growth, metastases, and sensitivity to treatment.[48,49,57,86,117]

Tumor heterogeneity is reflected at the clinical level by the predictably unpredictable nature of tumor growth. Patients can present with metastatic disease from a small or even undetectable primary tumor, whereas other patients have huge primary tumors that do not metastasize. A spectrum of outcomes may be seen among individuals with the same type, site, and stage of tumor. Some patients survive well in symbiosis with multiple primary tumors for years, whereas others succumb quickly to recurrences of small, putatively curable cancers.

The importance of clonal heterogeneity to tumor treatment and response has long been appreciated by medical oncologists but has received relatively little attention from radiation oncologists (who have historically considered differences in intrinsic radiosensitivity in neoplastic subpopulations too small to markedly influence treatment and because their focus has been on differences in radiosensitivity between normal and tumor tissues and on the influence of tumor microenvironment factors such as oxygenation[80,123]), and surgeons are even less cognizant of this important phenomenon.

As discussed below, tumors tend to stabilize their relative proportions and impose an equilibrium on the conglomerate population[76] both within and between cancer deposits (primary and metastases). Removal of a major clone by a cytoreductive treatment modality can permit the other subpopulations to proliferate unchecked and become dominant[6,36] (Fig. 13-2), and cytoreductive treatments (which shrink but do not totally eradicate a tumor) may stimulate cancer cell repopulation. Rapid tumor cell repopulation is currently thought to be a major limiting factor to obtaining cure in patients treated by RT and/or chemotherapy.[4,24,36] The diversified resurgent population is likely to be resistant to the treatment modality that removed the dominant clone initially.[36,115] In addition, some cancer cells appear to be intrinsically resistant to chemotherapy[11,15] or RT[52,111,112] a mechanism underlying the fact that such treatments are **cytoreductive** only; they do not kill all cancer cells because they kill a constant **proportion** rather than a constant **number** of cancer cells.[37] Thus, **cytoreductive** treatments can act as selection agents which can alter intra- and intertumoral "homeostasis," allowing aggressive variants to gain ascendancy. Shrinkage of a heterogeneous tumor may influence tumor/host interactions in positive or negative ways.

The concept of selection of aggressive variants is familiar to otolaryngologists in the context of the traditional dogma that verrucous carcinoma should not be radiated.[77] Presumably radiation of verrucous carcinoma can convert a benign-acting tumor which never metastasizes into an extremely aggressive variant which can spread widely to kill the host. In the present author's view, this phenomenon is not unique to verrucous carcinoma. **Selection mechanisms can act whenever cytoreductive treatments are applied to a heterogeneous tumor cell population.** The author has seen a number of instances of regrowth of T_1 glottic cancers (SCC) after RT—generally considered highly radiocurable—which resist repeated attempts at surgical salvage and eventuate in the patient's death. Interestingly, this pattern of cancer recurrence has not been seen (by the author) following initial surgical treatment (cordectomy or hemilaryngectomy).

HNC has been shown to be more heterogeneous than tumors from colon, breast, and non–small cell lung cancer, with a greater proportion of radioresistant subpopulations in HNC than in the other cancer types.[59] Such heterogeneity may be sufficient to explain the significantly decreased radiosensitivity often seen with recurrent head and neck tumors.[111] Evidence of heterogeneity in HNC also comes from studies on patients who have received chemotherapy.[23] **Thus, studies have specifically shown that HNC can be negatively influenced by treatments usually thought to benefit cancer patients.**

Another example of a potentially negative effect of treatment on tumor-host symbiosis is the **"tumor bed effect" of radiotherapy.** Not only can radiation treatment of heterogeneous tumors which possess intrinsically radioresistant cells result in the production of more radioresistant neoplasms, but radiation injury to **normal tissue** contiguous with heterogeneous neoplasms may play a major modulating role influencing the ultimate outcome of radiation treatment (the tumor bed effect).[59,65,74] The tumor bed effect—an effect on **normal** radiated tissue—is thought to reflect an altered hostile environment which can impact on an adjacent heterogeneous tumor by causing competition among neoplastic subpopulations for limited resources and nutrients. This produces a stimulation leading to extinction of minor subpopulations within the tumor, regardless of whether or not such populations are radioresistant.

The tumor bed effect can be a potent selecting agent. As the overall size of the tumor shrinks with radiation and the proportion of sensitive cells shrinks, the resistant subpopulation is no longer in the minority and therefore does not undergo selection and extinction and may gain ascendancy; this selects intrinsically aggressive and radioresistant cells for survival. Based on some mathematical models it is likely that such a radiation-induced selection process probably would be most effective at relatively low radiation doses, precisely in the range that fractionated clinical radiotherapy is delivered.[59]

Thus the effect of radiation on normal tissue stroma may provide a favorable environment for cancer cell regrowth while simultaneously producing a cytotoxic effect on the tumor. This is a mechanism whereby noncurative RT can result in a radioresistant tumor; growth of intrinsically radioresistant tumor subpopulations present in HNC can be favored during fractionated RT. Similar mechanisms may well operate after chemotherapy[58] or a combination of the two as well.

There may also be a "tumor bed effect" related to chemotherapy and surgery, but these remain to be characterized. Any time tumor cells are killed, lysis and release of cell-free factors occur, oxygenation levels of local tissue change, and scarring can affect the local milieu. All of these factors (and many other) can alter intra- and intertumoral interactions among heterogeneous tumor deposits to the benefit or detriment of the host. Thus, **all cancer treatments modulate tumor/host interactions,** a changing baseline with an impredictable outcome. The fact that cancer treatment often has a good result may relate more importantly to "tumor biology" factors than to treatment *per se,* especially when cytoreductive treatments are used which (by definition) do not kill all cancer cells. Many cancer theoreticians believe that attributing outcome to treatment is somewhat naive.[147,163]

As we have seen, the effects of treatment on a heterogeneous tumor population can enhance **or** suppress tumor growth because of the dynamic and changing equilibrium of complex tumor/host interactions. Currently available treatment modalities—surgery, radiation, chemotherapy—are acknowledged to be quite nonspecific, and hope for the future is that there will be an increasing role for **biologic therapy of cancer**—a modified form of immunotherapy including gene therapy—which will hopefully circumvent some of the problems of resistance of a heterogeneous cancer cell population to provide a more specific attack on cancer with fewer complications.[5,20] Again, such agents are **modulatory** (stimulatory **or** suppressive) and affect many biologic responses other than those associated with cancer growth. The end result depends on many endogenous relationships which are currently difficulty to characterize. Consequently, toxicities are presently significant.

Tumor-host interactions: interactions between primary and metastatic tumor deposits

A considerable body of experimental evidence supports the existence of mechanisms regulating total tumor mass within an individual organism.[32-34,40] In some nonimmunogenic tumor model systems with well-vascularized metastases (thereby excluding poor oxygenation and nutrition as reasons for growth retardation), the existence of a "tumor-related systemic growth-retarding factor" has been hypothesized. Nearly synchronous slowing of the growth rate of a primary tumor and its spontaneous metastases after the primary tumor reaches a critical size has been noted.[21] Sudden removal of a primary tumor's metastasis-inhibiting influence could explain the phenomenon of "metastatic explosion" which is occasionally noted after surgical excision of primary tumors. Based on tumor biology principles, release of subclinical metastases could equally follow cytoreductive therapy as well. It has been shown experimentally many times that irradiation can negatively influence the tumor-host interaction.[3,97] Irradiation of a primary tumor can be followed by growth of metastases larger than those which occur when the primary tumor is untreated.[108]

Concern that chemotherapy may increase metastatic rate has been noted in several reports in the HNC literature.[6,88] Although some studies of combination therapy have been interpreted to show meaningful reduction in the incidence of distant metastases (DMs) due to the addition of chemotherapy,[55] other authors have expressed concern that an alteration in the tumor-host interaction occurs after multimodality therapy which results in an increased incidence of metastases. It has been suggested that multimodality therapies might prove "double-edged swords"; while causing significant locoregional tumor regression they might promote frequent early DMs. Increased treatment has also been hypothesized to increase locoregional recurrence.[73] Such differing results in the clinical literature are more understandable based on the tumor biology/treatment factors discussed above. More treatment is not necessarily better.

The tumor-dormant state

The phenomenon of tumor growth appearing many years after apparently effective and permanent control of a cancer is attributable to regrowth of dormant tumor cells which have persisted in occult form for long periods of time in symbiosis with the host. Such tumor cells must have spread prior to removal of the primary tumor and lain dormant until "triggered" to regrow.[28,113] Pulmonary metastases in rats have been activated, leading to macroscopic disease when the hosts were immunosuppressed by whole body irradiation or thoracic duct drainage, suggesting immunologically

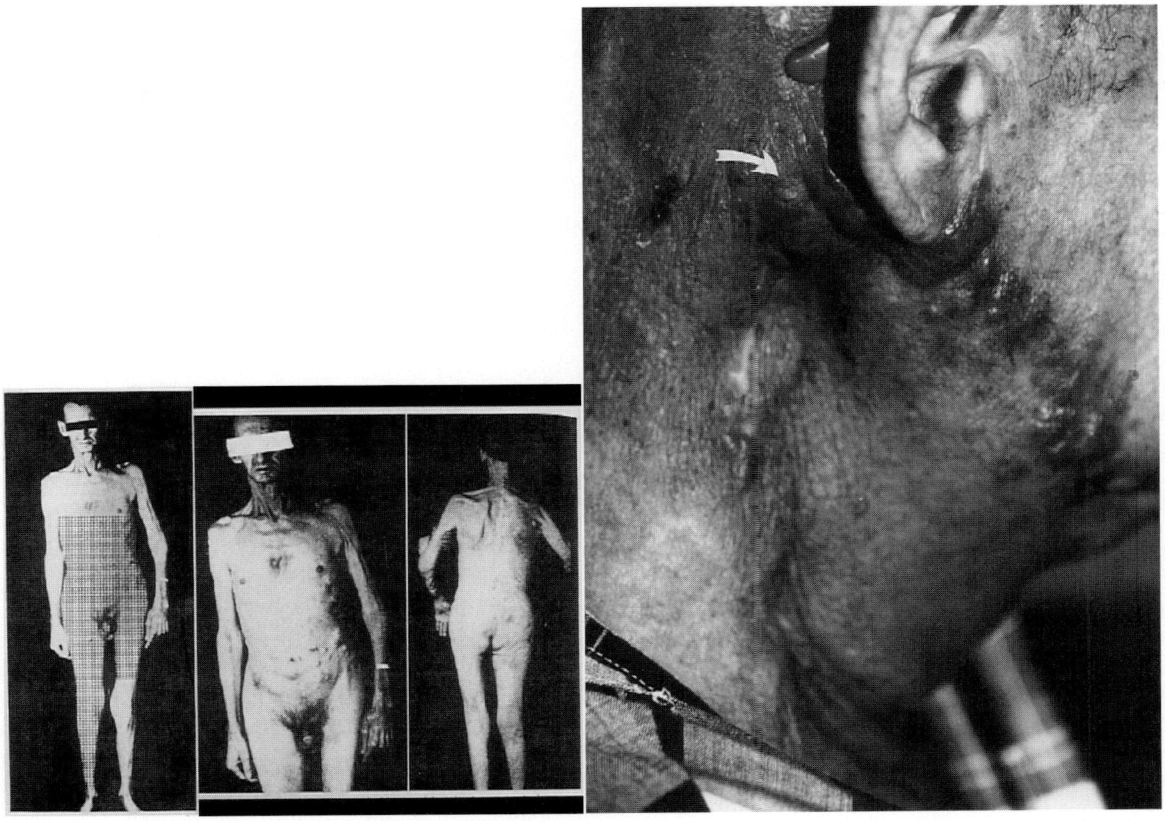

A

B

FIG 13-3
Examples of inflammatory oncotaxis: **A,** patient who was "cured" of laryngeal cancer by radiation five years prior required application of a body cast after trauma. When the cast was removed, multiple nodules of squamous carcinoma (which presumably had been dormant at distant sites in the patient's body) had developed in the distribution of the body cast. **B,** recurrent tumor outlining the margins of a radiation portal *(arrows)*. This suggests an altered interface between irradiated and nonirradiated tissue which may influence cancer regrowth, reminiscent of the tumor bed effect (see text).

mediated restraint of dormant tumor cells. Hormonal stimulation of dormant tumor cells has also been achieved.

There have been reports of the development of metastases after a long latent interval in cancer patients in areas of trauma; bruises, intramuscular injections (including dinitrochlorobenzene), distant skin graft donor sites, and other surgical wounds. For example, one patient "cured" of carcinoma of the larynx (5 years following radiation therapy) had a body cast applied for a spinal injury and subsequently developed SCC metastases in the skin underlying the cast (Fig. 13-3). At autopsy the patient did not have any locoregional tumor and cancer regrowth presumably represented reactivation of dormant tumor cells by trauma.[12] Tissue injury and inflammation can apparently enhance localization, implantation, and growth of circulating cancer cells at the site of the inflammatory response; a process known as "inflammatory oncotaxis."[19]

Tumor recurrence after long disease-free intervals implies either growth of dormant cells pre-existing at the points of trauma or an active attraction of dormant cells to these points from distant sources. Fisher[31] has suggested that some local cancer recurrences may actually represent this latter mechanism—"homing" of distant cancer cells to surgically traumatized areas rather than regrowth of cancer cells spilled or implanted in the wound during surgery.

It should be noted that surgery is not the only trauma-inducing mechanism; radiotherapy and chemotherapy can also cause inflammation and may significantly alter the tumor-host interaction by long-term exposure to tumor necrosis products. Although surgery under general anesthesia certainly can negatively affect the immune response,[45-47,75,79,81,85] surgery at least eliminates the bulk of tumor in a few hours.

CLINICAL ONCOLOGY—OVERVIEW

No one knows the best treatment for any size, site, or stage of head and neck squamous cell carcinoma (SCC) due to the lack of prospective randomized studies which have compared all three treatment modalities in a homogeneous patient group in one study. The (mainly retrospective) HNC literature is also confusing and contradictory because different end points are reported. All clinical oncologists are

> **Treatment Planning Considerations in Patients with Head and Neck Squamous Cancer**
>
> **Treatment/doctor factors**
>
> WHICH MD GETS THERE FIRST
> - Specialty bias vs multidisciplinary team
> - Referral patterns (competition, "cash flow")
> - Occasional vs frequent operator (medically inoperable/ technically unresectable)
> - Locally available expertise
>
> "FRESH" CASE VS PREVIOUSLY TREATED
> TREATMENT GOAL—CURE VS PALLIATION
>
> **Tumor factors**
>
> STAGE AND PRESENTATION
> - Anatomic site
> - Nodal/distant metastases
>
> HISTOPATHOLOGY
> - Tumor-host interface pattern
> - Lymphatic-vascular invasion
> - Interstitial spread, necrosis
>
> MULTIPLE PRIMARIES
> TUMOR-HOST RESPONSE TO PRIOR TX
> - Aggressiveness
> - Is the patient "beating the odds"?
>
> **Patient factors**
>
> - Genetic susceptibilities (clinical spectrum)
> - Age
> - Sex (hormones)
> - Habits:
>   diet
>   exercise
>   tobacco
>   alcohol
> - Attitude: "Will to live"
> - Support mechanisms
> - Socioeconomic status
>   Educational level
>   Access/use of medical care
>   Follow-up reliability
> - Intercurrent disease
> - Occupation/hobbies
> - Expectations/desires/fears preconceived notions; especially concerning various treatment modalities

ultimately interested in the survival of the patient. However, this is a very "contaminated" end point due to the many factors which impact on it (box above). Also, surgery and RT are locoregional treatment modalities (directed at the primary tumor and regional lymph node metastases) and do not affect (except possibly in a negative way—see tumor biology section above) the systemic component of the disease. Distant metastases are emerging as a more important limiting factor to cure[23,60,102,103] of HNC patients, since there is currently no reliably effective, curative treatment for systemic metastases. Thus, the end point of "control in the treated volume" is more appropriate for surgery and RT, especially when one is attempting to assess the impact of variations in locoregional treatment, such as comparing the outcome of radical versus conservation surgery[127] or assessing altered RT fractionation schemes. For example, in evaluating the validity of a modification of a traditional surgical procedure, one must look at the incidence of recurrent cancer adjacent to retained structures (as was done with conservation surgery for larynx cancer) rather than at survival *per se* since the latter end point is far removed from events that are occurring in the treated area. The radiotherapy literature reports "control in the treated volume," but the surgery literature focuses on survival. Therefore, because the wrong end result is reported (and because scientific trials are lacking), controversies persist concerning almost every question of interest to the HNC oncologist (see box on p 154).

The problem is further complicated by the fact that in order to accumulate data on these rare entities, treatment results of different cancer sites and stages are often lumped in discussions of "head and neck cancer," but this combines apples, oranges, and potatoes since the natural history of cancer in subsites of the head and neck is significantly different. These differences are obscured in such amalgamations. For example, larynx cancer has been the category of HNC traditionally used for investigation of altered treatment modalities (conservation surgery, additive chemotherapy) because endolaryngeal cancers have a favorable natural history, and, if the treatment under investigation fails, salvage of recurrent/persistent cancer with standard modalities (salvage surgery or RT) is often successful. But the natural history of laryngeal cancer differs significantly from other sites—pharyngeal wall, hypopharynx, oral cavity, sinus, etc.—and it is not valid, therefore, to extrapolate experimental data from one tumor site to others.[137,141] Similarly, data from different institutions cannot be lumped or rigorously compared (as is often done to get adequate numbers to support a point) because there is no control of the many factors which bias treatment selection.

Nevertheless, standard dogma which has emerged from the very flawed HNC literature has resulted in the following tenets which are generally accepted:

- Single modality surgery *or* RT results in equivalent survival for "early stage" (Stage I and II) HN SCC.
- For "advanced disease" (Stage III and IV) combination therapy is needed for any chance to control locoregional disease; a necessary (but not sufficient) prerequisite for ultimate cure of the patient.

It is important to note that the term "advanced HNC" (stage III and IV) applies to a very "mixed bag" of disease entities which differ in their natural history. For example, Stage III HN SCC could include a T_3N_0 glottic cancer and a T_1N_1 supraglottic cancer, either of which might be cured with single-modality treatment (including conservation surgery in some cases)! Thus, maintaining that all "advanced HNC" requires multimodality therapy (including chemotherapy) or that the treatment goal in these patients is palliation (often the goal of RT and chemotherapy) rather than cure (traditionally the goal of surgery) is not always valid.

Similarly, extending multimodality protocols to Stage II patients (T_2N_0) who are at low risk for regional or systemic disease presently appears even less appropriate. This is sometimes justified as an alternative to "mutilating surgery" but probably reflects lack of versatility on the part of the surgeon (e.g., unfamiliarity with partial laryngectomy procedures, etc.) more than a compelling need based on tumor biology.

Many controversies surround optimal **combination therapy** for advanced HNC, as discussed below. Unfortunately, there is no scientific trial which has shown that combination surgery plus postoperative RT is better than either alone as a single modality. However, it is so widely believed and intuitively logical that the combination is better, that this study probably cannot be done now since clinicians would consider it unethical. New, complex (chemotherapy, altered fraction RT,[110,114] biological therapy[5,78]) treatments are being piled on top of a baseline which has never been proved to be standard therapy, thus becoming progressively farther removed from a scientifically valid starting point.

Principles of combination therapy

1. Radiotherapy and chemotherapy are referred to as "cytoreductive" treatment modalities since they kill a constant **proportion** rather than a constant **number** of cancer cells, i.e., they reduce the number of cells in a cancer but never completely eliminate all cancer cells (log kill[37]). It is interesting that up-front chemotherapy cannot cure HNC alone and must always be "consolidated" with other treatment, whereas RT alone sometimes cures.

Locally advanced cancer of the head and neck may contain 10^{10} to 10^{11} (100 g) malignant cells. Even a 1 log reduction in cell member can lead to an impressive partial clinical response (PR) and a 2 to 3 log cell kill can be scored as a complete response (CR). Few pathologists can reliably detect the presence of one malignant cell among 1000 normal cells, and after a CR about 10^6 cells per gram of tissue remain since 1 g of tissue typically contains 10^9 cells.[98] The mechanism of action of surgery is quite different from "cytoreductive" therapies because surgery removes the "entire" tumor quickly, whereas cytoreductive modalities impact on the tumor-host over a prolonged period of time. This has implications for tumor response (cancer cell repopulation) as seen above.

2. An extremely important point (which is a major determinant of how multimodality treatment should be combined) is the fact that, when a cytoreductive treatment is applied, the tumor mass does not shrink in acentripetal manner to occupy a smaller cohesive central

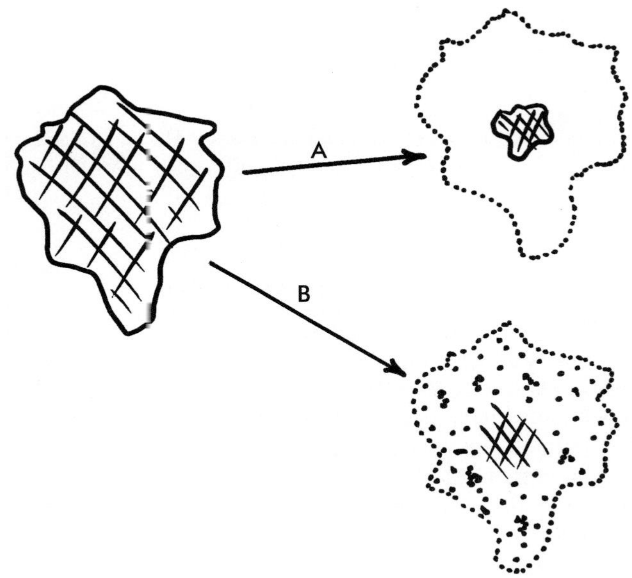

FIG 13-4
After cytoreductive treatment (radiation/chemotherapy) tumor does not shrink cohesively into a centripetal ball in the center of the field **(A)** but rather leaves discontinuous tumor foci throughout the entire field originally occupied by the tumor **(B)**.

tumor core. Rather, cancer cells remain diffusely dispersed throughout the entire field occupied by the original tumor (Fig. 13-4).[26,38,39,71,72,87,92,93,96] This is why the rule remains that, despite the extent of response to initial cytoreductive treatment, surgical margins cannot be decreased from those which would have been required initially,[96,98] regardless of tumor response to cytoreductive treatments. If the surgeon does not see the untreated tumor it is impossible to determine later what adequate margins should be, and in such a situation the surgeon must guess at the extent of the original tumor. **After any cytoreductive treatment, if surgery is required, it is difficult to determine an appropriate margin. Hence, locoregional recurrence is more likely than that in untreated patients (Figs. 13-10 and 13-11).**

3. In previously **untreated** patients, cancers usually have definable margins, spread tends to be by embolism (discontinuous spread of tumor cells or cell clumps) to regional lymphatics rather than by permeation (contiguous spread from primary tumor into adjacent soft tissue), and cancer spread along pathways of least resistance and adjacent fascial planes is somewhat predictable. In **previously treated** patients, however, such barriers and pathways are disrupted, patterns of spread are unpredictable, and permeation rather than embolism is the rule. In view of these factors, conservation surgery (radical excision of cancer which also preserves anatomy, structure, and function) is usually an option only in previously **untreated** patients (except for certain glottic cancer recurrences—see p. 160).

*References 26, 38, 39, 71, 72, 87, 92, 93, 96.

In **previously treated** patients, recurrent tumors typically present along deep fascial planes and are often perceived as a vague fullness which represents only the "tip of the iceberg." In this context, surgical excision—if any—must be more radical ("Halstedian"—see "History of surgical oncology" below), and even then success is unlikely due to the diffuse and difficult-to-define pattern of cancer persistence.

Formulating the initial treatment plan

Two basic tenets of clinical oncology are: (1) the first therapeutic attack on a cancer is the one most likely to control it, and (2) most patients with solid tumors (nonhematologic) who have been cured have had surgery as part of their initial treatment. It is seldom possible to surgically salvage recurrent HNC (with the exception of some glottic cancers), and, since the initial treatment plan usually determines the patient's outcome, decision-making at this stage must be taken very seriously. HN SCC is an aggressive disease and, as described above, previous treatment limits the efficacy of salvage surgery.

The literature is beginning to include a few articles which relate to the differences in specialty-related decision making.[58] One factor which is relevant here is the fact that radiotherapists and medical oncologists do not experience first-hand the difficulties encountered by the surgeon (especially in patients with recurrent cancer), whereas the surgeon is directly exposed to the complications of other treatments and patient complaints related to them.

Although there are limiting factors to patient survival which are beyond the control of the surgeon or radiotherapist (distant metastases, infraclavicular primaries), control of locoregional disease is a necessary prerequisite for ultimate cure. **The most reliable treatment for "advanced" HNC with curative intent in 1995 appears to be surgical excision followed by postoperative radiation.**

A treatment plan should be formulated which maximizes the chance of controlling cancer in the head and neck while optimizing function to achieve the best quality of remaining life. This may involve an attempt at organ preservation in one or more ways (see below), or, alternatively, a plan which includes total laryngectomy (rather than larynx-sparing surgery) might be the best option in patients who cannot tolerate aspiration. Use of cytoreductive therapy to avoid postoperative dysphagia is invalid since this is not the most reliable way to control HNC, and failure to control the primary tumor and/or sequelae of the treatment will also interfere with swallowing. Similarly, conservation surgery at the primary site is an especially attractive option in a previously untreated patient who presents with neck metastases, since overall survival is thereby limited by the likelihood of developing DMs and one desires to optimize the patient's function and appearance for remaining life.

Since surgery is critical for cancer control, it is extremely important not to eliminate patients as surgical candidates based on a superficial medical evaluation. The designation of a patient as **"medically inoperable"** should be **aggressively restricted** and the usual contraindication—cardiologic risk—should be corrected if possible (including bypass surgery) to allow an operation for HNC. Similarly, concluding that a patient is **technically unresectable** based on the radiologic appearance of the tumor is likely to deprive many patients of a potentially curative treatment plan. A head and neck cancer surgeon can greatly assist in accurate tumor staging. Unfortunately, who treats the patient is often an accident of referral patterns, and patients with HNC of all stages are now often initially referred to a chemotherapist and/or radiotherapist without involvement of a HNC surgeon until salvage treatment becomes necessary for persistent disease. The involvement of a surgeon at the time of initial treatment planning is essential and nonsurgeon specialists should not determine tumor resectability.

Defining treatment goals

An initial decision to make is whether the patient should be treated with **curative or palliative intent.** Certain sites of HNC are associated with such intrinsically poor prognosis that the goal from the outset is probably palliation (e.g., sinus cancer with positive nodes or postcricoid/cervical esophagus sites.) The concept of cure versus palliation also relates importantly to the previous treatment status of the patient, since patterns of cancer spread and recurrence differ significantly in patients who have not been previously treated in comparison with those who have been treated (see above). Deciding when the treatment goal should switch from cure to palliation can be difficult.[130,131,139,140] Prior treatment limits treatment options and salvage surgery is often associated with diminishing returns. However, there are exceptions. Multiple surgical attempts at cure are appropriate in patients with recurrent or multiple primary tumors who have never demonstrated positive cervical lymph nodes. A subset of such patients develops multiple (as many as 8 to 10) small primary tumors, and in this situation a surgical "whittling" approach (holding radiation in reserve) often works well.

Similarly, the patient should be given the benefit of the doubt if he or she is "beating the odds" and trying to act like a survivor. Anyone who works with cancer patients knows that some who present with apparently incurable disease survive, and, conversely, some patients with small primary tumors without evidence of metastases demonstrate an inexorable downhill course with death supervening rapidly. This clinical spectrum undoubtedly represents underlying factors which relate to tumor heterogeneity. For example, a patient who has undergone neck dissection and demonstrated many positive lymph nodes at the time of initial surgery, but who is still alive 5 years later, should be given the benefit of the doubt since that patient would have been expected to succumb within 1½ to 2 years if they were "following the rules."

With modern technology, chronologic age is not an absolute contraindication to aggressive treatment. A major operative procedure is not ruled out even if the patient has evidence of distant metastases, since palliative surgery can decrease the ulceration, bleeding, foulness, and, especially, the pain associated with recurrent HNC often without incurring unacceptable deterioration in function and esthetics.

In planning treatment, characteristics of the patient—as well as of the tumor—must be seriously considered, although this is not often emphasized (see box on p 158). Characteristics such as personal stability, family support mechanisms, motivation to cooperate in rehabilitation, educational level, etc., impact significantly on the outcome. Some patients who are poorly educated and fearful of the hospital setting (often related to ethnicity) may not be able to comprehend the nature of a surgical procedure being described or to cooperate adequately in their rehabilitation. Such patients might be best considered for nonsurgical treatment even if the goal thereby changes from cure to palliation.

Consistent with a basic human protective mechanism to avoid bodily injury, almost no patient would choose surgery if other treatments were available and equally effective. Nevertheless, for advanced and recurrent HN SCC, surgery provides the best chance for cure or palliation, and the **possible** complications of surgery are virtually **guaranteed** to occur if cancer in the head and neck is not controlled, resulting in airway and swallowing obstruction, altered speech, pain, bleeding, and foul odor.

It is likely that cancer specialists become somewhat inured to the morbidities associated with their own modalities; surgeons to cosmetic and functional disfiguration, radiotherapists to xerostomia, and chemotherapists to mucositis, nausea and vomiting, and death during nadir sepsis. Nevertheless, in the HNC literature, "mutilation" resulting from treatment is typically referred to only in the context of surgery; chemotherapy and radiation are generally thought to avoid such problems. One suspects that the perspective of the patient who undergoes any or all of these treatment modalities may be somewhat different than that of the treatment manager. For example, a tracheotomy and feeding gastrostomy are not usually mentioned as mutilations except when they are needed long-term postoperatively. Nevertheless, an increasing number of patients who have had cytoreductive treatment regimens are demonstrating a need for such appliances long-term as well. While these may not be considered significantly mutilating by clinicians, they may be considered very mutilating by patients—if they were asked.[69]

Conversely, total laryngectomy (TL) is suddenly considered very mutilating by nonsurgical clinicians, and the literature appears to condone virtually any other treatment as an alternative. This is confusing to surgeons, who for decades have managed patients—often with TL as the only treatment—and have seen long-term survival with an essentially normal life style, including return to the work place and (especially in the modern era) **excellent restoration of function** with voice prosthesis placement **despite removal of the entire organ.** One wonders how often patients who have had cytoreductive treatments return to adequate functioning in the work place. This is poorly documented in the literature. Many chemoradiotherapy studies which describe phase I and II trials—efficacy and toxicity studies—never mention the functional outcome of patients (voice quality, airway adequacy, deglutition).

Heroic attempts to preserve organs which have been significantly invaded by cancer with nonsurgical methods not only challenge oncologic principles—since increased locoregional failure is routinely seen with "organ preservation protocols"*—but is also "magical thinking." In 1955, Morfit wrote: "Loss of the larynx is admittedly a difficult thing to accept but is presumably preferable to dying from cancer. It must also be appreciated that by the time the diagnosis of cancer in this area is made, the tumor is well on its way to destroying the larynx anyway. It should not be necessary to state that unless the tumor is controlled, the larynx would eventually be totally destroyed in every case. Treatment of these lesions with irradiation carries with it the rosy dream of cure but is seldom realized. The concept of the word 'larynx' implies a functioning organ as well as an anatomic structure. If the cords are destroyed or the intrinsic musculature invaded by tumor so that no motion is present or if the airway is occluded and the cartilaginous structures are eaten away by a mixture of necrosis, infection and tumor, the structure is no longer fuller worthy of the term 'larynx' anymore than a gangrenous limb that will no longer bear weight and is threatening that patient's life by infection and sepsis is fully worthy of the term 'leg.'"[68]

Dogged adherence to cytoreductive modalities to avoid the apparent mutilation of surgery—a deeply ingrained concept especially among nonsurgical specialists (and probably among many otolaryngologists) as well as patients—seems odd when excellent function can be achieved even when the entire organ (larynx) is removed. Also, the option of using conservation surgery certainly exists for many sites of HNC as an alternative to total laryngectomy and other radical procedures (discussed below).

Having seen many patients treated initially with nonsurgical modalities and having treated many patients with operations which follow the principles of conservation surgery, the present author can attest to the fact that "mutilation" is neither an exclusive attribute of surgery nor does it necessarily follow all types of operations. As Morfits noted, when "advanced" cancer persists, the tumor-involved organ does not function normally. A typical scenario is to see a patient who has undergone cytoreductive therapy present with residual cancer, a whispered voice, difficulty handling secretions with aspiration pneumonia requiring placement of a tracheotomy and possibly a feeding gastrostomy, as well as (often intractable) pain. The ultimate mutilation is

*References 2, 10, 54, 84, 85, 94, 95, 116.

due to persistent cancer, and giving patients treatment which is less likely to control cancer than the standard best therapy (of course, we do not know what this is, unfortunately) may well be considered unconscionable in the absence of compelling evidence of increased effectiveness in locoregional control or survival.

It can be seen that many treatment-planning decisions involve ethical considerations which are difficult for the doctor alone to decide,[130,131,139,140,154] and such decisions should always be made in conjunction with the informed patient and family.

The individual treatment modalities: controversies

Radiation oncology. For Stage I and II HNC, the perennial argument of whether surgery or RT is the preferred modality usually favors RT, if only functional clinical considerations are taken into account; i.e., voice is better after radiotherapy than after hemilaryngectomy for $T_{1\text{-}2}$ glottic cancers, and, in some institutions in the USA and in many foreign countries, radical RT for all sites and stages of HNC (sometimes combined with brachytherapy) is standard treatment, with surgery held in reserve for "salvage" of persistent/recurrent disease.

In the minds of surgeons, complications of RT center around wound-healing problems encountered when surgery follows RT. One prospective randomized trial of preoperative versus postoperative RT in the 1980s was terminated early[101] because of prohibitive wound-healing complications in the patients who received surgery after preoperative RT. This problem is pervasive and is important to remember when evaluating use of other forms of preoperative treatment, especially combined chemoradiotherapy (see below).

There are other potentially negative side effects of RT on the tumor-host interaction, however, that go far beyond this rather superficial level of analysis, including profound, long-term systemic immunosuppression.[3,97] It is interesting to note that in the early days of tissue culture, adding radiated cells to culture enhanced the growth of tumor cells that otherwise would not "take" (presumably by acting as a nutrient feeder layer).[78] RT has been associated with an enhancing effect on local cancer and metastases.[73,108] Also, administering radiation to normal tissue may enhance growth of any cancer cells resident therein—"the tumor bed effect" (see Tumor heterogeneity section).

In contrast to the pervasive tendency to electively irradiate head and neck areas which may not need it (N_0 neck—see case example, below) is lack of awareness of the importance of extending a radiation portal to include a shaped field at the skull base for many sites and sizes of HNC (Fig. 13-5). The area of the retropharyngeal lymph nodes (RPLNs) adjacent to the internal carotid artery at the carotid canal is at risk for metastatic or direct-continuity spread from: (1) primary tumors of any size in the pyriform sinus, pharyngeal wall, paranasal sinuses and nasopharynx, (2) from large primary tumors in the oral cavity and oropharynx, and (3) in patients with bilaterally positive neck disease (retrograde aberrant flow to RPLNs). Few surgeons realize that standard RT technique for many HNCs is delivered to a square field (Fig. 13-5) at the skull base, which excludes the RPLN area. It behooves the surgeon to communicate information directly to the radiotherapist relating to the desired treatment portal postoperatively (including information gained intraoperatively) to assure that areas which need radiation are being included and that those which do not are excluded (although treatment specialty bias may determine the outcome—see sample case below).

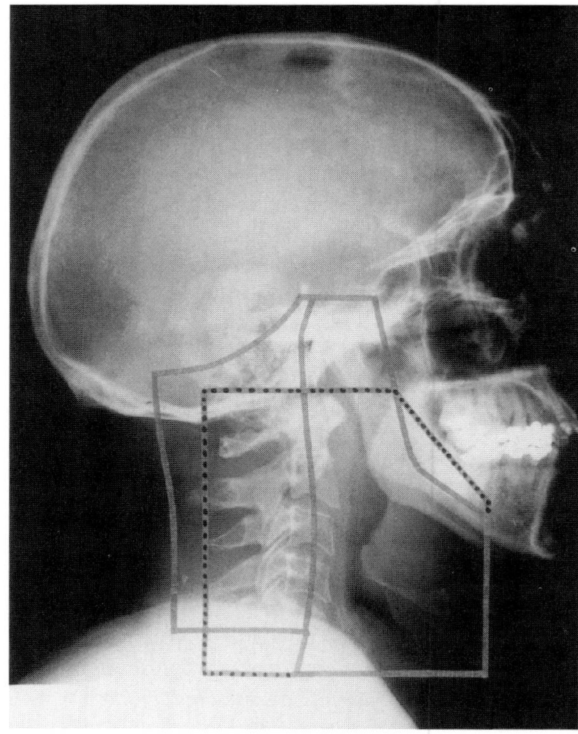

FIG 13-5
Appropriate radiotherapy portals for many sites and sizes of head and neck cancer require a shaped field which includes the skull base *(solid line)* in contradistinction to the usual square field used *(dotted line)*. Similarly the common practice of shielding the stomal tracheostomy site during postoperative RT undoubtedly accounts for a proportion of (often unresectable) stomal recurrence.

What is the role of RT in decreasing the risk of regrowth of cancer cells implanted during surgery? We have seen growth of cancer implants in the extended suture lines of skull-base operations at our institution, and RT portals may need to encompass the new wider surgical fields.

A variety of experimental RT protocols are being investigated. For example, a regimen of rapidly alternating multiagent chemotherapy and accelerated interrupted RT was tested in 19 patients with locally advanced SCC of the hypopharynx and upper esophagus.[104] Late complications occurred in 4 patients including laryngeal necrosis, pneumonia, esophageal stricture, and tracheoesophageal fistula. One patient died of nadir sepsis during treatment. One patient died of aspiration pneumonia. All of the partial responders relapsed and one complete responder relapsed, although mucosal toxicity was less than that was customary with radiation alone.

Wang[110] (1988) points out that in evaluating any new treatment modality, the concept of "therapeutic ratio"—the ratio of success to complications—must be constantly kept in mind. He also notes that dose-modification RT programs are being proposed by many radiotherapists, especially in response to regimens which include chemotherapy as an alternative. But many factors relevant to such alterations are unknown, including the effects of both acute and late responding tissues to multifractionated daily schemes.

Also, as noted above, some studies suggest detriment due to accelerated tumor repopulation.

Chemotherapy. Standard treatment for "advanced HNC" is generally considered to be surgery plus RT (without baseline studies which prove this). However, despite technical advances and refinements in both modalities, the overall survival rate for patients with HN SCC is estimated to have improved only about 11% over the past 30 years. Although reports from "state-of-the-art" institutions[103] indicate that locoregional disease is being controlled twice as well as in the past and that DMs are noted as sites of failure twice as often as heretofore (the incidence of second primaries has remained constant at about 15% overall), locoregional cancer failure is still the major limiting factor to survival in the HNC population.

In an effort to improve survival results, chemotherapy consisting of various combinations of drugs and regimens has been added to the management of "advanced" HNC in the neoadjuvant or induction ("up-front" before any other treatment) setting for the past 15 years. The reader is encouraged to review several excellent summary articles on this topic.[98,107,121,126]

Prior to the 1980s, chemotherapy—typically, single agent methotrexate—was used only in a palliative context to treat the patient (and the surgeon) with inoperable recurrent HN SCC.[125] Such treatment had few detectable side effects and was relatively benign, although it also had relatively little impact on the course of the disease. Otolaryngologists whose training occurred during a period when methotrexate was used in a such a context may still regard chemotherapy as a benign treatment, in comparison with the putatively more mutilating operations for HNC. (Morbidity related to the various treatments is discussed below.) However, it is important to realize that application of currently active drug regimens (cis-platinum and 5-fluorouracil; standard therapy = 3 cycles) to the fragile HNC population is associated with potentially life-threatening toxicities because of the frequently advanced age of HNC patients, their long-term exposure to the systemic effects of alcohol and tobacco, and frequent debilitation due to tumor interference with swallowing, airway, etc. The fact that more chemotherapy-related deaths are not reported in the literature—especially with current dose escalations—is a reflection of the tremendous effort devoted to managing these patients by dedicated head and neck medical oncologists at academic institutions (the source of most of the reports in the literature).[105] In treatment planning one must consider whether an equivalent level of care is available in the local community.

General conclusions about the role of **neoadjuvant** chemotherapy in treatment of HN SCC include[98,107]:

- Improved survival has not been demonstrated in any conclusive randomized studies.
- A decreased incidence of DMs ("meaningful systemic activity") has been repeatedly reported but, due to the specific natural history of HNC, this fact by itself will not translate into improved survival.
- Organ preservation has been shown to be feasible (see below).

Surgical oncology. Billroth stated that "in order to understand where we are and where we are going, one must be familiar with lessons from the past." This section will show how certain paradigms from the past have dictated the manner in which HNC and other solid cancers have been managed surgically and will outline the evolution of present conceptions concerning appropriate surgical management of cancer. Technical factors and patterns of cancer spread which relate to the primary task of cancer surgeon—removing the gross tumor with a margin of normal tissue—will also be discussed. Such an analysis shows how to avoid repeating mistakes made in the past.

Historical overview.—Surgery is the oldest method of cancer therapy and is the most frequently used and most successful method of treatment available today. More patients are cured of cancer by surgery than by any other single therapeutic modality. Nevertheless, the cure rates for the common neoplasms treated by operation alone have not changed much during the past 30 to 40 years, leading to use of combination therapies to hopefully enhance cancer control.[142]

The time-honored Halstedian paradigm for surgical treatment of cancer is based on the concept that cancer originates as a single cell mutation followed by progressive and unrestricted clonal expansion of uniform cells. As we have seen above, tumors are actually heterogeneous. Also, cancer was thought to be a local disease which spreads in an orderly fashion from the primary site to adjacent tissues and to regional nodes by **permeation** (spread in direct continuity between primary tumor and regional lymphatics), whereas spread to distant sites occurs through blood vessels. Such a paradigm dictates a surgical approach which removes the primary neoplasm and the regional lymph nodes *en bloc* with the aim of removing every cancer cell from the patient's body, attempting to improve results by developing progressively more radical operations to achieve a wider margin.

Advances in surgical technique, anesthesia, and supportive care permitted the development of ultraradical cancer operations in the 1940s and 1950s which extended surgery to its anatomic limits, including even hemicorpectomy in which the body was transected at the level of the umbilicus for neoplasms involving the lower half of the body. Since cancer was thought to spread by direct continuity, surgery for patients with advanced breast cancer in earlier decades sometimes included a fore-quarter amputation (resection of the arm at the shoulder) and/or incontinuity iliac crest resection since cancer in the hipbone was thought to originate by direct extension rather than by hematogenous metastasis.

Unfortunately, with few exceptions, such procedures did not significantly increase cure rates and, by the mid-1960s, the anatomic limits of cancer surgery had been reached and such supraradical operations were being restricted. Nevertheless, the concept that surgical cure requires removal of every last tumor cell persists today despite much evidence to the contrary. Studies on the "surgical personality" have shown that surgeons tend to resist change, persisting doggedly in a task using methods learned during residency. Thus, the Halstedian paradigm is still widely present in the surgical oncology community.

Several "alternative hypotheses" to the Halstedian have been developed based on more modern concepts of cancer spread, which give a different perspective on the appropriate context of cancer surgery (Table 13-1). First of all, the blood and lymphatic systems are not separate but are connected at multiple points to functionally constitute a single vascular system.[29]

Second, a consecutive series of well-designed, scientifically based, randomized prospective clinical trials started in the early 1970s (under the auspices of the National Surgical Adjuvant Breast Project—NSABP) have yielded much valuable information, and implications for other solid tumors such as HN SCC are obvious (although extrapolation of the conclusions to other tumor systems is not valid without corresponding clinical trials).[30,31] In the first trial, patients with early breast cancer without clinical evidence of regional lymphadenopathy were randomized to receive radical mastectomy (RM), total (simple) mastectomy (TM), or total mastectomy plus postoperative local-regional radiation (TM + RT) (Fig. 13-6). At 5 years, the incidence of distant disease in the three groups (those who had regional nodes removed, irradiated, or untreated) was similar. The time from operation to the detection of distant disease in each circumstance was not appreciably different. Overall survival of the three clinically node-negative groups did not differ significantly in frequency or in time from operation to death, indicating that the presence or absence of distant disease more closely correlated with patient survival than did the initial treatment failure site.

TABLE 13-1
Similarities and differences between the Halstedian and "alternate" hypotheses of tumor spread

Halstedian	Alternate
Tumors spread in an orderly defined manner based upon mechanical considerations	There is no orderly pattern of tumor cell dissemination
Tumor cells traverse lymphatics to lymph nodes by direct extension supporting en bloc dissection	Tumor cells traverse lymphatics by embolization challenging the merit of en bloc dissection.
The positive lymph node is an indicator of tumor spread and is the instigator of distant disease	The positive lymph node is an indicator of a host-tumor relationship which permits development of metastases rather than being the instigator of distant disease.
Regional lymph nodes (RLNs) are barriers to the passage of tumor cells	Regional lymph nodes are ineffective as barriers to tumor cell spread.
RLNs are of anatomic importance	RLNs are of biologic importance.
The blood stream is of little significance as a route of tumor dissemination	The blood stream is of considerable importance in tumor dissemination
A tumor is autonomous of its host	Complex host-tumor interrelationships affect every facet of the disease
Operable breast cancer is a local-regional disease	Operable breast cancer is a systemic disease.
The extent and nuances of operation are the dominant factors influencing patient outcome	Variations in local-regional therapy are unlikely to substantially affect survival.

Modified from Fisher B et al: The contribution of recent NSABP clinical trials of primary breast cancer therapy to an understanding of tumor biology—An overview of findings. *Cancer* 46:1009, 1980.

In clinically node-positive patients, there was no significant difference between those receiving RM and those with TM + RT with respect to total, local-regional or distant treatment failure, or survival. Whereas the combination of surgery and radiation reduced local recurrence, tumor-free survival was not appreciably affected. Although some patients who had TM alone required subsequent axillary dissection for delayed nodal appearance, these patients fared no worse than those in whom the axilla was treated initially.

The similarities in distant disease and survival rates and the relatively small increase in local-regional disease following TM compared with that following RM in node-negative patients were remarkable, considering that 40% of the RM patients were found to have histologically positive nodes in the removed axillary contents. Because the treat-

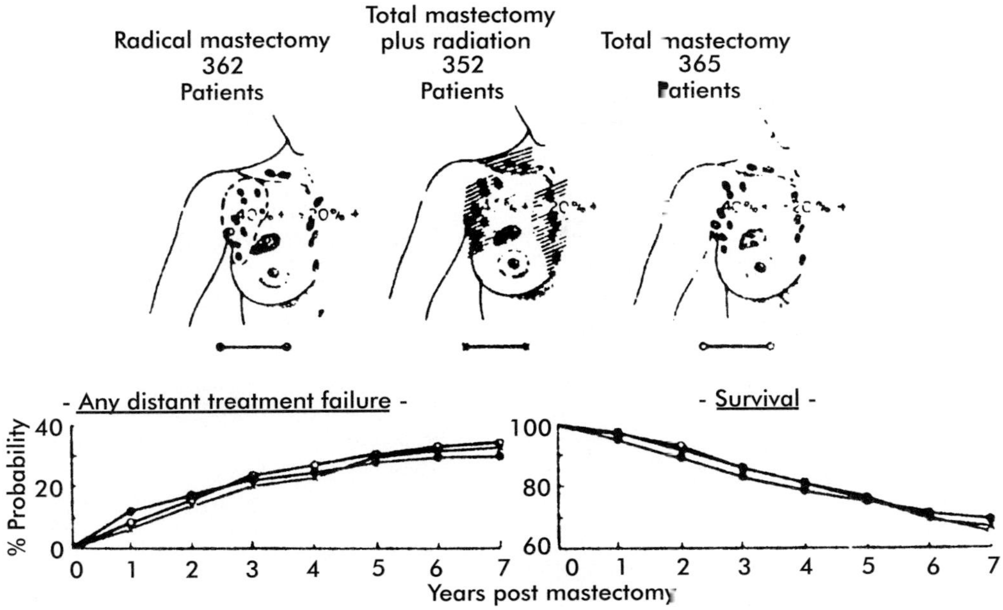

FIG 13-6
Similarity of treatment failure sites and survival in breast cancer patients with clinically negative nodes treated in three different ways: **1,** axilla dissected with radical mastectomy, **2,** axilla radiated, **3,** axilla observed. The type of treatment to the regional nodes did not influence distant treatment failure or survival.

ment groups were equivalent with respect to all parameters available for comparison owing to the prospective randomized format, it was expected that approximately 40% of women subjected to TM alone also had positive nodes that were untreated. Based on Halstedian concepts, such retained positive nodes could serve as a source of further tumor dissemination, resulting in an increase in distant treatment failure; yet patients who underwent TM alone had about the same incidence of distant disease and survival. Survival and recurrence in more than 2000 patients were independent of the number of axillary nodes removed. (Clinical practice currently includes routine axillary dissection to serve as a staging procedure to select breast cancer patients for adjuvant treatment).

Findings from a later NSABP protocol and a similar large trial reported from the Tumor Institute of Milan showed that, in pathologically node-positive patients who had RM and then received chemotherapy, there was a significant increase in disease-free interval over that observed in patients receiving no chemotherapy. This was the first demonstration of the ability of adjuvant systemic treatment to change the natural history of a solid tumor in humans. (A similar survival advantage has not been found in HN SCC patients.)

Because a large proportion of women operated upon for breast cancer develop metastatic disease regardless of the extent of locoregional surgery, it is apparent that the disease is often systemic at the time of surgery. In these cases, surgical therapy has limited effect on **survival,** although its utility in local palliation and hygienic control of disease should not be underestimated. These results have led to the growing opinion that tumor-free survival depends upon the biology of the tumor and not upon the extent of operation (see Table 13-1). The innate virulence of the neoplasm balanced against whatever defense reactions are excited in the host constitutes a biologic complex that determines the natural history and outcome of the process in the individual cancer patient.

In another "alternate" hypothesis of surgical oncology, Morton[70] extended Dunphy's ideas to conceptualize cancer surgery as a form of immunotherapy. The hypothesis was that surgery exerts its favorable influence on the tumor-host relationship primarily by removing the bulk of tumor, which lowers the level of systemic immunosuppression (specific and nonspecific) induced by the neoplasm.

A growing neoplasm is capable of evading immune attack by producing specific and nonspecific immunosuppression of the host's defenses, to enhance tumor growth. The magnitude of immunosuppression correlates with tumor burden and immunosuppression can be reversed by removing the neoplasm. Therefore, cancer surgery acts as immunotherapy because it removes the cancer cells that produce the immunodepression and allows the patient's immune response to recover. The chance of cure is greatest in patients with the least residual tumor (an argument for up-front surgery). Thus surgery, although possibly not curative in a classic sense, can decrease the patient's tumor burden to theoretically allow the host immune response to return to normal so that chemotherapy or immunotherapy may assist in overcoming minimal residual disease. One must assume

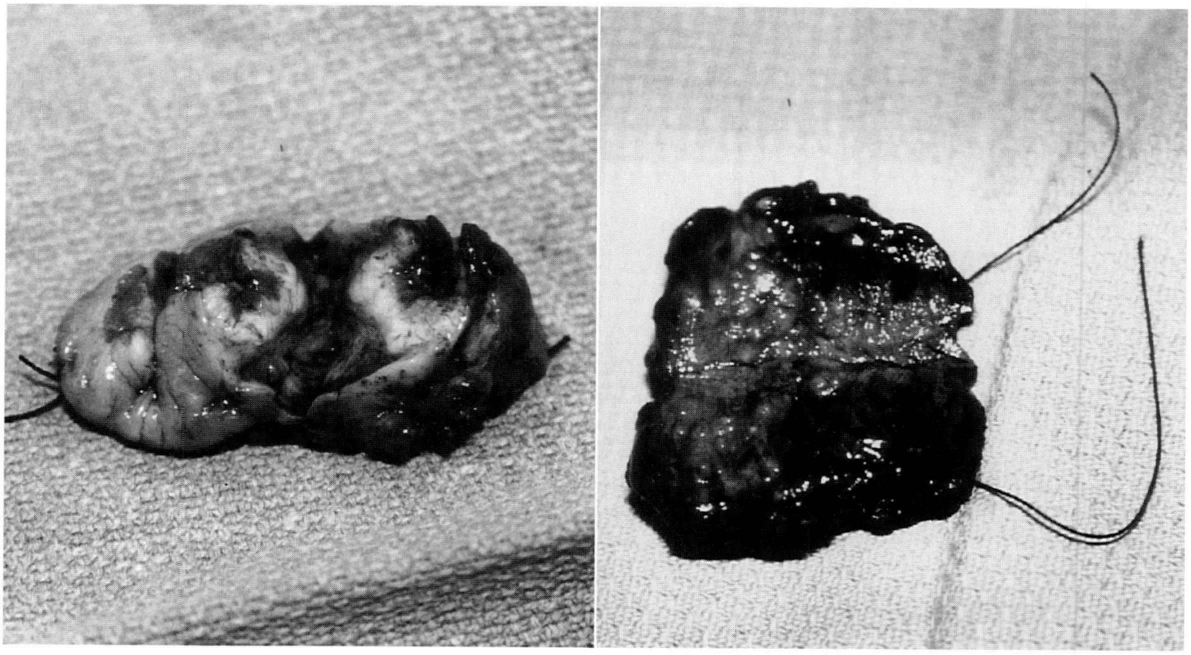

FIG 13-7
Adequate surgical excision of a head and neck cancer is more likely when the tumor has a well-defined pushing border **(A)** as opposed to a poorly defined margin **(B)**.

that apparently localized tumor is actually a manifestation of systemic illness whether or not the patient has overt metastases, and therapeutic advances will presumably come from combining surgery with the systemic treatment modalities (chemotherapy, immunotherapy, "biological" therapy) which, unlike surgery and radiation, are potentially effective against tumor cells that have already spread to distant sites.

The application of these principles has improved the results of surgical treatment for a wide variety of neoplasms such as osteo- and soft tissue sarcoma, breast cancer, lung cancer, melanoma, and ovarian cancer. It might be assumed that a wide *en bloc* resection is not particularly important in this paradigm. However, according to Morton, quantitative factors in the tumor-host relationship make this a false assumption which invites local recurrence at the site of an inadequate surgical procedure. Since it is impossible to know in any given patient how many tumor cells will be required for the induction of local tumor growth, the surgical procedure must have as its aim the removal of as many cancer cells as possible. If the surgical procedure removes the bulk of tumor leaving a "scattering" of 10^6 cells or less, the patient's immune defenses could theoretically "mop up after the surgeons knife."

Margins.—The present author's concept of limitations to cancer cure by surgery relate to the problems posed by discontinuous spread of cancer, which with HNC can occur at the primary site, in regional lymph nodes, and distantly. If all cancers spread cohesively outward with a well-defined, easily identifiable, pushing border they could be "easily" removed with good expectation of locoregional control (provided adequate excision was not limited by vital structures). Cancers with a well-defined, pushing border (Fig. 13-7, *A*) are much easier to excise with an adequate margin (which decreases the chance of local recurrence) than those with an ill-defined infiltrating border (Fig. 13-7, *B*). Previously untreated patients tend to have tumors with well-defined borders (although some tumors have naturally infiltrating borders), whereas previously treated patients (prior radiotherapy[9] and/or chemotherapy) have ill-defined tumor borders because of the mechanism of cancer shrinkage after cytoreductive therapy (described in the section on tumor biology), i.e., discontinuous cancer cell foci throughout the entire field originally occupied by the tumor. This is a major reason why salvage surgery is generally unsuccessful in comparison with "up-front" surgery. Even if the tumor was originally well circumscribed, it is converted to a diffuse interstitial pattern by cytoreductive treatment. A similar problem is seen with "extracapsular spread" of cancer from neck nodes.[8] Interstitial cancer spread is difficult for the surgeon to remove and is associated with locoregional cancer regrowth.[82] This helps explain why pathologically negative margins can be biologically positive, as demonstrated by cancer regrowth, even if circumferential mucosal margins are checked (Figs. 13-10 and 13-11). Cancer cells may not be visible to the pathologist if they are discontinuous and in small clumps. Margin assessment, even in previously untreated patients, is full of artifacts based on the nature of processing tissue. Typically, only four-quadrant mucosal margins and a few deep margins are cut. Obviously, cancer may be present subclinically in areas which are not sampled. Also the mucosal margins of a specimen can desiccate and contract against the primary tumor mass during transport, and, if cut in this condition, positive margins will be found more often than if the specimen is kept in saline and margins are cut by the surgeon at the time of excision. The present author always cuts surgical margins as soon as the specimen is removed and hemostasis is adequate. Surgeons have more of a vested interest in cutting negative margins than do surgical pathologists who are often unfamiliar with head and neck anatomy (especially residents-in-training).

The amount of tissue which constitutes an adequate margin varies with the site of the primary cancer. Tiny (1 to 2 mm) margins are adequate for glottic cancers, and, even when margins are positive at that site, cancer regrowth occurs only 18% of the time. Recurrent cancer after hemilaryngectomy can be salvaged 50% of the time with RT. In other sites, such as the tongue, the finding of discontinuous cancer cell clumps 1 cm away from the clinically detectable edge of the tumor has led Harrison to recommend wider margins (up to 2 cm) in this site.[43]

An important study showed that when margins of large head and neck mucosal cancers were examined completely in the manner of Mohs, that cancer cells were found, often discontinuously, at least 1 cm beyond the visible and palpable tumor edge in 70% of cases.[18] The pattern at the tumor-host interface (pushing/cohesive/continuous versus infiltrating/shattered/fragmented) has been emphasized in the Scandinavian literature[51] but not in that in the U.S. An infiltrating pattern at the tumor-host interface is associated with increased difficulty in performing adequate excision of primary tumors and with increased metastatic spread.[118] Of course, within a given tumor, the pattern at the interface with host tissue can vary.

Head and neck surgeons are constantly trying to balance adequate removal of cancer in the complex and compact anatomy of the head and neck with preservation of function, however, and do not have the leeway to remove large sections of an organ territory with impunity as in some other parts of the body. Dogmatic adherence to absolute extent of surgical margins as well as to the performance of traditional excisions must be modified if surgeons are to remain competitive in the modern "organ preservation" arena where function and quality of life are gaining increasing importance. Flexible combinations of various types of conservation surgery with radiotherapy to compensate for close margins are an option. For example, a large tongue tumor in a previously untreated patient which abuts the midline, if excised with a 2 cm margin, could result in a total glossectomy which is functionally devastating. However, if all gross tumor can be removed (essentially what HNC surgeons are doing most of the time anyway) with a hemiglossotomy, adjuvant radiotherapy could be delivered in the form of external beam plus brachytherapy to deliver a high dose to the remaining tongue.

Some articles in the literature have advocated re-excision of positive margins, and surgeons have gone so far as to leave a primary defect open until the permanent histopathology report is returned. One study using this approach showed only a 50% likelihood of finding cancer in additional excised margins, possibly because all cancer had been removed in the initial resection but more likely because the area of residual tumor was not actually re-excised.[56] During the time the wound has been left open, it has started to heal by contraction and secondary intention and migration of cells across the surface alters the area of the positive margin which may have moved significantly by the time of the re-excision. Even intraoperatively it can be difficult to identify the exact place at which a margin was sampled shortly before, unless the area is tagged with a suture.

Surgical technique is seldom emphasized as a factor in achieving negative margins. However, many of the primary tumors excised are vascular, and the excision is often performed in a bloody field with inadequate visualization of tumor margins. Therefore, surgical technique must be scrupulous, and anatomic dissection with hemostasis throughout is the technique most likely to avoid inadvertent "cut-through" of cancer, which may go unnoticed during rapid removal of a primary tumor if the field is obscured by blood.

Other factors within the control of the surgeon which are not measured by traditional margin assessment also influence the likelihood of locoregional cancer regrowth. For example, most of the primary tumors in the upper aerodigestive tract mucosa are ulcerated, and, during excision, exfoliated cancer cells carried on the surgeons gloves and instruments can contaminate normal tissue planes. Viable cancer cells can thereby be implanted anywhere in the area of dissection, and this is undoubtedly a source of tumor recurrence although it is impossible to identify the exact source of cancer cells which regrow to form a recurrence—incomplete excision, implantation of viable, exfoliated cancer cells,[1,42,109] regrowth of occult cancer in unexcised lymph nodes, etc.) Several maneuvers can decrease the likelihood of implanting viable cancer cells intraoperatively[14]:

- Excising the primary tumor as the initial step in the procedure through minimally elevated flaps rather than performing neck dissections first (as is traditional) decreases the likelihood of implanting exfoliated cancer cells from the primary in normal tissue planes. This is also a factor in surgery of N_0 neck(s). Does the risk of cancer regrowth from occult nodal disease warrant opening ipsilateral and contralateral neck planes to possible cancer cell implantation from the primary tumor?
- Change gowns, gloves, instruments and irrigate wound profusely with water to lyse any cancer cells in the surgical bed after removal of the primary tumor.

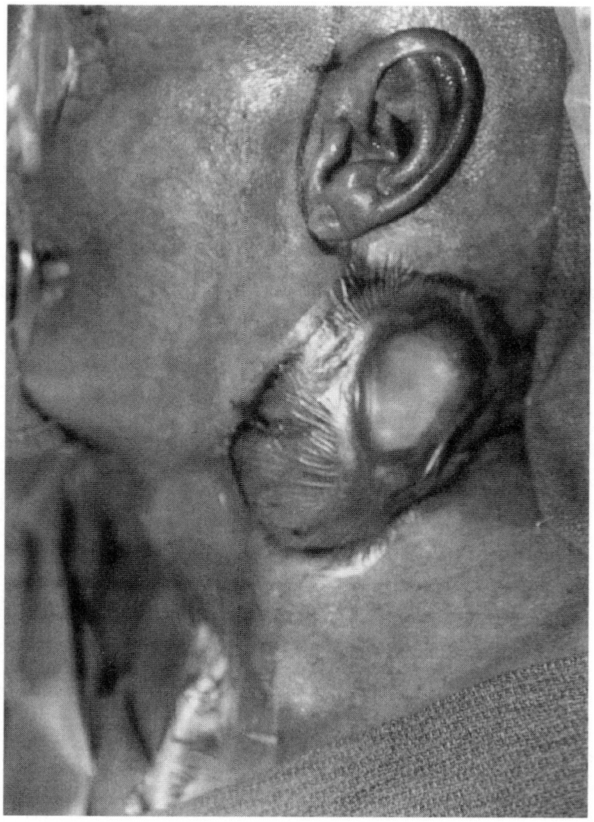

FIG 13-8
Method of protecting a tracheostome from exfoliated viable cancer cells: Tracheotomy site is covered with tegaderm immediately after the tracheotomy is placed and any tumor surfaces which might exfoliate cancer cells in the skin are similarly covered.

- After the primary tumor is removed with its exfoliating cancer cells and the wound has been irrigated, additional procedures such as neck dissections, placement of a percutaneous endoscopic gastrostomy (PEG), and tooth extractions can be performed, if indicated. (Passing an endoscope to perform a PEG past a primary tumor present in the mucosa of the upper aerodigestive tract risks implanting cancer cells at the G-tube site. This has been reported in the literature on multiple occasions, and some patients have died as a result of complications of gastrectomy for cancer in this site.)[64] Fresh tracheotomy sites should be protected (Fig. 13-8) to decrease the risk of touching the tissue with tumor-contaminated gloves and instruments, which is undoubtedly the source of many stomal recurrences (Fig. 13-9). Any discontinuous body area, such as one from which a distant flap is obtained, should obviously be operated as a separate clean field.

It is stated that, if patients are to receive cytoreductive treatment as the first treatment, the tumor margins should be tattooed. However, this only crudely marks two dimensions

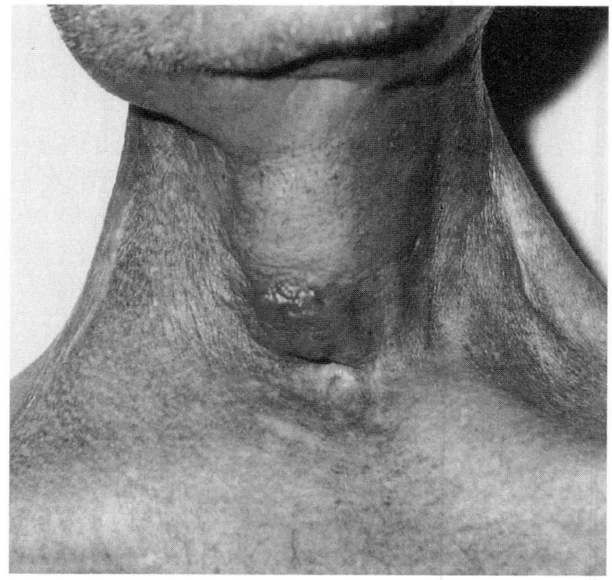

FIG 13-9
Example of recurrent cancer at a former tracheotomy site—possible regrowth of a tumor implant.

of the tumor along the mucosal surface and it is not possible to mark the third dimension—the deep margin.

The future of HNC surgical oncology.—Studies on "the surgical personality" show typical traits of intelligence, ambition, enterprise, and a need to achieve, control, resist change, and persist methodically and conventionally in a task. Such personalities must beware of opinion, inference, intuitively logical conclusions, circumstantial evidence, and tradition. It is time for surgeons to expand beyond the methodologic and philosophical confines of their training. Surgeons should remove a cancer rather than an organ.

Surgeons have failed to provide viable alternatives to the current trend to use cytoreductive modalities in organ preservation strategies. As has hopefully been demonstrated in this presentation, up-front conservation surgery gains immediacy not only from an oncologic and functional standpoint but also in the present socioeconomic milieu. In these days of capitation, surgeons must quickly become competitive in organ preservation strategies by "decapitating" fewer patients with "macho" operations. In untreated patients there are usually alternatives to traditional radical operations (the topic of a companion course, SL Collins, RW Bastian: Breaking the rules in head and neck cancer surgery), and, in previously treated patients, such operations do little good anyway, for the reasons cited above.

The only planned attempt in this direction is represented by several German surgeons who are currently viewed as a "fringe group" by most American HNC surgeons because their results seem too good to be true. The philosophy that ultraradical surgery for hypopharyngeal primaries with neck disease is not justified any longer considering the bad prognosis worldwide for these tumors has led German surgeons[22,90,91] to respond with "preservation of organs by renunciation of ablative surgical techniques," looking to improve the quality of remaining life. "Apart from survival times and local tumor control, the quality of life is considered to be increasingly more important. This is something that we as surgeons must consider in contemplating which procedures we use to prolong life meaningfully. The fact that the prognosis for hypopharyngeal cancer has improved very little over decades despite aggressive multimodality therapy indicates that there are absolute limitations to curability in this patient group."

This treatment plan has been in place since the 1980s and has focused on laser microsurgery with a goal of complete locoregional tumor control (often including postoperative RT and/or neck dissection or, more recently, multiagent chemotherapy instead of radiation for tumors not felt to be curable), and the majority of cases reported have involved tumors of the pyriform sinus.* ($T_{1\text{-}4}$;$N_{0\text{-}2}$).

These surgeons report amazingly good local control results despite the fact that the primary tumor is removed in a piecemeal way; progressively deeper slices are taken through the tumor until a negative margin is reached rather than attempting to cut at a negative margin initially. "The concept of minimally invasive therapy as represented in laser microlaryngeal surgery represents real progress in the treatment of tumors of the upper aerodigestive tract with respect to oncology, function."[50,53,90]

The use of cytoreductive treatments has been adopted not only by many medical and radiation oncologists in the community but apparently by many otolaryngologists, who now often refer cancer patients directly to one of these specialists rather than to another otolaryngologist who specializes in HNC surgery. Why is this? Possibly because of ego and/or because otolaryngologists trained in earlier decades were exposed mainly to traditional, radical operations for HNC which removed large organ territories and imposed significant cosmetic and functional mutilation on the patient with relatively poor cancer control rates. Also, they may not have seen the complications associated with modern chemotherapy (see above). The present author has seen many examples in which the patient died faster as a result of complications of initial chemotherapy or chemoradiotherapy than would have resulted from the cancer if left untreated. Even young, healthy patients have succumbed to treatment-related complications of cytoreductive therapy.

In many fields of solid tumor oncology, surgery is being investigated in a salvage context to debulk residual tumor after prior cytoreductive therapy.[41] Rosenberg states that this is only a viable option if there is additional effective adjuvant therapy available to control residual disease. Some currently propose to investigate HNC surgery in this context. This seems an incorrect sequence based on information presented herein. There is a long history of attempting other treatment before surgery to decrease the magnitude of operations for HNC. In the 1970s it was preoperative radiotherapy and in the 1980s it was preoperative chemotherapy. In the 1990s it is preoperative chemoradiotherapy.[59,66,106] In the future, biological response modifiers will undoubtedly be interdigitated in some manner. Based on the discussion presented so far, the reader should be able to realize that such a strategy is not likely to meet with success. Surgery after chemoradiotherapy is proving to be associated with prohibitive complications (see below) and is probably a dangerous exercise in futility (speaking from personal experience). Since I do not personally submit patients to induction chemotherapy or chemoradiotherapy if they are surgical candidates, such patients have been referred for persistent disease and I have not seen the original tumor prior to treatment, an additional and increasingly common problem since patients are more often being treated by chemotherapists or radiotherapists initially without the input of an experienced HNC surgeon. Attempting to dissect residual disease which is diffusely embedded in fibrotic tissue adjacent to the carotid artery and reconstructing the wound in a manner which will heal is extremely challenging, to say the least, and is seldom accompanied by the feeling that the residual cancer has been adequately removed at the end of the resection. Tumor typically recurs shortly thereafter in patients who have received prior radiation or chemoradiation (Figs. 13-10 and 13-11).

It is a dangerous precedent to allow surgery to become used in only a "salvage" treatment. Once surgery is given away in the initial treatment phase, it may be hard to get back, especially in these days of scrutinized medical resource allocation.

CASE EXAMPLE

Let's look at an example of how these aspects of tumor biology and clinical practice now combine in the more sophisticated evaluation of a common clinical problem in head and neck oncology: the delivery of elective neck irradiation (ENI) to one or both henminecks in a patient who does not otherwise require neck coverage in order to adequately treat the primary tumor. (This discussion does not relate to postoperative irradiation of the N_+ neck(s).)

Proposition

One or both sides of the N_0 neck should be irradiated to decrease the likelihood of later appearance of cancer arising in neck nodes, especially since this practice has no clinical detriment

This practice evolved from work in the 1970s on ways to combine initial surgery with postoperative irradiation, primarily originating from MD Anderson Hospital,[35] and there has been an increasing trend to use ENI to one or both sides of the patient's neck when the likelihood of occult

*N.B. The present author has recently completed work which shows that cancers of the posterior pharyngeal wall should no longer be considered to have such a dismal prognosis—if operated and radiated.

A 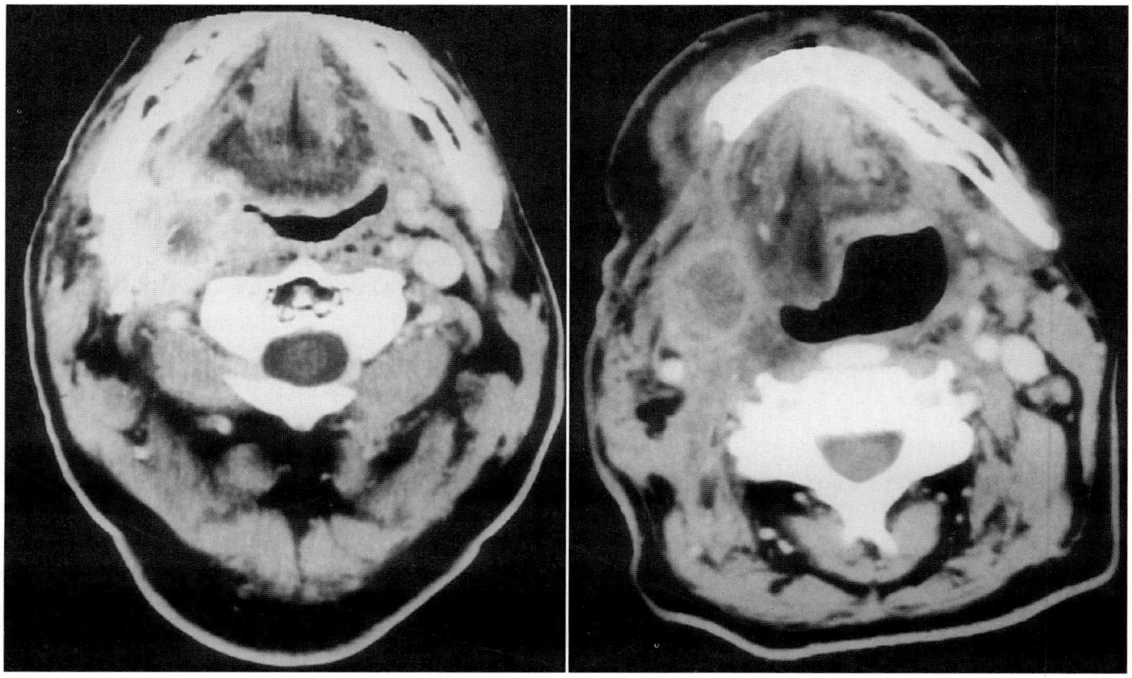 B

FIG 13-10
Recurrent mucoepidermoid carcinoma at base of tongue/parapharyngeal space with necrotic center (recurrent after radiotherapy) was excised and quickly regrew in the same location during postoperative re-irradiation. **B,** status post composite resection. This is an example of the difficulty in controlling recurrent cancer in a previously treated field. The cancer regrowth occurred within two months of the operation.

A 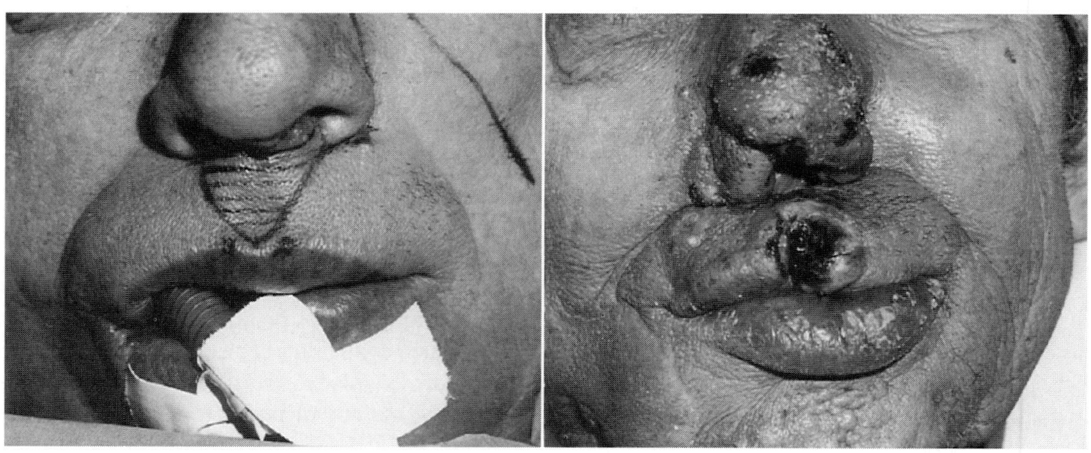 B

FIG 13-11
Surgical treatment of a nasal carcinoma (columella/pre-maxilla) after full-course radiotherapy. The extent of the excision was influenced by the reconstructive flap chosen and was inadequate for a recurrent cancer in a previously treated field, with predictably bad results **(B)**.

cancer spread to cervical nodes is estimated to be as little as 10% to 15%. The putative efficacy of ENI in this context derives from comparing the observed incidence of cancer growth in the neck to that which would be expected based on: (1) the incidence of occult disease found in elective neck dissection specimens and/or (2) a decrease in the development of cancer after ENI when compared with that in untreated necks which are observed and dissected therapeutically if cancer develops later.

There are many flaws in such a data base and in the underlying assumptions which presumably validate the utility of ENI, including nonstandard methods of examining neck dissection specimens for occult disease and the fact that it is never known whether occult disease was present in an individual patient. Thus, the end point evaluates a decrease in an event which might not have occurred. Another assumption in such a comparison is that all occult cancer will become clinically significant in the patient's life time, and there are many of other clinical situations (thyroid cancer, prostate cancer, data from the NSABP trial on breast cancer [see Fig. 13-6]) which suggest that this is not always the case.

The apparent lack of morbidity of ENI relates mainly to decreased soft tissue fibrosis—euphemistically referred to as "woody induration"—from that which occurs when therapeutic doses of radiation are delivered to the N_+ neck. In other words, ENI might help and it does not hurt when that single negative parameter is assessed. In fact, with skin-sparing techniques, underlying neck fibrosis may still be significant. And, of course, neck fibrosis increases over time even when elective doses (45-50 Gy) are delivered.

Another point in favor of ENI is the alleged need to decrease the likelihood of cancer growth in an N_0 neck contralateral to an N_+ neck, since ipsilateral neck treatment will result in lymphatic obstruction and cancer cells are more likely to be redirected to the opposite neck. In fact, the literature on the incidence of contralateral histologically positive occult disease associated with primary tumors of various sites and sizes is sparse, and there is virtually none which relates contralateral neck node development to ipsilateral cancer or treatment except at a theoretical level.[27]

Arguments **against** the use of ENI include:

- The difficulty in salvaging neck disease which may later arise in an N_0 neck which has been electively irradiated. Fibrosis in the neck soft tissues can interfere with early detection of recurrence, and when such recurrence develops the epicenter is typically along deep fascial planes with ill-defined borders—again, a situation difficult for surgeons to remove. Also, after delayed **therapeutic** neck dissection, more radiation cannot be delivered to control residual microscopic disease (if the neck proves to be technically resectable, which is not always the case). This aspect—that **recurrent disease in an electively irradiated neck cannot be reliably salvaged**—has not been emphasized in the literature.
- Treatment options for second primary tumors are diminished when wide-field RT has been applied to both sides of the neck in the treatment of the index cancer.
- No scientifically valid study shows compromised survival with watchful waiting of the N_0 neck with therapeutic treatment delivered if disease should develop later, versus elective treatment of the N_0 neck.
- There is significant morbidity related to delivery of irradiation, even at elective levels to a wide field which adequately covers all echelons of both hemi-necks. All of the major salivary glands are included in such radiation portals, and the profound xerostomia is a major (if not **the** major) complaint of patients who have had such treatment (try a scopolamine patch yourself for one day to get a hint of the discomfort to which these patients are subjected forever).
- Imposing such morbidity without a valid scientific reason for doing so (and no randomized trial comparing ENI vs elective neck dissection [END] vs observation vs delayed therapeutic neck dissection has ever been performed) could be considered bad treatment. Avoiding the morbidity pursuant to widefield ENI is especially relevant in patients with an overall limited prognosis (i.e., those with positive neck nodes—since this is a harbinger of the appearance of systemic disease within 1½ to 2 years of initial treatment). The survival of such patients is limited and adding to the morbidity of their remaining lifespan is not consistent with optimal quality of life.
- Xerostomia can "tip over" some patients who are eating well by mouth postoperatively to a status in which oral intake is impossible, thus further compromising quality of life by restricting the patient to tube feedings.
- Xerostomia also affects denture fit due to the lack of a moist interface, further compromising the pleasurable activities of chewing and swallowing.
- Because of quality of life considerations, some patients refuse **any** postoperative radiation and thereby deprive themselves of treatment which is presumably necessary to decrease the likelihood of cancer regrowth in an N_+ neck or at a primary tumor site with close or microscopically positive margins.
- The end point used to justify ENI is lack of appearance of neck disease. Since it is not known in an individual patient whether or not cancer was present in the neck, the assumption that 95% of the occult cancer present was controlled by ENI can be questioned, since this data was accumulated from single-institution historic comparisons or amalgamated multi-institution retrospective data, both of which are statistically invalid.
  When tumor biology processes such as the **tumor bed effect** and cancer cell dormancy (discussed above) are considered, one might equally well postulate that the effect of radiation on normal tissue might actually enhance growth of occult neck disease into clinically significant cancer! For example, if there had been a 1% incidence of **occult** cancer in the lymph nodes of the electively irradiated neck, finding a 5% incidence of **clinically detectable** neck cancer might reflect stimulated growth by RT on a heterogeneous tumor population, rather than decreasing the presumed incidence from 100% occult infestation to 95%. Since, by definition, it is not known whether or not cancer was present in an individual's neck, this explanation of the 5% incidence of clinically detected neck cancer after ENI is as valid as the traditional dogma.

As shown in this example, many clinical and tumor biology factors contribute to the morbidity of wide-field irradiation, most of which are not considered in daily treatment planning. Since such treatment actually has multifaceted morbidity, using it in the absence of a compelling scientific reason to do so is debatable.

An alternative to ENI is for surgeons to perform elective (functional) neck dissection(s) in N_0 neck(s) as a staging procedure (END).[7] If no positive nodes are found on careful histopathologic examination (surgeon dissects nodes from the fresh specimen in the operating room?) this can be a persuasive argument against postoperative RT. However, END is not without consequences to the patient. Not all surgeons who perform head and neck cancer surgery have the ability to quickly perform uni- or bilateral functional neck dissections without morbidity to the patient. General anesthesia time is increased, and this can be detrimental in the fragile HNC population. Also, a neck dissection opens previously uncontaminated tissue planes to potential implantation of cancer cells exfoliated from the primary tumor or contralateral positive neck nodes, especially if neck dissections are performed before removal of the primary tumor. (The present author removes the primary tumor initially through minimally elevated neck flaps to decrease the likelihood of this occurrence.)[14]

CONCLUSIONS

The information presented herein, derived both from the "tumor biology" and clinical arenas, allows deeper analysis of a number of the traditional controversies in HNC such as the relative merits of surgery versus RT as single modalities (see above example) and provides a conceptual framework showing how to combine the present treatment modalities to enhance their effectiveness and decrease their complications. Such information can be used by the reader to evaluate any current or future proposal in multimodality therapy for HNC.

During the past decade, clinical investigations of HNC have led to several new insights. Induction chemotherapy can result in high response rates and possibly a reduced incidence of DMs and laryngeal preservation in some cases. However, improved survival has not been achieved because of persistently high rates of locoregional failure. Concomitant chemoradiotherapy has been shown to improve locoregional control and possibly survival. The continued investigations of chemotherapy must strive for further improvement in the most relevant clinical endpoints: survival rates and the quality of life.

Controversy persists concerning the optimal way to combine the three major treatment modalities. In a commentary on the current status of chemotherapy for HNC, Taylor[98] promotes the use of adjuvant rather than neoadjuvant (up-front) chemotherapy after locoregional treatment. Some radiotherapists maintain that no regimen has replaced single modality radiotherapy as the "standard of care," and most would agree that the relative value of simultaneous versus sequential chemoradiotherapy also remains unsettled.

In the words of Tannock and Cummings from Princess Margaret Hospital in Toronto, ". . . the widespread adoption of neoadjuvant (induction) chemotherapy as a management strategy for locally advanced head and neck cancer seems to indicate a perverse willingness by many oncologists to ignore the results of clinical research. Any treatment that adds toxicity without benefit is bad treatment. Neoadjuvant chemotherapy for head and neck cancer is bad treatment, and until we have more effective drugs its use should be restricted to the research setting."[95]

Based on the concepts presented herein, an initial treatment plan which uses cytoreductive therapy (radiation/chemoradiotherapy) often wastes a surgical option which may be the patient's only chance for cure, especially in those who are not complete responders. New treatment combinations currently being suggested include using surgery to "debulk" the residual tumor core after cytoreductive therapy which uses chemotherapy and radiation simultaneously rather than sequentially and/or in rapidly alternating sequence including altered fractionation radiation schemes. The difficulties of such an approach, enumerated in this presentation, suggest that an alternative approach would be better: **use of surgery as the initial treatment followed by other modalities as adjuvant treatment(s) postoperatively, as indicated.** The initial surgical approach should be aggressive, although this does not necessarily equate with radical removal of large anatomic territories. As indicated elsewhere, the principle of conservation surgery for a variety of HNC sites should be the operating principle whenever possible. As pointed out in the section on surgical oncology, a surgeon's task is to remove all gross tumor with a boundary of normal tissue of some size. This can best be accomplished in a previously untreated patient in whom tumor boundaries are most easily detectable. Prior cytoreductive treatment instantly makes the surgeon's job more difficult, if not impossible, by obscuring the original tumor boundaries.

Initial conservation surgery is especially relevant in patients with positive neck disease who are at high risk to develop systemic cancer within the ensuing years, since preserving anatomy, structure, and function at the primary site can often optimize quality of remaining life.

It is unquestionably true that most patients who have been cured of solid tumors (including HNC patients) have had surgery as part of the **initial** treatment, and it is dangerous to eliminate this well-proved modality from the initial treatment plan, despite a seemingly pervasive tendency to do so. Most current "organ preservation" strategies substitute chemotherapy and/or radiation for surgery initially[116,126] not to improve survival rates, since surgery has never been exceeded in this regard, but to improve "quality of life" of cancer patients by decreasing the functional and cosmetic mutilation pursuant to surgery as widely perceived by patients, nonsurgical specialists, and probably many otolaryngologists.[61,62,67,78] The trade-off here is failure to control locoregional cancer with these less effective treatment modalities, and, as has been seen, function is not always improved when they are used.

Trotter noted that time-honored HNC operations are anatomic in design and were invented because they were easy for the surgeon to perform (total laryngectomy, total glossectomy, hemimandibulectomy), not because they were particularly suited to a specific cancer site or pattern of spread.[99,100] Such procedures tended to be unduly mutilating with respect to function and cosmesis and insufficiently radical with respect to cancer. HNC surgeons have been slow to provide alternatives to these traditional operations but must beware of losing their role in the initial management of HNC patients if they fail to provide suitable alternatives which are not perceived as mutilating. Many innovative operations can extend the principles of conservation surgery for laryngeal cancer to other HNC sites which leave patients relatively unscathed both functionally and cosmetically while removing the cancer in a manner which is at least as likely to achieve locoregional control as more radical and traditional procedures. Surgeons would be well advised to change their emphasis from the technical aspects of the field—undue emphasis on flap reconstruction, etc.—to providing more viable alternatives in the realm of ablative cancer surgery in order to allow conservation surgery to become the new neoadjuvant (up-front) treatment; a surgically based organ preservation strategy.

It is necessary to have an experienced HNC surgeon involved in the initial evaluation and treatment planning of the patient from the outset before seemingly "simple" cytoreductive treatment methods are chosen, since assuming that surgical salvage can be performed with useful results later for persistent/recurrent disease is a fallacy (Figs. 13-10 and 13-11). There is also no question that a number of patients are labeled "technically unresectable" on the basis of the appearance of their tumor on scan (CT/MRI) without the input of a trained HNC surgeon. A new category of "technical unresectability" (in addition to the traditional concept of operation being limited by the proximity of vital structures) is provided by patients who have had prior cytoreductive therapy (radical RT with or without chemotherapy), since the densely fibrotic tissue which results and the diffuse pattern of cancer spread within it effectively constitutes a "technically unresectable" barrier to effective surgical excision.

In a patient who for some reason (refusal of surgery?) is initially treated with a chemotherapy-based regimen, several points argue in favor of a sequential rather than simultaneous chemoradiotherapy approach, despite a current (unproved) trend to use the simultaneous combination in an attempt to achieve better cancer control. When chemotherapy is used alone initially, evaluation of tumor response can dictate the next step in the treatment. Additional treatment is always necessary since chemotherapy alone never cures HNC. If a complete response (CR) has occurred, the patient could proceed to radiotherapy, although treatment including surgery is always safest. If tumor persists following chemotherapy however, surgery should definitely be performed next, since radiation would still be available to potentially control any microscopic residual disease postoperatively. The operation should encompass the original extent of the tumor with an adequate margin, because after cytoreductive therapy tumor does not shrink into a cohesive central core but rather leaves diffuse cancer cell deposits throughout the field originally occupied by the tumor. If chemotherapy and radiation are given simultaneously and a less than complete response is achieved (as is likely), the opportunity for surgical salvage is essentially lost, with the possible exception of some endolaryngeal cancers.

In the strategy for combining multimodality therapy for HNC recommended here—initial use of surgery based on conservation principles (only widely applicable in **previously untreated** patients)—adjuvant treatment can then be added, as appropriate, postoperatively. For example, radiotherapy can be added for patients at risk of locoregional recurrence (positive neck nodes with extracapsular spread, close or microscopically positive margins), and/or a systemic modality such as chemotherapy—or in the future biologic therapy—could be given in an attempt to decrease the appearance of distant metastases, again in appropriate patients (N_+). The overall philosophy is the same as that in other organ preservation strategies—to decrease the magnitude of "mutilating" HNC operations—but the timing is different since surgery of a reduced scope is a viable option only in **previously untreated patients** with unaltered barriers to cancer spread and definable tumor boundaries. In this context, adjuvant cytoreductive modalities are used to combat minimal residual disease. With this strategy, oncologic and functional goals are likely to be better served and complications of the treatment minimized. This approach gains immediacy considering the fact that there is currently no evidence that neoadjuvant chemotherapy improves survival or locoregional cancer control or limits the need for subsequent aggressive surgery and that surgery following chemoradiation is fraught with life-threatening complications for the patient due to the difficulty of the dissection in fibrotic tissue and wound-healing complications.[16,17,81,83,100] When cytoreductive treatments are used initially in organ preservation strategies, the benefit accrues only to those who are complete responders. In others, radical surgery is not avoided and it becomes dangerous and essentially worthless because of use in the salvage context.

The fact that these issues have been on the minds of others[44,73] is attested by Spiro's recent Hayes-Martin lecture, "Less can mean more," in which a less mutilating approach to HNC surgery in selected patients was promoted toward the goal of enhancing quality of survival in HNC patients.[89] Examples given included fewer orbital exenterations in patients with sinus cancer, fewer composite resections for cancers abutting the mandible and involving the base of tongue, and fewer total laryngectomies. Spiro also noted the typical zeal for reconstruction demonstrated by surgeons and expressed the worry that the focus was being lost on when and when not to perform "high-tech" reconstructions in the enthusiasm for the various methods available. He noted that we currently lack evidence that free flaps offer a consistent advantage over primary closure and pointed out that, unless we move rapidly, "I fear that others will make treatment decisions for us based primarily on cost-effectiveness" since "clearly the era of surgical radicalism has ended."[66]

Will the technical capability to achieve wider surgical margins (e.g., skull base surgery) increase locoregional HNC cancer control? The answer to this question differs depending upon the context of treatment. In a **previously treated** patient in whom discontinuous cancer cell clumps contaminate the entire field occupied by the original tumor, one can extrapolate from the prior experience of surgical oncologists in attempting to remove large organ territories. This did not improve either survival or locoregional control. Wider surgical excision may have a function in improving locoregional control in a **previously untreated** patient, however.

In the final analysis, ". . . whatever may be our hopes about the discovery and the treatment for malignant disease of methods more specific and less harsh, the surgical operation must be admitted to be the most useful and trustworthy means we now possess."[99] Trotter's 1926 statement appears to be true even 70 years later.

REFERENCES

1. Ackerman LV: The implantation of cancer; an avoidable surgical risk? *Surgery* 37:341, 1955.
2. Adelstein DJ, Sharan VM, Earle AS, et al: Long-term results after chemoradiotherapy for locally confined squamous-cell head and neck cancer. *Am J Clin Oncol* 13:440-447, 1990.
3. Baskies AM: Radiation therapy: its effect on immunoreactivity. *Progr Clin Cancer* 8:215, 1982.
4. Begg AC, McNally NJ: A method to measure the duration of DNA synthesis and the potential doubling time from a single sample. *Cytometry* 6:620-623, 1985.
5. Boon T, Coulie P, Marchand M, et al: Genes coding for tumor rejection antigens: perspectives for specific immunotherapy. In DeVita VT Jr, Hellman S, Rosenberg SA, editors: *Important Advances in Oncology 1994*. Philadelphia, 1994, Lippincott, pp. 53-70.
6. Bourhis J, Wilson G, Wibault P, et al: Rapid tumor cell proliferation after induction chemotherapy in oropharyngeal cancer. *Laryngoscope* 104:468-472, 1994.
7. Byers RM: Modified neck dissection: A study of 927 cases from 1970-1980. *Amer J Surg* 150:414, 1985.
8. Carter RL, et al: Radical neck dissections for squamous carcinomas: pathological findings and their clinical implications with particular reference to transcapsular spread. *Int J Rad Oncol Biol Phys* 13:825, 1987.
9. Carter RL: Patterns and mechanisms of spread of squamous carcinomas of the oral cavity. *Clin Otolaryngol* 15:185, 1990.
10. Chauvel P, Lefebvre J-L, Luboinski B, et al: Follow-up of 408 clinically complete responders after neoadjuvant chemotherapy for head and neck carcinomas: a multicentric study of the GETTEC. Presented at the Third Intl. Conf. on Head and Neck Cancer. San Francisco, July 26-30, 1992, Abstr. 281, p. 120.
11. Childs S, Ling V: The MDR super family of genes and its biological implications. In DeVita VT Jr, Hellman S, Rosenberg, SA, editors: *Important Advances in Oncology 1994*. Philadelphia, 1991, Lippincott, pp. 21-36.
12. Cohen HJ, Laszlo J: Influence of trauma on the unusual distribution of metastases from carcinoma of the larynx. *Cancer* 29:466, 1972.
13. Collins SL. Controversies in the Management of Cancer in the Neck. In Thawley SE, Panje WR, editors: *Comprehensive Management of Head and Neck Tumors*. Philadelphia, 1987, Saunders, pp. 1386-1443. (2nd ed. in press, 1996.)
14. Collins SL: Decreasing the risk of implantation of cancer cells intraoperatively. *Laryngoscope* 103:825, 1993.
15. Cordon-Cardo C, O'Brien JP: The multi-drug resistance phenotype in human cancer. In DeVita VT Jr, Hellman S, Rosenberg SA, editors: *Important Advances in Oncology 1991*. Philadelphia, 1991, Lippincott, pp. 19-38.
16. Corey JP, Caldarelli DD, Hutchinson JC Jr, et al: Surgical complications in patients with head and neck cancer receiving chemotherapy. *Arch Otol Head Neck Surg* 112:437-439, 1986.
17. Croll GA, Gerritsen GJ, Tiwari RM, et al: Primary radiotherapy with surgery in reserve for advanced laryngeal carcinoma: results and complications. *Eur J Surg Oncol* 15:350-356, 1989.
18. Davidson TM: Mohs for head and neck mucosal cancer: report on 111 patients. *Laryngoscope* 98:1078, 1988.
19. der Hagopian RP, et al: Inflammatory oncotaxis. *JAMA* 240:374, 1978.
20. DeVita JT, Hellman S, and Rosenberg SA, editors: *Biologic Therapy of Cancer*. Philadelphia, 1991, Lippincott.
21. DeWys WD: Studies correlating the growth rate of a tumor and it's metastases, and providing evidence for tumor-related systemic growth-retarding factors. *Cancer Res* 32:374, 1972.
22. Eckel HE, Thumfart WF: Laser surgery for the treatment of laryngeal carcinomas: indications, techniques, and preliminary results. *Ann Otol Rhinol Laryngol* 101:113, 1992.
23. Ensley JF, Maciorowski Z, Hassan M, et al: Cellular DNA content parameters in untreated and recurrent squamous cell cancers of the head and neck. *Cytometry* 10:334-38, 1989.
24. Ensley J, Jacobs J, Weaver A, et al: Correlation between response to cisplatinum-combination chemotherapy and radiotherapy in previously untreated patients with squamous cell cancers of the head and neck. *Cancer* 54:811-814, 1984.
25. Farber E, Rubin H: Cellular adaptation in the origin and development of cancer. *Cancer Res* 51:2751, 1991.
26. Ferlito A: Histological classification of larynx and hypopharynx cancers and their clinical applications: pathologic aspects of 2052 malignant neoplasms diagnosed at the ORL Department of Padua University from 1966 to 1976. *Acta Otol Suppl* 342, 1976.
27. Fisch U: *Lymphography of the Cervical Lymphatic System*. Philadelphia, 1968, WB Saunders.
28. Fisher B, Fisher ER: Experimental evidence in support of dormant tumor cells. *Science* 130:918, 1959.
29. Fisher B, Fisher ER: Significance of the interrelationship of the lymph and blood vascular systems in tumor cell dissemination. *Progr Clin Cancer* 4:84, 1970.
30. Fisher B, et al: The contribution of recent NSABP clinical trials of primary breast cancer therapy to an understanding of tumor biology; an overview of findings. *Cancer* 46:1009, 1980.
31. Fisher B. Cancer surgery: a commentary. *Cancer Treat Revs* 68:31, 1984.
32. Fisher B, et al: Presence of a growth-stimulating factor in serum following primary tumor removal in mice. *Cancer Res* 49:1996, 1989a.
33. Fisher B, et al: Effect of local or systemic treatment prior to primary

tumor removal on the production and response to a serum growth-stimulating factor in mice. *Cancer Res* 49:2002, 1989b.

34. Fisher B, et al: Influence of the interval between primary tumor removal and chemotherapy on kinetics and growth of micrometastases. *Cancer Res* 43:1488, 1983.
35. Fletcher GH: Subclinical disease. *Cancer* 53:1274, 1984.
36. Fowler J: Rapid repopulation in radiotherapy: debate on mechanism, the phantom of tumor treatment; continually rapid repopulation unmasked. *Radiother Oncol* 22:156-158, 1991.
37. Goldie JH, Coldman AJ: A mathematical model for relating the drug sensitivity of tumors to their spontaneous mutation rate. *Cancer Treat Rep* 63:1727-1733, 1979.
38. Goldman JL, et al: Serial microscopic studies of radical neck dissections. *Arch Otol* 89:621, 1969.
39 Goldman JL, et al: The pathology of larynges and radical neck specimens in a combination radiation and surgery program for advanced carcinoma of the larynx and laryngopharynx. *Ann ORL* 754:313, 1966.
40. Gunduz N, et al: Effect of surgical removal on the growth and kinetics of residual tumor. *Cancer Res* 19:3861, 1979.
41. Hacker NF, Vanderburg EL. Debulking and intervention surgery. *Ann Oncol* 4:17-22, 1993.
42. Harris AH, Smith RR: Operative wound seeding with tumor cells: its role in recurrences of head and neck cancer. *Ann Surg* 151:330, 1960.
43. Harrison DFN: The questionable value of total glossectomy. *Head Neck Surg* 6:632, 1983.
44. Harrison DFN: Head and neck surgery in the 1980s: the role of more or less. In Chretien PB et al, editors: *Head and Neck Cancer, vol. 1.* St. Louis, 1985, C.V. Mosby, pp 27.
45. Harwood AR, Hawkins NV, Beale FA. Management of advanced glottic cancer. A ten-year review of the Toronto experience. *Int J Rad Oncol Biol Phys* 5:899-904, 1979.
46. Hattori T, et al: Experimental Studies on Operative Stress and Surgery for Cancer. *J Jap Surg Soc* 80:135, 1979.
47. Hattori T, et al: Enhancing effect of thoracotomy on tumor growth in rats with special reference to duration and timing of operation. *Gann* 71:280, 1980.
48. Heppner GH: Tumor heterogeneity. *Cancer Res* 44:2259-2265, 1984.
49. Heppner GH, Miller BE: Therapeutic implications of tumor heterogeneity. *Semin Oncol* 16:91-105, 1989.
50. Hirano M, et al: Pathologic study of carcinoma of the hypopharynx: implications for conservation surgery. *Ann ORL* 96:625, 1987.
51. Jakobsson PA, Eneroth GM, Killander D, et al: Histologic classification and grading of malignancy of the larynx. *Acta Radiol* 12:1, 1973.
52. Kasid U, Pirollo K, Dritschilo A, Chang E: Oncogenic basis of radiation resistance. *Adv Cancer Res* 61:195, 1993.
53. Kirchner JA: What have whole organ sections contributed to the treatment of laryngeal cancer? *Ann ORL* 98:661, 1989.
54. Kraus DH, Pfister DG, Harrison LB, et al: Larynx preservation with combined chemotherapy and radiation therapy in advanced hypopharynx cancer. *Otol Head Neck Surg* 111:31, 1994.
55. Laramore GE, Scott CD, Al-Sarraf M, et al: Adjuvant chemotherapy for resectable squamous cell carcinomas of the head and neck: report of Intergroup Study 0034. *Int J Radiat Oncol Biol Phys* 23:705, 1992.
56. Lee JG: Detection of residual carcinoma of the oropharynx, hypopharynx and larynx: A study of surgical margins. *Trans Am Assoc Ophthalmol Otolaryngol* 79:49, 1974.
57. Leith JT, Dexter DL: *Mammaliam tumor cell heterogeneity.* Boca Raton, 1986, CRC Press.
58. Leith JY, Falkner LE, Bliven SF, et al: Compositional stability of artificial heterogeneous tumors in vivo: use of mitomycin C as a cytotoxic probe. *Cancer Res* 47:2669-73, 1987.
59. Leith JT, Michelson S: Tumor radiocurability: relationship to intrinsic heterogeneity and the tumor bed effect. *Invasion Metastasis* 10:329, 1990.
60. Lindberg RD: Sites of first failure in head and neck cancer. *Cancer Treat Sympos* 2:21, 1983.
61. MacNeil BJ, Weichselbaum R, Pauker SG: Speech and survival. Trade-offs between quantity and quality of life and laryngeal cancer. N Engl J Med 305:982, 1981.
62. Maher E, Jefferis AF: Decision-making in advanced cancer of the head and neck: variation in the views of medical specialists. *J Roy Soc Med* 83:356, 1990.
63. Marcial VA, Pajak TF, Mohiuddin M, et al: Concomitant cisplatin chemotherapy and radiotherapy in advanced mucosal squamous cell carcinoma of the head and neck. Long-term results of the Radiation Therapy Oncology Group Study 81-17. *Cancer* 66:1861, 1990.
64. Meuer MF, Kenady DE: Metastatic carcinoma in a percutaneous gastrostomy site. *Head and Neck* 15:70, 1993.
65. Miles L, Hunter N, Peters LJ: Tumor bed effect; induced reduction of tumor radiocurability through the increase in hypoxic cell fraction. *Int J Radiat Oncol Biol Phys* 16:139-142, 1989.
66. Miller ML, Swartz WM, Miller RH, Harvey JM: Cost analysis of microsurgical reconstruction in the head and neck. *J Surg Oncol* 46:230, 1991.
67. Mohide EA, Archibald SD, Tew M, Young JE, Haines T: Postlaryngectomy quality-of-life dimension identified by patients and health-care professionals. *Am J Surg* 164:619, 1992.
68. Morfit HM: Surgical treatment of cancer of the extrinsic larynx and hypopharyngeal walls. *Surg* 37:229, 1955.
69. Morris J: Outcome following treatment for head and neck cancer: beyond clinical assessment. *Eur J Cancer* 27:675, 1991.
70. Morton EL. Changing Concepts of Cancer Surgery: Surgery as Immunotherapy. *AJS,* 135:367, 1978.
71. Norris CM Jr: Pathology of surgery after induction chemotherapy: an analysis of resectability and locoregional control. *Laryngoscope* 96:292, 1986.
72. Oloffson J, Van Nostrand WP: Growth and spread of laryngeal and hypopharyngeal carcinoma with reflections on the effect of preoperative irradiation: 139 cases studied by whole-organ serial sectioning. *Acta Otol* Suppl 308, 1973.
73. Papaionnou A: Hypothesis: increasingly intensive locoregional treatment of breast cancer may promote recurrence. *J Surg Oncol* 30:33, 1985.
74. Penhaligon M, Courtenay VD, Camplejohn RS: Tumor bed effect: hypoxic fraction of tumors growing in pre-irradiated bed. *Int J Radiat Biol* 52:635-641, 1987.
75. Pfister DG: In reply. *J Clin Oncol* 10:344, 1992.
76. Prehn RT: Tumor progression and homeostasis. *Adv Cancer Res* 23:203, 1976.
77. Proffitt, SD, et al: Origin of undifferentiated neoplasm from verrucous epidermal carcinoma of oral cavity following irradiation. *Cancer* 26:389, 1970.
78. Revesz L: Effect of tumor cells killed by x-rays upon the growth of admixed viable cells. *Nature* 178:139, 1956.
79. Roth JA, et al: Effects of operation on immune respose in cancer patients: sequential evaluation of *in vitro* lymphocyte function. *Surg* 79:486, 1976.
80. Sartorelli AC: Therapeutic attack on hypoxic cells of solid tumors: presidential address. *Cancer Res* 48:775-8, 1988.
81. Sassler AM, Esclamado RM, Wolf GT, et al: *Surgery after organ preservation therapy: analysis of wound complications. Arch Otol HNS* 121:162:1995.
82. Scanlon EF: The role of the fifth circulation in cancer dissemination. *AJS* 138:474, 1979.

83. Shamberger R: Effect of chemotherapy and radiotherapy on wound healing: experimental studies. *Recent Results Cancer Res* 98:17, 1985.
84. Shirinian MH, Weber RS, Lippman SM, et al: Laryngeal preservation by induction chemotherapy plus radiotherapy in locally advanced head and neck cancer: the M.D. Anderson Cancer Center experience. *Head Neck* 16:39, 1994.
85. Shochat SJ, et al: Evaluation of cellular immunity and adrenocortical activity in surgical patients. *J Surg Res* 26:332, 1979.
86. Skipper HE, Simpson-Herren L: Relationship between tumor stem cell heterogeneity and responsiveness to chemotherapy. In DeVita VT, Hellman S, Rosenberg SA, editors: *Important Advances in Oncology 1985*. p. 63. Lippincott, Philadelphia.
87. Skolnick EM, et al. Preoperative radiation of the larynx-analysis of serial sections. *Ann ORL* 79:1033, 1970.
88. Slotman GJ, et al: The incidence of metastasis after multi-modality therapy of cancer of the head and neck. *Cancer* 54:2009, 1984.
89. Spiro RH: Less can mean more. *Am J Surg* 166:322-325, 1993.
90. Steiner W: Therapy of hypopharyngeal carcinoma. In Johnson JT, Didolkar MS, editors: *Head and Neck Cancer Vol. 3* 1993, Elsevier Science Publishers. p. 101. Amsterdam.
91. Steiner W: Results after transoral laser surgery for hypopharyngeal carcinoma. Second World Congress on Laryngeal Cancer. Sydney, Australia, February, 1994, Abstract 0344.
92. Suit HD, et al: Intact tumor cells in irradiated tissue. *Arch Path* 78:648, 1964.
93. Tanner, NSB, et al: The irradiated radical neck dissection in squamous carcinoma: a clinico-pathological study. *Clin Otolaryngol* 5:259, 1980.
94. Tannock IF, Browman G: Lack of evidence for a role of chemotherapy in the routine management of locally advanced head and neck cancer. *J Clin Oncol* 4:1121-1126, 1986.
95. Tannock IF, Cummings BJ: Neoadjuvant chemotherapy in head and neck cancer: No way to preserve a larynx. *J Clin Oncol* 10:343-6, 1992.
96. Tannock IF: Is there evidence that neoadjuvant chemotherapy adds to radiation in limiting the necessity for aggressive surgery? In Johnson JT, Didolkar MS, editors: *Head and Neck Cancer vol. 3*. 1993, Elsevier Science Publishers.
97. Tarpley JL, et al: Prolonged depression of cellular immunity in cured laryngopharyngeal cancer patients treated with radiation therapy. *Cancer* 35:638, 1975.
98. Taylor IV: Why has so much chemotherapy done so little in head and neck cancer? *J Clin Oncol* 5:1, 1987.
99. Trotter W: The surgery of malignant disease of the pharynx. *Br Med J* 23:269, 1926.
100. Trotter W: Some principles in the surgery of the pharynx. *Lancet* 2:833, 1931.
101. Vandenbrouck C, Sandio H, LeFur R: Elective versus therapeutic radical neck dissection in epidermoid carcinoma of the oral cavity—results of a randomized clinical trial. *Cancer* 46:386, 1980.
102. Viadana E: The metastatic spread of "head and neck" tumors in men (an autopsy study of 371 cases). *Z Krebsforsch* 83:293, 1975.
103. Vikram B: Changing patterns of failure in advanced head and neck cancer. *Arch Otol* 110:564, 1984.
104. Vikram B, Malamud S, Gold J, et al: Chemotherapy rapidly alternating with accelerated radiotherapy for advanced carcinomas of the hypopharynx and upper esophagus: a feasibility study. *Head Neck* 13:415, 1991.
105. Vokes EE, Panje WR, Schilsky RL, et al: Hydroxyurea, flurouracil, and concomitant radiotherapy in poor-prognosis head and neck cancer: a phase I-II study. *J Clin Oncol* 7:761-8, 1989.
106. Vokes EE, Weichselbaum RR: Concomitant chemoradiotherapy: rationale and clinical experience in patients with solid tumors. *J Clin Oncol* 8:911-934, 1990.
107. Vokes EE, Haraf DJ, Weichselbaum RR, Brachman D: Induction chemotherapy: promises and limitations. In Johnson JT, Didolkar MS, editors: *Head and Neck Cancer vol. 3*. 1993, Elsevier Science Publsihers. Amsterdam.
108. von Essen, CF: Radiation enhancement of metastasis: a review. *Clin Expt Metas* 9:77, 1991.
109. Vujicic N, et al: The significance of cancer cells contaminating postoperative seroma. *Clin Expt Metas* 4:221, 1986.
110. Wang CC: The enigma of accelerated hyperfractionated radiation therapy for head and neck cancer. *Int J Radiat Oncol Biol Phys* 14:209, 1988.
111. Weichselbaum RR, Beckett MA, Schwartz JL, et al: Radioresistant tumor cells are present in head and neck carcinomas that recur after radiotherapy. *Int J Radiat Oncol Biol Phys* 15:575, 1988.
112. Weichselbaum R: Cellular and molecular aspects of human tumor radioresistance. In DeVita VT Jr, Hellman S, Rosenberg SA, editors: *Important Advances in Oncology 1991*. Philadelphia, 1991, Lippincott, pp. 73-80.
113. Wheelock ES, et al: The tumor dormant state. *Adv Can Res* 34:107, 1981.
114. Withers, HR: Biologic basis for altered fractionation schemes. *Cancer* 55:2086, 1985.
115. Withers H, Taylor J, Maciejewski B: The hazard of accelerated tumor clonogen population during radiotherapy. *Acta Oncol* 2:98, 1988.
116. Wolf GT, Fisher SG, Hong WK, et al: Induction chemotherapy plus radiation compared with surgery plus radiation in patients with advanced laryngeal cancer. VA Laryngeal Cancer Study Group. *N Engl J Med* 324:1685, 1991.
117. Woodruff MFA: Tumor clonality and its biological significance. *Adv Cancer Res* 50:197, 1988.
118. Yamamoto E: Mode of invasion in lymph node metastasis in squamous cell carcinoma of the oral cavity. *Head Neck Surg* 6:938, 1984.

SUGGESTED FURTHER READING

119. Awan AM, Vokes EE, Weichselbaum RR: Recent advances in radiation therapy for head and neck cancer. *Hematology/Oncology Clin N Amer* 5:635-655, 1991.
120. Bauer WC: Varieties of squamous carcinoma; biological behavior. *Front Rad Ther Oncol* 9:164, 1974.
121. Bosl GJ, Strong E, Harrison L, Pfister DG: Chemotherapy and the management of locally advanced squamous cell carcinoma of the head and neck: Role in larynx preservation. In DeVita VT Jr, Hellman S, Rosenberg SA, editors: *Important Advances in Oncology 1991*. Philadelphia, 1991, Lippincott, pp. 191-204.
122. Burns, L, Chase D, Goodwin JW: Treatment of patients with stage IV cancer: do the ends justify the means? *Otolaryngol Head Neck Surg* 97:8, 1987.
123. Bush RS, Jenkin RDT, Allt WEC, et al: Definitive evidence for hypoxic cells, influencing cure in cancer therapy. *Br J Cancer* 37(Suppl 3)302-326, 1978.
124. Cardinal CG, Yarbro JW: A conceptual history of cancer. *Semin Oncol* 6:396, 1979.
125. Choksi AJ, Dimery IW, Hong WK: Adjuvant chemotherapy of head and neck cancer: the past, the present, and the future. *Semin Oncol* 15:45, 1988.
126. Clark JR, Fallon BG, Frei III E: Induction chemotherapy as initial treatment for advanced head and neck cancer: a model for the multidisciplinary treatment of solid tumors. VT DeVita Jr, S Hellman, SA Rosenberg, editors: *Important Advances in Oncology 1987*. Philadelphia, 1991, Lippincott, p. 175.
127. Collins SL, Saunders VW Jr: Excision of selected intraoral cancers by use of sagittal inner table mandibulectomy. *Otolaryngol Head Neck Surg* 97:558, 1987.
128. Collins SL: Squamous Cancer of the Oral Cavity, Oropharynx and Pharyngeal Walls. In: Ballenger JJ, editor: *Diseases of the Nose,*

Throat, Ear, Head and Neck, ed 14. Philadelphia, 1991, Lee and Febiger, pp. 335-454. (2nd ed. in press, 1995.)

129. Collins SL: Diseases of the oral cavity and pharynx: malignant lesions. In Weisberger ED, editor: *Lasers in head and neck surgery.* New York, 1991, Igaku-Shoin, Chap 7B, pp. 121-144.
130. Conley JJ, et al: The meaning of life-threatening disease in the area of the head and neck. *Acta Otolaryngol* (Stockholm), 99:201, 1985.
131. Conley JJ: Have I Performed the Right Operation? *Arch OHNS* 112:385, 1986.
132. Duval MK, Healy MJ: Natural History and Effects of Treatment on Cancer of the Tongue. *Cancer* 9:1842, 1956.
133. Gilbert H, Kagan AR: Recurrence patterns of squamous carcinoma of the oral cavity, pharynx, and larynx. *J Surg Oncol* 6:357, 1974. (Critique of head and neck cancer literature reporting methods.)
134. Goepfert H, Schantz SP: Is it time for biologic staging of cancer? *Head Neck* 12:291, 1990.
135. Goepfert, H. Are we making any progress? *Arch Otol Head Neck Surg* 110:562, 1984.
136. Gordon-Taylor G: The incomputable factor in cancer prognosis. *Br Med J* 1:455, 1959.
137. Harrison DFM: Natural history of some cancers affecting the head and neck. *J Laryngol Otol* 86:1189, 1972.
138. Harrison DFN: Down with the dabblers. *Arch Otol Head Neck Surg* 114:809, 1988. (Letter to the Editor.)
139. Harrison DFN: Is surgery for the benefit of the patient or the surgeon? In Kagan AR, Miles J, editors: *Head and Neck Oncology: Clinical Management.* New York, 1989, Pergamon Press, Chap. 15, p 116.
140. Harrison DFN: 1990 Ogura Memorial Lecture: Moral dilemmas in head and neck cancer. *Laryngoscope,* 100:1191, 1990.
141. Jud MC: A study of the behavior of cancer of the head and neck during its late and terminal phases. *Am J Surg* 108:552, 1964.
142. Kallman RF, Southerland RM: Combined modalities. *Cancer Treat Sympos* 1:103-110, 1984.
143. Kirchner JA: Promising fields for investigation in laryngeal cancer. *Laryngoscope* 85:1709, 1975.
144. Larson DL, et al: Perineural lymphatics: myth or fact? *Am J Surg* 112:488, 1966.
145. Looney WB, Hopkins HA, MacLeod MS, et al: Solid tumor models for the assessment of different treatment modalities. *Cancer* 44:437-445, 1979.
146. Lore JM Jr: Dabbling in head and neck oncology (a plea for added qualifications). *Arch Otol Head Neck Surg* 113:1165, 1987.
147. MacDonald I: Biologic predeterminism in human cancer. *Surg Gynec Oncol* 90:443, 1951.
148. Broder S, ed: *Molecular Foundations of Oncology.* Baltimore, 1991, Williams and Wilkins.
149. Scanlon EF, Murtley SM: Basic science overview: the Process of metastasis. *Cancer* J 41:301-305, 1991.
150. Schipper H: Quality of life. meaning and measurement. In *Advances in Pain Research and Therapy, vol. 16.* New York, 1990, Raven Press, p 89.
151. Slaughter DP: Multicentric origin of intraoral carcinoma. *Surgery* 20:133, 1946.
152. Slaughter DP, et al: Field cancerization in oral stratified squamous epithelium-clinical implications of multicentric origin. *Cancer* 6:963, 1953.
153. Spratt JS Jr: Cancer: Do early diagnosis and treatment really help? How do we relate costs to benefit in cancer control? *Oral Surg* 45:220, 1978.
154. Stell PM: Can we afford to treat head and neck cancer? *Clin Otol* 12:321, 1987.
155. Sugarbaker EV: Cancer metastasis: a product of tumor-host interaction. *Curr Prob Cancer* 3:1, 1979.
156. Sugarbaker EV, et al: Observations on cancer metastasis in man. In *Tumor Invasion & Metastasis. Developments in Oncology vol 7.* Liotta LA, Hart IR, editors: Boston, 1982, Martinus Nijhoff Publishers.
157. Tannock IF, Rotin D: Keynote address: mechansims of interaction between radiation and drugs with potential for improvements in therapy. NCI monograph 6:77-83, 1988.
158. Tannock I: Important lessons learned from adjuvant and neoadjuvant studies. In Fee W, Goepfert H, Johns M, Strong E, Ward T, editors: *Head and Neck Cancer vol. 2.* Philadelphia, 1990, Marcel Decker, pp. 302-305.
159. Tannock IF, Hill RP, editors: *The Basic Science of Oncology.* 1987, Pergamon Press, New York.
160. Till, JE: Quality of life measurements in cancer treatment. In: DeVita VT, Hellman SA, Rosenberg S, editors: *Important Advances in Oncology, 1992.* Philadelphia, 1992, Lippincott, pp. 189-204.
161. Vokes EE, Weichselbaum RR, Lippman SM, Hong WK: Medical progress: head and neck cancer. *N Engl J Med* 328:184-194, 1993.
162. Weiss L: A pathobiologic overview of metastasis. *Semin Oncol* 4:5, 1977.
163. Williams, CT, editor: *Introducing new treatments for cancer: Practical, ethical and legal problems.* New York, 1992, John Wiley & Sons Ltd.

14

A Practical Approach to the Management of Oropharyngeal Cancer

Jack L. Gluckman, M.D.

Cancer of the oropharynx is relatively uncommon, with approximately 10,000 new cases being diagnosed in the United States each year.

Despite recent advances in diagnosis, surgical techniques, and ever-changing radiation and chemotherapy protocols, the selection of the ideal therapy for the patient with oropharyngeal cancer is as confusing today as it was 25 years ago. The disease is better understood, as are the needs of the patient, and yet this knowledge has not really as yet been translated into improved survival rates. This disappointment should not, however, deter the oncologist from aggressively treating these patients with all the resources currently available. If, in the final analysis, the patient cannot be cured but can be effectively palliated with an improved quality of life for their remaining days, this in itself is a laudable accomplishment. The basic premise of management is to maximize the results of treatment while minimizing the morbidity associated with the treatment.

THERAPEUTIC OPTIONS

Therapeutic options available to the physician are myriad but essentially can be categorized as follows: (1) surgery, (2) radiation, (3) combination surgery and radiotherapy, (4) chemotherapy as an adjunct to surgery and radiation therapy, and (5) symptomatic palliative therapy.

Each one of these modalities has its proponents and detractors, but, in the final analysis, because of the absence of any proved definitive approach, the oncologist should recommend the regimen with which he or she feels most comfortable and which seems best suited for an individual patient in an individual setting. This chapter reflects my personal philosophy and experience and should in no way be misconstrued as the definitive approach for these cancers.

FACTORS AFFECTING CHOICE OF THERAPY

Type of malignancy

Not all tumors that develop in the oropharynx are squamous cell carcinoma. A wide variety of benign and malignant tumors may arise in the oropharynx itself and in the parapharyngeal space with distortion of the lumen of the pharynx mimicking primary intrapharyngeal tumors.

Squamous cell carcinoma is the most common malignancy arising in the oropharynx. Although clinically this cancer is regarded as being more aggressive in behavior than oral cavity cancer, with a concomitant worse prognosis, this probably reflects the more advanced staging at the initial presentation because of late diagnosis.

Macroscopically, various types are described: superficial and exophytic, ulcerative and infiltrative, and fungating. The superficial spreading exophytic lesion is found most commonly on the soft palate and faucial arch. These lesions are frequently associated with areas of condemned mucosa and probably formed by coalescence of multifocal foci of cancer. They behave in a less aggressive manner with a low incidence of nodal metastases. On the other hand, ulcerative, infiltrative and fungating squamous cell carcinomas are more aggressive in behavior, with a higher rate of metastases and a more ominous prognosis.

Poor clinical prognostic indicators include tumor size, evidence of nodal metastases, and disease occurring in young patients who are nonsmokers and nondrinkers.

Several attempts to correlate histopathologic features with tumor behavior and survival have been made over the years. The classic Broders classification is of no value as a prognostic indicator. Conversely, the pattern of invasion at the host-tumor interface appears to be important. Carcinomas that invade in columns of small aggregates appear to have a worse prognosis compared with those that invade with a broad pushing border. In addition, frequency of mitoses, evidence of perineural invasion, and vascular invasion are important predictors of aggressiveness. Tumor thickness is an important negative prognostic indicator in advanced tumors, but its value in early cancers is less obvious.

In addition the search continues for significant biomarkers at a molecular level. Various oncogenes and DNA image analysis are all being evaluated with some encouraging results.

Lymphoepithelioma is regarded as variant of squamous cell carcinoma which arises from the faucial or lingual tonsils. It behaves somewhat differently from squamous cell cancer in that it has a propensity for early nodal and even distant metastases. Clinically this lesion is softer to palpation than squamous cell cancer. Histologically, it consists of nests of malignant epithelial cells with a background of lymphocytes scattered between the malignant cells. These tumors are exquisitely sensitive to radiation therapy which is the treatment of choice.

Verrucous carcinoma is an extremely well-differentiated carcinoma, characterized by slow growth and no propensity for regional or distant metastases. The treatment of choice for these lesions is surgical excision, although radiation can be successfully used if surgery is deemed inappropriate.

Tumors of minor salivary gland origin may arise in the oropharynx. These should be differentiated from tumors arising from the deep lobe of the parotid or de novo in the parapharyngeal space and distorting the oropharynx. Fifty percent to 70% of all minor salivary gland tumors are malignant. Of the malignant tumors, the most common is the adenoid cystic carcinoma, but other malignancies such as mucoepidermoid carcinoma, adenocarcinoma, acinic cell tumor, small cell tumor, and malignant pleomorphic adenoma all have been described. They usually develop as a painless submucosal mass, gradually increasing in size and become ulcerated only rarely. All, but particularly the adenoidcystic carcinoma, have a propensity for perineural spread and therefore great care should be taken to follow and biopsy any regional nerves to ensure adequate excision.

Hodgkin's and non–Hodgkin's lymphoma may arise in the tonsil and base of the tongue and should be strongly suspected in a unilateral enlargement of the tonsil, particularly if it is associated with large cervical nodes.

Sarcomas occasionally arise in the oropharynx.

Site of malignancy

Tonsil. The majority of oropharyngeal cancers arise in the tonsil or tonsillar fossa. As they enlarge, the tumor spreads superficially to involve the posterior-lateral pharyngeal wall and base of tongue and may extend inferiorly into the hypopharynx or superiorly to the nasopharynx. Deep extension can cause fixation to, or erosion of, the ascending ramus of the mandible or involvement of the pterygoid muscles causing trismus. Extension into the parapharyngeal space can result in perineural invasion of cranial nerves with extension to the base of the skull and involvement of the great vessels of the neck.

Base of the tongue. Cancer of the base of tongue may arise de novo or may be secondary to spread from regional areas (e.g., tonsil, anterior tongue, and supraglottic larynx). In any event, these lesions are associated with a poor prognosis because of late diagnosis, difficulty in determining the exact dimension, and the tendency to early bilateral regional metastases. As the tumor grows, it will spread deeply into the root of the tongue and into the pre-epiglottic space.

Palatine arch. Carcinoma of the anterior tonsillar pillar and soft palate usually presents as superficial spreading exophytic lesions in areas of condemned mucosa with multicentric cancers being a frequent associated finding. Generally, these tumors have a better overall prognosis but, if left untreated, will eventually infiltrate deeply and extend laterally to involve the lateral pharyngeal walls and the retromolar trigone.

Pharyngeal wall. Cancer of the posterolateral pharyngeal wall often presents late due to the relative lack of symptoms associated with early lesions. Interestingly, these tumors may attain considerable size before invading the underlying prevertebral musculature. This is fortunate, because, once this has been invaded, the tumor is unresectable and probably not curable.

Staging of the neoplasm

The superficial dimensions of the tumor are used for staging these cancers. While this is useful to some degree in predicting prognosis, it does not reflect tumor behavior and can be quite deceptive.

Presence of associated disease

Head and neck surgery, though complex in nature, in general does not result in a profound disturbance of body metabolism postoperatively. The patient who develops the cancer, however, is frequently poorly nourished and may have significant pulmonary, cardiovascular, and hepatic disease. If severe, these factors may preclude surgery from being a therapeutic option or may influence the type of surgery proposed (e.g., poor pulmonary reserve may necessitate a total laryngectomy in association with the glossectomy to prevent aspiration).

Psychologic attitude of the patient

The fear of cancer usually outweighs the fear of surgery or radiotherapy. This is, unfortunately, not always the case, and irrational fear may dictate a change in policy. Never force the patient into an option that is not requested or desired.

Attitude of family and support system

The family *must* be involved in the decision-making process. If they fail to live up to their obligations in aiding the patient's rehabilitation and acceptance back into society, the therapy will be judged a failure, no matter how successful it might appear to the oncologist.

Philosophy and experience of the oncologist

Each oncologist develops his or her own philosophy of management based on past experience and intuition in dealing with a particular oncologic problem in a particular setting. Until a fail-safe guaranteed "cookbook" cure for cancer is available, a diversity of opinion is to be expected and should, in fact, be encouraged.

Facilities available

It is a fact of life that many head and neck tumors are managed away from the "ivory tower" of academic institutions, where sophisticated backup and support systems are in place for the management of these patients. Not every oncologist has access to dedicated nurses, prosthodontists, social workers, speech therapists, and so forth. While a case can be made for the management of all these patients in a centralized tertiary setting, this is not the norm at present, and therefore the facilities available should be taken into consideration when making the decision to how best to treat the patient.

PATIENT EVALUATION

As already stated, the patient's general physical and emotional status must be assessed as part of the evaluation process and appropriate consultations obtained. Attention is then directed to the head and neck examination.

Every attempt should be made to delineate the exact extent of the tumor. A careful head and neck examination is essential. Not only should the primary tumor be assessed, but also one should also look for other signs which may aid in determining unexpected spread, e.g., trismus, limitation of tongue movement, cranial nerve involvement, particularly anesthesia in the distribution of the inferior alveolar nerve, and, of course, any palpable cervical metastases.

I order imaging only if specific questions must be answered. If I am concerned about mandible involvement, a Panorex or CT scan is performed. If prevertebral muscle involvement is suspected a CT scan or MRI is ordered. Base of skull erosion is evaluated by CT scan, whereas base of tongue extent is best assessed on MRI. In general, I do not routinely obtain imaging studies to evaluate the neck for nodal metastases, but, if one is obtaining the scan to answer specific questions regarding the primary tumor, the neck will obviously also be visualized.

If suspicion for distant metastases is great, e.g., multiple nodal metastases, biochemical abnormalities, and bone pain, a metastatic workup should be performed. I usually perform a CT scan of chest and abdomen and a bone scan. This is probably not very cost effective, but I have occasionally identified distant metastases not noted by more conventional investigations.

Examination under anesthesia should always be performed:

1. To permit more accurate evaluation of the tumor. This should include careful palpation particularly of base of tongue cancers which may have significant submucosal extension and posterior wall cancers to determine fixation to the underlying musculature.
2. Evaluation for multicentric cancers.
3. Allow for adequate biopsy of the cancer.

The tumor is then staged according to the American Joint Committee for Cancer Staging recommendations (1992).

RADIATION THERAPY

As surgical techniques for ablation and reconstruction have advanced, so too have radiotherapeutic techniques. As in surgery, the results of radiation vary according to the skill and experience of the radiotherapist and the facilities at his or her disposal. The results of radiation alone in the treatment of early lesions of the oropharynx are probably comparable with those obtained from surgery. This usually consists of delivering a dose of 60 to 70 Gy through a shrinking field to the primary lesion and both sides of the neck over the course of six to seven weeks. Alternatively, reduced external radiation can be combined with radium implants, thereby boosting the tumor dose. However, implants are difficult to insert in the oropharynx, although we have used these for more advanced base of tongue cancers with good local control. Alternate techniques to increase efficacy and minimize morbidity include submental boosts of external radiation, low-dose rate radiotherapy, and twice-daily radiation. As the stage of the tumor increases, it has been my experience that the efficacy of radiotherapy alone declines, and planned combined radiotherapy and surgery appears to offer a better chance for cure.

Radiation alone, therefore, may be used effectively in the following situations:

1. Small limited cancers.
2. Where surgery is contraindicated because of systemic disease.
3. If the patient refuses surgery.
4. For palliation in the extremely advanced tumor.

However, radiation should not be recommended with the vague notion that salvage surgery can always be used at a later stage if the disease should persist or recur. The success rate with surgical salvage after radiation for oropharyngeal cancer is extremely poor, and the surgery after high-dose curative radiation is associated with a significant morbidity rate.

Radiation itself is not without complications and may be associated with an significant sequelae in this area (e.g., xerostomia, loss of taste, mucosal ulceration, osteoradionecrosis, pharyngeal necrosis with fistula formation, and hemorrhage). The status of the teeth must be addressed *before* commencing radiation.

COMBINATION SURGERY AND RADIATION THERAPY

The concept of combined therapy for advanced cancer is based on the following philosophy:

The major reason for surgical failure is leaving residual viable tumor cells in the patient. This occurs because of unrecognized peripheral projection of malignant cells, undetected lymphatic or hematogenous metastasis, or the implantation of tumor during the surgery. Conversely, the major reason for radiation failure is the projection of tumor outside the treatment field or the presence of anoxic cells in the center of the neoplasm remaining untreated. Therefore, theoretically, planned combined radiation and surgery should serve to minimize the source of failure in each method.

Although it is strongly suggestive that combined therapy is the most effective treatment for advanced tumors and in my experience this is the case, it should be appreciated that there is no absolute supportive data for this concept.

In the 1970s, we, like others, used *preoperative* radiation usually consisting of 45 to 50 Gy, followed by a 4-week delay to allow the acute radiation reaction to subside before performing surgery. The rationale for this approach was that the tumor would be theoretically more radiosensitive if the blood supply was not compromised by the surgery and that radiation may seal off the lymphatics, thereby permitting subsequent surgical manipulation without fear of tumor seeding.

Over the past 15 years however, we have used *postoperative* radiation. The advantage is that the operative morbidity is significantly diminished, a slightly higher dose of radiation can be given, and there is less chance of inadequate resection because the margins are more clearly identified. The only disadvantage is that, if a surgical complication should occur, the radiation may be delayed sufficiently to become ineffective. Open wounds may, however, be irradiated without fear of worsening the situation and preventing healing.

ADJUNCT CHEMOTHERAPY

Chemotherapy has been used as a last resort for terminal cancer patients for many years, with its role being palliative in relieving pain and obstructive symptoms. The use of chemotherapeutic agents as an adjunct to both surgery and irradiation in the treatment of head and neck cancer continues to titillate the oncologist. Unfortunately, although many drugs have shown promise, there is still no definitive evidence that this approach has any influence on ultimate long-term prognosis. Whether adjunct chemotherapy will ultimately aid in the control of local disease or prevent tumor dissemination remains, as yet, unanswered.

As a result, at present, I do not routinely recommend the use of adjunct chemotherapy in the management of these cancers.

SURGERY

Historically, it should be appreciated that the reason radiation assumed a dominant role in the treatment of oropharyngeal cancers is because the oropharynx was felt to be inaccessible to adequate surgical resection. Today, however, a myriad of surgical approaches to lesions of the oropharynx have been described (Fig. 14-1):

1. Intraoral resection
2. Mandible-sparing procedures
   Lateral pharyngotomy
   Transhyoid pharyngotomy
3. Mandible-splitting procedures
   Lateral osteotomy
   Anterior osteotomy
4. Composite resection (jaw-neck procedure)

Which approach is optimal for a particular cancer is dependent on the site and size of the tumor and whether a concomitant lymph node dissection is needed.

Intraoral resection

Some cancers may be resected intraorally:

1. Superficial exophytic cancers, particularly arising from the posterior oropharyngeal wall and soft palate.
2. The "condemned mucosa," with multicentric lesions usually noted on the soft palate.

The excision can be accomplished using a scalpel, cautery, or carbon dioxide laser with equally good results. The

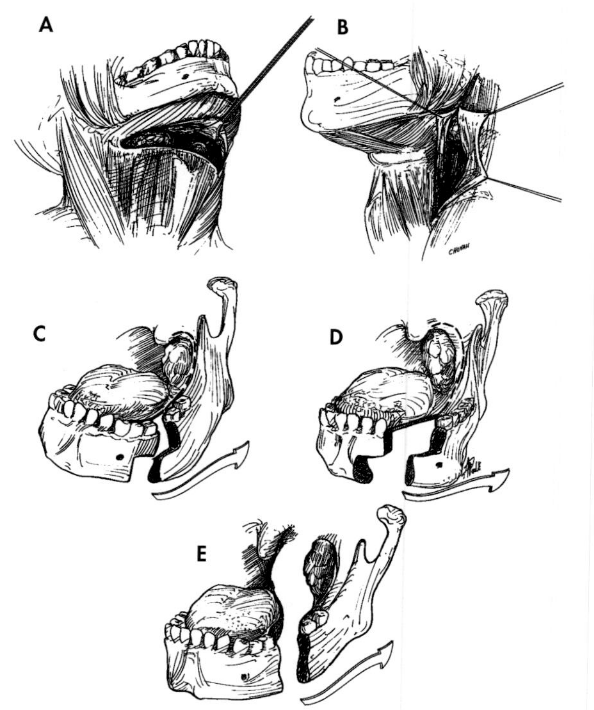

FIG 14-1
Surgical approaches to the oropharynx. **A,** Transhyoid pharyngotomy. **B,** Lateral pharyngotomy. **C,** Lateral osteotomy. **D,** Anterior osteotomy. **E,** Mandibulectomy. (From Gluckman JL: Current management of cancer of the oropharynx, *Oncology,* 4(4):23-29, 1990.)

CO_2 laser has some advantages, including improved hemostasis, less edema, and being more precise, but it is not essential for the treatment of these lesions.

Frozen section control should be performed, not only from the periphery but from the depth of the resection as well. I find the role of 1% toluidine blue most useful in defining the extent of resection.

After resection, the defect is usually allowed to heal by secondary intention. Other defects may be closed primarily by mobilizing the surrounding mucosa or using a split skin graft which should be quilted into position.

In general, think twice before attempting intraoral resection except in the most superficial of lesions. Particularly avoid the inclination to perform a tonsillectomy for squamous cell carcinoma apparently confined to the tonsil. Cancer does not obey normal tissue planes, and this operation can be regarded as at best a debulking procedure and at worst as opening tissue planes for further spread.

Mandible-sparing procedures

Transhyoid pharyngotomy (see Fig. 14-1, *A*). The transhyoid pharyngotomy is an excellent approach to lesions of the lower posterior oropharyngeal wall that are too large or too inferior to remove transorally. While one can enter the pharynx above the hyoid, I tend to remove the body of the hyoid as this greatly facilitates the procedure. Care is taken not to damage the superior laryngeal or hypoglossal nerves. The vallecula is entered, and an excellent view of the posterior pharyngeal wall is obtained. After resection, the wound is closed primarily. A temporary tracheostomy is performed, and the procedure can be combined with a neck dissection if indicated. This procedure gives an excellent cosmetic and functional result. Others have recommended this approach for tonsil and base of tongue cancers, but I believe this is too blind and limited an approach and better alternatives are available.

Lateral pharyngotomy (see Fig. 14-1, *B*). Lateral pharyngotomy is an excellent approach to moderately sized lesions on the posterolateral pharyngeal wall, provided they are small enough and inferior enough that adequate access can be attained without disrupting the mandible. Of course, if the lesion is large, the pharyngotomy may be extended superiorly and combined with a lateral mandibular osteotomy to improve access. This technique may be combined with a neck dissection. Key points in the technique are to enter the pharynx by retracting the thyroid ala medially and incising the mucosa of the upper pyriform sinus and extending the incision superiorly. The superior laryngeal and hypoglossal nerves must be identified and avoided. For practical purposes, I prefer not to split the mandible laterally and would rather combine it with an anterior osteotomy.

Mandible-splitting procedures

If the tumor cannot be readily accessed by working around the mandible, it may be necessary to split the mandible to obtain adequate exposure. After the resection and reconstruction have been completed, the mandible is reapproximated and plated into position. These osteotomies may be performed either anteriorly or laterally, although I almost never perform a lateral osteotomy. The indications for these procedures are moderately sized cancers of the tonsil, lateral pharyngeal wall, or base of tongue that are not in close proximity to the mandible or directly invading into the mandible itself.

Lateral osteotomy (see Fig. 14-1, *C*). Classically known as the Trotter's operation, this technique necessitates a stepped osteotomy of the body of the mandible with the exact site depending on the size and site of the tumor and the state of the patient's dentition. After the mandible has been splayed apart, the tumor is removed in continuity with the neck dissection and, after the appropriate reconstruction, the mandible is approximated using plates.

The major contraindication to this approach is, if postoperative radiation is used, as is frequently the case, nonunion may result. An anterior osteotomy, however, is out of the radiation field and not subject to this problem.

A further, if somewhat minor, sequela of this approach is that the inferior alveolar nerve is transected with resultant anesthesia in its distribution.

Anterior osteotomy (see Fig. 14-1, *D*). In my opinion, a more useful technique for splitting the mandible is the anterior osteotomy. Much discussion exists as to whether the osteotomy should be symphyseal or parasymphyseal or whether it should be straight or stepped. It is my opinion that the actual osteotomy is best performed in a stepped manner just anterior to the mental foramen, ensuring that the inferior alveolar nerve is preserved. I usually remove a tooth (lateral incisor or canine) to permit the osteotomy. The mandible is then swung apart after a release incision is made along the lateral floor of the mouth, leaving an adequate cuff of mucosa on the lingual surface of the alveolar ridge to allow primary closure or flap reconstruction. After the lesion has been excised and reconstructed, the mandible is reapproximated and plated. This obviously requires a lip-splitting skin incision.

In addition to the described indications, it is also an excellent approach to posterior pharyngeal wall and base of tongue cancers.

A variant of this technique is the median translingual pharyngotomy (median labiomandibular glossotomy), which also requires an anterior osteotomy. Instead of releasing the mandible along the lateral floor of mouth, the tongue is divided down the midline. This is useful as an approach to the posterior pharynx or resection of benign or low-grade malignancies of the base of the tongue. This approach results in minimal functional deformity but is used only rarely.

Composite resection (jaw-neck procedure) (see Fig. 14-1, *E*). Composite resection consisting of a neck dissection, together with partial mandibulectomy and incontinuity excision of the oropharyngeal lesion, has been and still is the cornerstone for the management of *advanced* cancer of the oropharynx. It is the technique of choice for extensive cancer with overt mandible involvement and in postradiation salvage situations in which the exact extent of the tumor is unclear. Although regarded as a very radical procedure, under the most ideal circumstances and with appropriate reconstruction, it may be associated with a very acceptable cosmetic and functional result.

The extent of the mandibulectomy varies depending on the clinical situation. If mandible is overtly involved, then a hemimandibulectomy is indicated, at least anterior to the mental foramen, in order to encompass the whole inferior alveolar canal. If the mandible is being removed because of close proximity, i.e., adherence to periosteum, then a smaller segment can be resected. A lip-splitting incision to improve access is of value, particularly for larger resections, but is not, in my experience, routinely necessary.

Technical points of interest are: While I try to pedicle the neck specimen on the angle and posterior third of the body of the mandible, I am not convinced incontinuity dissection is very important oncologically. Make sure the neck dissection is completely free from the carotid system before resection of the primary tumor is attempted. In advanced tumors in which there is a perception that the tumor has extended out into the submandibular triangle, it is better to perform the submandibular triangle dissection in continuity with the excision of the primary tumor rather than as part of the neck dissection.

After the anterior osteotomy has been performed, the posterior osteotomy is created horizontally below the notch, or the condyle may be divided just below the temporomandibular joint. Occasionally it may be necessary to disarticulate the temporomandibular joint to obtain an adequate margin. If reconstruction of the mandible is being contemplated, it is advisable however to perform a vertical osteotomy just posterior to the entrance of the inferior alveolar canal, leaving a 2 cm wide vertical strut of mandible to which a plate can be attached.

MANAGEMENT OF CERVICAL METASTASES

Controversy has always and will continue to rage as to how best to treat the neck in patients with cancer of the upper aerodigestive tract. Fifty-five percent to 75% of patients with oropharyngeal cancers have neck metastases at presentation, and approximately 20% have bilateral metastases. Therefore, the neck should be treated in some manner in all cases except in the smallest and most superficial cancers.

NO necks can probably be treated adequately using radiation or surgery, but, in my opinion, N1 to N3 nodal metastases should be treated surgically. Postoperative radiation, including both sides of the neck, should also given in advanced cancers. If bilateral metastases are present, simultaneous bilateral neck dissections are performed preserving one jugular vein.

The type of neck dissection to be performed is controversial. My inclination is to perform a modified radical neck dissection with sparing of the accessory nerve for N_0 and N_1 disease and radical neck dissection for more advanced nodal disease. I am not yet convinced that I am able to determine which patients that would do well with selective neck dissection.

RECONSTRUCTION

If there has been any advance in the past decade in the management of head and neck cancer, it has been in the realm of reconstruction. Adequate reconstruction is important not only from the aesthetic point of view but also, of course, is vital functionally. Poorly conceived reconstruction will result in significant alteration in speech, mastication, and deglutition. Never, however, should the resection be tailored to fit the preconceived reconstructive plan, because any compromise will result inevitably in recurrent cancer and subsequent death.

Healing by secondary intention

Small defects of the soft palate and posterior pharyngeal wall following intraoral resection can comfortably be allowed to heal in by secondary intention, particularly if the area excised is relatively superficial (e.g., mucosa and submucosa). This is frequently preferable to primary closure, especially if advancing the edges of the defect will lead to distortion of the pharynx.

Primary closure

Almost any defect in the oropharynx can be repaired by primary closure, however, the resultant distortion of the pharynx may be so significant that all the vital functions of the pharynx and, for that matter, the oral cavity are compromised. Small superficial and through-and-through defects are, however, quickly and easily managed in this way.

Primary closure was formerly the technique of choice following composite resection, because of its relative ease and because of the difficulties experienced in using a reliable flap. Indeed, one of the indications given for performing a partial mandibulectomy was not for oncologic reasons but to facilitate this closure! Today, it is a rare situation indeed that a primary closure is performed.

Free skin graft or dermal graft

Free skin grafts are extremely useful in closing defects of the posterior pharyngeal wall and may be maintained in position by means of a bolster or the quilting technique. The use of a bolster in the oropharynx will require a temporary tracheostomy, and, for this reason, quilting is preferable; however, it does not appear to fix the graft as well as a bolster.

Split-thickness graft reconstruction following a through-and-through composite resection can be used successfully. This method utilizes a large redundant pouch of either split-thickness skin or dermal graft that is sutured into the defect with a single layer of absorbably suture. This pouch is then packed with a bolster consisting of polymyxin B sulfate (Polysporin)–impregnated iodoform gauze. This results in a saliva tight anastomosis and minimal shrinkage. Intermaxillary fixation assists in graft immobilization, thereby improving graft take. While I have obtained good results using this technique and it certainly is quick and easy to perform, I believe a regional flap is probably preferable in the vast majority of cases.

Tongue flaps

Numerous tongue flaps are available for reconstruction of the oropharynx with the flaps being based either anteriorly or posteriorly. The advantages of the tongue flap are: (1) it has a rich blood supply that ensures viability even under the most adverse circumstances, and (2) no additional donor site defect is created.

The major disadvantage is that speech and deglutition will always be adversely affected to a greater degree than when other forms of reconstruction are used, and, given the current preoccupation with rehabilitation, it is probably better not to use these flaps unless no other alternatives are available.

Regional cutaneous and muscle flaps

Regional flaps were formerly the tissues of choice for reconstructing the pharynx. They have been surplanted largely by other flaps. There are two such flaps that I still use today:

The versatile *deltopectoral flap* remains an excellent means of reconstructing the oropharynx, particularly if the proximal pedicle is deepithelialized leaving a distal island of skin (Fig. 14-2). This allows the pedicle to be buried within the wound and eliminates the need for a second stage. I set the dermatome at 16 when the pedicle is deepithelialized to avoid compromising the blood supply of the flap. This gives a thin, soft pliable flap.

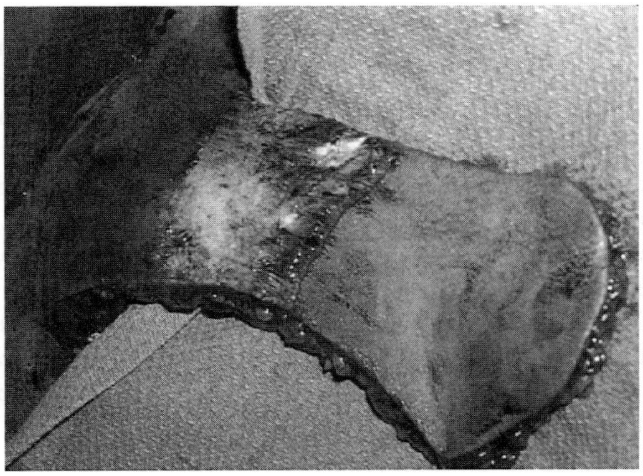

FIG 14-2
Deltopectoral flap with deepithelialized pedicle and distal skin paddle.

The *temporalis muscle flap* is easily harvested via a vertical incision in the hairline and is pedicled on the superficial temporal artery. The key is to elevate the flap as far posteriorly as possible. It is then brought into the pharynx under the zygomatic arch and sutured into the defect. A skin graft can be placed over the muscle but it is not usually necessary.

Myocutaneous flaps

In the past 15 years, myocutaneous flaps have gained increasing popularity as the definitive method of reconstruction of defects in the oropharynx. The pectoralis major, trapezius, sternocleidomastoid, and latissimus dorsi flaps all have a role. Of these flaps, the pectoralis major remains the most popular because of its reliability and ease of harvesting. The sternocleidomastoid is the least useful because of its rather tenuous blood supply as it is increasingly mobilized. In addition, it may well be oncologically contraindicated in patients who require a *radical* neck dissection for ablation of the tumor. The latissimus dorsi myocutaneous flap is not as popular as the pectoralis major flap since the patient must be repositioned intraoperatively.

The advantages of these flaps are that a large defect may be closed, and the bulkiness of the pedicle not only protects the carotid system but also camouflages the cosmetic defect created by the neck dissection and partial mandibulectomy. The bulkiness of the flap initially may be a problem impairing deglutition and even the airway occasionally, but this bulkiness always seems to settle with time.

Free flaps with microvascular anastomosis

Free flap reconstruction of the oropharynx has always been an attractive concept. The groin flap, dorsalis pedis flap, latissimus dorsi flap, radial forearm flap, and free jejunal graft have all been used with great success. Many of these flaps may be used not only alone but also combined with underlying bone to provide reconstruction of the mandible if indicated. The major advantage is the ability to harvest an almost limitless amount of tissue that can be used to close almost any defect. The disadvantages are that it is time consuming and it requires a two-team approach with personnel well trained in microvascular technique. The popularity of this technique will, therefore, always be limited because of the inconvenience and expense associated with this procedure. Where facilities for this technique do exist, however, it is a most attractive approach to reconstruction.

The free jejunal graft can be used as a patch graft for limited repair of the pharynx or as an intact tube for reconstruction following total laryngopharyngectomy for extensive tumors. The major disadvantage as a patch graft is that hypersecretion from the jejunum results in severe aspiration problems and therefore really should not be used in this situation. Conversely, it is an excellent technique for reconstructing the total laryngopharynx, with the ability to stretch

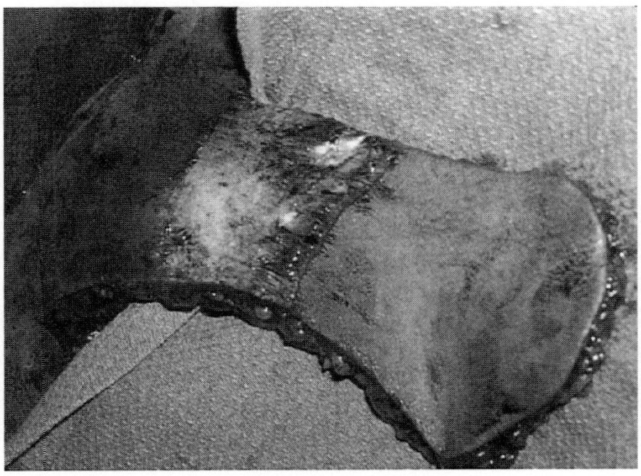

high up into the nasopharynx and low into the superior mediastinum. At this stage, the radial forearm flap is, for us, the most convenient and reliable free flap for reconstruction of partial oropharyngeal defects and most commonly used.

Reconstruction of the mandible

Significant controversy exists as to the indications for reconstruction of the posterior aspect of the mandible following composite resection. My philosophy is as follows:

In older edentulous patients, I do not reconstruct the resected mandible but merely insert a pectoralis myocutaneous flap. Cosmesis and function are good. If, however, the patient is younger and has full detention, I then reconstruct using a plate and pectoralis major myocutaneous flap (Fig. 14-3). I use a free flap to reconstruct the posterior mandible only in very young patients with a developing mandible. It involves too much effort and expense, and the advantages are marginal for the routine case.

PALLIATION

The management of the patient who is incurable because of either late presentation or failed therapy is a tremendous challenge to the oncologist. Every effort should be made to alleviate suffering and to allow the patient to spend his or her last days with dignity. The use of irradiation or chemotherapy to obtain tumor shrinkage or to alleviate pain should be considered. Tracheostomy or gastrostomy may be indicated. Placement in an institution even for short periods to relieve the burden on the relatives and friends may be necessary. The patient's pain medication must be constantly reevaluated to ensure that pain is controlled. No patient should die in pain.

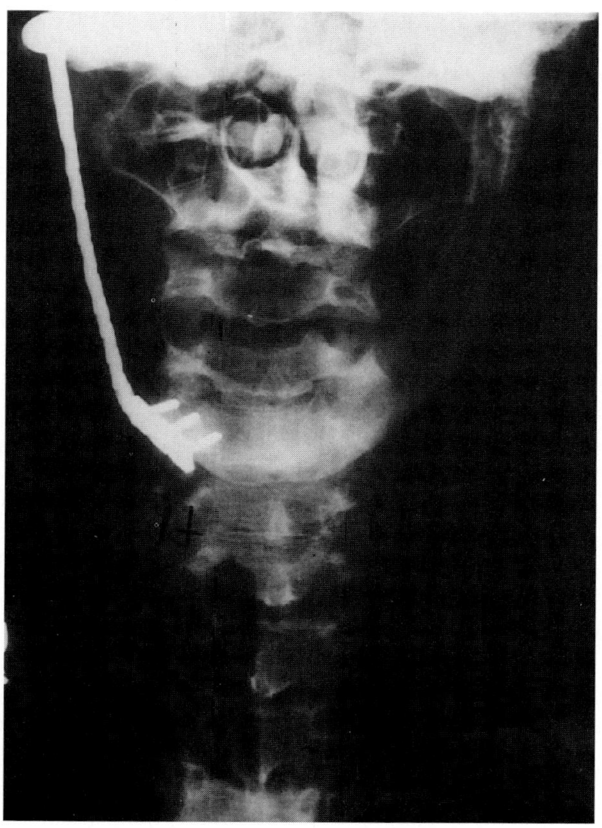

FIG 14-3
Plate reconstruction of the posterior mandible.

REHABILITATION

For too long, the exclusive objective of the surgeon was to cure the patient regardless of the cosmetic and functional sequelae. In recent years however, great emphasis has been placed on the total rehabilitation of the patient. The most important factor in achieving this is patient motivation. Without the patient desire to be rehabilitated, the oncologist and the rehabilitation team are helpless. Total rehabilitation is the function of a team of professionals, with the surgeon playing a lesser but coordinating role. Speech therapists, physical therapists, social workers, occupational therapists, prosthodontists, and nurses, together with the patient's immediate family, all are vital members of this team. A number of factors must be considered.

Cosmetic appearance

Since younger patients and more women are being treated for this disease, there is an increasing awareness of the cosmetic appearance after therapy. Although much of the surgery is mutilating to some degree, modern reconstructive modalities have been used to minimize the deformity created. As stated earlier, certainly the surgery should never be compromised in an attempt to minimize the defect created.

Speech

Dysarthria is a consequence of oral cavity and oropharyngeal resection, with the degree of tongue removal being the dominant factor in determining the severity of the speech defect. The articulation defect most apparent is in the formation of speech fricatives (e.g., this, that) that require lingual-dental approximation. Prevention by assuring that the tongue is not tethered by the interposition of flaps or grafts to provide more mobility is the best treatment. If a tongue tie does result, however, the problem can be improved by dividing the scar tissue by using a CO_2 laser. A speech therapist is invaluable in aiding these patients postoperatively.

Velopharyngeal incompetence due to removal of much of the soft palate is another cause of dysarthria. It has been my experience that prosthetic rehabilitation in the postoperative period affords the best relief.

Deglutition

If a large portion of the tongue has been removed and the remaining tongue is tethered, the posterior propulsion of food into the hypopharynx becomes awkward. The bolus has a tendency to be propelled down the side of the surgical defect and often directly into the larynx. This, combined with the denervated flap-covered portion of the pharynx, results in aspiration problems with all the sequelae of repeated lower respiratory tract infections, fear of eating, and debility. Most patients can be trained to correct this problem by swallowing therapy. Rarely, a cricopharyngeal myotomy may be useful as a secondary procedure if the swallowing problem continues. Velopharyngeal incompetence with reflux in food through the nose is helped by the use of a dental appliance.

Mastication

In patients on whom partial mandibulectomy has been performed, the mandible is frequently deviated by scarring, resulting in interference with mastication.

Prevention is vital, and undoubtedly the best prophylactic measure is the judicious use of flap reconstruction to prevent scarring and tethering of the mandibular remnant. In addition, reconstruction of the mandible using bone or plating, particularly if the ipsilateral temporomandibular joint has not been disturbed, may further improve this situation.

Psychosocial functioning

Too often insufficient attention is devoted to the tremendous psychologic adjustments the patient has to make, with attention zeroing in on his or her physical adjustments. The emotional status of the patient in the postoperative period is important. The patient is frequently depressed, and this depression interferes with motivation for physical rehabilitation. An experienced and understanding nursing, medical, and paramedical staff is, therefore, important in aiding the patient to overcome this problem. If necessary, psychiatric guidance should be sought.

In addition, there may be a change in the relationship to the immediate family, particularly because of fear of rejection. Adequate family counseling is vital. The patient and family must learn to accept the situation and make the necessary alterations in life style to compensate for the particular disability.

RECOMMENDED READING

Christopoulos E, Carrau R, Segas J, Johnson JT, Myers EN, Wagner RL: Transmandibular approaches to the oral cavity and oropharynx: a functional assessment. *Arch Otolaryngol Head Neck Surg* 118:1164-1167, 1992.

Gluckman JL, Thompson R: Cancer of the oropharynx. In Paparella M, Shumrick DA, Gluckman JL, Meyeroff W, editors: *Otolaryngology,* vol 3. Philadelphia, 1991, WB Saunders.

Komisar A: The functional result of mandibular reconstruction. *Laryngoscope* 100:364-74, 1990.

Komisar A, Warman S, Danziger E: A critical analysis of immediate and delayed mandibular reconstruction using A-O plates. *Arch Otolaryngol Head Neck Surg* 115:830-833, 1989.

McConnel FM, Teichgraeber JF, Adler RK: A comparison of three methods of oral reconstruction. *Arch Otolaryngol Head Neck Surg* 113:496-500, 1987.

Pauloski BR, Logemann JA, Rademaker AW, et al: Speech and swallowing function after anterior tongue floor of mouth resection with distal flap reconstruction. *J Speech Hear Res* 36:267-76, 1993.

Urken ML: Functional evaluation following microvascular oromandibular reconstruction of the oral cancer patient: a comparative study of reconstructed and non-reconstructed patients. *Laryngoscope* 101:935-950, 1991.

Zieske LA, Johnson JT, Myers EN, Schramm VL, Wagner R: Composite resection reconstruction: split thickness skin graft—a preferred option. *Otolaryngol Head Neck Surg* 98:170, 1988.

15

Interdisciplinary Management of Surgical Parathyroid Disease

Phillip K. Pellitteri, D.O., K. Thomas Robbins, M.D., F.A.C.S., and Wolfgang Dillman, M.D.

The recorded history of hyperparathyroidism in modern medicine is relatively recent. Sir Richard Owen, a renowned British anatomist and curator, is generally acknowledged as being the first to describe the existence of the parathyroid glands in 1852.[16] This discovery occurred subsequent to the death of the Zoological Society of London's Indian rhinoceros, the postmortem of which was conducted by Owen and subsequently reported to the Zoological Society. In 1877, the Swedish histologist, Ivar Sandstrom, reported the existence of distinct glandular tissue adjacent to the thyroid in a dog.[14] Over the subsequent two years, similar findings in other small mammals led to the search for, and ultimate discovery of, a similar organ in humans (glandulae parathyroideae), which Sandstrom reported on in 1880.

The earliest reports of clinical hyperparathyroidism involved bone disease, or osteitis fibrosa cystica, as termed by von Recklinghausen.[11] These reports, however, did not associate the characteristic changes in bone from hyperparathyroidism with parathyroid gland abnormalities. It wasn't until Erdheim, a Viennese pathologist, discovered parathyroid gland morphologic and histologic abnormalities in diseased patients with bone disease that an association between osteomalacia and parathyroid gland function was suspected.[4] Numerous reports of this association followed, leading to Mandle's historic removal of a parathyroid tumor from a crippled TRAM conductor in 1924,[7] thus ushering in the surgical treatment of parathyroid disease.

From its inception, the quest for information on parathyroid dysfunction has involved many disciplines, including anatomy, physiology, pathology, and the surgical application of the principles accumulated from these basic sciences. Accordingly, the management scheme for treating parathyroid disorders should be no different. Ideally, a clinic setting for treatment of parathyroid disease would involve surgeons, endocrinologists, and pathologists, all of whom concurrently evaluate the patient and offer expertise in developing a comprehensive management plan. The authors' advocate such a unified setting, termed an interdisciplinary head and neck endocrine clinic, whereby the evaluation of a combined head and neck endocrine team provides comprehensive care to patients and creates an educational forum for exchange of information between disciplines.

HYPERPARATHYROIDISM: CLASSIFICATION, ETIOLOGY, EPIDEMIOLOGY

Hyperparathyroidism results from excessive production of parathyroid hormone which may be caused by tumor or hyperplasia of the parathyroid glands. Parathormone acts directly on bone tissue to increase remodeling and release calcium into the extracellular fluid. It also acts at the level of the kidney to increase 1,25-dihydroxy vitamin D which results in the increased absorption of calcium by the gut.

Primary hyperparathyroidism

Primary hyperparathyroidism results from hyperfunctioning parathyroid glands without the influence of a proved physiologic stimulus. Parathyroid hormone secretion is elevated, and, consequently, patients are rendered hypercalcemic. The incidence in patients greater than 50 has been variably determined to be approximately 4 to 6/1,000, with female to male ratios varying from 2:1 to 4:1.[3] This incidence appears highest in postmenopausal women over 65 years old.

The prevalence in making the diagnosis of primary hyperparathyroidism has increased, primarily as a result of widespread use of routine blood chemistry screening in ambulatory and hospitalized patients over the last three decades. The usual offending lesion in primary hyperparathyroidism is the parathyroid adenoma, occurring in a solitary manner in approximately 80% of patients with primary hyperparathyroidism in large studies (Table 15-1).[19] Hyperplasia has been judged to occur in approximately 20% of patients, the chief cell variety being more common than the clear cell. The incidence of multiple adenomas is low, occurring in approximately 1% to 2% of patients with hyperparathyroidism. Some of these may actually represent nodular hyperplasia.[5] Carcinomatous parathyroid glands inducing hyperparathyroidism is a rare event, occurring in less than 5% of patients with hyperparathyroidism.

Secondary hyperparathyroidism

Secondary hyperparathyroidism refers to hyperparathyroidism and resultant sequelae occurring as a consequence of chronic renal failure. This occurs as a result of increased parathyroid hormone secretion and parathyroid hyperplasia in renal failure patients, the stimulus for which remains unclear. Evidence indicating stimulation of parathyroid tissue, with or without hyperplasia, has been uniformly demonstrated in patients with long-standing renal failure.[12] As suggested by one study, approximately 70% of patients maintained on dialysis require parathyroid surgery following a median of approximately six years on dialysis.[10] The parathyroid lesion noted in renal failure patients may vary from hyperplasia to pseudoadenomatous hyperplasia to nodular transformation.[9]

HYPERPARATHYROIDISM: CLINICAL CHARACTERIZATION, EVALUATION, MANAGEMENT

Presentation

Most patients treated for hyperparathyroidism over recent years have not manifested symptoms related to the disease. The usual presenting abnormality in these patients is an abnormally elevated serum calcium detected on routine blood chemistry screening. There are, however, "silent" sequelae of hyperparathyroidism which may be present in asymptomatic patients, notably renal stones.

A large number of organ systems potentially may be involved in primary hyperparathyroidism. Historically, greater than 50% of patients developed renal symptoms manifested by nephrolithiasis and nephrocalcinosis. This decreased markedly to approximately 4% following the widespread use of screening tests for serum calcium levels.[6] Symptoms associated with urolithiasis include renal colic, hematuria, and polyuria. Abnormalities of the skeletal system in the form of osteitis fibrosa cystica, once a common malady in primary hyperparathyroidism, is now rarely encountered (less than 10%). These changes include subperiosteal erosion of the distal phalanges, bone wasting and softening, and chondrocalcinosis as a result of bone demineralization. Those postmenopausal women exhibiting early signs of osteoporosis are at greatest risk for developing more severe bone disease and resultant sequelae, i.e., pelvic and vertebral fractures.

Hypertension may occur in association with primary hyperparathyroidism in as many as 50% of patients. Convincing evidence for a pathogenetic mechanism does not exist, however, and parathyroidectomy results in decreased blood pressure in only a small number of patients.

Hypercalcemic syndrome occurring as a result of hyperparathyroidism includes polydipsia and polyuria, anorexia, vomiting, constipation, muscle weakness, fatigue, mental status changes, and skin abnormalities. Those patients with severely elevated calcium levels may present with marked mental status changes or coma, so-called hypercalcemic crisis, requiring intensive medical therapy for stabilization.

Gastrointestinal disorders which may occur in hyperparathyroidism include acid peptic disease, pancreatitis, and cholelithiasis. Those patients with MEA Type I, exhibiting the Zollinger-Ellison syndrome, have the highest incidence of peptic ulceration.

Diagnosis

The diagnosis of primary hyperparathyroidism rests on the establishment of excessive parathyroid hormone secretion in the setting of hypercalcemia. Hypercalcemia is a prerequisite sign in primary hyperparathyroidism, which represents one of several disorders in the differential diagnoses of an elevated serum calcium level (box on p. 191). Primary hyperparathyroidism may be borderline, resulting in a marginal elevation of serum calcium, frequently with few or no symptoms. Serial determinations of serum calcium may be required to demonstrate the presence of hypercalcemia. In this setting, the diagnosis of primary hyperparathyroidism may be confirmed through the use of parathyroid hormone radioimmunoassay (RIA). RIA is used to measure biologically active or intact PTH, through the determination of the active amino fragment of PTH. The relationship between primary hyperparathyroidism and other

TABLE 15-1
Pathologic classification of parathyroid lesions in 1076 patients[19] with primary hyperparathyroidism (in %)

Adenoma	
Single	84
"Double"	2
Lipoadenoma	<1
Hyperplasia	
Chief cell	9
Clear cell	2
Familial hyperparathyroidism	
MEA I (gastrinoma, insulinoma, prolactinoma)	
MEA II (pheochromoceptoma, medullary carcinoma)	
Carcinoma	3

Data drived from Watson-*Clin Endocrinol Metab* 3:215, 1974.

etiologies of hypercalcemia, with reference to serum calcium, PTH, and associated electrolyte levels, is illustrated in Table 15-2. Malignancy (excluding parathyroid carcinoma), with or without bone metastasis, is a frequent cause of hypercalcemia. Local mechanisms in the form of osteolytic bone lesions are responsible in patients with bone metastasis. The etiology for elevated calcium levels in patients without metastasis is more vexing and may involve humoral factors or elements produced by solid tumors themselves. Those tumors known to be associated with hypercalcemia include adenocarcinomas of the lung, pancreas, kidney, ovary, and breast, all of which may be associated with bone metastasis. Malignancies primarily involving bone, which may induce hypercalcemia, include multiple myeloma, leukemia, and lymphoma. In most circumstances, the level of biologically active PTH is normal or reduced in the hypercalcemia of malignancy, and the presence of an ectopic PTH-like substance is yet to be determined in patients with these tumors. Hypocalciuric hypercalcemia represents a specific form of familial hypercalcemia which, in general, follows a relatively benign course. Measurements of biologically intact PTH have not proved fruitful in this disorder, and the differentiation from asymptomatic primary hyperparathyroidism may be difficult in the absence of familial occurrence. The differentiation is based on sensitive measurements of circulating amino fragment PTH in the absence of decreased urinary calcium excretion for patients with enlarged parathyroid tissue and primary hyperparathyroidism. Other abnormalities representing infrequent etiologies for hypercalcemia and which may be excluded on a clinical basis include those noted in the left box below.

Once the diagnosis of primary hyperparathyroidism is established, the decision exists as to whether imaging studies to localize the offending adenoma should be carried out. The necessity of localization procedures is questionable and ultimately rests with the surgeon's personal preference. A consensus conference conducted by the NIH regarding the management of primary hyperparathyroidism stated that preoperative localization studies prior to initial surgery are not indicated. This recommendation is based predominantly upon a 90% to 95% rate of cure at initial exploration performed by an experienced surgeon. Further, according to the NIH investigation, these preoperative studies do not prevent unsuccessful explorations, shorten operative time, or prevent complications. Advocates of preoperative localization studies dispute these claims, indicating that these studies are instrumental in directing the exploration to one side of the neck rather than initial bilateral exploration. The experience and philosophy of each individual surgeon concerning the use of localization studies will be different. The authors advocate the use of such studies, the methodology of which will be presented further in this discussion.

Several invasive and noninvasive imaging techniques are currently available for localization of enlarged parathyroid tissue. High-resolution real-time ultrasonography is a reliable and accurate method for imaging parathyroid adenoma and represents the noninvasive procedure of choice for localization of these lesions. The accuracy of this method ranges from 75% to 95% and, unlike other cross-sectional techniques such as CT and MRI, is operator and technology dependent. Ultrasonography usually does not image normal parathyroid tissue. Adenomas appear as marginated

Etiologies for Hypercalcemia

Endocrinopathies

Thyrotoxicosis
Adrenal insufficiency
Pheochromocytoma

Medication

Thiazides
Vitamin A, D
Milk alkali syndrome
Lithium

Malignancy

Granulomatous disease

Sarcoidosis

Miscellaneous

Immobilization
Acute renal failure
Familial hypercalcemic
Aluminum hypocalciuria

Hyperparathyroidism

Primary
Secondary
"Tertiary"

TABLE 15-2
The relationship between serum Ca^{++}, P and PTH levels and urinary Ca^{++} in disorders producing hypercalcemia

	Ca^{2+}	P	PTH	Urine Ca^{2+}
Hyperparathyroidism (50% of all cases)	↑	↓	↑	↑
Malignancy (solid tumors)				
Local osteolytic	↑	—	↓	↑
Humoral	↑	—	(↓)	↑
Hematologic	↑	—	↓	↑
Familial hypocalciuric hypercalcemia	↑	—	— (↑)	↓

hypoechoic soft tissue masses whose echogenicity is lower than that of neighboring thyroid tissue. Their size and shape are variable, and they may present uncommonly as hyperechoic complex masses.

In general, hyperplastic glands are less echogenic than are adenomas, however, given a wide spectrum of adenoma echogenicity, differentiation may be difficult without enlargement of multiple glands in hyperplasia. A number of elements pose problems in the use of ultrasonography for localization of parathyroid tumors. Although high-resolution real-time ultrasound may be commonly found in large tertiary centers, its use may not be practical in the community. An experienced ultrasonographic technician and radiologist are important for the performance and interpretation of the study. Ectopically located adenomas which may be obscured by a hollow viscus (trachea, esophagus) or those located in the mediastinum are not imaged by ultrasound because of acoustic shadowing. Coexisting nodular thyroid disease poses a problem in detecting adenomas, especially those located posterior to the thyroid gland in the superior position. Another problem which exists in ultrasonographic detection of parathyroid tissue includes localization of minimally enlarged glands, which may prove difficult to differentiate from adjacent native tissues.

Nuclear imaging using combination radionuclides and subtraction scanning techniques represents a valuable modality in evaluating parathyroid disease. The radionuclides used have traditionally been a combination of technetium pertechnetate and thallium 201 chloride. The method is based upon the differential uptake of these materials by both thyroid and parathyroid tissue. Thyroid tissue will accumulate both technetium and thallium, while parathyroid tissue uptakes only thallium. Administration of thallium alone produces a dual image of both parathyroid and thyroid tissue. Subtraction scintigraphy is applied with administration of technetium, which is taken up only by thyroid and produces an enhanced image of thyroid tissue. The combined technetium/thallium image of the thyroid gland is subtracted out, leaving only the thallium-enhanced image of the parathyroid tissue. In differentiating normal from enlarged glands, normal sized glands are usually too small to be detected by the subtraction technique. However, large glands and, in particular, adenomatous glands can be visualized readily. Hyperplastic glands may be seen to a lesser extent than adenomas. Subtraction may not be required for mediastinal glands, which should be distinct following thallium administration alone. The sensitivity for localization of adenomas in this technique is approximately 90% and is somewhat lower for hyperplastic glands.[20] Coexisting nodular thyroid disease, goiter, and previous central neck surgery may affect the specificity and sensitivity of this technique. In particular, previous neck exploration for adenoma may significantly decrease the sensitivity for localizing adenomas prior to re-exploration.[21]

Technetium sestamibi is an isonitrile radiopharmaceutical of technetium 99m originally developed for nuclear studies of myocardial function. Incidentally, sestamibi was noted to concentrate in thyroid and abnormally enlarged parathyroid tissue with a differential retention of the radiotracer between these tissues. This has allowed enlarged parathyroid tissue to be accurately imaged following intravenous administration of sestamibi, with retention of the tracer in parathyroid adenoma and washout from normal thyroid gland. Nuclear scintigraphic images are obtained at ½ hour, 2 hours, and 3 hours following injection to allow for adequate washout from thyroid tissue and delayed retention in abnormal parathyroid tissue. This method has demonstrated a sensitivity for localizing parathyroid adenoma exceeding 95%.[1]

When localization is desired preoperatively and either ultrasound or scintigraphy (or both) does not succeed in finding a mass, MRI represents the next imaging step. With improved technology and high resolution of soft tissue using head and neck surface coils, this modality offers high-contrast detection of abnormal parathyroid tissue. In general, parathyroid adenomas will demonstrate high-signal intensity on T2-weighted images which will allow optimal contrast and resolution against surrounding soft tissues such as thyroid gland and lymph nodes. Lesions as small as 0.5 cm. have been localized using high-field strength units in combination with head and neck surface coils.[15] Factors which mitigate against initial use of MRI as a localizing modality include high cost and the compliance of patients who may be claustrophobic.

The authors advocate the use of high-resolution ultrasonography as a preoperative localizing technique and employ it according to the algorithm in Fig. 15-1. We find it to be a rapid, noninvasive, and efficacious method by which to localize parathyroid adenomas which additionally carries with it a high sensitivity in our experience.[13] A prerequisite, as stated earlier, is the availability of the proper technology and expertise in performing and carrying out the procedure. Failing the availability of these, we recommend subtraction scintigraphy or sestamibi imaging as the localization modality of choice because of its relative low cost, reliability, and high compliance. We reserve MRI for those situations in which either ultrasound or scintigraphy fails to localize the offending adenoma.

In general, the decision to use localizing studies prior to initial exploration rests with the individual surgeon, according to that person's experience with these modalities, personal preference, and medical profile of the patient to be explored.

Therapy

Surgical exploration of the neck with removal of the offending adenoma, or subtotal parathyroidectomy in the case of MEA, represents the only effective treatment for primary hyperparathyroidism. There are situations, however, which require pre-emptive medical stabilization through management of hypercalcemia in preparation for surgery.

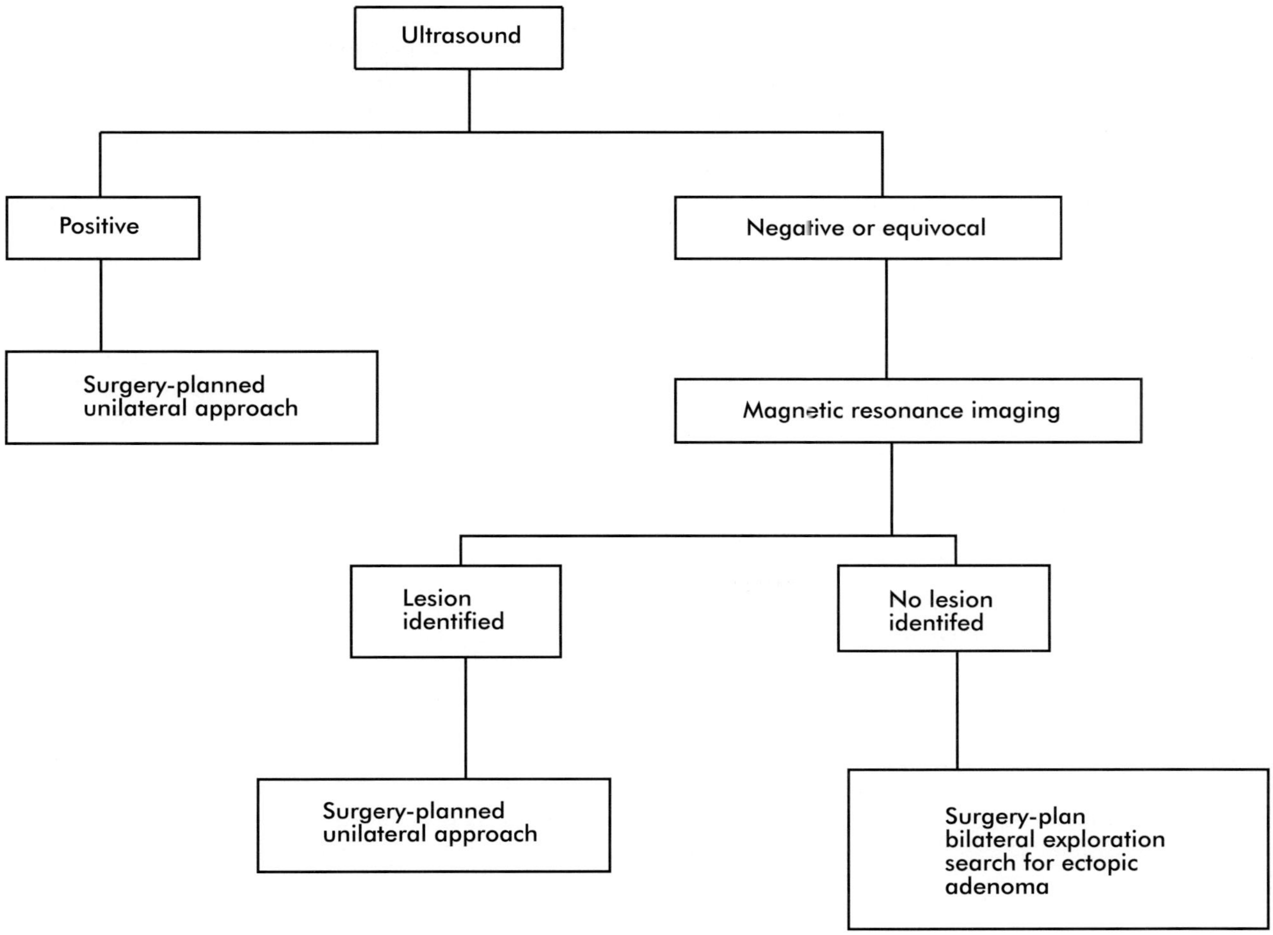

FIG 15-1
Algorithm for preoperative imaging in primary hyperparathyroidism. (From Weinberger MS and Robbins KT: Diagnostic localization studies for primary hyperparathyroidism: a suggested algorithm. *Arch Otol-Head Neck Surg,* vol. 120, no. 11:1187-1189, Nov. 1990. Copyright 1994 by the American Medical Association. By permission.)

Medical management of hypercalcemia. Patients who may require medical stabilization of conditions unrelated to hyperparathyroidism prior to definitive surgery or those in whom hyperparathyroidism is secondary to chronic renal failure will need adequate management of symptomatic hypercalcemia. Those patients manifesting symptoms of mental derangement such as confusion, somnolence, or coma and those in whom the risk of cardiac dysrhythmia is high should receive aggressive hydration and diuresis with furosemide. Up to 8 to 10 l of isotonic saline may be administered over a 24-hour period with concurrent administration of furosemide to produce such a diuresis with resultant elimination of calcium. Patients for whom stabilization of other medical conditions requires a more prolonged period of time can be administered mithramycin to lower serum calcium and reduce accelerated bone loss. Mithramycin may be given at a dose of 25 mcg/kg intravenously in a 4 to 6 hour infusion in one administration. The effect is a rapid decline in serum calcium level over a 1 to 3 day period. This dose may be repeated twice; however, renal and platelet function must be determined prior to repeat administration.

Patients with elevated serum calcium levels without overt symptoms may be medically followed while surgery is planned or contemplated. Adequate hydration should be encouraged with acceptable levels of exercise and avoidance of immobilization. Hypertension as a result of hypercalcemia should be treated. Administration of oral phosphates is not recommended in that the shift in calcium will result in an increased stimulation of parathormone production. Women should receive estrogen replacement if they are postmenopausal, whether or not they have already manifested signs of osteoporosis or bone loss. In general, 20% to 30% of asymptomatic patients with primary hyperparathyroidism become symptomatic within five years.

Surgical management of hyperparathyroidism—preoperative preparation. The decision to perform surgical exploration in the medically stable patient with primary hyperparathyroidism is predicated upon the potential development of complications secondary to prolonged hypercalcemia and the long-term benefit of surgery. In general, patients should be assessed for the risk of developing long-term complications on the basis of disease progression in terms of time and extent. Patients who have manifested complications at the time of diagnosis or those previously diagnosed who now develop initial complications over a short interval since diagnosis are at significant risk of developing further problems.

Patient age should not be an absolute determinant of candidacy for surgery; rather, general medical condition and potential for active living will play a greater role in determining candidacy. In general, those younger patients who have more potential exposure to hypercalcemia are placed at greater risk for developing complications.

The severity of hypercalcemia represents a consideration in the decision to perform surgery. Most surgeons and endocrinologists consider a serum calcium level greater than 11.5 to 12.0 mg/dl an indication for surgery. Special emphasis should be given for surgical consideration in postmenopausal women, independent of the severity of hypercalcemia and/or absence of symptoms. Women in this category are at greatest risk for developing long-term skeletal complications such as hip and vertebral fractures secondary to osteoporosis.

Patients in whom surgery may be delayed in lieu of close follow-up for medical reasons or patient choice include: those patients who are asymptomatic and without risk factors and those with mild disease (serum calcium less than 11.5 mg/dl) and no symptoms.

The second major factor to be considered in determining the need for surgery is potential long-term benefit and opportunity for cure. In 85% to 90% of patients, primary hyperparathyroidism is a result of a single adenoma. Exploration and removal of the adenoma is curative in greater than 90% of cases, and thus the long-term benefit and potential for cure is high in these patients. Hyperplasia of all four glands is the etiology in approximately 8% to 10% of cases of primary hyperparathyroidism. Surgery in these patients involves subtotal parathyroidectomy, the amount of parathyroid tissue left remaining ultimately deciding the long-term benefit of surgery. Because of the variable amount of tissue remaining and thus variable activity, the curability is less reliable than that in those situations involving adenoma. Patients in this category have cure rates significantly reduced from those in patients with single adenomas.[2]

A history of prior exploration without success, especially when performed by an experienced surgeon, portends a significantly reduced potential for cure following re-exploration. In general, the cure rate following re-exploration for persistent hypercalcemia drops to approximately 60% to 70%. An important distinction in evaluating unsuccessful initial exploration is whether hypercalcemia is *persistent* following surgery or normalizes postoperatively and subsequently *recurs* six months or more postoperatively. The former implies the high probability of a missed abnormal gland (adenoma) and represents the most frequent indication for reoperation, while the latter implicates multiple gland disease (hyperplasia) or the development of carcinoma.[8,17] Parathyroid carcinoma, although rarely (1% or less) a cause for primary hyperparathyroidism, represents a potential etiology for recurrence. Patients with persistent or recurrent hyperparathyroidism are at increased risk for complications associated with reoperation, including: recurrent laryngeal nerve injury with resultant vocal cord paralysis/paresis and postoperative hypoparathyroidism and hypocalcemia.

Thus, the long-term benefit of surgery and potential cure in these patients is significantly different than that for patients without prior exploration. The decision to re-explore must be viewed in light of the severity of disease, the patient's medical condition, and the potential for successful surgical management of the lesion, i.e., missed adenoma versus hyperfunctioning multiple glands. In general, greater consideration for medical follow-up is appropriate for selected patients in this category.

Once the decision to explore the neck has been made, a localization study may be performed if desired. Our preference is to perform preoperative high-resolution ultrasonography in an effort to localize the offending adenoma as outlined in Fig. 15-1. We advocate this approach on the basis of several factors: (1) localization of suspected pathology directs the surgeon to a specific side, thereby avoiding mandatory bilateral exploration, (2) our experience with this localizing modality has yielded a high sensitivity in detecting pathology, and (3) failure to demonstrate pathology raises the surgeon's suspicion of the possibility that ectopic disease or hyperplasia may be present. If high-resolution ultrasonography fails to identify an obvious adenoma, an MRI may be used to localize the lesion if this preoperative step is desired. Preoperative localization becomes important when dealing with patients with significant medical problems who are at increased risk for cardiopulmonary complications under general anesthesia. By directing a planned unilateral exploration, it is possible to reduce overall general anesthesia time, thus reducing the risk of potential complications. One of the authors (PKP) utilizes nuclear scintigraphy with sestamibi technetium for preoperative localization in the presence of clinically apparent nodular thyroid disease. This is due to the observation that, despite the accuracy of high-resolution ultrasonography to detect enlarged parathyroid tissue, the adjacent nodular thyroid gland makes differentiation of parathyroid tissue (especially in the superior gland location) very difficult.

Surgical management of hyperparathyroidism—operative philosophy. It is not the intent of this presentation to discuss the specific nuances of surgical technique; however, several points germane to the philosophy of a planned unilateral approach following localization may be illustrated. In performing unilateral exploration, access is gained into the viscerovertebral angle or that area medial to the carotid sheath, lateral to the trachea, and posterior to the thyroid lobe. Following division of the middle thyroid vein, medial mobilization of the thyroid lobe allows blunt dissection of areolar tissue in the viscerovertebral angle. This permits visualization and/or palpation of enlarged parathyroid tissue without much dissection and resultant staining of the tissues with blood. Often these maneuvers will allow the surgeon to identify both the abnormal gland and the remaining single normal gland by scrutinizing the expected anatomic locations. Once identified, the abnormal gland is removed and sent for pathologic analysis. A search is made to identify the second gland on the same side; if found, it is biopsied for pathologic determination. If the enlarged gland is reported as abnormal and the second gland normal, the procedure is terminated. If, however, the second gland is not identified and the enlarged gland is abnormal, the contralateral side is explored in the same manner as that used in the first. An attempt is made to localize either or both of the two contralateral glands. Once parathyroid tissue is identified, biopsies are obtained until normal parathyroid tissue is encountered.

If the second gland on the side explored first is found to be abnormal, all four glands must be identified and biopsied in preparation for subtotal parathyroidectomy. The distinction between adenoma and hyperplastic parathyroid tissue may be difficult or impossible on frozen section analysis; therefore, the surgeon cannot rely on single gland analysis for determinative therapy.

Re-exploration following parathyroidectomy. In patients requiring re-exploration, localization studies are mandatory. We advocate a series of evaluations prior to undertaking surgery. Preliminary evaluation rests upon the scrutiny of the first operative procedure with special attention to number of glands identified, biopsy results, and which glands were removed. As specified previously, it is critical to determine if hypercalcemia is persistent (missed adenoma) or recurrent (hyperplasia). We perform noninvasive localizing studies first, usually with technetium/thallium subtraction or sestamibi uptake. This may be combined with MRI and/or ultrasound in cases in which equivocal results are obtained with scintigraphy. Usually, the accumulated results of these studies will yield localization. It should be noted that the majority (90%) of missed adenomas reside within reach of exploration conducted through a cervical incision (Fig. 15-2). Localization studies in re-exploration cases serve to limit dissection in uninvolved regions distorted by fibrosis and scarring, thereby reducing the possibility of recurrent laryngeal nerve injury and troublesome bleeding.

When noninvasive studies to identify the location of the lesion fail, the authors proceed to invasive venous sampling for PTH levels. This technique rapidly measures increased levels of PTH emptying into the thyroid and thymic venous plexus in an effort to localize the general anatomic region of the lesion. This procedure requires an experienced radiographer and the ability to rapidly assess venous samples for PTH levels.

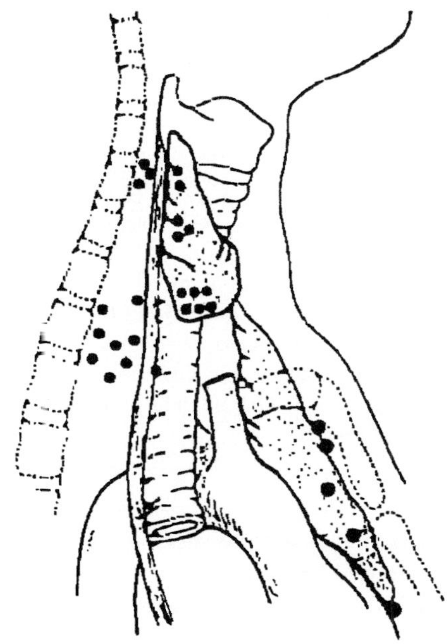

FIG 15-2
Location of missed parathyroid adenomas following initial exploration for primary hyperparathyroidism. (From Brennan MF, Doppman JL, Marx SJ, et al: Reoperative parathyroid surgery for persistent parathyroidism. *Surgery:* 83;669-676 1978.)

If a cervical site is not identified by localizing studies, a mediastinal site must be considered. Prior to contemplating mediastinal exploration via sternotomy, it is helpful to identify a candidate lesion. The mediastinum is best evaluated by MRI in this situation. Digital subtraction angiography has been used in such cases with success; however, performance of the technique requires a skilled interventional radiologist and may be fraught with severe neurologic complications, i.e., embolic CVA.[18]

Postoperative evaluation. It is rare to encounter postoperative symptomatic hypocalcemia, especially in cases in which successful unilateral exploration has been performed. In those instances in which symptomatic and prolonged hypocalcemia occurs following exploration, supplementation should ensue while the patient remains hospitalized. The response to symptomatic hypocalcemia is determined by the level of serum calcium and severity of symptoms. In patients developing acute severe symptoms including tetany, steps in replacement may be followed as in box on p. 196. Calcium gluconate, 10 cc. of a 10% solution, is administered intravenously over 10 minutes. A continuous intravenous administration is then started consisting of 10 ampules of 10% calcium gluconate (930 ml of elemental calcium) in 1 l of normal saline solution. This is given over 6 to 8 hours at approximately 2 mg/kg/hr. Periodic serum calcium, phosphorus, and magnesium determinations are obtained-from the arm opposite the intravenous site. The process may

Postoperative Calcium Supplementation

Replacement

Acute to severe symptoms
I.V. over 10 min, Ca^{2+} gluconate 10 cc of 10% solution
Continuous IV, dilute 10 ampules, 10% calcium gluconate (930 mg, elemental calcium) in 1 L NS or glucose
Give over 6 to 8 hours (2 mg/kg/hr)
Check Ca^{2+}, P, Mg (draw blood from other arm)
Repeat IV calcium, if required
If calcium continues to decrease after IV is stopped, consider starting on 1.25 OH Vitamin D, e.g., 250 ng, 1.25 OH D every 12 hr

be repeated again and, if hypocalcemia is recalcitrant, 1.25 dihydroxyvitamin D_3 may be started. Starting dose for 1.25 vitamin D is 250 ng every 12 hours.

For asymptomatic patients in whom serum calcium levels dip below 7.0, a single intravenous administration of calcium gluconate may be considered prior to beginning oral calcium supplementation if calcium levels remain low or if mild symptoms are present (digital/perioral paresthesias). Our choice for oral administration is calcium carbonate, 500 to 1000 mg tablets, 2 tablets three times per day which may be continued for 2 to 4 weeks postoperatively and gradually reduced according to periodic calcium determinations.

CASE PRESENTATIONS

Case 1

A 35-year-old black woman presents with a history of episodic renal lithiasis over the past six years. Her serum calcium is 11.5 mg/dl and serum PTH is 550. She has no other systemic complaints and has no history of bone pain or hypertension.

This patient has symptomatic hyperparathyroidism with mild elevation of serum calcium and a history of renal stones. She is at high risk for development of further problems from prolonged hypercalcemia. High-resolution ultrasonography of the central compartment is performed in an effort to localize the suspected adenoma.

The ultrasonographic evaluation demonstrates a suspicious area of nodularity posterior to the left thyroid lobe at the mid pole level.

The findings on ultrasonography are indicative of a left superior parathyroid adenoma. Unilateral exploration on the left is accomplished. A nodule 1.2 cm × 1.0 cm × 1.1 cm is noted posterior to the thyroid lobe superior to the inferior thyroid artery. A frozen section is performed yielding the report abnormal parathyroid tissue: adenoma vs. hyperplasia. A single small gland is identified in the inferior position—biopsy yields normal suppressed parathyroid tissue.

The procedure is thereby terminated. Twelve hours postoperatively the serum calcium is 9.0 mg/dl. Further decreases are noted to 8.2 mg/dl at 24 hours and 7.5 mg/dl at 36 hours postoperatively. The patient, however, remains asymptomatic.

Despite a falling serum calcium, the patient remains asymptomatic. No supplementation is administered, and within 48 to 72 hours the patient's serum calcium returns to normal. Final pathology demonstrates parathyroid adenoma.

Case 2

A 65-year-old previously healthy white woman presents with a serum calcium of 10.8 mg/dl on routine screening examination. Follow-up serum calcium levels are noted to be 10.9 mg/dl and 11.2 mg/dl, respectively. An intact PTH is determined to be 200 and 280 on serial evaluations. The patient is healthy with the exception of mild arthritis felt to be degenerative in nature and mild osteoporosis. There is no history of renal calculi, hypertension, arrhythmia, or muscle weakness.

This patient has asymptomatic hyperparathyroidism with mild elevation in serum calcium. Although asymptomatic at present, she has risk factors which predispose her to long-term problems secondary to her disease. These include osteopenia from degenerative joint disease and osteoporosis. Surgical therapy is recommended in light of the potential benefit of resection and the prospect of cure and subsequent significant disease-free life span. Medical therapy with estrogen administration, hydration, and mild diuresis with adequate physical activity may be used as a temporizing measure.

An MRI of the neck is obtained by the referring endocrine specialist. This demonstrates a 1.0 cm nodule in the left superior thyroid lobe and a 0.5 cm nodule just posterior to the right thyroid lobe. On physical examination, there are no obvious neck masses. Because of the equivocal findings on MRI, bilateral exploration is planned and undertaken. Findings demonstrate a left superior thyroid nodule and right inferior thyroid nodule. Both right inferior and superior parathyroid glands are identified and biopsied yielding normal parathyroid tissue. No visible left parathyroid glands are noted.

The suspected adenoma is not apparent. A systematic approach is undertaken to locate the missing glands. The thymic tongue is located on the left and followed—carefully dissecting within the tissue and palpating for nodularity. The superior thyroid pole is mobilized and the undersurface of the pole, adjacent to the esophagus, is scrutinized. The inferior thyroid artery is identified and traced to the carotid sheath. Any tributaries, especially those descending, may be associated with an ectopic superior gland.

During exploration of the left viscerovertebral angle and tracing of the inferior thyroid artery, a large oblong encapsulated mass is noted plunging posterior to the carotid sheath resembling a lipoma. Frozen section of this mass demonstrates lipoadenoma.

Parathyroid lipoadenoma represents approximately 1% of all adenomatous parathyroid lesions. Resection of the lesion in this case should be curative in that no other enlarged/abnormal parathyroid tissue was identified. The inability to locate the second gland on the left in this situation is inconsequential.

Case 3

A 38-year-old white woman, who is six months status postparathyroid exploration with excision of presumed right parathyroid adenoma, presents with recurrent hypercalcemia. During initial surgery, two normal glands were identified and biopsied. Final pathology in the resected adenoma yielded the finding of *normal tissue*. Postexploration the patient's serum calcium declined and remained stable over 6 to 8 weeks but had gradually increased to preoperative levels and is now 11.6 mg/dl. Intact serum PTH level is 350. The patient has a history of renal calcinosis for the past five years but is otherwise asymptomatic.

Although the patient has recurrent hypercalcemia following exploration, she is presumed to have a missed adenoma rather than hyperplasia on the basis of the presence of histologically normal *parathyroid glands. A possible exception would be the presence of parathyroid carcinoma, but this is unlikely. A localizing study should be performed. Our recommendation is to perform a combination of studies in an effort to accumulate data so that an accurate prediction of the location of the lesion may be attained. The most important lesion to identify or rule out is a mediastinal adenoma.*

An MRI scan of the neck is performed which is suboptimal secondary to patient compliance. The patient undergoes a technetium/thallium subtraction scan together with angiography and venous sampling for intact PTH levels. The subtraction scan demonstrates increased uptake in the left lower neck, and venous sampling yields increased intact PTH levels from the left thymic plexus.

These data indicate that the lesion resides in the inferior left central neck compartment. Re-exploration through a repeat cervical incision is recommended.

During re-exploration, a large left paraesophageal parathyroid adenoma is noted and removed. Autotransplantation of a devascularized left parathyroid gland to the left sternomastoid muscle is accomplished. There is a rapid decline in serum calcium postoperatively with 12-hour serial determinations of 9.2 mg/dl, 8.0 mg/dl, and 6.8 mg/dl. Shortly before the last level is measured, she develops perioral tingling and digital cramping. Physical examination demonstrates a brisk Chvostek sign.

The patient has acute symptomatic hypocalcemia secondary to iatrogenic hypoparathyroidism. Treatment begins with administration of intravenous calcium gluconate 10 cc of a 10% solution over 10 minutes. This may be combined with a continuous IV calcium gluconate infusion administered over 6 hours. Oral calcium supplementation, calcium carbonate, 625 mg × 2 three times per day should be started if serum calcium declines again following intravenous administration. Autotransplanted parathyroid tissue may be expected to function within 12 weeks postoperatively. The temptation to begin vitamin D therapy with oral supplementation of calcium should be tempered by the prospect of retarding return of parathyroid function. Serum calcium levels may be monitored 2 to 4 weeks after hospital discharge and, if appropriately elevated, supplementation can be weaned. It is important to measure serum phosphorus and magnesium levels during management of acute hypocalcemia.

Case 4

A 77-year-old black woman presents with mental status changes, hypertension, and hypercalcemia. She has a history of peptic ulcer disease. Her serum calcium is 14 mg/dl and intact serum PTH is 630. A metastatic disease workup is negative.

This women has moderate to severe symptoms of hypercalcemia secondary to hyperparathyroidism. Medical stabilization should be accomplished and should include adequate hydration coupled with furosemide diuresis and treatment of hypertension. The patient will require neck exploration for primary hyperparathyroidism. A localizing study is recommended.

High-resolution ultrasonography is performed yielding suspected nodular thyroid disease involving both thyroid lobes as well as a questionable nodule adjacent to the thyroid in the right lower neck.

Because of the nodular thyroid abnormalities, clear discrimination of a parathyroid abnormality cannot be accomplished by ultrasound alone. Nuclear scanning is recommended to support the findings on ultrasound.

Technetium/thallium subtraction scanning demonstrates a suspected parathyroid adenoma adjacent to the left inferior thyroid pole. Neck exploration is performed demonstrating nodular thyroid disease and a hard fibrotic gray mass adjacent to the right lower thyroid pole.

Parathyroid carcinoma is suspected from the gross findings. Biopsy should be obtained, although, if suspicion is high for carcinoma, wide resection of the mass with contiguous adjacent tissues and ipsilateral thyroid lobectomy should be performed. A serum calcium level of this degree may have offered a clue to the diagnosis with parathyroid carcinoma demonstrating markedly high levels of hypercalcemia.

Final pathology yields the diagnosis of parathyroid carcinoma. There is no overt neck metastasis on clinical examination. Calcium levels returned to normal approximately 72 hours postoperatively. Adjuvant therapy is considered.

In general, most cases of parathyroid carcinoma follow a slow indolent course of growth. Morbidity usually results from sequelae of severe hypercalcemia rather than meta-

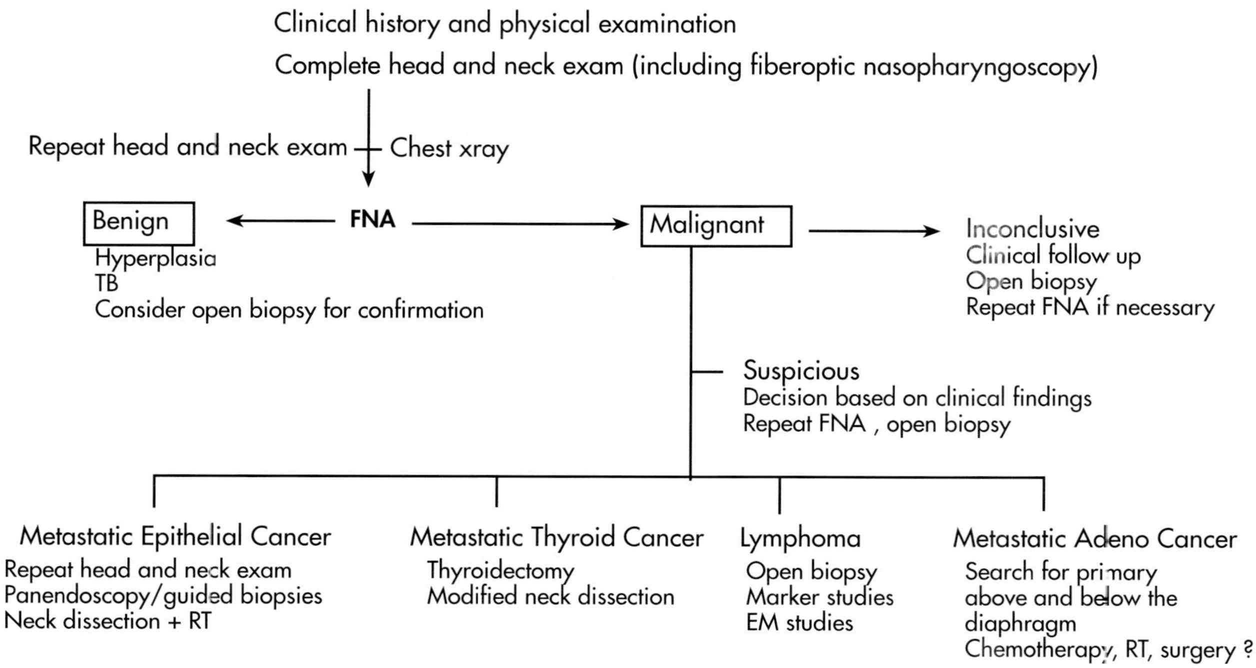

FIG 16-1
Algorythmic approach to cervical lymphadenopathy.

Possible Adverse Consequences of Untimely Lymph Node Biopsy

Spread of the tumor
Infection, cellulitis, delay in treatment
Improper incision for biopsy
Primary remains undetected and untreated
Patient feels adequate treatment is given
Loss for follow-up

Patient's symptomatology including sore throat, weight loss, cough, and hemoptysis are very important. The tumors in the posterior triangle generally originate from primary into the nasopharynx or skin tumors in the scalp area. The presence of bilateral metastatic disease generally indicates primary in the midline. The possible sites of the location of the primary lesions are shown in Table 16-2.

SEARCH FOR PRIMARY

A thorough and detailed examination of all the possible areas in the head and neck should be performed. Occult primary tumors are commonly missed in the nasopharynx, base of the tongue, laryngeal aspect of the epiglottis, and pyriform sinus. Obviously, these areas need special attention. Fiberoptic examination of the nasopharynx should be performed routinely. Fiberoptic telescopes are of immense

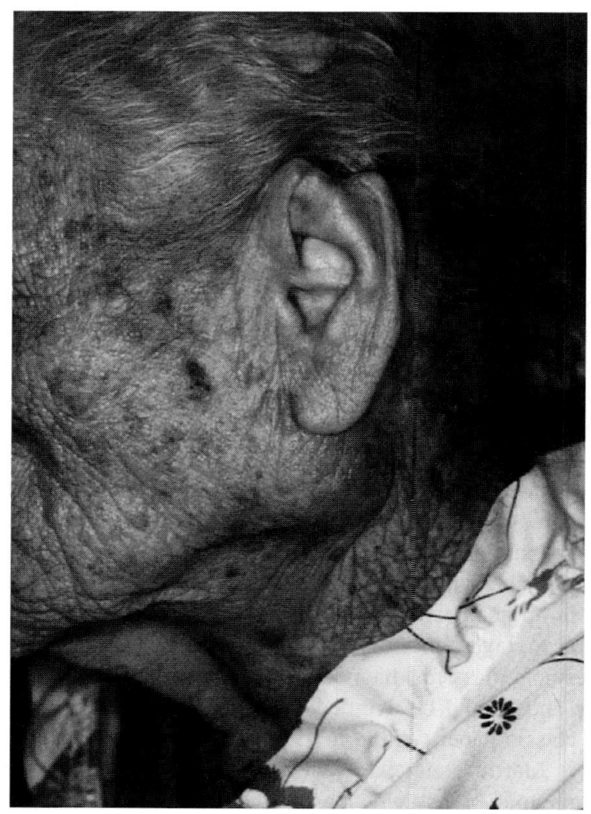

FIG 16-2
Presentation as left retromandibular mass—metastatic squamous carcinoma from previously treated cancer of the ear

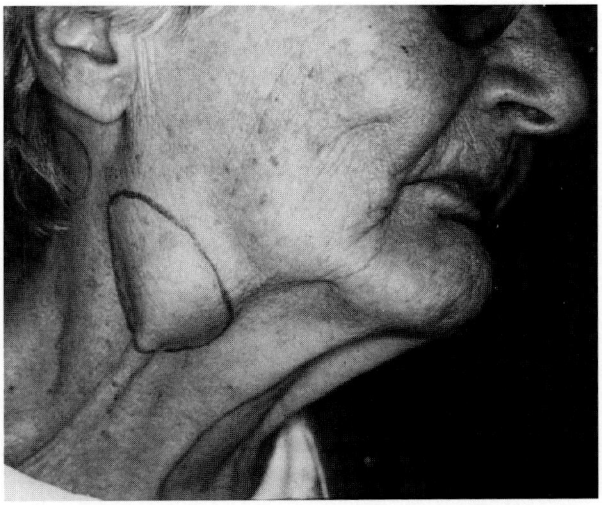

FIG 16-3
Classical jugulodigastric mass—in 75-year-old woman metastatic carcinoma with unknown primary.

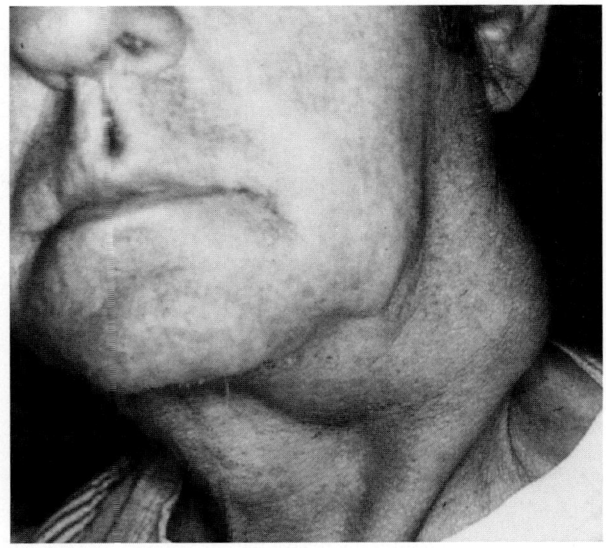

FIG 16-4
Large N_3 left neck metastatic tumor—unknown primary.

TABLE 16-1
Supraclavicular nodes and sites of primary tumors

Metastatic squamous cell carcinoma	Metastatic adenocarcinoma
Above clavicle	Above clavicle
Hypopharynx	Minor salivary tumors
Cervical esophagus	Thyroid
Below clavicle	Below clavicle
Esophagus	Breast
Lung	Lung
Cervix, uterus	Stomach
Urothelium	Pancreas
Anal canal	Ovary
	Prostate
	Colon

TABLE 16-2
Sites of metastatic nodes and possible primary sites

Region	Primary site
Submental	Lip, floor of mouth, tongue
Submandibular	Lip, tongue, floor of mouth, gum
Parotid nodes	Upper lip, skin of face and temple; metastatic melanoma
High jugular nodes	Oropharynx, base of tongue, nasopharynx
Mid-jugular nodes	Larynx, hypopharynx, thyroid
Low jugular nodes	Hypopharynx, esophagus, thyroid, lung, breast; structures below diaphragm
Posterior triangle nodes	Nasopharynx, scalp tumors

help in evaluating the entire laryngopharynx. Examination of lymph nodes in other areas such as axilla and groin should be completed to rule out lymphoma and generalized lymphadenopathy (Figs. 16-3 and 16-4).

RADIOGRAPHIC STUDIES

A chest x-ray is routinely performed for any parenchymal lesion, pleural effusion, or widening of the superior mediastinum. Esophagogram is usually of little help in evaluation of an unknown primary, however, if the patient gives a history of persistent weight loss or dysphagia, it is of paramount importance to search for possible esophageal carcinoma. In addition, x-rays of the paranasal sinuses are rarely helpful since the metastatic cervical lymphadenopathy from the primary in the paranasal sinus is quite rare. CT scan of the neck provides accurate assessment of the extent of the metastatic disease in the neck and is also helpful in evaluating the nasopharynx and retropharyngeal lymph nodes. Additional workup in search of primary tumor in the lung, esophagus, and GI tract or kidneys is not recommended at this point in the initial evaluation of the patient. Such tests may be performed if the FNA was definitely diagnostic of metastatic adenocarcinoma.

EXAMINATION UNDER ANESTHESIA

Examination under anesthesia (EUA) and random biopsy have become pivotal in the evaluation of unknown primary. EUA is especially very important for evaluating the base of the tongue and all the areas of the upper aerodigestive tract. The endoscopy should include nasopharyngoscopy, la-

Differential Diagnosis of Metastatic Undifferentiated Tumor

Lymphoma
Metastatic oat cell tumor
Kaposi's sarcoma
Merkel cell tumor
Eccrine carcinoma
Metastatic seminoma—germ cell tumor
Medullary carcinoma
Esthesioneuroblastoma
Amelanotic melanoma
Anaplastic carcinoma

ryngoscopy, pharyngoscopy, and esophagoscopy. The question about bronchoscopy and bronchial washings remains controversial. If the chest x-ray remains absolutely normal and the metastatic lymph node is not in the supraclavicular region, a lung primary is not likely. Bronchoscopy and bronchial washings will therefore contribute little and generally can be avoided. Blind biopsy, which used to be performed routinely, is very important in the evaluation of specific regions and difficult areas such as nasopharynx. With the routine use of fiberoptic telescope, the nasopharynx can be evaluated much better. Instead of performing routine blind biopsies of multiple areas of the upper aerodigestive tract, we generally perform "directed" or "guided" biopsies from the suspicious areas or the regions that are most likely to yield malignant pathology. The abnormal or irregular mucosa should obviously be biopsied. Sampling of the base of the tongue and nasopharynx is still a common practice. Unilateral tonsillectomy is practiced by some, however, in the absence of obvious clinical abnormality, it is generally not helpful.

PATHOLOGY

The most common pathology is generally metastatic squamous cell carcinoma, which is quite easy to diagnose on routine histology. Metastatic adenocarcinoma may present high or low in the neck. The metastatic adenocarcinoma in the upper portion of the neck may be from primary tumor in the salivary glands or of minor salivary gland origin. Metastatic adenocarcinoma in the supraclavicular region may originate from the thyroid or other regions below the clavicle. Metastatic undifferentiated tumor may be confused with a host of differential diagnoses which are depicted in the box above. The experienced pathologist will be able to confirm the diagnosis with special stains, marker studies, and immunoperoxidase stains.[2] The pathologist will also be able to help the clinician by studying the histologic features of the tumor to determine the possible primary site such as nasopharynx-lymphoepithelioma, lung, breast, kidney, prostate, and colon. Feinmesser[5] reported the role of polymerase chain reaction (PCR) in needle biopsies for the presence of EBV genome. Of 11 informative specimens, 3 were positive and 8 negative for PCR. All the patients negative for EBV had nonnasopharyngeal primaries, while 3 with positive EBV by PCR were noted to have nasopharyngeal primaries subsequently.

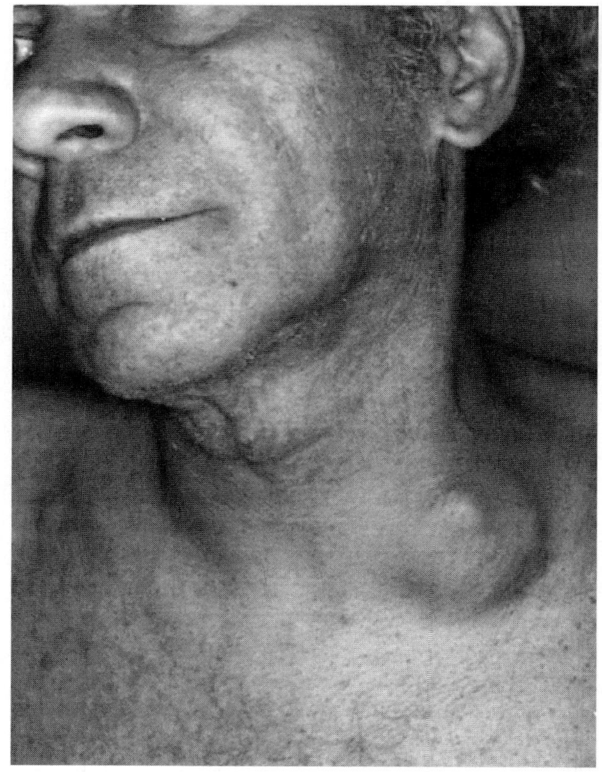

FIG 16-5
Left supraclavicular mass—biopsy positive for prostae specific antigen (PSA), metastatic prostatic carcinoma.

Many other tests may be of help in evaluating an unknown primary, such as a PSA stain of the neck mass (for prostatic tumor, Fig. 16-5) thyroglobulin, and calcitonin stain and EB virus titer may be indicative of nasopharyngeal primary if it is very high.

TREATMENT

The treatment of metastatic cancer of unknown primary origin in the neck consists of multimodality therapy which includes surgery and RT.[10] There are no prospective trials of the role of chemotherapy in the management of this disease except in patients with distant metastasis. The experience obtained from other chemotherapeutic trials in the head and neck reveal that there is no role of chemotherapy in the definitive management of this disease. de Braud[4] et al have reported their experience of 41 patients treated by chemotherapy along with surgery and radiation therapy.

Their results appear encouraging. Harper et al[6] reported their experience of 69 patients treated by radiation therapy with or without neck dissection. Mucosal site failures were noted in 12%. In-field mucosal failures decreased from 19% to 7% by increasing radiation dosage from 4500 to 6000 cGy.

The mainstay of treatment revolves around surgery or RT. Patients presenting with metastatic cancer in the supraclavicular region with a high possibility of primary below the clavicle are generally not recommended for neck dissection unless there are compression symptoms or fungation in the neck.

Bataini et al[1] reported a series of 138 patients with metastatic epidermoid carcinoma of unknown origin. These patients had either surgery and postoperative RT (48 patients) or RT only (90 patients). All patients received RT to the presumed occult sites. Forty-five percent of the patients had unilateral adenopathy. Patients who had initial surgery had a recurrence of 17% and a survival rate of 53%. Only 4% of the patients developed overt cancer at the occult site in the first 5 years. The authors recommended combination of surgery and RT whenever possible. They recommended prophylactic radiation of the occult site to be individualized according to the location of the cervical nodes; a dose of 5,000-6,000 cGy was recommended.

Spiro[12] reported a 74% survival rate in patients with N1 disease after radical neck dissection, whereas a 5-year survival rate of patients with N2 and N3 disease was 41%. Since the last publication by Spiro in 1983, the experience of Memorial Hospital was updated by Davidson et al.[3] This third report from Memorial Sloan-Kettering Cancer Center analyzes patients with unknown primary of whom 73 had squamous cell carcinoma. Seventy-one percent of the patients still presented with advanced metastatic cancer in the neck N2 and N3. Surgery included comprehensive neck dissection in 59 (81%), and adjuvant RT was implied in 54 (83%) of surgically treated patients. The subsequent identification of primary in the head and neck was noted in 9 patients (12%) including 4 of 11 (36%) who did not receive adjuvant RT and 5 of 54 (9%) who did receive RT ($p = 0.038$). The neck control rate was 74%, which shows considerable improvement when compared with the previous experience in 1983 in which the control rate was 50%. The control rate was much better in patients with extensive neck disease. Unfortunately, however, the cumulative survival rate at 5 years was 45%, which was not significantly different from that in the previous reports. Spiro et al[1] also reported survival difference between various tumor histologic types treated by neck dissection. For anaplastic or undifferentiated carcinoma, the 5-year survival was 53%, for epidermoid carcinoma, 48%, for metastatic melanoma, 20%, and for metastatic adenocarcinoma, 0%.

In a patient with metastatic carcinoma with unknown primary, whether the patient should have a standard neck dissection or modification is controversial. Generally, a classical radical neck dissection is recommended in almost all patients, except in select circumstances, especially when a patient presents with a single metastatic node in the anterior triangle or submandibular region. The only modification one would consider under these circumstances is comprehensive neck dissection, Level I-V, with preservation of the accessory nerve. The optimum radiation field for treatment of metastatic carcinoma in the neck is also controversial. A wide range of treatment volumes and techniques have been used. The choices represent a balance between the need to include the known area of disease and the likely occult primary site. The incidence of morbidity increases with increasing radiation volumes and fields. Xerostomia poses a major concern. The issue about including or excluding the nasopharynx in radiation portal has become a very controversial topic. Even though there is no definitive data, it appears that most would be willing to include the nasopharynx in the postoperative RT of such patients. The survival rate reported by Spiro and Bataini indicates that aggressive treatment of the neck can yield long-term survival in patients with epidermoid, anaplastic, or undifferentiated carcinoma. Radical neck dissection appears to be the treatment of choice for occult metastatic disease. M.D. Anderson Hospital recently reported a series of 157 patients with epidermoid carcinoma, the over-all five year survival was 55%.[13] Primary was manifested in 16% of the patients, and distant metastases were noted in 13% of the patients. The management of the primary detected in the follow-up after initial definitive treatment of an unknown primary depends on the location and size of the primary lesion.

METASTATIC ADENOCARCINOMA

This pathologic variety presents a separate and difficult problem—metastatic nodes in the supraclavicualr region, especially Virchow's nodes, with primary site in the lungs or below the diaphragm. Metastatic adenocarcinoma is generally considered a systemic disease with poor prognosis. Surgery and neck dissection are reserved only for patients with fungating tumors or with pressure effects. Chemotherapy and RT are considered to be the best modalities available at this time for patients with metastatic adenocarcinoma. There is considerable controversy regarding the extent of workup, which includes GI series, bronchoscopy, bronchial washings, ERCP, CT scan, barium enema, colonoscopy, and intravenous pyelography. The role of surgery is limited to very select circumstances, when the nodal disease is limited to the middle or upper portion of the neck, where the primary may be originating in the salivary glands.

In a recent report from M.D. Anderson Hospital on metastatic adenocarcinoma to the neck, the mean survival was 17 months and the median survival was 8 months. The survival was 20% for 2 years and 9% for 5 years.[7] There was increased survival associated with unilateral neck involvement ($p = 0.001$) and disease limited to nodes above the cricoid cartilage ($p = 0.007$).

Unknown Primary—Prognostic Factors

1. Site of metastasis
   Jugulodigastric vs posterior triangle vs supraclavicular
2. N Status - N_1, N_2, N_3
   Single/multiple nodes
   Unilateral/bilateral
3. Pathology
   Type of tumor
   Extracapsular spread
4. Previous open biopsy
5. Appearance of subsequent primary

TREATMENT FAILURE

The primary site is discovered after treatment in approximately 20% of the patients. In patients who failed treatment, 50% will demonstrate uncontrolled disease in the neck or primary region and the remaining 50% will have distant metastases. In patients treated with radiation as part of the definitive therapy, the incidence of appearance of primary tumor is reduced to 4% to 14%. The prognostic factors in the management of unknown primary include the site of the metastatic disease, the N status, unilateral or bilateral neck node metastasis, pathologic type of the tumor and extranodal spread, history of previous open biopsy, and appearance of subsequent primary (box above).

The prognosis for patients with primary tumors that are located after initial treatment is generally worse than that for those in whom the primary cancer remains indeterminate. The possibility of a subsequent appearance of occult primary tumor decreases with time. If tumors above the clavicle become manifest, they will usually do so within the first two years. Most of the primary lesions below the clavicle become manifest during the first year.

REFERENCES

1. Bataini JP, Rodriquez J, Jaulerry C, et al: Treatment of metastatic neck nodes secondary to an occult epidermoid carcinoma of the head and neck. *Laryngoscope* 97:1080-1084, 1987.
2. Batsakis JG: The pathology of head and neck tumors: the occult primary and metastases to the head and neck, part 10. *Head Neck Surg* 3:409, 1981.
3. Davidson B, Spiro RH, Patel S, Patel K, Shah JP: Cervical Metastases of Occult Origin: The Impact of Combined Modality Therapy. *Am J Surg* 168:395-399, 1994.
4. de Braud F, Heilburn LK, Ahmed K, et al: Carcinoma of the unknown primary metastatic to the neck: advantage of aggressive treatment. *Cancer* 54:510-515, 1989.
5. Feinmesser R, Miyazaki I, Cheung R, et al: Diagnosis of nasopharyngeal carcinoma by DNA amplification of tissue obtained by fine needle aspiration. *N Engl J Med* 326:17-21, 1992.
6. Harper CS, Mendenhall WM, Parsons JT, et al: Cancer in neck nodes with unknown primary site: Role of mucosal radiotherapy. *Head Neck* 12:463-469, 1990.
7. Lee NK, Byers RM, Abruzzese JC, et al: Metastatic adenocarcinoma to the neck from an unknown primary source. *Int J Surg* 162, 1991.
8. Martin HE: Untimely lymph node biopsy. *Am J Surg:* 102:17, 1961.
9. Martin H, Romieu C: The diagnostic significance of a "lump in the neck." *Postgrad Med* 11:491-500, 1952.
10. Shah JP: The unknown primary: surgical treatment. In Chretian PB, Johns ME, Shedd DB, et al, editors: *Head and Neck Cancer,* vol 1. St. Louis, 1985, Mosby, pp. 289-300.
11. Shaha AR, Webber C, Marti J: Fine needle aspiration in the diagnosis of cervical lymphadenopathy. *Am J Surg* 152:420-423, 1986.
12. Spiro RH, DeRose G, Strong EW: Cervical node metastasis of occult origin. *Am J Surg* 156:441-446, 1983.
13. Trevino, RJ: Food Allergies and Hypersensitivities. In Donald PJ, Gluckman, JL, Rice, DH, The sinuses. Raven Press, NY., 1995:123-132.
14. Wang RC, Goepfert H, Barber A, et al: Unknown primary squamous cell carcinoma metastatic to the neck. Arch Otolaryngol *Head Neck Surg* 116:1388-1393, 1990.

17

Tracheostomal Stenosis following Laryngectomy

Mark K. Wax, M.D., F.A.C.S., B. Joseph Touma, M.D., and Hassan H. Ramadan, M.D.

Laryngectomy for carcinoma of the larynx has been performed since it was first described in the late 1800s. Stell reviewed the literature and verified that Billroth did the first total laryngectomy for recurrent carcinoma following a hemilaryngectomy.[12] Securing the tracheal stump to the cervical skin was first described by Soillis-Cohen in 1892.[12] Although this development greatly facilitated the care of the laryngectomy patient, it brought about the development of the postoperative stomal stenosis. Since than the complication of tracheostomal stenosis has plagued both surgeons and patients.

A reduction of the tracheal lumen by 50% in all diameters will result in a 75% reduction in the cross-sectional surface area. [1] Patients who have a normal pulmonary reserve and pulmonary function will be able to maintain a normal tolerance for exercise. Unfortunately, the majority of patients requiring laryngectomy will have some form of chronic obstructive pulmonary disease. These patients will experience a significant respiratory impairment. Not only will their exercise tolerance be markedly decreased, but their ability to function in a normal setting will also be affected. Patients with emphysema who require positive expiratory pressure or patients who have a chronic productive cough may in fact exhibit respiratory insufficiency or even hypoxia at rest. Thus, an inadequate tracheostoma may very well functionally disable the patient.[1]

In order to overcome this functional debility, the patient is required to wear a laryngectomy tube or stent. To the patient, wearing of the tube entails cosmetic, physiologic, and psychological problems. Cosmetically, wearing of a stent or tube is just another of the many stigmas associated with having lost their larynx. While many patients accept the loss of speech, the stigmata of having a permanent tracheostomy tube is hard to overcome. Psychologically, the patient becomes dependent on the tube/stent. Knowing that their airway could be lost if the stent were to fall out, patients often become quite nervous and fixated as to the position and condition of their stent. Many of our patients must travel great distances for their care since their primary care physician is unfamiliar with the placement and care of the stents. Thus, not only is the patient obsessed with the condition of the stent, but the referring physician, if he is not an otolaryngologist, often panics at any problem with the stoma. Tracheostomy tubes or stents require frequent removal and cleaning in order to maintain adequate hygiene. Many patients who have had a laryngectomy find the removal and reinsertion of this tube to be quite onerous. The manual dexterity may, in fact, be beyond them. Repeated removal and insertion of the stent contributes to irritation of the tracheostoma. The newer soft sialastics stents have removed much of the mucosal problems of the past. Previously, a stainless steel or plastic type laryngectomy tubes was used. These often times caused irritation and sometimes ulceration of the overlying tracheal mucosa. This would then cause mucosal erosion, exposure of perichondrium, increased inflammation, necrosis, and increased scarring with more stenosis. Bleeding as well as tracheal irritation with constant coughing were problems that were also frequently seen. Another problem encountered is formation of crusts if the stents are not cleaned. These crusts cause irritation, promote coughing, as well as harbor a bad odor (Figs. 17-1 and 17-2).

Perhaps, most importantly, is that the stenosed tracheostoma precludes against the insertion of a tracheoesophageal voice prosthesis. While some authors[11,15] have described ingenious methods of incorporating a tracheoesophageal puncture device with a stent, often the two are incompatible.

The authors would like to thank Lillian J. Lawson for her technical assistance in the preparation of this manuscript and Pavlina Vagoun-Gutierrez for her artistic assistance.

A

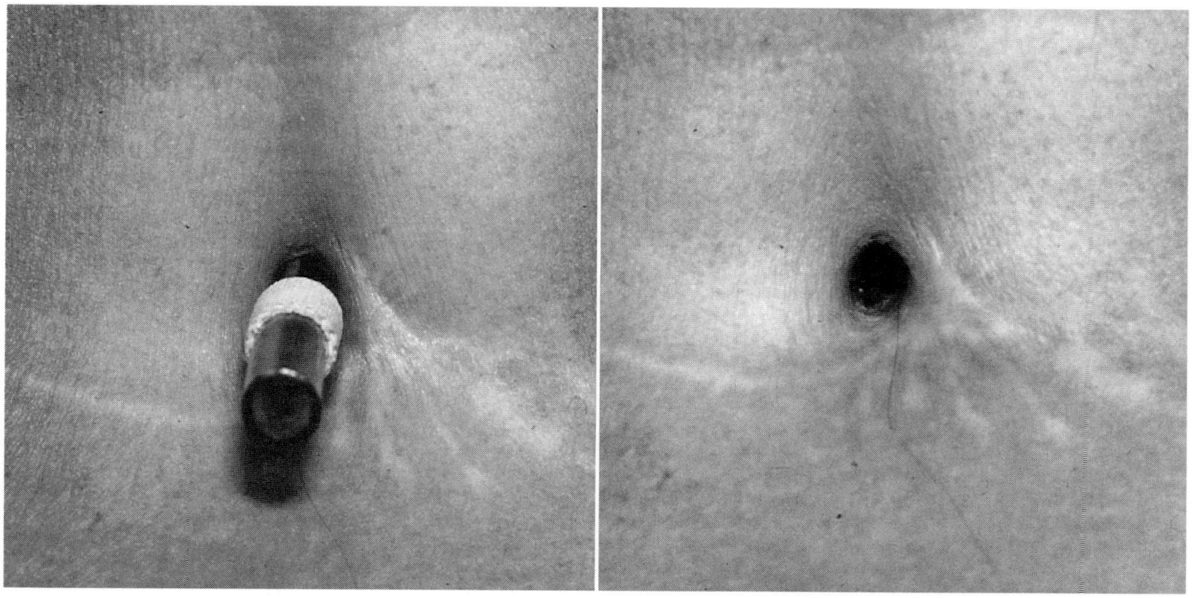

B

FIG 17-1
This woman demonstrates a stenotic stoma that requires wearing a homemade stent. **A.,** With stent in place. **B,** With stent out.

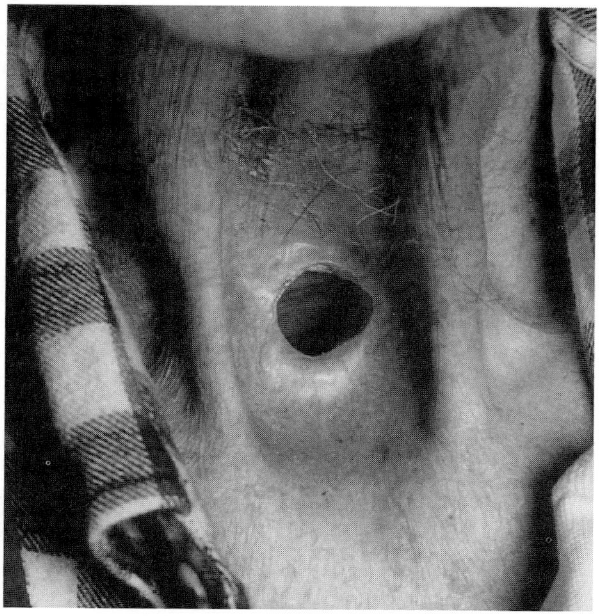

FIG 17-2
An adequate tracheostoma.

In order to rehabilitate our laryngectomy patients to the best of our ability, we must be able to provide them with an adequate stoma. Many factors have been implicated and examined in the etiology of tracheostomal stenosis. By far the most important factor is that of formation of the stoma at the time of the initial surgery.[13] We will review etiologic factors in the ensuing chapter.

DEFINITION

The incidence of tracheostomal stenosis following total laryngectomy varies depending upon the criteria used to define it. We have chosen to define a patient with tracheostomal stenosis as being anyone that requires wearing a stent in their tracheostoma for longer than three months following surgery. Furthermore, any patient who requires revision surgery for whatever reason is also considered to have a stenotic stoma. The majority of patients at our institution will wear some form of stoma vent upon discharge from the hospital. This stoma vent stays in an average of less than one month. Most of our patients travel great distances and are followed up on monthly intervals. If they are uncomfortable with not wearing a stent on discharge, they are given one until their next visit. Occasionally, they do not return until two months following discharge. Referring physicians are unwilling to remove the stent until they are seen by us. In our experience, only the occasional patient requires a stent for up to three months. Any patient who required stenting for greater than three months ultimately required revision.[13]

INCIDENCE

The incidence of stomal stenosis is reported as varying from between 4% to 42%,[5,13,14] (Table 17-1). One of the first articles on the subject in this country, by Langenbrunner and Chandler,[7] reported an incidence of 34%. Yonkers and Mercurio,[14] also from America reported, an overall incidence of 42%. Meanwhile Balle and Bretlau[2] from Denmark had reported an incidence of 41% prior to these previous two studies. Prior to these three reports, there was

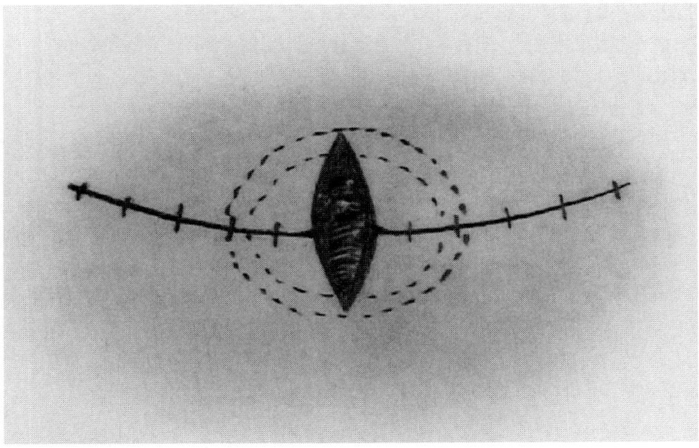

FIG 17-3
This artist representation depicts a verticle slit type of tracheostomal stenosis.

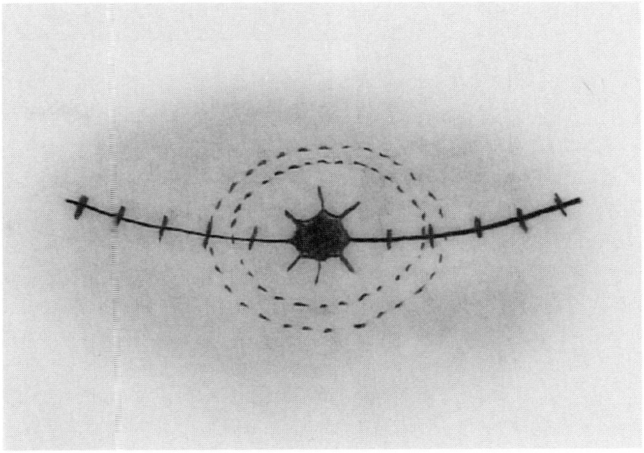

FIG 17-4
This artist representation depicts a concentric type of tracheostomal stenosis.

TABLE 17-1
Incidence of postlaryngectomy tracheostomal stenosis and the effect of closure at the time of initial surgery

			Stomal technique (% stenosis)			
			Circle	Bevel	Plastic	
Authors	Year	#Patients	No %	No %	No %	Overall stenosis #3 (%)
Griffith and Luce[4]	1982	99	56 (71)	20 (15)	13 (8)	22
Yonkers and Mercurio[14]	1983	107	—	Not ment oned	—	42
Lam et al[6]	1983	141	—	116 (31)	25 (4)	26
Balle and Bretlou[2]	1985	36	36 (55)	—	—	55
Kuo et al[5]	1994	207	—	—	207 (13)	13
Wax et al[13]	1994	105	9 (75)	70 (33)	26 0	28

little in the literature on the incidence of this problem. Most literature has dealt with the management of the patient who had suffered a tracheostomal stenosis. In 1985, Griffith and Luce[4] reported an overall incidence of 22%. They concluded that the technical construction of the stoma was the most important determinate of the incidence of tracheostomal stenosis. A simple circle or straight transection of the trachea had the highest incidence (29%) of stenosis which could be markedly reduced with a bevel technique (15%). A primary plastic or flap interposition construction yielded the lowest incidence at 8%. A recent report by Kuo et al[5] demonstrated a stomal stenosis rate of 13%. Their technique utilized a plastic type of closure. A review of 106 patients undergoing laryngectomy at our institution[13] revealed that the overall incidence of tracheostomal stenosis was 28.4%. Patients undergoing laryngectomy in the latter part of the study (1991 onward) all underwent a plastic closure with insertion of an advancement flap into the trachea. None of these 28 patients subsequently developed a stenosis. This was significantly at $p < 0.05$.

It would appear that with careful attention to detail at the time of the construction of the original stoma the tracheostomal stenosis rate should be under 5%.

CLASSIFICATION

In 1962,[8] Montgomery described three forms of tracheostomal stenosis:

The Vertical Slit (Fig. 17-3)
The Concentric (Fig. 17-4)
The Superior Shelf (Fig. 17-5)

Subsequently, few authors have subdivided their stomal stenosis into these categories. In Yonkers' and Mercurio's[14] discussion, 60% of the stenosis were concentric, 30% were vertical, and only the rare one was a superior shelf. Superior shelf and vertical stenosis are primarily technical and anatomic in origin. Vertical stenosis is felt to be due to tenting of the head of the sternocleidomastoid muscle. Superior shelf stenosis is secondary to an abnormal band of tis-

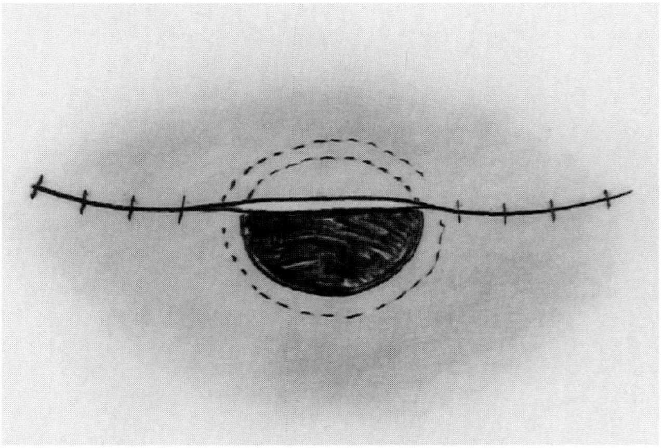

FIG 17-5
This artist's representation depicts a superior shelf type of tracheostomal stenosis.

sue from the superior cervical flap. In our experience, both vertical and superior shelf stenosis are exceedingly rare. Only two patients in our series were classified as having a superior shelf stenosis. Both of these patients functioned quite well with an electrolarynx and did not require stomal stenting. However, as they desired tracheoesophageal punctures, they required revisions for technical reasons. The superior shelves were the result of nonaggressive defatting of the superior flap. This was easily revised and a tracheoesophageal puncture placed. Another possible cause of a superior shelf is redundant cervical skin. Removal of this at the time of the stomal construction will prevent the stenosis. We have not encountered a patient with a vertical slit type of stenosis to date. The lack of a vertical slit stenosis is due to the technical construction of the stomas. Following Montgomery's[8] description of the vertical slit stenosis secondary to sternocleidomastoid or thyroid pathology, a better understanding of the role of these structures in the etiology of the stenosis was defined. Thus, most authors, in order to overcome the possibility of vertical stenosis, construct the stoma routinely with maximal lateral suturing. In patients with prominent sternocleidomastoid heads, the muscle can be divided to prevent this type of stenosis. An abnormally large thyroid lobe can be resected. Care in suturing the remaining thyroid lobe near the stoma also prevents this type of problem. At our institution, the majority of stenosis, has been concentric stenosis.

ETIOLOGIC FACTORS

In general the factors that contribute to the formation of tracheostomal stenosis may be divided into preoperative, intraoperative, and postoperative (Table 17-2).

Gender, radiotherapy, method of construction, placement of stoma, myocutaneous flap, and tracheoesophageal fistula formation have all been found in various reports in the literature to contribute to stomal stenosis. The contribution of various factors from our series is reviewed in (Table 17-3).

TABLE 17-2
Possible etiologic factors in the formation of tracheostomal stenosis

Period	Factors
Preoperative	Gender
	Race
	Keloid
	Radiotherapy
	Steroid usage
	Chemotherapy
Intraoperative	Neck Dissection
	Construction
	Circle
	Bevel
	Plastic
	Placement
	Inside incision
	Outside incision
	Myocutaneous flap
	Tracheoesophageal fistula
Postoperative	Infection
	Fistula
	Radiation
	Tracheoesophageal fistula

Gender

It has been suggested that women, due to their smaller tracheas, have a higher incidence of tracheostomal stenosis. Lam et al[6] and Kuo et al[5] failed to establish a significant difference in the incidence of stenosis among women. However, the study by Nigam[10] compared the cross-sectional area of the stoma in relationship to gender. They were able to demonstrate a large difference in the cross-sectional area of the stomas between men and women which, while not significant, did approach significance. In the Nigam[10] study, the numbers were quite small, and in the other two studies the population base was Chinese, which may have predicated against determining a significant affect. Experience at our institution[13] demonstrated a 46% incidence of stenosis in females versus a 22% incidence in males ($p < 0.05$) (Fig. 17-6). Anatomically, women have a smaller cross-sectional area to the trachea compared with men. This predisposes them to smaller tracheostomas. It is the decrease in cross-sectional area of the stoma that causes symptomatology. Since males have an inherently larger trachea, a reduction in the size of the stoma that would be unnoticeable and asymptomatic in the male is highly symptomatic in the female.

Since 1991, when we started to use a plastic type of closure for our tracheostomas, we have not had any women

TABLE 17-3
Etiologic factors implicated in tracheostomal stenosis

Factor	No. patients	Tracheal stenosis	
Sex			
Male	74	16 (21.6%)	
		$p < 0.05$	
Female	28	13 (46.4%)	
Radiotherapy			
Preoperative	29	6 (20.7%)	
Postoperative	42	14 (33.3%)	NS
Both	2	0 (0%)	
None	28	9 (32.1%)	
Chemotherapy			
Preoperative	5	0 (0%)	
Postoperative	14	5 (34.7%)	NS
Both	0	0 (0%)	
None	82	24 (29.3%)	
Stoma site			
Incision Site	85	23 (27.1%)	
Caudal to Incision Site	17	6 (34.3%)	NS
Closure			
Circle	8	6 (75%)	
Bevel	70	23 (32.9%)	
		$p < 0.05$	
Plastic	24	0 (0%)	
Neck dissection			
Unilateral	29	10 (34.5%)	
Bilateral	37	5 (13.5%)	NS
None	36	14 (38.9%)	
Steroid use	12	2 (16.7%)	NS
Fistula	29	9 (31.0%)	NS
Infection	33	11 (33.3%)	NS

develop stomal stenosis. Kuo et al[5] were unable to establish a significant difference in the incidence of stenosis based on gender. Like Kuo et al,[5] we employ a plastic type closure on a routine basis. However, one must always be aware that, since this trachea is smaller in women, attention to detail and technique is warranted.

Radiotherapy

Radiotherapy may contribute to poor wound healing secondary to the obliterative vasculitis and ischemia that it induces. Yonkers and Mercurio,[14] as well as Griffith and Luce,[4] found that postoperative radiotherapy was associated with a higher incidence of stenosis than preoperative radiotherapy. In all of these patients, concentric scarring was the underlying etiologic factor. With the advent of organ preservation and the increased utilization of radiotherapy as a primary modality for treating laryngeal carcinoma, more and more laryngectomies will be performed in the postradiated field. Our experience, as well as that of others, has been that, with good attention to detail and the use of a plastic type closure, the incidence of stomal stenosis should be minimal.

Neck dissection

There has been some suggestion that a unilateral or no neck dissection may predispose the patient to development of a stomal stenosis.[5,6,8,9] A radical neck dissection may theoretically decrease this incidence due to the removal of a prominent head of the sternomastoid muscle. These prominent heads of the sternomastoid muscle contribute to the development to the vertical stomal stenosis as described by Montgomery.[8] If, during the formation of the stoma, we find the heads of the sternocleidomastoid muscle to be prominent, then division of part of the muscle is performed. Recent experience, both by Kuo et al[5] and us,[13] has failed to support the allegation that modified neck dissection with preservation of the sternomastoid muscle predisposes to stomal stenosis.

Stomal placement

One of the variables in the technique of fashioning the stoma consists of whether to place the stoma within the main incision or in an inferior position (Fig. 17-7). Placement inferior to the main incision requires a separate stab incision through the lower cervical skin flap. Most authors in this country prefer to place the stoma in the main incision site. At our institution, 83% of stomas were placed in the main incision while 17% were placed below it.[13] The overall rate of stenosis was similar in both groups. Reasons for placement of the stoma in either site are usually surgeon's preference. Nigam et al[10] analyzed 61 patients undergoing laryngectomy. Thirty-five patients had stomas formed via a separate stab incision through the inferior cervical flap, while 26 patients had the stoma incorporated into the main incision. Sixteen of the thirty-five (42%) patients with the stoma formed separate to the main incision required usage of a stomal button or tube, whereas only one patient with a stoma formed in the main incision required a button or tube. On measuring horizontal, vertical, and cross-sectional area stomas that were incorporated into the main incision were significantly larger than stomas that were separated (cross-sectional area 190 mm vs 98 mm).[2] Placement of the stoma through a separate stab incision in the neck requires resection of a circular or oval patch of skin. This new stomal site will be predisposed to circular contraction as the wound heals. This in turn will lead to a circumferential stenosis. Placing the stoma in the main incision allows the lateral forces exerted by the main incision to help keep the stoma patent. Since the forces are directed both laterally and superiorly, there is a tendency in the well-constructed stoma to keep it open. Another option in the formation of the stoma that is inferior to the main incision is to break up the suture line by insetting skin flaps. This may decrease the incidence of stenosis.

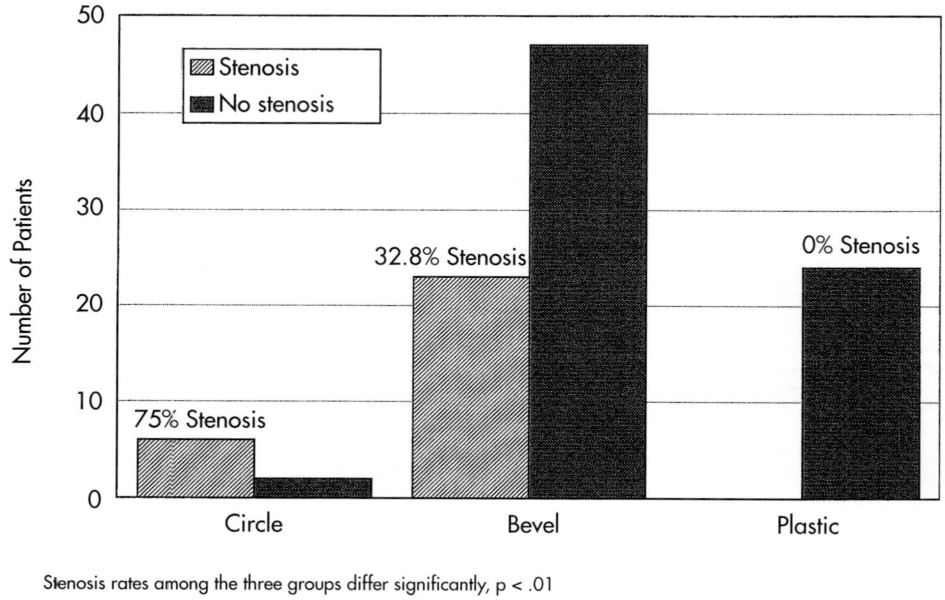

FIG 17-9
The technical construction of the stomal at the time of initial surgery is the most important factor in determining the final stenosis rate. Circular and bevel constructions yield a significantly higher stenosis rate than a plastic type closure.

secondary repair following dehiscence of the stoma four days after the primary surgery. Neither of these patients underwent a plastic type closure.

All patients who undergo myocutaneous flap reconstruction will have a large bulge of muscle where the pectoralis major turns over the clavicle. This never interferes with stomal function. Patients with this form of reconstruction do tend to wear their stomal stents for longer periods of time (3 months) when compared with patients without this form of reconstruction.

The myocutaneous flap may be utilized to reconstruct the pharyngeal defect or help form the stoma. When used to assist in the construction of the stomas, the muscle is usually used with a skin graft. We would expect that there would be tremendous contracture as the muscle atrophies. The numbers in the literature are too small to allow conclusions to be drawn. In instances in which the muscle is used to help construct the stoma, we would expect a higher incidence of stoma, especially in women with the smaller tracheas. When the flap is utilized to reconstruct only the pharynx, there would be a minimal effect on the stoma.

Experience with free flaps in this area, while common, is rarely commented on. We have had experience with patients undergoing jejunal reconstruction of total pharyngeal defects and rectus abdominous reconstruction of total laryngectomy/glossectomy defects. None of these patients experienced stenosis.

Tracheoesophageal puncture

Rehabilitation of patients who have had a laryngectomy often involves placement of a tracheoesophageal puncture. This may be performed primarily or secondarily. Patients who undergo secondary tracheoesophageal puncture may or may not require tracheostomal revision at the time of placement of the puncture. Very rarely has there been a report of stomal stenosis following secondary tracheoesophageal puncture. Most reports concern themselves with the incidence of stomal stenosis in patients undergoing primary tracheoesophageal puncture. A review by Kuo et al[5] demonstrated a 19% incidence of stomal stenosis in patients undergoing primary tracheoesophageal puncture versus 6% in patients who did not. This was significant at $P < 0.05$. In controlling for other etiologic factors such as gender, previous tracheostomy, radiotherapy, wound infection, anastomotic leakage, and tracheostomal infection, there was still a significant difference. The exact reasons are unknown. The actual technique used in creation of the tracheoesophageal puncture does provide more trauma to the airway. This in turn leads to increased inflammation with an increased chance of stenosis. Certainly the benefits of primary tracheoesophageal puncture outweigh the possible draw backs.

Since placement of a tracheoesophageal puncture is quite common, one should plan for this when constructing the tracheostoma. If one plans to use a local flap to break up the suture line, it is best to leave the posterior mucosal wall intact. A lateral or inferior flap is best. Insetting of skin into the posterior wall contributes to an increased technical difficulty in placing the puncture.

Infection/fistula

Infection of the mucocutaneous junction between the cartilage of the trachea and the cervical skin flap may lead to

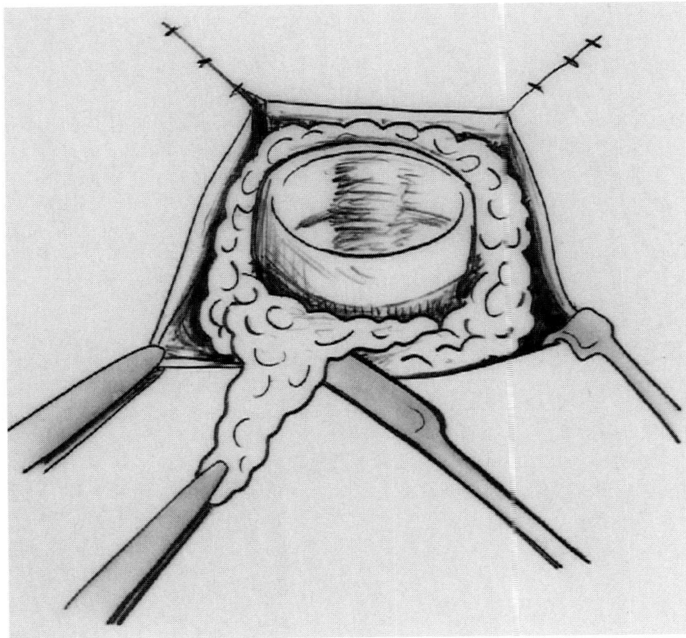

FIG 17-10
Fat is debulked from the inferior cervical skin flap.

the formation of granulation tissue. This results in healing by secondary intention. The subsequent fibrosis and contracture predispose to stenosis at the stomal site. Furthermore, the development of a tracheoesophageal fistula with subsequent constant soiling of the wound edges will also lead to a delay in primary healing. It has been suggested by a number of authors[13,5,14,4,6] that infections or fistula contribute to an increased incidence of tracheostomal stenosis. This has not been substantiated in recent literature.[13,5] In two series there was no correlation between the development of tracheostomal stenosis and patients who developed infection or fistulas. The majority of fistulas heals spontaneously, only occasionally requiring some form of myocutaneous flap closure. In both of these series all patients had some form of plastic closure at the time of reconstruction. Most likely it is the initial formation of a large tracheostoma that prevented the subsequent formation of a stenosis.

Miscellaneous factors

Keloid formation has been hypothesized to contribute to the incidence of tracheostomal stenosis. While mentioned in the literature, very few articles actually report on the true incidence.[9] In fact, in a review of the literature we were unable to detect a substantiated incidence. Theoretically, patients who are keloid formers should be at increased risk of keloid formation due to the extent and contamination of the wounds at the time of laryngectomy. However, this is a very rare occurrence.

Steroid usage,[9,13,14,15] by contributing to poor wound healing and increased incidence of both local and systemic infection, would theoretically contribute to an increased incidence of stomal stenosis. This has not been substantiated in the literature.

Occasionally, stomal stenosis will be the presenting sign of recurrent tumor. However, only rarely does the stomal stenosis predate the diagnosis and development of the stomal recurrence.

Chemotherapy[13] is being utilized more often as an organ preservation technique. General surgical literature would tend to show that the administration of chemotherapy does not contribute to an increased incidence of wound and healing problems. However, in debilitated patients with a contaminated field such as those having undergone laryngectomy, the prior administration of chemotherapy will certainly contribute to decreased healing. This in turn may contribute to an increased incidence of stomal stenosis. Only one series in the literature[13] has researched this factor, and in it the authors were unable to ascribe a higher incidence, perhaps due to small numbers.

TECHNIQUE

The technique that we utilize to construct the tracheostoma is as follows: Subcutaneous tissues of the lower apron flap are thinned and excessive tissue is removed (Fig. 17-10). The superior cervical skin flap is trimmed if it is felt to be excessive. Rarely is this necessary. An advancement rotation flap is fashioned from the lower cervical skin flap (Fig. 17-11). This flap is 3 to 4 cm long and 1 cm in width at its base. It is fashioned in such a way so as to allow ro-

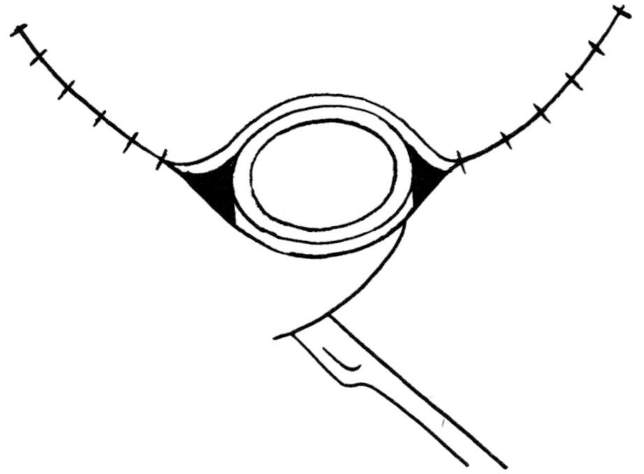

FIG 17-11
An advancement rotation flap is fashioned from the lower cervical skin flap.

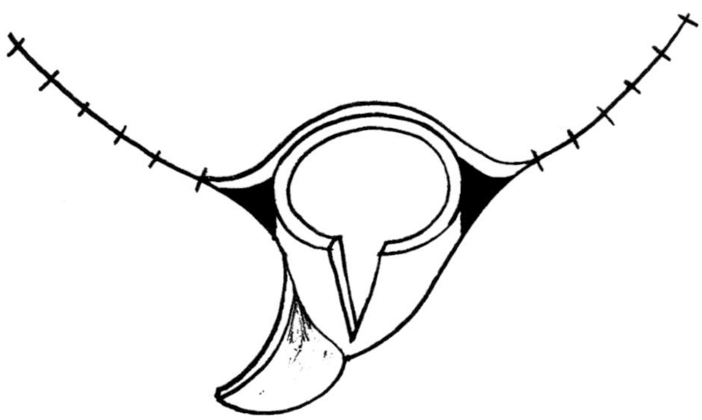

FIG 17-12
The anterior trachea is divided through two tracheal rings. The edges are splayed open to form a V.

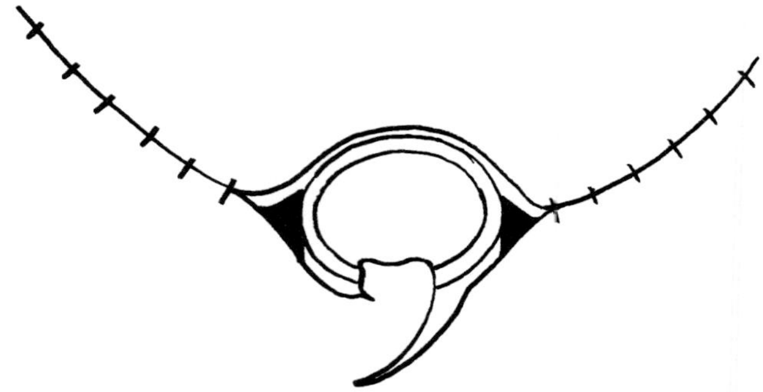

FIG 17-13
Rotation advancement flap is then inset into the depths of the trachea and secured with 0-nylon via bolsters.

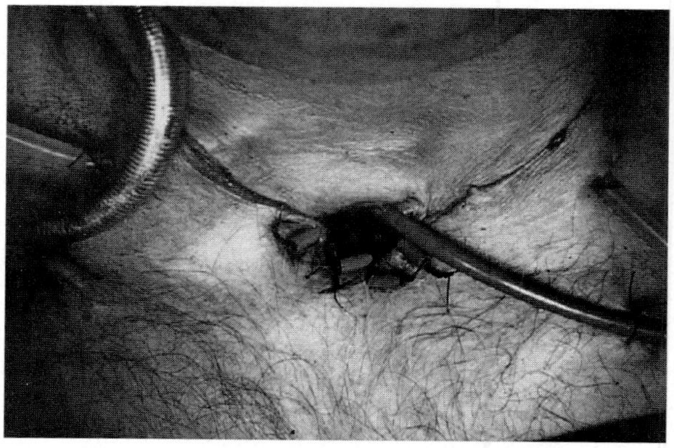

FIG 17-14
A well-formed stoma with a primary tracheoesophageal puncture is demonstrated.

tation into the trachea without tension. Anteriorly, the trachea is then divided through two tracheal rings in an inferior fashion. The edges of the trachea are splayed open to form a V (Fig. 17-12). The rotation advancement flap is then inset into the depths of the trachea and secured with 0 nylon via bolsters. The bolsters are formed from 14 gauge red rubber catheters (Fig. 17-13). The tracheostoma is then closed under slight tension to laterally dilate the trachea, with 0 nylon sutures fashioned in a way to provide coverage of the exposed cartilage. The anterior two-thirds of the trachea is secured to the skin of the lower cervical flap, utilizing a vertical-type mattress stitch in the flap and a simple stitch through the trachea encompassing a cartilaginous tracheal ring. Only a single layer closure is performed. This ensures coverage of the exposed tracheal cartilage. Occasionally a small shelf of skin is seen in the postoperative phase, but this has not proved to be a problem. The mucosa of the posterior wall is closed in two layers using an absorbable 3-0 vicryl suture with a simple stitch. Immediate tracheoesophageal puncture may be utilized with this technique (Fig. 17-14). Utilizing this technique, we have been able to decrease our rate of tracheostomal stenosis in the last twenty-eight patients to 0%.

MANAGEMENT OF STENOSIS OF THE TRACHEOSTOMA

Even with exemplary preoperative planning, good surgical technique, and an experienced surgeon, stenosis of the tracheostoma following laryngectomy will still occur in the occasional patient. Stomal stinting or dilation of the tracheostoma is not practical. Consequently, surgical revision is the optimal treatment.

Correction of the stoma stenosis will depend on addressing the same factors that must be addressed during the construction of the stoma during the laryngectomy.

The usual etiologic factors that cause stomal stenosis are excessive scar tissue in a concentric fashion or excessive fat or skin around the stoma. If aggressive defatting of the superior or inferior cervical skin flaps is not performed at the time of the initial surgery, these flaps may be bulky and protrude into the stomal airway. Revision is often simple and involves removal of this excessive tissue with reformation of the stoma.

Concentric scarring of the stomal is best approached by

surgically resecting the fibroptic tissue and reconstructing the stoma. Resection of the scar tissue and simple reconstruction will lead to a reformation of a stenotic stoma, since nothing has been done to address the underlying factors. A measure to break up the suture line is mandatory if one wishes to prevent recurrence of the stomal stenosis. Many methods have been described to prevent restenosis of the stoma. A review of the literature and our own experience would suggest that any form of insetting of skin flaps into the trachea will prevent recurrence of the stenosis. We prefer not to inset a posteriorly based skin flap into the mucosa. Current rehabilitation involves tracheoesophageal fistula formation, and it is not optimal to disrupt the skin mucosal suture line posteriorly. Consequently, most of our efforts have been directed at interposing skin into the tracheal part of the suture line. This can be done in the form of a Z-plasty, simple rotation advancement flap, or any one of a multitude of ways.

Our preferred method for revision of the tracheostoma is to advance and rotate two flaps laterally into the trachea after it is divided through one or two rings. With this technique we have met with success in 90% of our stomal stenosis.

SUMMARY

Tracheostomal stenosis is a frustrating problem for the patient and surgeon. It is associated with a multitude of problems. With good surgical technique and attention to detail, the incidence of stomal stenosis can be drastically reduced from 40% to 50% to less than 5%. Gender, primary tracheoesophageal puncture, use of pectoralis major myocutaneous flaps in reconstruction, formation of the stoma, and plastic closure have all been found to significantly contribute to the incidence of stomal stenosis. In the unfortunate patient who does develop a tracheostomal stenosis, the approach to reconstruction of the stoma following resection of the fibrotic scar tissue should be the same as that when one fashions a primary stoma. Adequate debulking and defatting of the skin flaps should be undertaken. Excess skin should be trimmed, and, finally, insetting of a skin flap through the mucosa of the trachea should be performed.

REFERENCES

1. Bain J: Late complications of tracheostomy and prolonged endotracheal intubation. *Int Anesthesiol Clin* 10:225-244, 1972.
2. Balle VH, Bretlau P: Tracheostomal stenosis following total laryngectomy. *Laryngol Otol* 99:577-580, 1985.
3. Clairmont AA: Tracheostoma construction during laryngectomy: techniques to prevent stenosis. *J Laryngol Otol* 92:75-78. 1978.
4. Griffith GR, Luce EA: Tracheal stomal stenosis after laryngectomy. *Plastic Reconstruct Surg* 70:684-698, 1982.
5. Kuo M, Ho CM, Wei WI, et al: Tracheostomal stenosis after total laryngectomy: an analysis of predisposing clinical factors. *Laryngoscope* 104:59-63. 1994.
6. Lam KH, Wei WI, Wong J, et al: Tracheostome construction during laryngectomy—a method to prevent stenosis. *Laryngoscope* 93:212-215, 1983.
7. Langenbrunner DJ, Chandler JR: Tracheostomal stenosis: causes and correction. *South Med J* 61:838-842, 1968.
8. Montgomery WW: Stenosis of tracheostoma. *Arch Otolaryngol* 75:76-79, 1962.
9. Myers EN, Gallia LJ: Tracheostomal stenosis following total laryngectomy. *Ann Otol Rhinol Laryngol* 91:450-453, 1982.
10. Nigam A, Campbell JB, Daggapta AR: Does the location of the laryngectomy stoma influence its ultimate size? *Clin Otolaryngol* 18:193-195, 1993.
11. Schueitzer VG, Rosi HD, Mohr R: Tracheostomal stenosis: a new prosthetic technique for postoperative stenting in postlaryngectomy stomal revision and in permanent tracheostomy. *Laryngoscope* 95:736-737, 1985.
12. Stell, PM: The first laryngectomy. *J Laryngol Otol* 89:353. 1975.
13. Wax MK, Touma BJ, Ramadan HH: Tracheostomal stenosis following laryngectomy: incidence and predisposing factors. *Otolaryngol Head and Neck Surg*, In press, 1994.
14. Yonkers AJ, Mercurio GA: Tracheostomal stenosis following total laryngectomy. *Otolaryngol Clin North Am* 16:391-405. 1983.
15. Yoshida GY, Hamaker RC, Singer MI, et al: Primary voice restoration at laryngectomy: 1989 update. *Laryngoscope* 99:1093-1095.

Part Four

Laryngology

18

Evaluation and Management of Chronic Aspiration

Andrew Blitzer, M.D., D.D.S., Yosef P. Krespi, M.D., Jonathan E. Aviv, M.D., and Isaac Eliachar, M.D.

Aspiration, or contamination of the airway with saliva, secretions, or food material may produce life-threatening pulmonary disease. Aspiration causes approximately 50,000 deaths per year in stroke patients alone. Intermittent or persistent aspiration may cause symptoms including cough, intermittent fever, recurrent tracheobronchitis, atelectases, pneumonia, and/or empyema. The pulmonary disease may be associated with weight loss, cachexia, and dehydration. In many cases the aspiration is caused by laryngeal dysfunction, allowing pulmonary contamination with swallowed material. In other cases, the aspiration is caused by a dysfunction of the oral, pharyngeal, or esophageal phases of swallowing. In some cases the aspiration is caused by a combination of laryngeal and swallowing dysfunction. Geriatric patients are more likely to have aspiration, since muscle weakness causing mechanical disability and neurologic impairment are more common in this group. Therefore, with an ever increasing aging of our population, these disabilities will be on the rise, with an associated increase in pulmonary disease and death. The approach to evaluation and management of these disorders should necessarily be based on an understanding of the underlying functional impairment.

PULMONARY CONSEQUENCES OF ASPIRATION

Normal individuals, aspirate small amounts of secretions during sleep, but they are easily able to clear the airway. Viral infections, ethanol ingestion, and altered states of consciousness may increase the amount of the aspirate, decrease the response, and therefore increase the severity of the tracheobronchial and pulmonary response. The quantity and frequency of aspiration increases with mechanical impairment of the larynx and pharynx, neurologic impairment, and decreasing levels of consciousness.[8,14,35,57]

The pulmonary response to small quantities of aspirated material may vary according the amount of aspirate, the pH of the aspirate, and the underlying status of the pulmonary, cardiovascular, and immune systems. With larger amounts of aspirated material, especially with a low pH, an intense bronchospasm is usually produced, as well as severe injury to the pulmonary capillary endothelium and the epithelium of the distal airway (Mendelson's syndrome).[51] The resultant injury causes hypotension, hypoxia, hypercarbia, and pulmonary edema and may result in death. When small solid particles are aspirated, they may obstruct bronchi, causing a secondary pneumonia and possible empyema. Larger particles may completely obstruct the airway, causing death. A chest x-ray of these individuals shows scattered irregular densities or occluded segment and most often shows involvement of the lower lobes, especially the right. The upper lobes may be involved in patients who remain supine.[1,6,20,34]

Aspiration related to neurological dysfunction

Disorders of the nervous system may result in significant dysfunction of the larynx and/or produce swallowing disorders. These are more common in the elderly, who are more likely to develop disorders of the neuromuscular system related to vascular or degenerative diseases.

Changes in the cortex, including stroke, drug-induced changes, seizure disorders, infection, tumors, and/or trauma often lead to laryngeal dysfunction, swallowing disorders, and consequent aspiration. More diffuse brain lesions can cause increased intracranial pressure that may produce altered levels of consciousness, stupor, or coma. These more diffuse processes include neoplasia, hematoma, abscess, massive infarction, meningitis, encephalitis, cerebritis, degenerative diseases—including Jacob-Creutzfeldt disease or adrenoleukodystrophy—, excess ingestion of alcohol, narcotics, or barbiturates, and increased or decreased serum calcium, sodium, or glucose. Aspiration and pharyngeal dysfunction may also produce laryngeal dysfunction, swallowing disorders, and aspiration, as seen in the extrapyramidal syndromes of Parkinson's disease, Huntington's disease, myoclonus, and tardive dyskinesia. The motor neuron disorders, including progressive spinal muscle atrophy (PSMA), progressive bulbar palsy (PBP), amyotrophic lateral sclerosis (ALS), and poliomyelitis, tend to produce severe laryngeal and pharyngeal dysfunction. Aspiration may be produced in disorders of transmission at the neuromuscular junction such as myasthenia gravis and the Eaton-Lambert syndrome. Peripheral nerve disorders, such as Guillain-Barre syndrome, or primary muscle disorders, such as muscular dystrophy, poliomyelitis, or metabolic myopathies, may also cause aspiration or swallowing disorders.[15]

SWALLOWING MECHANISMS

Swallowing is a synchronized, coordinated system of voluntary and involuntary muscle contractions and relaxation which results in the movement of a bolus of material in the oral cavity, past the laryngeal inlet, and then into the esophagus. When these events are disordered, aspiration, choking, nasal reflux, or regurgitation will occur.

In the oral phase of swallowing (voluntary), the tongue prepares the bolus for swallowing by mixing the food with saliva and sorting out the big particles that need to be chewed again. The the tongue then compresses the bolus against the palate, shaping it and coating it with mucus. The bolus is then squeezed into the oropharynx. The soft palate is elevated, separating the nasopharynx from the oropharynx, which prevents nasal reflux. When the bolus reaches the vallecula, the larynx is elevated, and the involuntary portion of the swallow is initiated.[27]

The pharyngeal phase of swallowing occurs after the bolus has passed the faucial pillars. Respiration is inhibited during this involuntary phase of swallowing. Once the bolus reaches the oropharynx, the tongue base first moves posteriorly, the epiglottis is tipped posteroinferiorly, and the larynx is raised by the supraglottic musculature. The bolus is diverted posterolaterally by the epiglottis away from the airway. The bolus then descends into the hypopharynx, with the airway protected by the epiglottis, collapse of the aryepiglottic folds and false cords, and the closure of the vocal cords.[1,4,27,58]

The esophageal phase of swallowing begins as the bolus passes through the upper esophageal sphincter. Problems may occur if the upper esophageal sphincter (the cricopharyngeus muscle) fails to open or the esophagus fails to contract. In 1958, Kirchner[38] studied the function of the cricopharyngeus muscle in dogs using endoscopy, radiographic studies, and pressure recordings. He found that the horizontal fibers of the cricopharyngeus were functionally different from those of the inferior constrictor, which is composed of the oblique fibers and the thyropharyngeus. The cricopharyngeus was found to be contracting during the relaxation phase. The tonic contraction is mediated by vagal fibers which provide tonic stimulation for contraction via lower motor activity.[77,84] After the pharyngeal phase of swallowing, the cricopharyngeus muscle relaxes, allowing passage of the bolus, and then contracts to a pressure equal to or greater than the resting pressure.

The nerve fibers supplying the cricopharyngeus arise in the vagal nuclei and pass without synapse to the motor end plates via the vagus nerve. The motor end plates are cholinergically mediated through nicotinic junctions. The tonic contraction is neurogenic, while central inhibition is responsible for the relaxation during swallowing.[23] The cricopharyngeus normally exerts a pharyngeal pressure of 15 to 23 mm Hg and must be overcome by the hypopharynx to induce the opening of the upper esophageal sphincter. Conditions which damage vagal fibers and interfere with the relaxation of the cricopharyngeus, such as basilar artery thrombosis, may cause cricopharyngeal achalasia, dysphasia, and aspiration. Neuropathic and myopathic processes may produce a relative cricopharyngeal achalasia, dyssynchrony, and dysphagia.

Evaluation of swallowing function

In order to decipher the cause of dysphagia, each phase of swallowing must be evaluated. The evaluation should begin with a complete history and physical examination, including fiberoptic laryngoscopy. This direct view of the larynx and pharynx during swallowing can identify any defects in the larynx, pooling of secretion in the hypopharynx, and any mass lesions that may be causing obstruction.

The radiographic evaluation must include a modified barium swallow or "cookie swallow," in which a video tape is made so that the study can be replayed at various speeds to identify subtle changes within the phases of the swallow. Small amounts of barium of different consistencies are given to the patient, who is kept in a natural upright position, to best assess the oral and pharyngeal phases of the swallow. The swallowing effort can be analyzed for adynamic areas, relative or true obstructions, and dysynchrony. The patient's position can also be changed to see in which position his swallowing is best. Assessment of aspiration can also be performed in regard to consistency of the bolus, the position of the patient, and any other associated dysfunction.[48,49]

Ultrasonography may be useful in studying the oral phase of swallowing but cannot be used for the pharyngeal or esophageal phases due to interference of the cervical spine. This study is noninvasive and safe and can be repeated on regular intervals without harm to the patient[69,72] CT and MRI scans can be used to detect brain stem or cortical lesions which may be the etiology of a neurologic dysfunction producing dysphagia. Radionuclide scans have also been found useful in the evaluation of the patients who have dysphagia and aspirate. A radioactive bolus, usually composed of ^{99}Tc sulfur colloid, is fed to the patient. The swallow is recorded with gamma scintillation camera as the bolus passes from the oropharynx to the esophagus. The pharyngeal transit time, clearance rate, and degree of aspiration can easily be quantified.[72]

Multiple port manometry, in which simultaneous pressure measurement can be taken in the pharynx, cricopharyngeus, and esophagus, is a useful way of identifying subtle failures of pressure generation or hyperfunction of the sphincter. Manometry does not, however, yield any information about aspiration. Therefore, manometry and videofluoroscopy have been used together, as reported by McConnel et al,[50] for the accurate evaluation of dysphagia and aspiration.

Analysis of the saliva can sometimes help determine the etiology of an oral phase dysfunction. Salivary samples can be collected from the parotid and submandibular glands and analyzed for quantity and chemical composition.[75]

Laryngopharyngeal sensory testing is an exciting new avenue for evaluating the causes of aspiration. The sensory apparatus can be tested utilizing a pressure and duration controlled puff of air delivered to the anterior wall of the pyriform sinus (the area innervated by the superior laryngeal nerve). The air puff is delivered from an internal port of a flexible fiberoptic laryngoscope made especially for this purpose (Pentax Precision Instrument Corporation, Orangeburg, New York). To determine an individual's sensory pressure threshold, air pressure is varied according to the psychophysical method of limits, while the duration of the air puff is held constant at 50 msec.[5]

The testing is carried out after a patient has had the opportunity to read a description of apparatus and procedure then given the opportunity to feel an air puff on the cheek and comment on the sensation. The floor of the nose is then anesthetized with 1% xylocaine with epinephrine 1:100,000 that is placed on a cotton-tipped applicator and inserted 1 cm from the nasal vestibule. Next, the flexible laryngoscope is inserted into the nasal passage and the patient is given a 1 minute rest period to adapt to the laryngoscope and prepare for testing. Testing begins by orienting the subject to the supraglottic stimulus with a suprathreshold stream of air for 5 seconds. After a 15-second rest period, presentation of air puffs begins. Six blocks of stimulus administration trials are given in which a threshold is obtained for each block. One stimulus is presented per trial. Trial duration is approximately 10 seconds with a ten-second intertrial interval. The air puff is administered after a verbal announcement of the beginning of the trial, at a random time from 2 to 8 seconds within the 10-second trial interval. Three blocks of descending pressure stimulus presentations and three blocks of ascending pressure stimulus presentation are randomly ordered for each subject. Within a block, air puffs are presented in sequential steps of 10 test unit changes (each unit is equivalent to $7.5 \times 10 \cdot 3$ mm Hg)—from subliminal to supraliminal for ascending blocks and from supraliminal to subliminal for descending blocks. A detection response occurs when the subject raises a hand within 2 seconds of actual stimulus presentation. A 30-second rest period separated the blocks. The mean of the lowest detected pressures from the six blocks is used as that subject's sensory threshold. Both the right and left sides of the pharynx and supraglottic larynx are studied.[5]

Treatment for swallowing disorders

The treatment for swallowing disorders should address the underlying defect and/or to help provide compensatory activity. Swallowing therapy can be of benefit in some of these individuals. In patients who still cannot swallow, gavage feeding can be taught which will bypass the oral phase. Some patients additionally have velopharyngeal insufficiency which allows for rhinolalia and nasal reflux. If very symptomatic, treatment can be offered ranging from a prosthetic appliance, which will elevate the soft palate, soft palate or posterior pharyngeal wall augmentation, or pharyngeal flaps.

The epiglottis is useful but not crucial in swallowing, as is evidenced by the swallowing abilities of patients after epiglottectomy or supraglottic laryngectomy. Treatment of a combined oral and pharyngeal phase defect in swallowing may include gavage or nasogastric tube feedings. Some patients with nasogastric tubes continue to aspirate a reflux of material around the tube. These patients may need a gastrostomy, and/or tracheostomy, and/or other laryngeal and pharyngeal procedures to prevent life-threatening aspiration.[48,49,70]

Swallowing therapy should be individualized based on observations during swallowing efforts and on video recording of the swallowing efforts during modified barium swallow. The consistency, head position, neck position, the method of food introduction, the quantity of food, and other parameters of swallowing can be assessed and modified for each patient to allow the maximum swallowing situation for that patient.[49]

Some patients who have oral phase defects may benefit from the use of dental prostheses. Some types of obturators or guide bar appliances can be used to direct food away from nonfunctional areas of the mouth, and allow the more functional areas to deal with the ingested food material. The construction of such an appliance is based upon the functional deficits detected on clinical examination and the modified barium swallow. The benefit of such an appliance can be documented on a repeat modified barium swallow. Adjustments to the appliance can be performed based on this follow-up study.[22,82]

Management of disabilities of the pharyngeal phase of swallowing are usually related to the cricopharyngeus muscle. Patients who have true cricopharyngeal achalasia or relative cricopharyngeal achalasia are often aided with a cricopharyngeal myotomy. Cricopharyngeal myotomy is the treatment for true cricopharyngeal achalasia or relative cricopharyngeal achalasia and the associated dysphagia and aspiration. It is not, however, a cure all for dysphagia attributable to a variety of neurologic conditions, as some authors suggest. Patients who have difficulty in all phases of swallowing from generalized mechanical failure related to such conditions as ALS, brain stem stroke, or myopathies have limited or no benefit from cricopharyngeal myotomy.*

Esophageal dysmotility may be improved in some cases with medical therapy. Peristalsis is mediated through vagal cholinergic fibers. The peristalsis can be abolished with curare and succinylcholine in the proximal esophagus and by atropine in the distal esophagus. Most of the esophageal motility research has addressed increasing the pressure of the lower esophageal sphincter for the treatment of gastroesophageal reflux. Two agents commonly used to increase contractility of the esophagus are bethanechol (which increases esophageal contractility but also increases the production of gastric acid) and metoclopramide (a potent antiemetic which has been found additionally to increase contractility without increasing gastric acidity).[26,66] The effect of these or other agents on the upper esophagus and upper esophageal sphincter are still not precisely known. In patients who have diffuse esophageal spasm, the use of a histamine blockers in conjunction with calcium channel blockers such as nifedipine or diltiazem (although not FDA approved for this purpose) has been shown to be effective in some cases.[18]

Patients with Parkinson's disease may also present with swallowing disorders. These patients have been found to have a lengthened oral phase of swallowing related to lingual dysmotility, a lengthened pharyngeal phase with vallecular stasis, and a lengthened esophageal phase due to dysmotility. These finding are not seen in patients with essential tremor. Poor motility and decreased sphincter pressure is also commonly found in diabetic patients.[66]

Severe esophageal dysmotility may also be found in patients with acute and chronic changes from caustic ingestion. Caustic agents may also lead to aspiration due to decreased sensation and fibrosis. These changes may be irreversible and difficult to treat. In severe cases, it may be necessary to bypass the esophagus with a gastric pull-up or interposition of small or large bowel.

LARYNGEAL INCOMPETENCE

The occurrence of aspiration does not necessarily mean laryngeal dysfunction. During the pharyngeal phase of swallowing, the larynx is elevated, the tongue base is moved posteriorly, the epiglottis and aryepiglottic folds close over the glottic inlet, the vocal cords close, and the bolus is pushed posteriorly into the food passage. If some of the material remains in the hypopharynx when the larynx descends and the vocal cords open, it may run into the airway producing a cough or soilage of the airway.

In the normal larynx, unilateral sensory stimulation will evoke reflex adduction of the vocal cords. The sensory signal is carried via the superior laryngeal nerve, and the bilateral motor response is carried via the recurrent laryngeal nerves. If there is a decreased or absent sensory signal, foreign material in the supraglottis and glottis may escape detection and fail to trigger laryngeal closure. Without laryngeal closure, swallowed material may spill through the glottis until it is detected by sensory fibers of the recurrent laryngeal nerve which provides sensation over the undersurface of the vocal cord and subglottis. If the vagal sensory fibers are also disabled, a cough may not be initiated, and the foreign material will descend into the tracheobronchial tree until it provokes a response from the vagal tracheal fibers which has considerable crossover.

Aspiration may also occur due to mechanical or neuromuscular impairment of the vocal cords. When a unilateral vocal cord paralysis prevents complete glottic closure, the airway may become soiled during a swallow. The cough reflex is also diminished since it becomes much harder to build up an adequate amount of subglottic pressure without forcing the paralyzed cord open.

Mechanical disabilities such as congenital abnormalities, anatomic changes due to trauma, or deficiencies due to surgery or loss of vocal cord volume may leave an open glottis and lead to aspiration. Traumatic dislocation of the cricoarytenoid joint may also predispose a patient to aspiration when the vocal cord is fixed in a relatively open position.[47,68]

Evaluation of laryngeal dysfunction

Indirect laryngoscopy and fiberoptic laryngoscopy should be performed at rest and during function in patients who have an open glottic chink, hoarseness, and intermittent aspiration to determine the etiology. The movement (including tremors, twitches, and other unusual movements) and the coordination of the vocal cord activity can be evaluated visually. In addition, the use of a stroboscope will slow the motion to allow for evaluation of very rapid, unusual, or uncoordinated movements. Electromyography of the larynx will provide electrical evidence of early neuromuscular change such as patterns of denervation, reinnervation, tremor, myoclonus, and myopathy.[13]

Electroglottography and photoglottography have also been used to study characteristics of the vocal cord movement. Electroglottography is based on the change in electrical potentials from the motion of the vocal cords, as measured by surface electrodes. Photoglottography is based on the change of transglottic transmission of light by the opening and closing of the vocal cords. In cases in which a brain stem or central etiology for the laryngeal dysfunction is being considered, electroencephalography, brain stem–evoked response audiometry, and CT and MRI scans are often essential.[33]

*References 3, 9, 19, 43, 53, 56, 62, 67, 73, 81.

Treatment of aspiration and laryngeal incompetence

Once the etiologic evaluation is complete and a presumptive diagnosis has been made, a treatment plan can be constructed. The therapeutic plan should be based on the patient's underlying disease, the likelihood for recovery, general medical status, quality of life issued, severity of the aspiration, and laryngeal incompetence.

Patients who chronically aspirate copious secretions may warrant a separation of the airway and food passages. Tracheotomy is the most commonly used method of providing this separation. The airway can be secured utilizing a tracheostomy tube with a cuff. The tracheotomy tube cuff will keep secretions or food substances from entering the airway. It will also provide access for good pulmonary toilet. Suctioning of secretions above the cuff is necessary to prevent soilage of the airway upon cuff deflation. Tracheotomy is a short-term solution only, since, with time, pressure from the cuff will produce tracheomalacia and an inability to obtain an effective seal, allowing continued airway soilage. Therefore, other solutions are necessary for long-term disability.[17,30,29]

Glottic prosthesis. A glottic stent is an attempt to separate the food and air passages without the use of an inflated cuffed tracheotomy tube, much like a cork in a bottle. The prosthesis can be prefabricated or custom made and is placed in the larynx endoscopically, usually held in place with transcutaneous sutures, and can be removed if the patient improves. The patient has a tracheotomy for an airway. The problems with this technique have been related to local inflammation, discomfort, scarring at the glottic level, and the leak of fluid around the prosthesis due to an ineffective seal.[80]

A new type of stent has recently been described by Eliachar et al.[28] It is made of a soft silicone material which minimizes local tissue inflammation, discomfort, and scarring. It easily contours to prevent leakage around the stent. Since it is hollow and soft, it has a superior slit which allows phonation through the tube while maintaining a seal in the glottic opening. The stent is placed through the tracheostomy over a Yankower suction tip and is held in place by an external adjustable tab.

Vocal cord augmentation. A noncompensated open glottic chink due to anatomic deficiency, mechanical impairment, or a neuromuscular disability should be corrected if symptomatic. In 1911[16] Bruning reported moving a paralyzed vocal cord toward the midline using an injection of paraffin. Paraffin was found to produce granulomas and was abandoned, but other materials were tested including glycerine, cartilage, bone dust, and Tantalum. Tantalum and glycerine and then Teflon and glycerine were first used by Arnold[2] in 1962. Lewy et al[45,61,65] have since reported successful treatment of vocal cord paralysis using Teflon injection. Teflon is injected into the larynx during a direct laryngoscopy using local anesthesia so that the airway and voice can be constantly assessed. Injection of Teflon in the vocal cord has also be performed in selected patients percutaneously via the cricothyroid membrane, as recently reported by Ward.[79]

Once injected, Teflon is difficult to remove from the larynx, therefore judicious use is imperative, since, if Teflon is accidently placed in the vocalis muscle, it will produce a change in the resonant characteristics of the vocal cord. In addition to medializing the paralyzed vocal cord, Teflon can be used to augment some vocal cord deficiencies. Teflon, a silicone product, is not currently available in the U.S. for injection. An alternative to Teflon is fat injection, which is not permanent but can medialize the vocal cord for a year or more.[26,31,63,64]

In patients who have had recurrent laryngeal nerve trauma or brain stem stroke, in which there is a possibility of return of function, glycerine or gelfoam injection can be used for medialization for a limited time until the material is resorbed.[65] If function does not return and the patient again becomes symptomatic, the vocal cord can be medialized with a more permanent material.

In patients with larger laryngeal defects, augmentation with autogenous costochondral, nasal septal or thyroid cartilage, or alloplastic materials may be safer and more effective. In 1952, Meurmann first described a technique in which cartilage was placed submucosally through a midline thyrotomy. This technique was later refined by others.* Recently, Isshiki described several different procedures for modifying the laryngeal framework, including a medialization laryngoplasty (type I) for voice improvement and correction of glottic incompetency to avoid aspiration in cases of vocal cord paralysis.[36,37,39] In this procedure a window is created in the thyroid ala, and the paralyzed vocal cord is medialized using cartilage or alloplastic material inserted via the window. Other authors have devised their own modifications of this technique, achieving good results.[24,40,59]

The implant procedure can be combined with a vocal fold adduction procedure, as described by Isshiki and later by Koufman, to provide good posterior laryngeal closure.[36,39]

Glottic and supraglottic laryngeal closure. An adequate separation of the food and air passages may be provided by closing the larynx. This avoids tracheal damage from a constantly inflated cuffed tracheotomy tube and creates a potentially reversible situation if the patient recovers laryngeal and pharyngeal function.

In 1975, Montgomery[54] described a glottic closure procedure performed through a median thyrotomy in which the mucosa of the vocal cords is stripped bilaterally and figure of eight suture is placed to close the glottis and allow fibrous union of the vocal cords. This technique allows adequate separation of the air and food passages with a permanent tracheotomy. The problems associated with this pro-

*References 44, 52, 60, 71, 78.

cedure are: the patient cannot phonate the seal may pull apart before healing and leak posteriorly if the vocal cords are functional preoperatively. The procedure is potentially reversible, but laryngeal webs are often difficult to correct, leaving vocal cords with significant scarring and poor phonation.

An alternative to closure of the larynx at the glottic level is a closure of the supraglottis. This is advantageous because it causes no scarring in the area of the vocal cords. In 1972, Habal et al[32] described a two-layered horizontal closure of the supraglottis via a pharyngotomy. The epiglottis, aryepiglottic folds, arytenoids, and interarytenoid area are then incised and the tip of the epiglottis is then folded over the arytenoids and sutured in place. Patients are unable phonate and breathe through a tracheotomy tube. As reported by Strome and Fried[74] in 1983, the procedure is reversible. In some cases recurrent aspiration occurs, perhaps due to the suture line opening posteriorly from the spring of the epiglottic cartilage. In 1983, a vertical supraglottic closure was created by Biller et al[10] to avoid the posterior opening and leave a small opening at the top. With an opening at the level of the tip of the epiglottis, aspiration does not occur but phonation is possible in some patients. This authors have used this closure with excellent results successfully in several patients with intractable aspiration. Patients can often again eat, and some can speak.

Laryngeal diversion

In 1975, Lindeman[46] described a procedure to separate the air and food passage in a reversible fashion without damage to the laryngeal structures. In this procedure the trachea is separated at the third or fourth tracheal ring, with the distal portion brought out and sewn to the neck skin. The proximal tracheal stump and larynx are sewn to a small opening in the esophagus. This procedure allows all material entering the larynx to exit into the esophagus with a complete separation of the airway. Phonation cannot occur following this treatment. If the patient recovers function, the procedure is reversible. Lindeman reported two such reversals of his procedure. This author has used this technique many times with success.[12,83] Lindeman[46] and Baron and Dedo[7] reported the creation of a blind end pouch of the proximal trachea in patients who had high tracheostomies. Another approach to the patient with a very high preliminary tracheostomy was described by Krespi et al.[41] Their modification included saving the mucosal lining as a superiorly based mucosal flap and cartilage resection from the cricoid cartilage and the first and second tracheal rings. An esophagotomy is made at the level of the first tracheal ring and the tracheal mucosal flap is sutured to the esophagotomy. Tucker[76] devised an alternative diversion technique in which both the proximal and distal trachea stumps are diverted to the anterior cervical skin, thereby creating a double-barrelled tracheostoma. The proximal trachea is brought out to the skin through a split in the sternocleidomastoid muscle. This maneuver supposedly compresses the trachea, minimizing leakage of aspirated material to the skin. This procedure has the obvious disadvantage of draining corrosive substances to the cervical skin.

Partial cricoid resection

Krespi et al[42] have recently described a technique for use in patients who develop postoperative aspiration after head and neck cancer resections. At the time of surgery, a submucosal dissection of the posterior aspect of the cricoid is performed and a large segment of the center of the posterior cricoid lamina is removed. This, in conjunction with a cricopharyngeal myotomy, leaves a large hypopharyngeal portal for secretions and food and decreases the anteroposterior diameter of the larynx. Patients require a permanent tracheotomy, but phonatory capability remains. Another alternative to this procedure was described by Biller and Urken[11] for patients who have continued aspiration after supraglottic laryngectomy. Vertical cuts are made in half of the cricoid cartilage allowing for a collapse of the hemilarynx, thereby decreasing the space available for airway soilage. Some patients continue to have a functional airway.

Laryngectomy. The oldest treatment for life-threatening aspiration has been a total laryngectomy. Total laryngectomy provides a permanent cutaneous tracheostoma and a permanent separation of the airway and food passage, but it eliminates phonation or the possibility of reversal in patients who might recover some or all of the function.[55] Some suggest that laryngectomy, particularly a narrow-field laryngectomy, is still indicated in patients with poor prognoses or associated medical problems.[21]

CONCLUSION

Chronic recurrent aspiration and swallowing disorders may become life threatening. Techniques have been developed to allow thorough evaluation to identify which of the diverse etiologies is causing the disability. There is an eclectic group of therapeutic modalities to allow better laryngeal and swallowing function. Many innovative surgical procedures are available to compensate for some of the functional deficits. If the patient recovers from the underlying disability, some of the procedures can be reversed. In the future it may be possible to use more sophisticated nerve grafting or electronic microcomputerized laryngeal pacing to allow return of laryngeal and pharyngeal function. Continued research in these areas will allow physicians to treat disorders leading to life-threatening aspiration more effectively.

REFERENCES

1. Ardan GM, Kemp FH: The protection of laryngeal airway during swallowing. *Br J Radiol* 25:406-416, 1952.
2. Arnold GE: Vocal rehabilitation of paralytic dysphonia. *Arch Otolaryng* 76:358-368, 1962.
3. Asherson N: Achalasia of the cricopharyngeal sphincter. *J Laryngol Otolog* 64:747-758, 1950.
4. Atkinson M, Kramer P, Wyman SM, Ingelfinger FJ: The dynamics of swallowing. I. Normal pharyngeal mechanisms. *J Clin Invest* 36:581-588, 1957.

5. Aviv JE Martin JH, Keen, MS, et al: Air pulse quantification of supraglottic and pharyngeal sensation: a new technique. *Ann Otol Rhinol Laryngol* 102:777-780, 1993.
6. Awe WC, Fletcher WS, Jacob SE: The pathophysiology of aspiration pneumonitis. *Surgery* 60:232-239, 1966.
7. Baron BS, Dedo HH: Separation of the larynx and trachea for intractable aspiration. *Laryngoscope* 90:1927-1932, 1980.
8. Bartlett JG, Gorbach SL: The triple threat of aspiration pneumonia. *Chest* 68:560-566, 1975.
9. Begley MD: Cricopharyngeal Achalasia. *J Coll Radiol,* 6:138-141, 1962.
10. Biller HF, Lawson W, Baek S-M: Total glossectomy: a technique of reconstruction eliminating laryngectomy. *Arch Otolaryngol,* 109:69-73, 1983.
11. Biller HF, Urken M: Cricoid collapse. a new technique for the management of glottic incompetance. *Arch Otolaryngol,* 111:740-741, 1985.
12. Blitzer A: Evaluation and management of chronic aspiration. *NY State J Med.* 87:154-160, 1987.
13. Blitzer A, Lovelace RE, Brin MF, et al: Electromyographic findings in focal laryngeal dystonia (spastic dysphonia). *Ann Otol Rhinol Laryngol* 94:591-594, 1985.
14. Bonano PC: Swallowing dysfunction after tracheostomy. *Ann Surg* 174:29-33, 1970.
15. Brin MF, Younger D: Neurologic disorders and aspiration. *Otol Clin NA* 21:691-701, 1988.
16. Brunings W: Uber eine neue behandlungsmethode. *Verh Deutche Laryngol* 18:93-151, 1911.
17. Bryant LR, Tinkle JK, Dubiler L: Tracheal damage from cuffed tracheostomy tubes. *JAMA* 215:625-628, 1971.
18. Buchin PJ: Swallowing disorders: diagnosis and medical treatment. *Otolaryng Clin NA* 21:663-667, 1981.
19. Calcaterra TC, Kadell BM, Ward PH: Dysphagia secondary to cricopharyngeal muscle dysfunction: surgical management. *Arch Otolaryng* 101:726-729, 1975.
20. Cameron JL, Reynolds J, Zuidema GD: Aspiration in patients with tracheostomies. *Surg Gynecol Obstet* 136:68-70, 1973.
21. Cannon CR, McLean WC: Laryngectomy for chronic aspiration. *Am J Otolaryng* 3:145-149, 1982.
22. Chalian VA, Drane JB, Standish SM: *Maxillofacial prosthetics: multidisciplinary approach.* Baltimore, 1971, Williams Wilkins Co.
23. Christenson J: *Innervation and function of the esophagus.* In Stipa S, Belsey RHR, Moraldi A, editors: Medical and surgical problems of the esophagus. (London, 1981 Academic Press) pp 14-16.
24. Cummings CW, Purcell LL, Flint PW: Hydroxylapatite laryngeal implants for medialization: a retrospective analysis. *Ann Otol Rhinol Laryngol* 102:843-851, 1993.
25. Dedo HH, et al: Intracordal injection of Teflon in the treatment of 135 patients with dysphonia. *Ann Otol Rhinol Laryng,* 82:661-667, 1973.
26. Diamant NE: In *Normal esophageal physiology.* In Cohen S, Soloway RD, editors: *diseases of the esophagus.* New York, 1982, Churchill Livingstone, pp 1-33.
27. Didio LJA, Anderson MC: *The "sphincters" of the digestive system.* (Baltimore, 1968, Williams Wilkins Co.)
28. Eliachar I, Roberts JK, Hayes JD, Tucker HM: A vented laryngeal stent with phonatory and pressure relief capability. *Laryngoscope* 97:1264-1268, 1987.
29. Fearon B, McDonald RE, Smith C: Airway problems in children following prolonged endotracheal intubation. *Ann Otol Rhinol Laryngol* 75:975-986, 1966.
30. Fee WE, Ward PA: Permanent tracheostomy: a new surgical technique. *Ann Otolaryng* 86:635-638, 1977.
31. Ford CN: *Laryngeal injection techniques.* In: Ford, CN, Bless DM, editors: Phonosurgery: assessment and surgical management of voice disorders. New York, 1991, Raven Press Ltd, pp 123-141.
32. Habel MB, Murray JE: Surgical treatment of life endangering chronic aspiration pneumonia. *Plast Recon Surg,* 49:305-311, 1972.
33. Hanson DG, Gerratt BR, Ward PH: Glottographic measurements of vocal dysfunction: a preliminary report. *Ann Otol Rhinol Laryngol* 92:413-420, 1983.
34. Hawkins DB: *Noninfectious disorders of the lower respiratory tract.* In Bluestone CD, Stool SE, editors: Pediatric Otolaryngology. Philadelphia, 198[illegible], WB Saunders Co, pp 1265-1269.
35. Huxley EJ, Viroslav J, Gray WR, Pierce AK: Pharyngeal aspiration in normal adults and patients with depressed consciousness. *Am J Med* 64:564-568, 1978.
36. Isshiki N: Recent advances in phonosurgery. *Folia Phoniatrica* 32:119-154, 1980.
37. Isshiki N, Okamura H, Ishikawa T: Thyroplasty type I (lateral compression) for dysphonia due to vocal cord paralysis or atrophy. *Acta Otolaryngol* [illegible]0:465-473, 1975.
38. Kirchner JA: The motor activity of the cricopharyngeus muscle. *Laryngoscope* 68:1119-1159, 1958.
39. Koufman JA: *Laryngoplastic phonosurgery.* In Johnson JT, et al, editors: *Instructional courses.* Am Acad Otolaryng–Head and Neck Surgery. St. Louis, 1988, CV Mosby Co, pp. 339-352.
40. Koufman J: Laryngoplasty for vocal cord medialization: an alternative to Teflon. *Laryngoscope* 96:726-731, 1986.
41. Krespi Y, Quatela VC, Sisson GA, Som ML: Modified tracheoesophageal diversion for chronic aspiration. *Laryngoscope* 94:1298-1301, 1984.
42. Krespi Y, Sisson G: Management of chronic aspiration by subtotal and submucosal cricoid resection. *Ann Otol Rhinol Laryngol* 94:580-583, 1985.
43. Lebo CP, Sang K, Norris FH: Cricopharyngeal myotomy in amyotrophic lateral sclerosis. *Laryngoscope* 86:862-868, 1976.
44. Levine HL, Tucker HM: *Surgical management of the paralyzed larynx.* In Bailey B, Biller HF, editors: Surgery of the larynx. Philadelphia, 1985, WB Saunders Co pp 117–147.
45. Lewy RB: Glottic rehabilitation with Teflon injection—the return of voice, cough, and laughter. *Acta Otolaryngol* 58:214-222, 1964.
46. Lindeman RA: Diverting the paralyzed larynx: a reversible procedure for intractable aspiration. *Laryngoscope* 85:157-180, 1975.
47. Litton WB, Leonard JR: Aspiration after partial laryngectomy: cineradiographic studies. *Laryngoscope* 79:887-907, 1969.
48. Logemann JA Bytell DE: Swallowing disorders in three types of head and neck surgical patients. *Cancer* 44:1095-1105, 1979.
49. Logemann J: *Evaluation and treatment of swallowing disorders.* San Diego, 1983, College Hill Press.
50. McConnel FMS: Analysis of pressure generation and bolus transit during pharyngeal swallowing. *Laryngoscope* 98:71-78, 1988.
51. Mendelson CL: Aspiration of stomach contents into lungs during obstetrical anesthesia. *Am J Obst Gyn* 52:191-205, 1946.
52. Meurmann Y: Operative mediofixation of the vocal cord in complete unilateral paralysis. *Arch Otolaryngol,* 55:544-553, 1952.
53. Mills CP: *Dysphagia in pharyngeal paralysis treated by cricopharyngeal sphincterotomy.* Lancet 1:455-457, 1973.
54. Montgomery WW: Surgical laryngeal closure to eliminate chronic aspiration. *N Engl J Med* 292:1390-1391, 1975.
55. Montgomery WW: *Total Laryngectomy.* In Montgomery WW, editor: Surgery of the upper respiratory system. Philadelphia, 1973, Lea Febiger, pp 484-496.
56. Montgomery WW, Lynch JP: *Oculopharyngeal muscular dystrophy treated by inferior constrictor myotomy.* Trans AAOO 75:986-993, 1971.
57. Nahum AM, Harris JP, Davidson TM: The patient who aspirates—diagnosis and management. *J Otolaryngol* 10:10-16, 1981.
58. Negus JE: The second stage of swallowing. *Acta Otol* 78(suppl):78-82, 1949.
59. Netterville JL, Stone RE, Luken ES, et al: Silastic medialization and

arytenoid adduction: the Vanderbilt experience. A review of 116 phonosurgical procedures. *Ann Otol Rhinol Laryngol* 102:413-424, 1993.
60. Opheim O: Unilateral paralysis of the vocal cord. *Acta Otolaryngol* 45:226-230, 1955.
61. Rontal E, Rontal M, Morse G, Brown EM: Vocal cord injection in the treatment of acute and chronic aspiration. *Laryngoscope* 86:625-634, 1976.
62. Ross ER, Green R, Auslander MD, Biller HF: Cricopharyngeal myotomy: management of cervical dysphagia. *Otolaryngol Head Neck Surg* 90:434-441, 1982.
63. Rubin HJ: Intracordal injection of silicone in selected dysphonias. *Arch Otolaryngol* 81:604-607, 1965.
64. Rubin HJ: Misadventures with injectable polytef (Teflon). *Arch Otolaryngol* 101:114-116, 1975.
65. Schramm VL, May M, Lavorato AS: Gelfoam paste injection for vocal cord paralysis:temporary rehabilitation of glottic competence. *Laryngoscope* 88:1268-1273, 1978.
66. Schulze-Delrieu K: *Esophageal pharmacology.* In Cohen S, Soloway RD, editors: *Diseases of the esophagus.* New York, 1982, Churchill Livingstone, pp. 35-49.
67. Seaman WB: Cineroentgenographic observations of the cricopharyngeus. *Am J Roent Radium Sher Nucl Med* 96:922-931, 1966.
68. Sessions DG, Ogura JH, Cralsky RH: Late glottic insufficiency. *Laryngoscope* 85:950-959, 1975.
69. Shawker T, Sonies B, Stone M: Real-time ultrasound visualization of tongue movement during swallowing. *J Clin Ultrasound* 11:485, 1983.
70. Shedd DP, Scatliff JA, Kirchner JA: A cineradiographic study of postresectional alterations in oropharyngeal physiology. *Surg Gynecol Obstet* SGO 110:69-89, 1960.
71. Smith GW: Aphonia due to vocal cord paralysis corrected by medial positioning of the affected vocal cord with a cartilage autograft. *Can J Otolaryng* 1:295-298, 1972.
72. Sonies BC, Baum BJ: Evaluation of swallowing pathophysiology. *Otolaryng Clin NA* 21:637-648, 1988.
73. Stevens KM, Newell RC: Cricopharyngeal myotomy in dysphagia. *Laryngoscope* 81:1616-1620, 1971.
74. Strome M, Fried MP: Rehabilitative surgery for aspiration. *Arch Otolaryng* 109:809-811, 1983.
75. Stuchell RN, Mandel ID: Salivary gland dysfunction and swallowing disorders. *Otolaryng Clin NA* 21:649-661, 1988.
76. Tucker HM: Management of the patient with an incompetent larynx. *Am J Otolaryng* 1:47-56, 1979.
77. Van Overbeck JJ, et al: Cricopharyngeal myotomy in pharyngeal paralysis, cineradiographic and manometric indications. *Ann Otol Rhinol Laryngol* 88:596-602, 1979.
78. Waltner JG: Surgical rehabilitation of voice following laryngofissure. *Arch Otolaryngol* 67:99-101, 1958.
79. Ward PH, Hanson DG, Abemayor E: Transcutaneous Teflon injection of the paralyzed vocal cord: a new technique. *Laryngoscope* 95:644-649, 1985.
80. Weisberger EC, Huebsch SA: Endoscopic treatment of aspiration using a laryngeal stent. *Otolaryngol Head Neck Surg* 90:215-222, 1982.
81. Wilkins SA: Indications for the section of the cricopharyngeus muscle. *Am J Surg* 108:533-538, 1964.
82. Wurster CF, Krespi YP, Davis JW: Combined functional oral rehabilitation after radical cancer surgery. *Arch Otol* 111:530-533, 1985.
83. Yarington CT, Linderman RC, Sutton D: Clinical experience with the tracheoesophageal anastomosis for intractable aspiration. *Ann Otol Rhinol Laryngol* 85:609-612, 1976.
84. Yoshida Y: Localization of efferent neurons innervating the pharyngeal constrictor muscles and the cervical esophagus muscle in the cat by means of horseradish peroxidase method. *Neurosci Lett,* 10:91-95, 1981.

19

Evaluation and Management of Unilateral Vocal Fold Paralysis

Maisie L. Shindo, M.D., and Peak Woo, M.D.

Phonation is dependant on highly coordinated activity of the laryngeal muscles which requires both anatomic and neurophysiologic integrity. An immobile vocal fold may be a manifestation of several different disease entities. As such, neurologic disorders of central and peripheral etiology, muscular disorders, and anatomic abnormalities such as ankylosis must all be considered and systematically evaluated. It is important to accurately identify the etiology and the residual pathophysiology so that treatment can be planned rationally. An understanding of neurolaryngology and a systematic, logical approach to evaluation and treatment of vocal fold paresis will improve treatment outcome. This chapter will review: (1) the relevant neuroanatomy and neurophysiology of the larynx, (2) the causes and pathophysiology of vocal cord paralysis, (3) a variety of state-of-the-art diagnostic modalities that are currently used to aid in diagnosis and treatment planning, and (4) the surgical treatment modalities for unilateral paralysis, their relative advantages and disadvantages, and treatment selection.

ANATOMY

The evaluation and management of laryngeal paralysis requires a thorough knowledge of the laryngeal biomechanics, laryngeal neuroanatomy, and physiology of vocal fold movement. Vocal fold movement is controlled by groups of laryngeal musculature that exert different vectors of forces on the arytenoid cartilage. These muscles consist of a group of adductors—the thyroarytenoid, lateral cricoarytenoid, and interarytenoid—and the sole abductor, the posterior cricoarytenoid. The cricothyroid muscle increases the tension of the vocal cords, though it may function as an abductor during stressed respiration. All of the muscles are paired and receive innervation separately from each side, except the interarytenoid muscle which is a single muscle that receives bilateral innervation.

The essential functions of the larynx are respiration, phonation, protection of the airway, and cough production. The vagal nervous system controls the functions of the larynx by providing motor innervation to the laryngeal musculature and carrying sensory fibers from the larynx. Laryngeal motor fibers arising from the cerebral cortex and midbrain pass caudally to the lower pontine levels as part of the pyramidal tracts, enter the medulla, and terminate in various motor nuclei within the nucleus ambiguous. Before entering the medulla, some of these fibers decussate, giving bilateral innervation to the nucleus ambiguous. As its name implies, the nucleus ambiguous is a motor nucleus without clearly defined boundaries containing motor neurons to the larynx, upper cervical esophagus, and pharynx. Nerve fibers arising from the nucleus ambiguous form the peripheral vagus trunk and exit the skull through the jugular foramen. In addition to containing motor fibers to the laryngeal, pharyngeal, and upper esophageal musculature, the vagus nerve also carries sensory (visceral afferent) fibers from these sites. These sensory fibers terminate in the nucleus solitarius in the brain stem. Immediately below the jugular foramen, the vagus nerve swells to form the nodose ganglion. The superior laryngeal nerve arises just inferior to the nodose ganglion. It branches into an external branch, that innervates the cricothyroid muscle, and an internal branch that carries sensory fibers from the supraglottic larynx. The cell bodies for these sensory fibers are located in the nodose ganglion. The vagus nerve continues its course in the neck along the carotid arteries and terminates in the chest as recurrent laryngeal nerves (RLN). On the right the RLN courses anteriorly to the subclavian artery, loops around it, and courses cephaladly in the tracheoesophageal

Causes of Vocal Cord Paralysis

- Surgery
- Neoplastic processes
  - Bronchogenic/lung cancer
  - Thyroid cancer
  - Laryngeal cancer
  - Cancer of the upper esophagus
  - Mediastinal lymphoma
  - Paragangliomas
- Trauma
- Neurologic diseases
  - Parkinson's disease
  - Multiple sclerosis
  - Myesthenia gravis
  - Cerebrovascular accident
- Inflammatory
  - Intubation
  - Rheumatoidal arthritis
  - Gastroesophageal reflux
  - Chronic nasogastric tube
- Idiopathic

Iatrogenic Causes of Vocal Cord Paralysis

- CVP placement
- Carotid endarterectomy
- Cervical laminectomy
- Pneumonectomy
- Esophagectomy
- Radical neck dissection
- Thyroidectomy
- Zenkers diverticulectomy
- Skull base surgery
- Glomus vagale resection
- Carotid body resection
- Open heart surgery

groove to enter the larynx. On the left, the RLN courses anteriorly to the aorta, loops around it, and courses cephaladly in the tracheoesophageal groove to enter the larynx. The RLN branches into abductor and adductor branches to innervate these respective groups of muscles.

DIFFERENTIAL DIAGNOSIS

Laryngeal paralysis is a symptom, not a disease. Therefore, a diligent search for the etiology of the paralysis is essential. The causes of laryngeal paralysis are listed in the box above. In many cases, the cause of vocal fold paralysis is evident, for example, from penetrating neck trauma, thyroid cancer, or surgery—most commonly thyroidectomy. In a number of cases, even after an extensive search, the etiology is unknown and a viral neuritis is thought to be the cause.

When the vagus nerve or its branches are injured, wallerian degeneration occurs and results in a flaccid paralysis of the vocal fold. Similarly, injuries to the cell bodies in the nucleus ambiguous from a vascular insult, trauma, and neoplastic and degenerative processes of the central nervous system will result in a flaccid paralysis. Although injury to the peripheral Xth nerve and its lower motor neurons typically results in flaccid paralysis, upper motor neuron lesions may also manifest as vocal fold paresis or paralysis and should be considered in the differential diagnosis.

Iatrogenic injury to the Xth nerve and its branches remain one of the most common causes of vocal cord paralysis. The box above right lists some of the common procedures and surgeries which can result in vocal cord paralysis. Peripheral vagal nerve injury may occur by a variety of mechanisms. Neoplasms along the long course of the Xth nerve may affect its function by compression or direct invasion. Cancers of the thyroid, esophagus, lung, and metastatic carcinomas to the neck and base of skull are common causes of vocal cord paralysis and should be ruled out prior to considering symptomatic treatment. Rarely, primary tumors affecting the Xth nerve, such as vagal schwannomas and glomus vagale tumors, may cause flaccid paralysis. Peripheral neuropathy due to chemotherapeutic agents (vincristine), diabetes, renal failure, and dialysis may affect Xth nerve function. Viral inflammation (postpolio syndrome, Guillan Barré syndrome) may also affect Xth nerve function. Cardiovascular diseases may cause paralysis of the left vocal cord by compression or stretch injury. Cardiomegaly, aneurysm, mitral stenosis, and cardiac surgery are some specific causes.

Inflammatory etiologies include rheumatoid arthritis, endotracheal intubation, chronic nasogastric tube, and gastroesophageal reflux. Cricoarytenoid arthritis due to rheumatoid arthritis manifests during the inflammatory period as an erythematous, immobile joint. Later, the presence of an affected immobile joint can best be confirmed by diagnostic laryngoscopy and palpation of the joint. Posterior glottic stenosis or web should be suspected in patients with a recent history of prolonged intubation and head injury. In patients with prolonged nasogastric tube use, erosion of the posterior cricoid lamina by the nasogastric tube resulting in injury to the PCA muscle along the posterior cricoid plate has been described.

Laryngeal trauma may result in fracture of the thyroid lamina or cricoid ring, dislocation of the arytenoid cartilage, or blunt injury to the recurrent laryngeal nerve, all of which can result in flaccid vocal folds. Arytenoid dislocation can also result from endotracheal intubation. The diagnosis of arytenoid dislocation is made by a combination of careful indirect endoscopic examination, CT scan of the larynx, and direct laryngoscopy with palpation.

Various central nervous system disorders may affect vocal fold movement. These disorders include amyotrophic lateral sclerosis, syringobulbia, poliomyelitis, multiple sclerosis, Shy-Drager syndrome, and Parkinson's disease. Bulbar and pseudobulbar palsy may also manifest with flaccid vocal folds and dysphonia. Neuromuscular diseases and diseases of muscle may result in flaccid dysphonia. Myasthenia gravis is a disease of neuromuscular junction resulting in progressive flaccid weakness with voice use. Bilateral vocal fold weakness, incomplete adduction, incomplete abduction, bowing, and loss of rapid diadochokinesis characterize this muscular disorder and should be evaluated by enzyme testing and tensilon test. Other muscular disorders such as muscular dystrophy, myositis, and dermatomyositis may affect muscles of the larynx and pharynx preferentially.

Idiopathic vocal cord paralysis is a term used for those cases of vocal cord paralysis in which a specific etiology cannot be identified. As such, idiopathic vocal cord paralysis is a diagnosis of exclusion and is to be made only after all other diagnostic tests have been completed. Idiopathic vocal cord paralysis is considered a mononeuropathy, possibly related to viral inflammation. Spontaneous recovery can be expected in most cases of idopathic vocal cord paralysis. If vocal cord function does not return after a reasonable period of time, usually 4 to 6 months, a diligent search for the etiology should continue.

CLINICAL EVALUATION

A systematic approach should be taken in the evaluation of the patient with an immobile vocal fold. A thorough history, physical, endoscopic, and flexible examination of the vocal fold movement, and stroboscopic examination of the vibratory pattern of vocal folds are essential. Radiographic evaluation of the neck and chest should be done if the etiology is not obvious. If indicated, operative endoscopy, laryngeal electromyography, and objective testing of vocal function should be performed to assess nerve integrity, determine prognosis for return of function, and assess treatment results.

History

A general medical history should be attained, including questions regarding prior intubation, heart disease, medications, and systemic medical illnesses, such as rheumatoid arthritis, diabetes mellitis, renal failure, and neurologic disorders. Inquiries should be made regarding antecedent viral illness. The history should also include a review of the onset and duration of the dysphonia.

The voice in vocal cord paralysis is typically characterized as breathy hypophonia with little fluctuation. Fluctuations in voice quality suggest paresis. Some patients with paresis do not complain of voice difficulties until the end of the day after heavy usage. The voice complaints of patients with vocal cord paralysis is typically one of a weak, soft voice which is difficult to project beyond a whisper. Patients complain of difficulty in being heard in a crowded environment such as a party or restaurant. Some patients complain of dyspnea, while others complain of the need to strain when speaking. These complaints correspond directly with the physiologic findings of high air leakage during phonation, shortened phonation time, and loss of high-frequency acoustic energy associated with the breathy voice.

Complaints of swallowing difficulties are common. Although many patients with vocal cord paralysis do not have overt aspiration, some notice that extra care is necessary to prevent aspiration of liquids. Patients with high vagal injury have pharyngeal paralysis and are much more debilitated by aspiration than those with unilateral vocal cord paralysis. Aspiration of liquids may occur early in the course of recurrent laryngeal nerve injury, however adequate compensation and improvement is seen over time in most patients. Patients with advanced age, cancer, weight loss, and prior prolonged intubation are at greater risk for aspiration than young neurologically intact patients with ability to compensate. Cough and dyspnea are also frequent complaints. The cough is ineffective and sometimes leaves the patient with residual excess phlegm and a sensation of the need to continually cough. Dyspnea on exertion may be present in patients with unilateral paralysis but is much more severe in those with bilateral nerve injuries.

When possible, the level of the injury or lesion should be localized, as it has prognostic and therapeutic implications. When the lesion is high in the jugular foramen or at the exit of the Xth nerve from the base of skull, branches to the pharynx, superior laryngeal nerve and the recurrent laryngeal nerve will be affected. Patients with this type of lesion often have severe aspiration, breathy dysphonia, and levator palatine weakness. Isolated injury to the external (motor) branch of the superior laryngeal nerve, usually caused by trauma or iatrogenic injury, results in a reduction in the pitch range of the voice, but aspiration and dysarthria are rare. When the recurrent laryngeal nerve is affected, the voice will be breathy and hoarse. Vocal fold position helps in the differential diagnosis but is by no means diagnostic. In differentiating a flaccid lower motor neuron lesion from an upper motor neuron injury, it is important to assess the quality of the voice and look for evidence of other multisystem involvement.[1] Patients with supranuclear lesions, such as Parkinson's disease, often present with hypophonia and difficulty in producing voicing after voiceless consonants. Similarly, dysarthria and poor breath support are overt comorbid processes in the voice production of patients with bulbar and pseudobulbar lesions. Swallowing function is often affected more than voice in patients with bulbar lesions. This is in contrast to the peripheral nerve palsies which affect voice but in general spare articulation and swallowing. Table 19-1 lists some common central nervous disorders and their findings.

Physical examination

A thorough head and neck examination is essential. This should include assessment of the cranial nerves II to XII, examination of the neck and thyroid landmarks, and maneuvers designed to assess laryngeal function. The neck and

TABLE 19-1
Central and neuromuscular system diseases affecting vocal fold movement

Disorder	Features	Voice characteristic
Parkinson's disease	Fading with tremor Onset of voice difficult Rapid glottal stops difficult	Reduced intensity and "range"
Shy-Drager syndrome	Slow dysarthric speech Hypotension, apnea, autonomic symptoms, bilateral abductor paralysis	Slow speech, reduced intensity, unintelligible
Amyotrophic lateral sclerosis	Spastic and flaccid picture Asymmetric movement of vocal folds Velopharyngeal insufficiency	Hoarseness or harsh wet voice Hypernasal with poor articulation
Multiple sclerosis	Fluctuation in symptoms Intermittent spasticity or flaccidity Other sensory or motor involvement	Variation on rate of speech, disrupted spastic voice, tremor
Upper motor neuron atrophy	Swallow affected, muscle wasting, aspiration, stridor	Voice weak, dysarthric breathy
Myasthenia gravis	Fatigue of voice with use small muscle affected, i.e., eye	Hypophonia, breathy, voice fluctuations

larynx should be carefully palpated to evaluate cricothyroid contraction with phonation, assess laryngeal elevation with each swallow, assess voice improvement with various head positions and neck turning, and determine the degree of voice improvement with medial compression testing. Medial compression testing has been advocated to predict whether medialization laryngoplasty will result in a better voice. Voice improvement with neck turning and position may indicate that such patients will improve with speech therapy. Assessment of vocal function with the help of a speech language pathologist may reveal a particular pitch range that gives the patient an optional voice. Such "better" voice may then be used by the patient with appropriate training by the speech language pathologist.

Endoscopy is essential for visual documentation of vocal fold movement. Multiple techniques are available to perform such endoscopy. Mirror examination is simple and easy but often fails to detect fine details which are better revealed by fiberoptic examination with or without video. Rigid indirect telescopic examination of the vocal folds affords an excellent view of the vocal folds but has poor capability to assess motion of the vocal cord apparatus in the natural state. Therefore, paresis and compensatory changes of the vocal tract mechanism is often not appreciated by rigid endoscopic examination of the vocal folds. The preferred method is to use the rigid telescope to assess lesion and anatomy, while flexible endoscopy is used to assess motion and vocal function. Rigid endoscopic examination should assess the normal capability of the vocal folds to change length with increasing pitch and assess the vocal folds for ulcerations and structural abnormalities which are easily missed by the flexible fiberoptic examination. Flexible examination of the larynx is done with a standard set of vocal maneuvers which tests voice and other vegetative functions of the larynx. Specifically, the larynx is examined during sustained vowel phonation as well as during running speech, readings of a rainbow passage, whistle, cough, and swallow. Flexible laryngoscopy is also used to assess palatal function and the nasopharyngeal port if such documentation is necessary or desirable. The vocal fold position in unilateral vocal cord paralysis can be quite variable. The arytenoid is often rolled forward and the vocal process may be anywhere in the paramedian to abducted position. With phonation, the contralateral innervated vocal cords may overcompensate and cross the midline. Vocal fold length comparisons show the denervated vocal cord to be shorter than the innervated side during inspiration. With phonation, the innervated side will shorten and adduct to match the shortened denervated cord. If there is excessive contraction by the innervated side, the paralyzed side will appear longer than the innervated side during phonation and shorter during inspiration. Such compensatory gestures of the larynx and pharynx are common in patients as they try to produce better phonation. These findings on fiberoptic laryngoscopy may show anterior posterior supraglottic squeezing, ventricular phonation, and pharyngeal constriction with laryngeal elevation. Abnormal pitch elevation with habitual phonation in falsetto is a common finding in many patients with vocal cord paralysis.

Flexible video laryngoscopy is used to assess: (1) the closure of the glottis, (2) extent of pharyngeal compensation, (3) false cord medialization, and (4) extent of spontaneous movements. During the flexible video examination, estimates of the phonation time, maximum phonation decibel output, and fundamental frequency may be made. With modern endoscopy equipment, estimates of statistics such as decibel and frequency output may be directly displayed on screen.

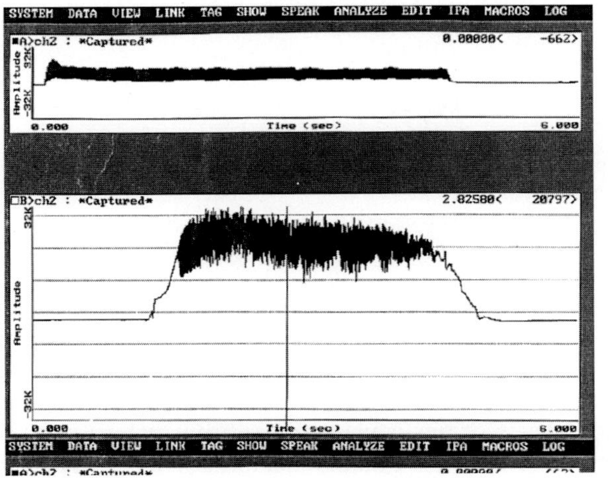

FIG 19-1
Air flow signal of normal phonation (top) contrasted with vocal cord paralysis (bottom). There is shorter phonation time, with greater unmodulated flow in the paralysis case.

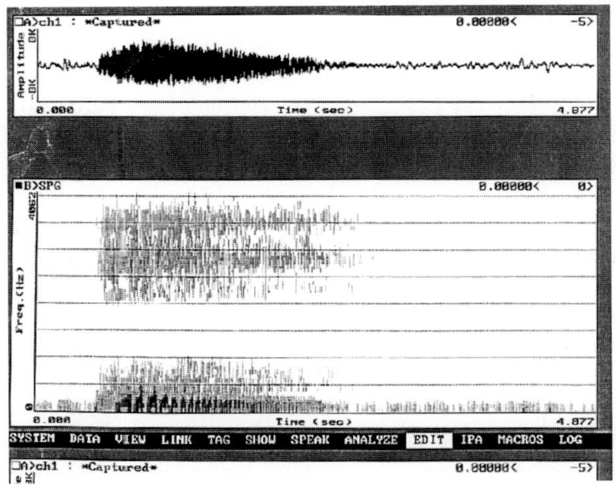

FIG 19-2
Acoustic signal (top) and spectrum (bottom) of breathy phonation in vocal cord paralysis. Note the short phonation time, the small amplitude of the acoustic signal, and the tapering of the acoustic signal over time. On the spectrum, there is lack of high frequency energy and well-defined formant energy.

Objective testing

A variety of objective tests can be used to assess the breathy voice quality, glottic configuration, vibratory characteristics of the vocal folds, and degree of muscle denervation. These objective tests are important for both assessment and documentation.

1. *Laryngeal function studies.* Breathy voice quality in vocal cord paralysis is associated with reduced phonation time, need for frequent inhalations during conversational speech, and increased mean air flow rates (Fig. 19-1).[21] Airflow measures show increase in the mean flow rates and an increase in glottal leakage flows. Measures of the efficiency of airflow conversion shows reduction in the AC/DC flow ratio. Analysis of the frequency component of airflow signal shows increase in the turbulent energy and a decrease in the harmonic energy. With surgical rehabilitation, phonation time, mean flow rates, and other aerodynamic factors revert toward a more normal value.
2. *Acoustic measures.* These studies show several common features. Besides the reduction in phonation time, there is reduction in the dynamic range both in loudness and frequency.[7] Spectrogram analysis shows loss of high-frequency energy and loss of higher formant peaks on the spectrogram. Fig. 19-2 demonstrates these changes. Increase in the signal to noise ratio, increase in the aperiodicity, jitter, and shimmer are other features common to the voice of patients with vocal cord paralysis.
3. *Glottography.* Electroglottography has only limited clinical application at this time in the diagnosis of vocal fold paralysis, although it has research applications in understanding vibratory functions of the vocal fold. In general, there is a short contact period, prolonged open period, and a reduced rate of vocal fold opening and closing velocity. Photoglottography complements the electroglottography finding by providing some information on the pattern of vocal fold function during the opening period.[6] Unfortunately, at this time neither of these tests can be used to determine the etiology.
4. *Videostroboscopy.* By direct inspection of vibratory behavior of the vocal folds using videostroboscopy, dennervation pattern and early reinnervation can be differentiated. Glottal configuration during phonation can also be appreciated better with stroboscopy. Typical patterns of vocal fold closure include mid cord gap, posterior gap, and level differences between the vocal folds. The stroboscopic examination often shows incomplete closure, prolonged open phase, amplitude reduction, asymmetry, and loss of mucosal wave. Phase differences between vibration of the vocal folds will show the innervated vocal fold to open earlier than the denervated vocal fold. The denervated vocal fold often show a "flag in the breeze" floppy appearance. With early reinnervation, there is reversal of many of these findings before gross movement restoration. This is correlated with improved voice.
5. *Electromyography (EMG).* Assessment of the innervation status of the intrinsic laryngeal muscles with EMG is important for both diagnosis and determination of prognosis.[15,17] Neuropathic disorders and myopathic disorders are differentiated by monopolar needle EMG examination of the intrinsic laryngeal muscles as well as limb muscles. Diagnosis of vocal cord paralysis versusankylosis can be differentiated using electromyography. The differentiation of vagal paralysis, superior laryngeal paralysis, and recurrent nerve paralysis can also be differentiated by testing the thyroarytenoid and the cricothyroid muscles sequentially. Electrical patterns are analyzed for spontaneous and evoked activity. The presence of polyphasic giant potentials indicates denervation and

TABLE 19-2
Substances used for vocal cord injection

Substance	Duration of medialization	Indications	Contraindications
Teflon	Permanent	Permanent paralysis	Mobile vocal cords
Gelfoam	4 to 8 weeks	Temporary paralysis	None
Collagen	Some resorption over the first 3 months, stablizes over a year	Temporary or permanent paralysis	Hypersensitivity to collagen
Fat	Variable from 2 months to permanent	Temporary or permanent paralysis	None

subsequent reinnervation. Electrical silence and spontaneous discharge of low-voltage fibrillation potentials are evidence of dennervation with poor reinnervation. Recruitment patterns during voluntary activity such as phonation and cough give an estimate of the degree of voluntary activity in the particular muscle of interest. In general a three- to five-fold difference between maximal recruitment pattern and minimal voluntary recruitment activity can be expected in normal muscles.

Diagnostic imaging

CT scan with constrast from the base of the skull to the chest, which includes the jugular foramen, thyroid gland, root of the neck, and the carina, should be attained to investigate the cause of unexplained vocal fold paralysis. When it is necessary to assess the level differences between the vocal folds and endoscopic evaluation is not possible, a fluoroscopic examination in the AP plane or tomography of the larynx in the AP plane during phonation can offer additional information. MRI of the brain and neck structures are indicated in selected patients as indicated by history and physical examination. In cases of laryngeal trauma, including intubation injury, thin-cut CT scan of the larynx (2mm cuts) should be obtained to search for evidence of arytenoid dislocation and/or laryngeal fracture.

Operative laryngoscopy

Occasionally the etiology of vocal fold immobility is not clear even after office examination and radiographic investigation. In such patients operative laryngoscopy may be warranted. Operative laryngoscopy is done to rule out laryngeal pathology and to evaluate esophageal pathology which may mimic vocal cord paralysis. In addition, examination of the posterior cricoid plate, palpation of arytenoid motion, and examination of the integrity of the cricoarytenoid joint are best done under operative conditions.[20]

MANAGEMENT

The management options includes observation, speech therapy, and surgical intervention. The choice of therapy in the management of unilateral vocal cord paralysis is determined by the degree of functional deficit, the etiology, and the prognosis for recovery. It is important in the management of vocal cord paralysis to have an appreciation of the wide variety of functional deficits with which patients may present. A functional rating should be noted on the initial presentation and followed. Many patients with unilateral VCP will have improvement of the voice over time as the contralateral vocal cord compensates and, therefore, do not require surgical intervention. Most of the improvement is noted over the first 3 to 6 months. Typically, the voice stabilizes but remains weak. Occasionally, the voice will become more diplophonic and hoarse. This has been attributed to vocal fold atrophy and the effect of asymmetric mass. The voice fluctuates with use and is typically better early in the day before heavy use. Speech therapy is important to educate the patient regarding vocal mechanisms that improve voice quality as well as prevent the development of potentially harmful vocal habits from compensatory efforts. Speech therapy can help with breath control and management. In helping the patients to explore areas of voice which can be produced with the greatest ease, functional improvement can be obtained without surgery. Reduction of hyperkinetic and hyperadductive compensatory gestures before and after surgery can help to improve the surgical result. Speech therapy cannot be used to rehabilitate the aphonic patient. It cannot be used to reduce breathy voice to a significant extent and it cannot be expected to correct level differences due to vocal fold atrophy. By using a variety of speech therapy techniques such as vocal range exercises, hum, aspirate voice, trill, valsalva, and other voice awareness programs, the speech therapy is usually complete after 8 weeks. Speech therapy is used together with surgical treatment. In many patients, sufficient improvements may be obtained to avoid surgery.

In considering treatment options for the patient with vocal cord paralysis, it is important to consider the needs of the patient, the natural course of the disease, and the expected result from each type of therapy. The indications for surgical intervention are aspiration, disabling breathy hypophonia, and inability to produce an effective cough.

The options for surgical intervention are medialization and reinnervation. Medialization can be accomplished through vocal cord injection, medialization laryngoplasty (thyroplasty), or arytenoid adduction. Substances that are currently used for vocal cord injection are Teflon, gelfoam,

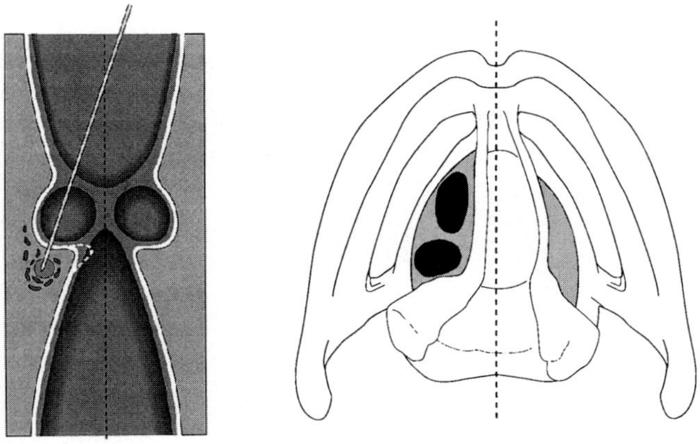

FIG 19-3
Technique of vocal cord injection.

collagen, and autologous fat.* The surgical technique, indications, and contraindications for each of these substances are listed in Table 19-2. The injection is accomplished through direct laryngoscopy by injecting the substance using a Bruning syringe. Except for collagen, the substance should be injected into the thyroarytenoid muscle. The recommended sites of injection are shown in Fig. 19-3. Conversely, collagen should be injected just lateral to the free edge of the vocal cord rather than into the thyroarytenoid muscle.[5] When collagen is injected into muscle, the effects last several months for only, however, injecting it into the Reinke space results in maintenance of the medialization for a longer period of time (up to a year). Potential complications of vocal cord injection include failure to achieve the desired voice result, airway obstruction, and Teflon granuloma. Failure to achieve a good voice may be due to any of the following reasons: overinjection, underinjection, decreased vibration of the vocal cord due to mass effect, and failure to close the posterior glottic chink. Airway obstruction is rare and usually results from injetion into the subglottic space.

Medialization laryngoplasty (ML) and arytenoid adduction (AA) are external approaches for medialization of vocal cords. ML is accomplished by excising a rectangular window of cartilage from the thyroid lamina at the level of the true vocal cords and placing an alloplastic implant to push the vocal fold medially (Fig. 19-4). The size of the window varies from 3 mm to 6 mm × 10 mm to 13 mm. The superior border of the window is determined by a horizontal line drawn from the midpoint of the thyroid notch and the inferior border and paralleling the inferior border. The anterior border of the window is placed approximately 6 mm to 8 mm from the midline to avoid injury to the anterior commissure. A 4 mm to 5 mm strut of cartilage is usually left inferiorly. Silastic is the most commonly used substance for ML, though the use of other preshaped implants has also been re-

*References 5, 9, 12, 14, 16.

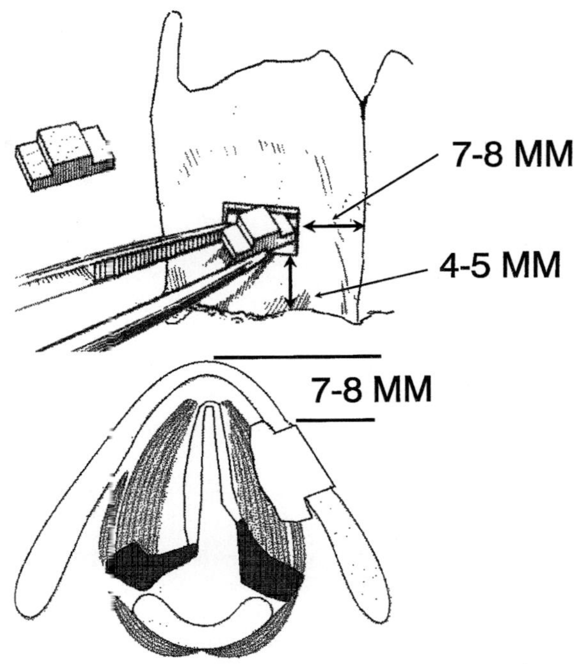

FIG 19-4
Technique of medialization laryngoplasty (thyroplasty).

ported recently.* The best results with ML are obtained when the glottic gap is along the mid portion of the cord. It is difficult to correct a large posterior gap or a vocal cord that lies at a lower level with ML. Complications of ML include implant extrusion, airway obstruction, wound infection and fistula formation.[8,11,18] Implant extrusion usually occurs intralaryngeally through the ventricle. This can be avoided by not placing the implant too anteriorly where it can come in close proximity to the ventricle.

To perform AA, the posterior border of the thyroid lamina is exposed and the cricothyroid joint is separated. The muscular process of the arytenoid cartilage is identified and a 3-0 nylon suture is placed through it. Using a straight needle, the suture is then passed through the thyroid lamina near its anterior inferior border and tied. This rotates the vocal process medially toward the midline to medialize the vocal cord (Fig. 19-5). Since the procedure is performed under local anesthesia with intravenous sedation, the patient can be asked to phonate to confirm good medialization when the suture is tied. AA is ideal for correction of a glottic gap involving the posterior and mid-cord. ML may need to be performed in conjunction with AA to correct very large gaps. Complications of AA include slipped-suture, airway obstruction, wound infection, and fistula formation.[8] One case of carotid artery injury has been reported

*References 2, 8, 10, 11, 13, 18

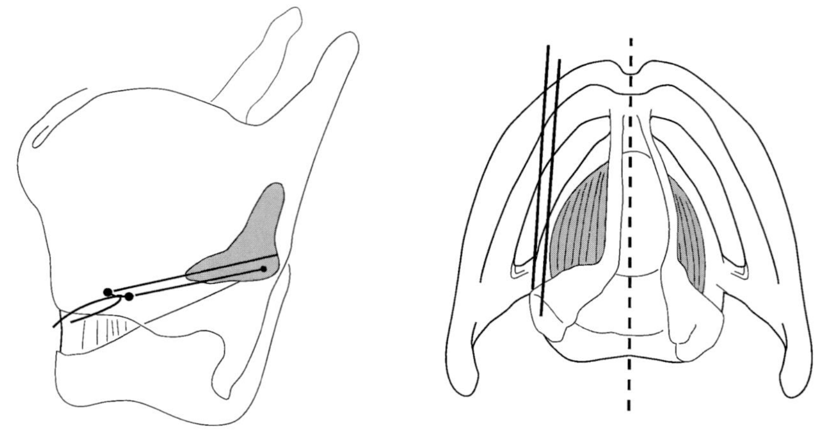

FIG 19-5
Technique of arytenoid adduction.

with this procedure that was performed in an irradiated patient.

Various reinnervation procedures have be advocated for rehabilitation of the paralyzed larynx.[3,19] The ultimate goal of reinnervation is to restore purposeful movement, adduction during phonation or swallowing, and abduction with inspiration. However, purposeful movement does not always occur even if the laryngeal muscles are successfully reinnervated. The most likely reason for failure to restore purposeful movement is nonselective reinnervation of the adductor and abductor muscles, resulting in cancellation of the vectors of pull on the arytenoid cartilage—a phenomenom termed "laryngeal synkinesis."[4] Nevertheless, even if purposeful movement is not restored, muscle bulk and normal joint position can be maintained with reinnervation. For unilateral paralysis, reanastomosis of the RLN, selective reanastomosis of the abductor and adductor branches of the RLN, ansaomohyoid neuromuscular pedicle implantation onto the thyroarytenoid muscle, and ansa cervicalis-RLN anastomosis have been performed in human subjects with variable success.

The decision regarding when to surgically intervene depends on the degree of functional deficit, etiology of the paralysis, and prognosis for recovery. It is important to remember that the resting position of a paralyzed vocal cord can change with time depending on the degree of muscle atrophy and the ultimate resultant vector of muscle pull on the arytenoid cartilage. Atrophy of the TA muscle may result in progressive bowing of the vocal cord. Conversely, should spontaneous reinnervation occur, the vocal fold may shift back toward the midline even if movement is not restored. With early surgical intervention the vocal fold may either be overmedialized or undermedialized in a year. Therefore, if the patient does not have a significant functional deficit, surgical intervention for voice improvement should be postponed for at least 6 months even if the paralysis is permanent. Certainly, early surgical intervention is indicated when severe functional disability exists, such as aspiration, ineffective cough, disabling breathy hypophonia, as evidenced by phonation time of less than 5 seconds, high mean flow rates exceeding 250 cc/sec, or reduced maximal decibel output (<75 dB). Surgical therapy at 6 months to 9 months after injury is indicated in patients who demonstrate evidence of denervation or little activity on EMG and have had a poor response to a reasonable trial of speech therapy.

Selection of the appropriate procedure is based on prognosis for recovery and glottic configuration. Patients in whom the paralysis resulted from transection of the vagus or RLN are treated with definitive, permanent procedures, such as AA, ML, Teflon injection, or ansa-RLN reinnervation. ML and Teflon injection are best for mid cord paralysis, as correction of posterior gap is difficult with these procedures. A large posterior gap is best treated with AA. Some surgeons perform ML first, assess the quality of the voice intraoperatively and proceed with AA if necessary. Others perform AA first if there is a large posterior gap and then proceed with ML if there is residual mid-cord gap. Either approach is reasonable. Vagal paralysis usually results in a posterior gap as well as different cord levels and, therefore, is generally best treated with AA. In most cases of vagal paralysis, ML needs to be performed in conjuction with AA to maintain adequate medialization of the mid-cord. If functional recovery is expected and the patient requires medialization for functional problems, injection of Gelfoam, collagen, or fat or performing a potentially reversible procedure such as ML are indicated. The role of autologous fat injection is unclear at this time since the duration of medialization is quite variable. It appears that it can be used at least for temporary paralysis. It can also be attempted in cases of permanent paralysis, however, resorption is likely to occur. Further studies are needed to investigate various techniques of harvesting and processing to improve the survival of the fat.

Though these static medialization procedures offer a significant improvement in the intensity of the voice, the patients should be warned that the voice probably will not be normal. Static procedures may not always restore symmetrical mucosal wave. Early postoperative voice quality is usually diplophonic, harsh, high pitched, and gravelly. It is frequently strained, especially in patients who have had longstanding paralysis. It is likely that most of these patients have developed mechanisms to compensate for the breathy hypophonia. It is well recognized that the paralyzed vocal fold is often shortened, probably due to the scar contracture, and the normal vocal fold will shorten and hyperadduct to attain approximation with the paralyzed vocal fold. Such compensatory mechanisms persist following medialization. Therefore, speech therapy is an essential component in the management of vocal cord paralysis, both preoperatively and postoperatively.

REFERENCES

1. Aronson AE: *Clinical Voice Disorders*. Organic Voice Disorders: Neurologic Disease, Chap 5. New York, 1985, Thiem Medical Publishers.
2. Cummings CW, Purcell LL, Flint PW: Hydroxylapatite laryngeal implants for medialization. preliminary report. *Ann Otol Rhinol* 102:893-851, 1993.
3. Crumley RL: Update: Ansa cervicalis to recurrent laryngeal nerve anastomosis for unilateral laryngeal paralysis. *Laryngoscope* 101:384-387, 1994.
4. Crumley RL: Laryngeal synkinesis: it's significance to the laryngologist. *Ann Otol Rhinol Laryngol:* 98:87-92, 1989.
5. Ford CN, Bless DM: Clinical experience with injectable collagen for vocal fold augmentation. *Laryngoscope* 96:863-869, 1986.
6. Hanson DG, Garratt BR, Karin RR, Berke GS: Glottographic measures of vocal fold vibration: an examination of laryngeal paralysis. *Laryngoscope* 98:541-549, 1988.
7. Hirano et al: Acoustic analysis of pathological voice. *Acta Otolaryngol* (Stockh) 105:432-438, 1988.
8. Kaufman JA, Isaacson G: Laryngoplastic phonosurgery. *Otolaryngol Clin N Am* 24:1151-1177, 1991.
9. Lewy RB: Teflon injection of the vocal cords: complications, errors, and precautions. *Ann Otol Rhinol Laryngol* 92:473-474, 1983.
10. Maves MD McCabe BF, Gray S: Phonosurgery: Indications and pitfalls. *Ann Otol Laryngol* 98:577-580, 1989.
11. Netterville JL, Stone RE, Lken ES, et al: Silastic medialization and arytenoid adduction: The Vanderbilt experience. A Review of 116 Phonosurgical Procedures. *Ann Otol Rhinol Laryngol* 102:413-424, 1993.
12. Mikaelian DO, Lowry LD, Sataloff RT: Lipoinjection for unilateral vocal fold paralysis. *Laryngoscope* 102:495-500, 1991.
13. Montgomery WW, Blangrund SM, Varvares MA: Thyroplasty: a new approach. *Ann Otol Rhinol Laryngol* 102:571-579, 1993.
14. Sadek SAA, Nassar WY, Tobias MA: Teflon injection of the vocal cords under general anesthesia. *J Laryngol Otol* 101:695-705, 1987.
15. Schaefer SD: Laryngeal electromyography. *Otolaryngol Clin of North Am* 24:1053-1057, 1991.
16. Schramm VL, May M, Lavorato AS: Gelfoam paste injection for the vocal cord paralysis: temporary rehabilitation of glottic incompetence. *Laryngoscope* 88:1268-1273, 1978.
17. Simpson DM, Sternman D, Graves WJ, Sanders I: Vocal cord paralysis: clinical and electrophysiologic features. *Muscle and Nerve* 16:952-957, 1993.
18. Tucker HM, Wanamaker J, Trott M, Hicks D. Complications of laryngeal framework surgery. *Laryngoscope* 103:525-528, 1993.
19. Tucker HM: Reinnervation of the unilateral paralyzed larynx. *Ann Otol Rhinol Laryngol* 86:789-790, 1977.
20. Tucker H: Vocal cord paralysis: etiology and management. *Laryngoscope* 90:585-590, 1980.
21. Woo P, Colton R, Brewer D, Casper J: Functional staging for vocal cord paralysis. *Otolaryngol Head Neck Surg* 105:440-448, 1991.

20

Clinical Voice Evaluation: A Practical Approach

Gayle E. Woodson, M.D., F.A.C.S., F.R.C.S.(C) and Thomas Murry, Ph.D.

A variety of methods is currently available for assessing vocal function, and technical advances are steadily continuing. The incorporation of this technology into a clinical practice requires knowledge of the physiology of normal and disordered phonation, comprehension of exactly what the equipment is measuring, and understanding how to apply measurements in the management of voice disorders. Patients who present with vocal problems vary greatly in symptoms and underlying pathophysiology. Objective voice measures are useful only if the specific parameters measured are relevant to problems of the individual patient.

Acquisition of equipment for a voice clinic should be based on the specific requirements of the practice, taking into account the clinical problems of the patient population and the objective measures which will enhance the management of those patients. Much more important than the equipment is the ability of the practitioners to interpret the information derived from using the instrumentation and to apply it appropriately in planning management.

In general, the *diagnosis* of a vocal problem is made on the basis of a history and physical examination. Listening to the patient and performing office endoscopy are integral components of this examination. Objective vocal function tests primarily serve to *quantify* the degree of vocal impairment and to *document* the response to treatment. There is *no standard battery of tests* analogous to audiometry. Relevant parameters can be chosen which are sensitive to the patient's presenting symptoms and which provide information about underlying pathophysiology. These measures can be compared with reported norms to establish functional status. The greatest utility is in documenting changes over time and with treatment for the individual patient

Modes of assessment can be grouped into the following categories:

Perceptual: Listening to and judging the voice
Visual: Observing laryngeal morphology and movement
Acoustic: Analyzing physical properties of sound
Aerodynamic: Measuring air pressure and flow
Glottographic: Electronic measures of vocal fold vibration

This chapter will address current technology for voice evaluation, beginning with a brief review of relevant vocal physiology. As previously mentioned, diagnosis is usually achieved by perceptual and visual means. Acoustic measures identify and quantify physical properties of the voice, but they do not distinguish well between causes of voice disorders. Aerodynamic measures provide objective information on pathophysiology and hence give more insight into etiology. Glottography is still relatively undeveloped as a clinical tool but can provide information about vocal fold movement and contact which is complementary to the other measures.

VOICE PHYSIOLOGY

A firm grasp of vocal physiology is crucial to the interpretation and application of data from a voice laboratory. One must understand how normal voice is produced in order to comprehend what is measured and why, as well as to utilize abnormal data in planning treatment.

Components of speech

The human voice which we hear during speech or singing is not equivalent to the sound which is produced at the level of the glottis. That sound is modified significantly by the resonance of structures in the vocal tract. To understand the significance of resonance, consider that the same sound source (lips and mouthpiece) generates the sound of the trumpet, french horn, and tuba. The characteristic quality and pitch of each of these instruments is determined by the resonant properties of the body of the instrument.

One implication of this is that when we analyze the sound of the voice, we do not obtain direct information

Components of Speech

Phonation
Passive vibration of the vocal folds, powered by exhaled air
Resonance
Alteration by vocal tract of the spectral composition of the voice by selective enhancement or damping of component frequencies
Articulation: The shaping of sounds into words

Voice Pathophysiology

Expired airflow
The voice may be weak due to inadequate lung power (low flow, low pressure)
Vocal fold approximation
Too tight—strained or strangled voice (high pressure, low flow)
Too loose—breathy, weak voice (low pressure, high flow)
Normal vibratory property of the vocal fold
Too stiff or stuck to underlying muscle—increased effort and hoarseness (high pressure, variable flow)
Control of vocal fold length and tension
No variability—monotonous voice
Spasmodic motion—pitch breaks, voice breaks
Tremor—wobbly voice

about what is happening at the level of the glottis. Acoustic analysis of the voice provides information about the integrated function of the vocal tract as a whole. Another implication is that hoarseness is not always the result of glottal pathology but occasionaly stems from altered resonance.

Articulation adds another level of complexity to speech production. The formation of vowels and consonants during connected speech requires rapid laryngeal adjustments, which can overly tax a marginal vocal apparatus. Patients who can produce a reasonably normal isolated vowel sound may not be able to sustain that vocal quality during conversational speech. Examples of this would include patients with mild spasmodic dysphonia or with marginally compensated vocal fold paralysis. In cases such as these, adequate characterization of the functional deficit requires analysis of samples from connected speech. It is also common for patients with dysarthria to refer to the problem as hoarseness, even when the phonatory mechanism is normal (box above).

Requirements for phonation

Sound is produced by the larynx when appropriate conditions are met to induce oscillations in the laryngeal mucosa. The physical requirements for normal phonation include breath support, approximated vocal folds normal vibratory properties of the mucosa, and control of vocal fold length and tension (box above right).

Phonation cannot occur without exhaled air to set the vocal folds in oscillation. Inadequate airflow results in a weak voice. Normal vital capacity and tidal volume are in excess of requirements for casual conversation and so respiratory disorders do not present as speech problems. In problems such as emphysema or asthma, pulmonary function must be significantly impaired before everyday speaking is affected, usually manifested by low volume and inability to complete normal phrases in one breath. More commonly, breath support in speech is compromised by faulty technique.

Vocal folds must be apposed very precisely to permit oscillation. If they are pressed together, excessive pressure is required to induce vibration. The patient subjectively notes increased effort in speaking and frequently the voice fatigues easily. The voice sounds strained or strangled, and aerodynamic measures will demonstrate low airflow and high subglottic pressure.

Conversely, if the glottis is too loose, a larger flow of air will be required to induce oscillation. The patient feels short of breath during speaking and is not able to say many words on a single breath. The voice will be weak and often breathy. If the glottal gap is significant, the patient can only whisper. Aerodynamically, pressure is low and flow is increased.

Stroboscopy and high-speed photography both demonstrate that the mucosa on the edge of the normal vocal fold undulates through an impressive range of motion during phonation. The mucosa has a amplitude of vibration much greater than that of the underlying muscle, because the two components are separated by a specialized layer of connective tissue, with stratified concentrations of elastin and collagen. The capacity of the vocal fold mucosa to vibrate may be impeded by any scarring to the underlying muscle or by edema in the submucosal space which tenses the mucosa. Mass lesions or hyperplasia of the epithelium also impair vibration.

The normal voice is not monotonous. Variations in pitch and intensity add dimensions to spoken communications. Such inflection requires, among other things, adjustments in the length and tension of the vocal folds. Instability in this control system, such as tremor or spasmodic movements, can be manifest by a "wobbly" voice, with pitch breaks or oscillation.

Listening to the patient

Listening to the patient is the first step in voice evaluation. It is often possible to make a working diagnosis within minutes, based on the sound of the voice and the patients description of the problem. However, it is *very* important

Symptoms Perceived as Hoarseness

- Raspy voice
- Volume Loss
- Breathiness
- Abnormal pitch
- Vocal fatigue
- Pain on speaking
- Increased effort
- Glottic tightness
- Unstable pitch
- Pitch breaks
- Resonance changes
- Tremor
- Dysarthria

to establish the patient's specific complaint rather than to focus on what sounds most abnormal at first listening. For example, a patient with abnormal pitch may not be presenting because of the deep voice but with some other problem, such as vocal fatigue or low volume. Many different problems may be perceived by the patient as hoarseness. The pathophysiology can usually be deduced on the basis of the specific difficulties. The patient should be questioned carefully to determine which of the following specific problems have been encountered.

PERCEPTUAL ANALYSIS

Perceptual voice assessment is an essential component in the evaluation of voice disorders. Patients come to the doctor because they *perceive* hoarseness, and a patient who is improved according to laboratory tests but who still sounds just as hoarse is not really improved (box above). However, a major limitation of perceptual analysis is that it is subjective. It is difficult to make comparisons between centers, or even between patients. Also, perceptual analysis does not provide information about what the patient is feeling during speech. Increased effort, even if the voice sounds normal, will be perceived by the patient as hoarseness, and will in fact often lead to easy vocal fatigue.

Scale

The vocal qualities commonly referred to in most systems of perceptual analysis include: Pitch, Loudness, and Quality. Quantification of perception requires a rating scales. The Voice Committtee of the Japan Society of Logopedics and Phoniatrics has proposed the GRABAS Scale (Table 20-1), rating each parameter on a 4 point scale.

TABLE 20-1
GRABAS scale

G, Overall grade of hoarseness	0 = Normal
R, Rough	1 = Mild
B, Breathy	2 = Moderate
A, Asthenic	3 = Severe
S, Strained	

VIDEOENDOSCOPY

The practice of laryngology has been tremendoulsy advanced by developments in optics and low light level cameras. This has dramatically increased the ability to evaluate the anatomy and physiology of the vocal mechanism. Not only can a magnified and brighter view be obtained, but the image can be recorded or photographed. This enhances diagnositic capability because the record can be reviewed repeatedly and viewed by consultants. An objective record is also provided for monitoring the progress of the disorder or the patient's response to therapy. Therefore the most crucial acquisition of any voice clinic is an effective system for videolaryngoscopy.

Telescopic laryngoscopy

Transoral examination by a rigid rod with a quartz lens system provides a magnified and clear view. Most commonly, a 70° or 90° viewing angle is used to examine the larynx. This is the best technique for demonstrating laryngeal morphology and documenting even minute laryngeal lesions.

Use of a telescope has limitations, particularly in some patients. The mouth must be opened widely with the head extended, and strong traction must be applied to the tongue. Thus, the larynx cannot be viewed during speech tasks or swallowing. Also, hypopharyngeal anatomy is somewhat distorted by this tongue position. The examination is uncomfortable, and the vast majority of patients require topical anesthesia to prevent gagging and choking. In many patients, the examination is not anatomically feasible because of such problems as a large tongue, overhanging epiglottis, long soft palate, or redundant pharyngeal walls.

Fiberoptic laryngoscopy

Flexible laryngoscopy via the nose is possible in nearly all patients. With topical nasal anesthesia, there is minimal discomfort. The endoscope does not interfere with laryngeal and pharyngeal motion, thus the larynx can be viewed during a variety of activities, such as quiet breathing, speech, cough, and valsalva. Pathologic movement, such as spasm or tremor, can be identified easily. In nonorganic voice disorders, maladaptive postures and compensatory hyperfunction during speech are evident. This is important not only for diagnosis but also for planning voice therapy. Flexible endoscopy has also been used in biofeedback therapy.

A limitation of flexible laryngoscopy is that the image is not as bright and clear as that obtained with a telescope. The image is small and grainy, and resolution is not sufficient to detect fine detail. Stroboscopy can be performed with a flexible scope, but, because the light level is very low, documentation requires a very sensitive camera.

Stroboscopy

This instrument senses the fundamental frequency of the voice and drives a flashing light at or near the fundamental frequency of the voice, to *simulate* either a slow motion view of vocal fold vibration, or an image in one phase of the vibratory cycle. The slow motion mode permits assessment of the mucosal wave, which may be impaired by scarring, edema, and/or subtle defects in the mucosa. Stroboscopy also demonstrates the pattern of glottic closure and indicates the probable underlying mechanism for faulty closure. For example, incomplete or brief glottal closure may result from vocalis muscle atrophy, posterior laryngeal edema, or faulty vocal technique. Each of these has a characteristic endoscopic appearance.

Stroboscopy is not, however, the *sine qua non* of vocal assessment. It often makes little contribution to patient management, because observation with continuous light clearly establishes the diagnosis. Stroboscopy cannot be used when voice is too unstable to drive the strobe generator, as in many cases of laryngeal paralysis or vocal fold scarring, or in spasmodic dysphonia.

The chief indication for stroboscopy is in searching for an explanation of why a glottis, which appears grossly normal under continuous light, is incapable of producing a normal sound. Subtle edema may restrict the motion of the mucosa. Submucosal cysts have a characteristic appearance on stroboscopy, analogous to a beach ball under a fluttering beach towel. The submucosal mass can be discerned because the overlying tissue does not participate in undulation during the mucosal wave. Scarring may not distort the vocal fold at rest, but, by tethering between the free edge of the mucosa and the underlying muscle or ligament, it will become manifest as an adynamic segment of the mucosal wave during stroboscopy.

Stroboscopy can also be helpful in determining whether a vocal fold lesion is potentially invasive. A small superficial lesion will appear to ride on the mucosal wave. However, an epithelial lesion which is bulky or which invades submucosal tissue will dampen or abolish the wave.

Although vocal nodules are often quite easy to diagnose, stroboscopy can be very helpful in patient management. Nodule diathesis, or subtle swelling of the nodule area, may be apparent only during stroboscopy. Detection of early or incipiently recurring nodules can direct voice therapy to avert progression of the dysphonia. Some nodules appear to be on the superior surface of the vocal fold and may not appear to contact during normal phonation. In such cases, stroboscopy may reveal contact of the nodule areas during specific speaking and singing modes, such as falsetto or shouting. These obervations are very helpful in directing therapy.

Requirements for Recording

High-quality tape recorder and microphone
Quiet or soundproof room
Constant mouth to microphone distance
Standard protocol, including a variety of tasks.
- *Sample*
  - Name and date
  - Conversational speech
  - Reading or monologue
  - Counting
  - Sustained phonation

Because of the high cost of stroboscopy and the limits to its indications, it is not essential to the general otolaryngologist. However, it is not possible provide comprehensive voice care without access to the information provided by stroboscopy.

High-speed video

This technology is not yet commercially available for routine clinical use. A rapid sequence of images, in the range of 2000 per second, provides detail similar to that observed by the more expensive and labor intensive technique of high-speed motion pictures. One system, developed in Japan, uses a chip in a 35-mm camera body to digitally aquire the images. Data are then downloaded into a computer to display the images, either simultaneously as a composite picture or as an animated sequence. Another option is a high-speed video camera with recording on tape. High-speed video has the potential to be extremely useful clinically. Because it provides a real slow motion view (not averaged), it can be used in all patients, even those whose voices lack sufficient periodicity to drive a stroboscope. After the technology becomes commercially available, it is likely to become more affordable and eventually become a valuable clinical tool.

VOICE RECORDING TECHNIQUE

Audio tape recording provides a permanent record of vocal function, which can be compared from visit to visit, before and after surgery, and before and after therapy. As such, it is the most important mode of documentaion in voice care. It is strongly recommended that a voice recording be made before embarking on any therapy, particularly surgery.

Because this is an important record and potentially a legal document, high-fidelity equipment is essential (box above). The entire system is as good only as the weakest link; therefore all components (recorder, microphone, and tape) should be of equivalent quality, with compatable frequency response characteristics. It is imprudent to couple an inadequate microphone to and expensive recorder. Recordings may be stored on a variety of media, including analog audio or video tape, digital audio tape, or direct computer storage.

ACOUSTIC ANALYSIS

Physical measures of sound are objective but must be validated to prove that the parameters measured are relevant to the acoustic signals which are perceived to be abnormal. The data are useful only in so far as they ultimately relate to the sound of the voice or the ease with which the patient speaks.

There is still no test battery for the voice which is analogous to the audiogram for hearing. The sound waves in a voice recording can be analyzed by a variety of methods and several are in wide use. The availability of relatively low-cost PC-based systems has increased the frequency of clinical use. However, acoustic parameters are frequently measured and reported with little consideration as to whether the measures are relevant to the voice problem being studied.

What does acoustic analysis tell us? The acoustic signal of the voice is not a simple sine wave, but a complex wave form which varies in regularity. Therefore, measures of pitch and loudness do not completely describe the sound. We do not know exactly what the brain attends to in perceiving voice quality, but regularity (periodicity) and spectral characteristics are important. Clinically used parameters describe these dimensions of vocal sound mathematically.

A complex wave, such as the sound of the voice, can be mathematically described as a composite of sine waves of varying frequency. In a completely periodic wave, all frequencies above the fundamental frequency (F_0) are integer multiples of F_0, termed harmonics. Lack of periodicity is perceived as noise and can be described as frequencies between the harmonics. A Fourier analysis is a computational means of breaking a complex wave into its components. Such an analysis permits identification of F_0, harmonics, and noise frequencies.

In the voice, the harmonics which are generally attributed to the resonant frequencies of specific structures in the vocal tract are referred to as formands, and denoted "F," followed by a subscript. Thus, the fundamental frequency is F_0, the first harmonic is F_1, and so on. The sound wave generated at the larynx is best described as a ramp or sawtooth wave. Transmission of sound through the vocal tract, with its characteristic resonant properties, alters the sound by enhancing the resonant frequencies. Vowel sounds are primarily determined by the relative amplitudes of formand frequencies.

The following measures are commonly reported in voice literature and have practical applications in voice analysis.

Fundamental frequency

This is the number of glottic cycles (opening and closing) per second. Higher frequency is perceived as a higher vocal pitch. Slower vocal fold vibration (low frequency) is perceived as a lower pitch.

Perturbation measures

The vocal folds always open and close with some degree of irregularity. Some means of fundamental frequency identification is required in order to evaluate regularity of vibration (periodicity). Measures which quantify variability are listed:

Shimmer—cycle to cycle variability in amplitude (loudness)
Jitter—cycle to cycle variations in frequency (pitch)
Standard deviation of the fundamental frequency—variation in pitch over many glottal cycles
Voice break factor—voiceless intervals per second

Shimmer is usually expressed as a percentage. Jitter may also be expressed as a percent, but it is frequently measured in milliseconds. Standard deviation is a statistically derived value.

Spectral analysis

The amount of acoustic energy can be determined as a function of frequency to describe the spectral structure of a sound. The distinctive character of a sound derives from its harmonic structure and well as from nonperiodic sound components. The pattern of spectral composition of each individuals' voice contributes greatly to the identification of a speaker. Mimic's are skilled in adjusting the vocal tract to transform voice quality. Within speakers, harmonic structure is an important variable in speech production. Vowel sounds are distinguished on the basis of harmonic stucture. Accordingly, the vocal tract adjusts during speech to enhance certain regions of the spectrum.

Because spectral structure varies greatly with the vowel being produced, it is clear that, if spectral analysis is to be used clinically, then the vowel to be uttered in the samples to be analyzed must be controlled. Commonly used parameters of spectral characteristics are listed:

Power spectral analysis—a sample is analyzed and sound pressure level is plotted across frequencies.
Sonagraph—plots frequency and intensity against time for a speech sample; this graph allows a qualitative appreciation of the signal to noise ratio and allows easy identification of voice breaks.
Signal to noise ratio—the amplitude of periodic vibration in a sound, divided by the amplitude of noise; this correlates roughly with the overall perception of hoarseness.

AERODYNAMIC MEASURES

Aerodynamic measures are not used as commonly as acoustic measures, because fewer commercial systems are available and because data acquisition is more complex. However, measurements of airflow and air pressure provide much useful clinical information. These measures not only describe laryngeal function quantitatively but also identify pathophysiology. This can be extremely helpful, not only in documenting changes but also in planning treatment.

Maximum phonation time (MPT)

This is the maximum time that a patient can sustain a vowel after maximal inhalation. It is technically not *really* an aerodynamic measure, since it measures time rather than pressure or flow. However, it is easy to measure, requiring only an ear and a stopwatch, and is an indirect measure of glottic competence. If the vocal folds are not close enough together, excessive airflow is required for phonation, and MPT is shortened because the patient runs out of air quickly. MPT varies significantly with different levels of sound pressure, pitch, and quality of the vowel utilized. A standardized procedure can reduce the variablilty. MPT is a valuable clinical parameter, particularly when equipment for true aerodynamic measurement is not available.

Mean phonatory airflow

The volume of expired air during a phonatory segment, divided by the elapsed time interval, yields the average airflow. It is important to select a stable segment of a vowel. Usually, a sustained phonation is selected, but information can also be derived from vowel segments in connected speech. The latter option, while a bit more involved and subject to variation, probably yields more valid information about vocal function. Mean phonatory airflow is increased with glottic incompetence, such as laryngeal paralysis, abductor spasmodic dysphonia, or vocal fold tissue deficit. However, airflow also increases with patient effort to produce a louder volume or more forceful voice. A low airflow may indicate either increased glotal resistance (as in adductor spasmodic dysphona) or inadequate expiratory effort, both of which can be due to either organic or functional causes. Therefore information on driving pressure is frequently required to draw any meaningful conclusions about aerodynamic measures.

"AC" airflow, the rapid changes in airflow with the vibratory cycle, can be analyzed to derive information about vocal fold vibration. This requires a very sensitive transducer, such as that which accompanies the Rothenberg mask.

Instrumentation for phonatory airflow

The rate of air escape through the mouth during phonation is relatively easy to measure but requires one of the following items of equipment: body plethysmograph, magnetic induction, spirometer, hot wire anemometer, and pneumotachograph.

Body plethysmography provides an excellent extrapolation of lung volume changes over time. This permits computation of airflow and does not interfere with airflow from the mouth during phonation. However, it is expensive and cumbersome, requiring considerable space. It is not satisfactory for sensing rapid changes in airflow.

Induction plethysmography (respitrace) utilizes magnetic coils around the chest and abdomen to determine changes in lung volume. Like body plethysmography, it does not require anything around the mouth. However, calibration is difficult, thus the technique is subject to error. It is not sensitive to rapid flow oscillations.

The hot wire anemometer has a rapid response, with essentially no interference with airflow, and is extremely sensitive to rapid changes in airflow. However, data are relative values, not real airflow rates, this it cannot be used to determine mean airflow rate or to calculate volume.

The pneumotachygraph, essentially an electronic spirometer, is the instument used most commonly to measure phonatory airflow. It is compact and measures real airflow rates. However, it adds some resistance to expired airflow. Some units have a sufficiently rapid response to measure the "AC" component of airflow, for example, the Rothenburg mask.

Subglottic pressure

Subglottic pressure is the force resulting from expiratory effort and laryngeal resistance. It can provide invalulable information about the amount of force required to induce oscillation in vocal fold mucosa. Because it is a resultant force, determined by upstream resistance and downstream effort, it must be interpreted in the context of airflow and sound pressure level. In a normal larynx, both airflow and air pressure increase as a louder voice is produced (assuming constant resonance). Glottic overclosure will result in low airflow, despite a high expiratory effort level and high subglottic pressure. Conversely, very stiff vocal folds require high pressure to oscillate to produce phonation. In such a case, if the vocal folds are appropriately approximated, both airflow and pressure will be elevated.

In clinical settings, subglottic pressure during phonation is most commonly determined by noninvasive measures, extrapolating from oral pressure at a point in time when the vocal folds are determined to be *open*. This is not practical in situations in which a stable phonatory segment is difficult to achieve, such as spasmodic dysphonia or vocal fold scarring.

Pressure can also be determined invasively, by introducing a pressure transducer by one of these routes: transglottal tracheal catheter (via nose or mouth), percutaneous tracheal puncture, or esophageal balloon or solid-state transducer.

Laryngeal resistance is an important concept in assessing vocal function, but it cannot be directly measured. It must be calculated from measurements of pressure and flow and cannot be determined in isolation from upstream resistance. Further, although it is greatly affected by stiffness of the vocal folds, the net value is not an inherent physical property of the glottis. Laryngeal resistance varies profoundly with the degree of glottic closure during phonation. Finally, even assuming constant glottal closure, resistance is not constant or even linear across frequency and amplitude of phonation.

Laryngeal efficiency is a parameter defined as sound pressure level divided by laryngeal resistance. This is an appealing concept in theory, because it is an attempt to determine how much sound output the larynx can generate from a given input of energy. There are, however, a number of factors which conspire to make this an unreliable measure. First of all, it is subject to all of the limitations of laryngeal resistance measurement, since it is derived from this parameter. As mentioned above, laryngeal resistance is not a constant, but varies with laryngeal motor activity and frequency and amplitude of vibration. Second, sound pressure level of the voice is not determined solely by laryngeal output but is profoundly affected by upstream resistance and resonance of the vocal tract. The parameter, laryngeal efficiency, could be more accurately termed vocal efficiency, since it assesses the entire mechanism. Interpretation of the variable must be tempered by awareness of its vagaries.

GLOTTOGRAPHY

Vibration of the vocal folds is extremely rapid, and it is often difficult in a clinical setting to determine whether or not the pattern of vocal fold vibration is abnormal in a given patient. Stroboscopy is very useful in patients with regular vocal fold vibration, with sufficient sound output to drive a stroboscope. However, it generates only an average pattern of movement during several cycles not a true description of movement. Movement can be directly observed only by high-speed cinematography, a technique which is far too cumbersome and expensive even for most research applications, let alone the clinic.

Two electronic measures, electroglottography (EGG) and photoglottography (PGG), have been developed to indirectly sense vocal fold contact and contact. They provide very accurate information, and EGG is a very effective signal for triggering a stroboscope. But, at present, there is insufficient experience to validate the extensive clinical application of these tools.

Electroglottography (EGG) assesses changes in vocal fold contact over time by measuring electrical impedence across the neck at the level of the glottis. This is accomplished by passing a weak electric current between two metal plates placed on the skin overlying each thyroid ala. Impedance is greatest when the glottis is open and drops when the vocal folds touch. As the vibratory cycle progresses, an increasingly larger surface area of the vocal fold edges come into contact and impedance drops accordingly. Impedance is not affected by changes in distance between separated vocal folds, and therefore it provides information only about the closed phase of the glottic cycle. Qualitatively, one can observe the signal and make subjective judgements about patterns of closure. It is not a *direct* measure of vocal fold contact, and so one can use the signal quantitatively only to determine the temporal relationship of vibratory events. When combined with data from photoglottography, parameters can be calculated which provide much useful information.

Photoglottography (PGG) measures light transmitted across the glottis, as sensed by a phototransducer placed on the skin overlying the trachea. This signal is directly proportional to the area between the vocal folds. Because it provides temporal information about vocal fold vibration during the open phase of the cycle, photoglottography is complementary to electroglottography. A simultaneous plot of both signals allows recognition of significant events in the vibratory cycle.

Calculated parameters

These values change with volume and frequency in the normal larynx, and data must be interpreted in the context of acoustic parameters.

$$\text{Open quotient} = \frac{\text{duration of open phase}}{\text{duration of closed phase}}$$

Inadequate closure during phonation will increase the open quotient. Pressed phonation will decrease the open quotient.

$$\text{Speed quotient} = \frac{\text{opening time}}{\text{closing time}}$$

Stiff vocal folds require greater subglottic pressure and will open more slowly, but snap together rapidly, resulting in a decreased speed quotient. Flaccid folds are easily displaced but return to midline more slowly, so the speed quotient is decreased.

ARCHETYPICAL CASES

Here are some examples of the clinical utility of vocal analysis.

Unilateral laryngeal paralysis classically presents with a breathy weak voice. However, symptoms vary widely, depending on patient compensation, and whether or not the lesion is complete. Some patients have gross laryngeal incompetence and are aphonic and aspirate during swallowing, while other patients speak and swallow so nearly to normal that no therapy is needed. Vocal function assement can aid in treatment decisions and monitor the effectiveness of therapy.

Perceptual—breathy, strained voice and brief phrases indicate glottal incompetence.

Videoendoscopy—flexible endoscopy allows accurate assessment of glottic configuration and residual vocal fold motion, to determine best mode of therapy.

Objective measures

F_0

Usually lower in males, higher in females (may be higher due to compensatory falsetto)

Jitter

Increased

Shimmer

Increased

S/N ratio

Decreased

Mean air flow

Increased

Subglottic P

Decreased

Maximum phon time

Decreased

Comment: Acoustic measures may remain abnormal after surgery or speech therapy have restored glottic competence as documented by aerodynamic measures. In such a situation, surgical attempts to further medialize the vocal fold are unlikely to be beneficial and may be detrimental.

Vocal nodules or polyps can produce vocal problems by interfering with glottal closure, limiting vocal fold vibration, or by a combination of these. Most vocal nodules are treated with voice therapy rather than surgical removal because they are generally the result of faulty vocal technique or poor vocal hygiene. Most polyps require surgical removal but may sometimes respond to voice therapy. Voice assessment can guide these clinical decisions.

Perceptual assessment—Hoarse, rough voice

Endoscopy—Rigid endoscopy is best for morphologic diagnosis of the lesion. Stroboscopy demonstrates the extent to which the lesion interferes with vibration and/or glottic closure and may reveal submucosal lesions. Flexible endoscopy may reveal abusive vocal posture, amenable to voice therapy.

Objective measures

F_0

Usually lower

Jitter

Increased

Shimmer

Slightly increased

S/N ratio

Decreased

Mean air flow

Normal or increased

Maximum phon time

Normal or decreased

Spasmodic dysphonia produces a severe vocal handicap. Botulinum toxin has proved very effective in improving voice and speech function. Diagnosis is clincal, but objective measures are important in determining the dose of toxin to be used, to assess results, and detect the need for futher injection.

Perceptual—Strained-strangled voice, voice breaks, vocal tremor

Endoscopy. Flexible laryngoscopy is required to assess laryngeal behavior during connected speech, to document adductor and abductor spasm, and to detect hyperfunction of extrinsic laryngeal muscles and/or tremor of the pharynx and soft palate. Rigid endoscopy may be helpful to rule out a morphologic lesion. Stroboscopy is usually not practical or helpful.

Objective measures:

F_o

Normal or slightly decreased

Jitter

Increased

Shimmer

Normal or increased

S/N ratio

Decreased

Mean air flow

Decreased (adductor) or increased (abductor)

Maximum phon time

Variable

Voice breaks

Present

Speech rate

Decreased

Comment: Successful treatment with botulinum toxin therapy reduces vocal effort and eliminates voice breaks but commonly does so at the expense of vocal power. Acoustic measures may remain quite abnormal, with the exception of the voice break factor. Aerodynamic measures are very useful in determining optimal dosage and route. The optimal dose is that which results in maximal decrease in voice breaks, without elevating phonatory airflow above normal. Persisting voice breaks, with normal or decreased airflow, indicates the need for a higher dose.

Functional dysphonia is faulty vocal technique which results in hoarseness and/or vocal fatigue. This can be the underlying cause of recurrent laryngitis or vocal fold lesions. It may also occur as maladaptive compensation for a laryngeal lesion. Diagnosis is based on flexible endoscopy and external examination of the neck during connected speech. Most commonly, hyperfunction is involved, with elevation of the larynx, anterior-posterior compression, and/or false vocal fold closure. Voice therapy is directed at correcting specific malfunction, with guidance from aerodynamic measures.

Perceptual
Hoarse, effortful voice
Endoscopy Flexible endoscopy identifies specific dysfunction for therapy planning, patient eduation, and possibly biofeedback; rigid endoscopy and stroboscopy are indicated to rule out underlying organic lesion.
Objective measures
F_o
Decreased
Jitter
Increased
Shimmer
Normal
S/N ratio
Decreased
Mean air flow
Variable
Maximum phon time
Variable

SUMMARY

Clinical management of voice disorders has been greatly advanced by the availability of new technology for evaluation. The cornerstone of diagnosis is still the history and physical examination. There is no vocal equivalent of the audiogram, but objective measures are invaluable indetermining the severity of the problem, planning therapy, and determining the effects of therapy. Effective use of these data requires thorough understanding of the physiologic correlates of what is being measured. The field of vocal assessment is still rapidly developing, and the validity of much existing technology remains to be established, especially for the abnormal voice. New approaches are likely to emerge which will futher enhance our understanding of voice and extend our healing capability.

SUGGESTED READING

1. Baken RJ: *Clinical Measurement of Speech and Voice*. 1987, College-Hill Press.
2. Cooper JA: *Assessment of Speech and Voice Production:* research and clinical applications. NIDCD Monograph Proceedings of a Conference, September 27-28, 1990.
3. Hanson DG, Gerratt BR, Ward PH: Glottographic measurement of vocal dysfunction: a preliminary report. *Ann Otol Rhinol* 92:413-420, 1983.
4. Hirano M: Objective evaluation of the human voice: clinical aspects. *Folia Phoniatrica* 41:89-144, 1989.
5. Zwirner P, Murry T, Swenson M, Woodson G: Effects of botulinum toxin therapy in patients with adductor spasmodic dysphonia: acoustic, aerodynamic and videoendoscopic findings. *Laryngoscope* 102:400-406, 1992.

Part Five

Otology

21

Who's afraid of the facial nerve?

Kedar Karim Adour, M.D.

ABSTRACT

Facial paralysis is frightening to the patient and to the physician (Fig 21-1). This fear often leads to unnecessary, expensive tests and, at times, to inappropriate treatment. A systematic guide for evaluating patients with facial paralysis is offered which includes completion of a medical history and physical examination and selection of laboratory, x-ray, magnetic resonance imaging (MRI), and prognostic electrical testing. Nuances of differential diagnosis and use and interpretation of electroneurography and maximal stimulation testing (MST) are discussed. A newly revised method of recording and predicting prognosis using the Hilger H3 Nerve Stimulator and MST is given. Guidelines for frequency of follow-up visits, need for consultation, and treatment are offered. The objective of this text is to instill confidence in the treating physician, which in turn will reassure the patient and reduce the cost of evaluation without sacrificing sound medical judgment. Medico-legal implications will be considered, and case studies will illustrate the course.

Key words
electric testing
facial nerve
facial paralysis
pathophysiology
herpes simplex
treatment

Reprint requests: Kedar Karim Adour, M.D., Department of Head and Neck Surgery, Kaiser Permanente Medical Center, 280 West MacArthur Blvd, Oakland, CA 94611-5693.

Acknowledgement: The Medical Editing Department, Kaiser Foundation Research Institute, provided editorial assistance.

Juan Domingo provided original illustrations: Figs. 21-7 and 21-9 through 21-12 inclusive. Burroughs Wellcome provided funding and double-blind samples of Zovirax and placebo.

Terminology for electrical tests

Minimum Nerve Excitability Test = NET
Maximal Stimulation Test = MST
Electro*neuro*graphy = ENOG*
Synonyms
Electro*neurono*graphy, first used by Fisch.
Evoked electromyography, suggested by May, abbreviated EEMG.
Neuromyography, suggested by Adour, abbreviated as NMG.

PART I—HISTORICAL COMMENT

Before 1931, patients with Bell's palsy were most often evaluated and treated in the departments of neurology and physical medicine.[116] Treatments were empiric and usually reserved for those with delayed recovery. In 1931, Arthur Duel, on the basis of collaborative work with Sir Charles Ballance,[32] performed the first facial nerve decompression for Bell's palsy. The operation, suggested by Ney in 1922[113] and Martin in 1931,[93] was based on the assumption that entrapment of the facial nerve in the temporal bone caused the paralysis. The primary-ischemic theory of pathogenesis postulates dysfunction of the autonomic nervous system. This dysfunction could produce arteriolar spasm and thrombosis in the vessels supplying the nerve within the rigid bony fallopian canal; the theory was not widely accepted.[82] Later, the secondary-ischemic theory[37,38] suggested that primary inflammatory, viral,† or immunologic edema‡ causing disturbance of the microcirculation leads to loss of nerve conductivity. Both concepts suggest that these processes lead to anoxia, followed by compensatory dilation of the

*To standardize, *ENOG* will be used for electroneurography and all synonyms.
†References 4, 9, 12, 14, 47, 52, 53, 55, 66, 88, 103, 119, 123, 126.
‡References 1, 31, 38, 39, 78, 79, 90, 104.

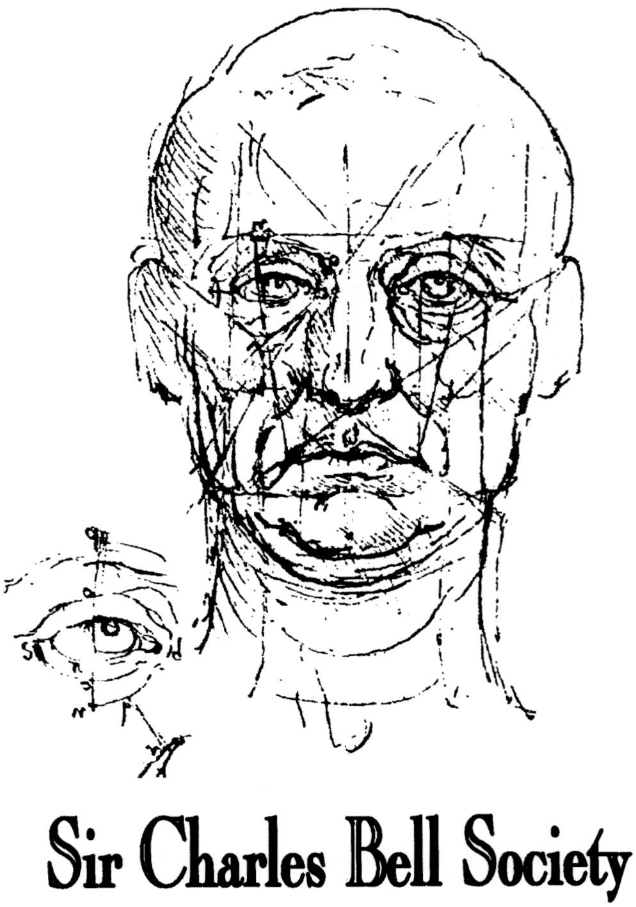

FIG 21-1
Sir Charles Bell Society Logo.

vessels and transudation, further increasing the vascular compression effect. The goal of treatment would be to reduce the compressive effect and break the vicious cycle of damage to the facial nerve. Bell's palsy became a surgical disease.[75-77,106,145]

Bell's palsy became synonymous with the term idiopathic facial paralysis, defined as unilateral facial paralysis of unknown cause. Because other diseases of the temporal bone, such as acute and chronic otitis media and primary and secondary tumors were known to cause facial paralysis, Bell's palsy was a diagnosis of exclusion. Once possible surgical treatment for Bell's palsy was developed, otologists became more interested in the disease, stating they were qualified to make accurate diagnosis and could institute appropriate treatment.[19] Today, the preponderance of Bell's palsy research is performed by otologists.* But even though otologists were highly qualified to make the exclusionary diagnosis of Bell's palsy, serious questions arose about patient selection as well as about timing and extent of surgical facial nerve decompression.[19]

Patient selection

The natural history of Bell's palsy was such that most patients recovered without treatment.[116,117] Thus, selection of patients for surgical treatment caused a major dilemma for the otologist. Methods were needed for determining which patients were at risk for nerve degeneration (denervation) and subsequent delayed poor recovery. In the early years, the decision to perform facial nerve decompression was based on faradic-galvanic muscle stimulation test results.[107,108] The loss of brisk response to faradic stimulation and its replacement by prolonged, sluggish response to galvanism was labeled the reaction of degeneration.[54] Lack of galvanic response was a contraindication for surgery.

In the 1950s, it was suggested that clinical testing based on the differential of the faradic-galvanic response might not be reliable.[42,109,121] Because electrical tests were unreliable, the decision to operate was based upon clinical experience (empirical indication).[75-77] Factors such as presence of pain at onset and poor muscle tone were stressed as indicators of poor prognosis. Patients with these clinical signs were considered for facial nerve decompression. The 1960s were influenced by Richardson's and Wynn Parry's work in 1957 on electrodiagnosis.[121] Campbell[42] and Laumans[85] standardized facial nerve testing using nerve excitability, and Hilger[67] designed the portable facial nerve stimulator. For facial nerve testing, the stimulating electrode producing a square wave measured in volts or mAmp was placed over the facial nerve trunk, and threshold intensity producing a visible muscle contraction was recorded. This procedure was called the minimal nerve excitability test (NET). Percutaneous nerve excitability testing became the standard for patient selection for surgery, although disagreement about interpretation existed. Campbell[42] stated that a difference of 2 mAmp between the affected and unaffected side should be used as the criterion for decompression. Alford[27,28] suggested a 3-mAmp difference, and Jongkees[77] used a 3.5-mAmp difference to select patients for treatment. Because of this lack of agreement in interpretation, a modification was suggested[95] using maximal stimulation (MST) of peripheral facial nerve branches to yield more accurate and earlier assessment of denervation.[16,97,101]

Salivary flow testing to predict prognosis was heralded by Magielski and Blatt[89] as a "practical and invincible guide to deciding for or against surgical decompression of the facial nerve." Performing the test was technically difficult, time consuming, uncomfortable for the patient, and never gained popularity.

Determination of denervation by NET results relied on visual assessment of muscle motion and was considered only partially reliable.[96,101] To obviate interpretation errors, Esslen,[56,57] working with Fisch,[58] devised electroneurogra-

*References 3-10, 13-16, 28, 30, 45, 50, 62, 64, 71, 78, 79, 147.

phy (ENOG) to produce a recorded measurement of facial compound summation muscle action potential (CAP). Electroneurography was suggested as the "gold standard" among electrical tests used for patient selection for surgery.[60,61,80,100,138]

Timing of surgery

Although some agreement existed that electrical testing was a good method of patient selection for surgery, disagreement was wide on when to perform surgery. Ballance and Duel[32] operated when persistent absence of faradic response existed but did not define how long the condition should exist before it was termed persistent. Lack of galvanic response was a contraindication for surgery.

Morris[108] defined persistent as 3 to 4 weeks after faradic response was lost. He added that decompression was indicated when faradic response was lost and clinical improvement ceased. He further suggested operating between 6 and 12 weeks after palsy onset, when evidence of voluntary motion was absent and reaction of degeneration was present. Tumarkin[145] advised early surgery but did not define early, although he probably meant before 2 months. In the 1940s, Lathrop[84] suggested decompression for any patient after 3 months without recovery and response to faradic stimulation.

In the 1950s, Cawthorne,[43] who became a leading advocate of facial nerve decompression, operated 1 month after palsy onset when faradic stimulation was lost. Jongkees[75-77] stressed decompression within 12 weeks of onset when reaction of degeneration was present. Kettel[82] summarized the philosophies of his contemporaries and avoided strict guidelines for timing of decompression.

In the 1960s, results of percutaneous NET continued to determine timing of surgery. The role of surgery was to prevent facial nerve denervation and to operate on patients who had impending denervation. Prediction of impending denervation was performed on the basis of test result differential between affected and unaffected side, and daily electrical tests were advocated. Decompression became a surgical emergency when test results became abnormal.

The concept of impending denervation has continued through the 1970s and 1980s, and it was agreed that surgical intervention after complete loss of electrical excitability was not indicated.[57-60] Currently, the most popular concept for timing of surgery is based on a differential of 90% in recorded ENOG compound summation muscle action potential of affected and unaffected side occurring within 2 weeks of paralysis onset.[59,60]

Extent of surgery

The intratemporal facial nerve is divided into 5 segments (Fig. 21-2). The meatal portion traverses the internal auditory meatus. The labyrinthine segment begins as the nerve enters the fallopian canal, then extends to and includes the geniculate ganglion. The horizontal segment begins just posterior to the geniculate ganglion and extends to the ampullary end of the horizontal semicircular canal. The pyramidal segment lies between the horizontal segment and the vertical segment, intimately related to the inferior surface of the horizontal semicircular canal and the superior-posterior wall of the middle ear. Finally, the vertical segment begins below the posterior end of the horizontal semicircular canal, ending at the stylomastoid foramen. Another portion of the facial nerve, the *iter chordae posterius,* represents the bony passages surrounding the facial nerve, where the chorda tympani nerve enters the middle ear space. During the past six decades, each of these segments has been implicated as a crucial area causing entrapment of the facial nerve in Bell's palsy.

*References 60, 61, 80, 100, 138.

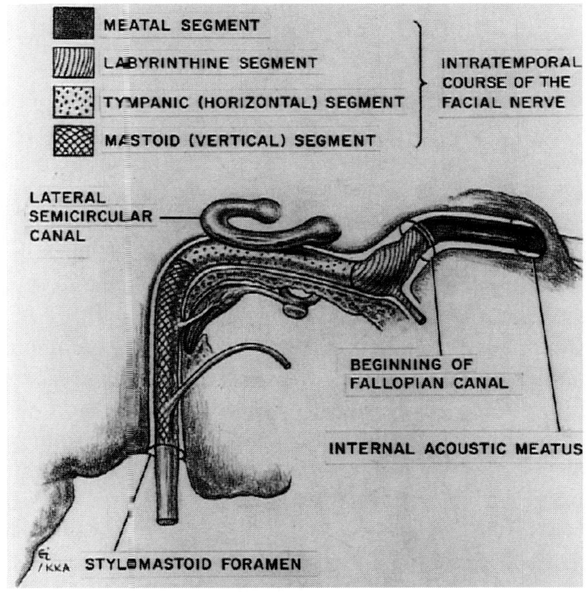

FIG 21-2
Drawing showing the anatomic divisions and relationships of the facial nerve from the internal auditory canal to the stylomastoid foramen. (Reproduced by permission of the editor and publisher from Adour KK: *Facial Nerve Testing and Evaluation.* In House JW, O'Connor AF, editors. Handbook of neurotological diagnosis. New York, 1987, Marcel Dekker, 175-219.)

When the operative treatment of Bell's palsy was first introduced in 1932, Ballance and Duel[32] proposed decompression of the distal 1 cm of the facial nerve at the stylomastoid foramen. They emphasized that removal of less than one half of the outer bony wall was sufficient and that no effective decompression occurred until the fibrous sheath was slit. Tumarkin[145,146] disagreed with the concept of unroofing the fallopian canal and performed a simple mastoidectomy; he ablated the stylomastoid artery to diminish tympanic vascular compression. In 1938, Morris[107] suggested that the entire lower half of the facial nerve should be decompressed; in 1939, Tickle[140] decompressed the entire vertical segment.

With the advent of the acoustic impedance measurement of Metz,[105] the operating microscope, and Tschiassny's[143,144] topographic diagnosis, otologists were theoretically able to pinpoint the site of compression. Surgery should be performed only when the site of the lesion was surgically accessible. For Cawthorne,[43] surgical treatment was permissible in the area from the face to the geniculate ganglion. In contrast to Ballance and Duel,[32] Sullivan and Smith[132] advocated removal of two thirds of the circumferential bony canal as far as surgically possible and posterior incision of the sheath to protect arcading arterioles. Lewis[86] developed the facial recess approach to the horizontal and geniculate portion of the facial nerve and questioned the reliability of accurate localization of the site of lesion. Lewis[86] also advised the endaural approach, used copious irrigation to cool the nerve, removed the thin bone from the perineurium with a pick and dental excavator, and slit the sheath of the posterior surface to protect the arterioles. Shambaugh[128] insisted that only the vertical segment be decompressed and that the ossicles not be disturbed. Jongkees[75] stressed decompression of the vertical and pyramidal segments.

The middle cranial fossae approach to the internal auditory canal was devised by House[69] in 1961, making it possible to decompress the entire facial nerve. In the early 1970s, Fisch and Esslen[57-60] advocated total facial nerve decompression and showed swelling in meatal and labyrinthine segments. In the late 1970s, Fisch[60] (published 1981), on the basis of these surgical findings, believed that decompression of only meatal and labyrinthine segments was necessary and began facial nerve decompression at the internal auditory canal through the middle cranial fossa approach. This concept persisted throughout the 1980s until gadolinium-enhanced magnetic resonance imaging (MRI) showed inflammatory response in multiple areas of the facial nerve in the fallopian canal.[78,94,148] Using MRI findings, studies are underway to determine if extent and location for surgery can be more accurately assessed.

Present status of surgery

Laboratory and clinical studies have established that Bell's palsy is a viral, autoimmune, demyelinating disease, probably caused by herpes simplex virus,* and recent research shows efficacy of treatment with the antiviral agent acyclovir (Zovirax, Burroughs Wellcome Co, Research Triangle Park, NC; Adour KK, unpublished data, 1994). The selection of patients, timing of surgery, and extent of surgical decompression may become moot. The words of Jongkees in the 1960s[76,77] that surgery cannot benefit a viral disease gain further validity in the 1990s. The primary role of the otologist in treatment of Bell's palsy is again as it was in the 1930s—to rule out other diseases as cause of paralysis.[102]

*References 9, 103, 112, 131, 152.

PART II—CLINICAL MANAGEMENT

When Sir Charles Bell[34] (1821) first showed that the facial nerve is a motor nerve, unrelated to sensory innervation of the face, he named it the nerve of respiration. He had noted that after cutting the facial nerve of his laboratory animal, the jackass, the nasal ala on the affected side collapsed and did not flare with respiration. The observation was correct, but the conclusion was erroneous. Since then, all cases of facial paralysis have tended to be labeled Bell's palsy. Bell's palsy has also been synonymous with and defined as idiopathic facial paralysis affecting only the facial nerve within the confines of the temporal bone. This, in association with outdated erroneous data found in the biomedical literature, often leads to unnecessary costly diagnostic tests[70] and extensive, potentially life-threatening surgical procedures.[58,92,99]

Recent observations have clarified this misconception. Bell's palsy is the clinically evident aspect of cranial polyneuritis[10,14,124,125] probably caused by herpes simplex virus (HSV-1). Neutralization antibody to HSV-1 reactivation in Bell's palsy indicates HSV-1 as causative.[153] The T-lymphocyte changes suggest an autoimmune reaction, and T2-weighted gadolinium-enhanced MRI has shown regions of increased signal intensity, indicating inflammation, in the brain stem as well as the intratemporal course of the facial nerve. The clinical, neurologic, laboratory, and immunologic similarities between Bell's palsy and known manifestations of reactivated neurotropic HSV-1 in cranial ganglia support the diagnosis.[33,111,149,150] Further, 30 years ago, Dalton[47] postulated that Ramsay Hunt syndrome[74] (herpes zoster cephalicus)[35] represented a more florid form of Bell's palsy. Cranial polyneuritis due to herpes zoster virus (HZV) is differentiated from that due to HSV-1 by increased severity of symptoms, presence of ear vesicles, and rising antibody titer to herpes zoster virus.* A zoster-like form of Bell's palsy exists without vesicles or rising titer to herpes zoster virus.[26] Patients with this syndrome have a higher risk of nerve degeneration.[26,51,129]

Formerly, we[17] suggested that the term idiopathic facial paralysis be replaced with Antoni's palsy in honor of the man who, in 1919, correctly labeled the disease as acute infectious polyneuritis cerebralis acusticofacialis.[29] Substituting the eponym Antoni's palsy emphasized that the diagnosis was *not* a diagnosis of exclusion. Because Bell's palsy can display the initial symptoms and signs of mononeuritis of the facial nerve or as polyneuritis, a more appropriate term is mononeuritis multiplex.

*References 26, 40, 41, 122, 129, 151.

DIAGNOSIS

Obtaining an accurate medical history and performing a complete physical examination often can yield sufficient information to provide diagnosis or suggest which diagnostic tests are needed.* However, complacency and reassurance alone by the physician must be condemned.

Cases of cranial polyneuritis of herpes simplex (Antoni's palsy) are similar in history, natural course, and outcome. Onset of paralysis is often preceded by a viral syndrome. Symptoms and signs during the early phase of facial paralysis include facial numbness, epiphora, pain, dysgeusia, hyperacusis (dysacusis), and decreased tearing.[98] Facial numbness indicates an affected trigeminal nerve because no somatic sensory fibers have been found in the facial nerve. The pain is often retroauricular, indicating inflammation of cervical 2 or 3, but can and does radiate into the face (cranial V) or into the neck and arm (cervical 4, 5, and 6). Dysgeusia (aberrant taste) suggests dysfunction of the geniculate ganglion, which contains the cell bodies of the chorda tympani nerve and is probably the site of reactivation of the herpes simplex virus. These symptoms are usually unilateral but can be contralateral. The hyperacusis is better labeled as dysacusis because it reflects intolerance to noise and not more acute hearing. Dysacusis is not related to stapedial muscle paralysis and probably represents loss of inhibition to the cochlea.[14] After evaluating more than 4000 patients who had all forms of facial paralysis, we concluded statistically that the presence of dysgeusia or dysacusis in a patient with acute facial paralysis is sufficient for a definitive diagnosis of cranial polyneuritis (Antoni's palsy).[24]

Physical findings can include inflammation of fungiform and circumvallate papillae of the tongue as well as hypoesthesia of cranial nerves V and IX and of cervical 2. Motor paralysis of branches of the vagus nerve are seen as unilateral shift of the palate or shortening of one vocal cord with rotation of the posterior larynx to the affected side.

Thus, Antoni's palsy (Bell's palsy) can be diagnosed when facial paralysis is peripheral in origin, systemic disease is not evident, the history is of acute onset, and concomitant sensory cranial polyneuritis is evident. The disease is expressed as viral sensory polyganglionitis with secondary autoimmune demyelinization, and the motor nerves are affected as they traverse the affected sensory ganglions. No further diagnostic tests are needed. The diagnosis must not be made when symptoms have been slowly progressive or when evidence of cerebral vascular accident exists (Fig. 21-3).

Pathophysiology of Antoni's palsy

When a patient recovers from a primary herpes simplex virus infection, the virus subsides to latency in the trigeminal and other cranial and spinal sensory ganglia.[33,111,150] Through a method not yet elucidated, the virus is reactivated and replicates within the ganglion cells, where it is protected from the circulating antibodies. During replication, local damage to the ganglia causes hypofunction of these nerves clinical symptoms are hypoesthesia of the face, pharynx, and head and neck. The virus then passes down the axons to induce radiculitis and passes up the nerve to the brain stem to induce local meningoencephalitis evidenced by increased protein in the cerebrospinal fluid and lymphocytic pleocytosis. This inflammatory response has been shown by gadolinium-enhanced MRI.[78,141,148]

At this point, two events occur: the virus infects Schwann cells in the affected nerve, causing inflammation, and because the virus accumulates a protein coat from the nerve cells as it extrudes through their membrane, a damaging autoimmune response to nerve cell membrane ensues. Lymphocytic infiltration of the peripheral nerve fiber follows, which leads to fragmentation of myelin with demyelinization and causes chromatolysis of the facial nucleus cells. This circumstance impairs the nerve cells but leaves them potentially retrievable, provided the distal disease process resolves. Inflammatory edema cannot exert sufficient compression to prevent the nerve from firing. Inflammatory edema is possible only when intra-arteriole pressure is greater than pressure in the surrounding tissue. Suprasystolic pressure is necessary to cause a compression great enough to stop the nerve action potential. The paralysis is caused by segmental demyelinization and not by compression.

When the inflammation and autoimmune reaction does resolve, remyelinization ensues, and functional muscle innervation is re-established. The degree and rate of recovery depend directly on the degree and rate of damage.

Topographic diagnosis is unreliable (Fig. 21-4). The facial nerve carries three types of nerve fiber: branchial motor, visceral motor, and visceral sensory. Topographic diagnosis is founded on this anatomic and physiologic anatomy of the facial nerve.[143,144] The particular motor, sensory, and secretory deficits which result from facial paralysis supposedly depend on extent and site of the lesion. But the validity of topographic test results has been shown by many researchers and clinicians to be completely unreliable.[13,44,128,142] Gadolinium-enhanced MRI shows that multiple sites of demyelinization can exist from the brain stem to the periphery. The inflammation and demyelinization occur horizontally and not perpendicular to the facial canal. Topographic diagnostic test results are thus useful only to supplement other diagnostic information: they are partial indicators of severity and therefore are relative indicators of prognosis.[7, 22,73, 81]

Audiometry and stapedial reflex. A pure-tone audiogram must be recorded for all patients with facial paralysis. If the hearing is normal or if symmetric sensorineural

*References 10, 14, 17-24, 91.

Diagnostic Pearls

When should you question the diagnosis of "mononeuritis multiplex" formerly called Bell's palsy and Ramsay Hunt syndrome?

when partial facial paralysis:
--does not resolve in 3 to 6 **WEEKS**.
--is accompanied by electrical evidence of nerve degeneration:
-Maximal Stimulation Test(MST)indicates moderate to severe decrease in muscle motion in one or more branches
-Global MST less than 3.
-electromyographic fibrillation (denervation) potentials are present.
--is accompanied by ipsilateral hearing loss.

when any facial paralysis is accompanied by evidence of chronic otitis media, or history of previous ear surgery.

when total facial paralysis is present:
--with **NO** return of facial motion within 4 months.
-even with total loss of nerve excitability shown by ENOG or Global MST, 99.9% of all Bell's palsy or Ramsay Hunt Syndrome will regenerate with mid-face contracture with synkinesis; earliest sign of regeneration is the return of the stapedial reflex; next earliest sign is evidence of mouth motion with voluntary forced closure of the eyes (synkinesis).
--with electrical evidence of nerve degeneration that resolves **WITHOUT** mid-face contracture with synkinesis.
-facial nerve degeneration with regeneration in Bell's Palsy or Ramsay Hunt syndrome is followed by the sequelae of mid-face contracture with synkinesis.

Note: Progressive facial paralysis during weeks or months is not Bell's palsy.
--damage to the nerve is complete by day 14 in Bell's palsy but not until day 21 in Ramsay Hunt syndrome.

when recurrent ipsilateral facial paralysis is accompanied by electrical evidence of nerve degeneration and recovery **BUT NOT** by contracture with synkinesis in 4 months.

Other Pearls

Measurement of the stapedial reflex is "otologic electromyography." Clinical total facial paralysis with intact stapedial reflex is a partial paralysis and return of the stapedial reflex 3 weeks post onset indicate good prognosis. The Global MST score allows you to predict rate and degree of recovery.

Question the validity of Bell's palsy treatment results where the number of patients showing electrical evidence of nerve degeneration does not equal the number of patients with contracture with synkinesis.

FIG 21-3
When should you question the diagnosis of "mononeuritis multiplex," formerly called Bell's palsy and Ramsay Hunt syndrome? (Adapted and reproduced by permission of the publisher from Adour KK: *Bell's Palsy: Contemporary Perspectives on Etiology and Management.* In UC Otolaryngology Update, 1994, November 3-5, 1994. San Francisco, California. University of California, San Francisco, 1994.)

hearing loss exists, speech discrimination and brain stem–evoked auditory response tests are not indicated to assess the paralysis. In a research setting, evoked auditory response can yield information which confirms that the brain stem is affected in some cases of acute facial paralysis with normal hearing,[65] but the finding has no therapeutic or prognostic significance.

Of all the topographic tests, the stapedial reflex test is the most objective and reproducible. The accuracy of stapedial reflex testing in determining site of lesion is suspect, but the prognostic value is unquestioned. If the stapedial reflex remains intact, it indicates incomplete paralysis and excellent prognosis. If the stapedial reflex is absent but returns before day 21, the prognosis is improved. We refer to the stapedial reflex as the otologist's electromyography.[17,44] The stapedial muscle is the first muscle innervated by the facial nerve and is the first muscle to show reinnervation.

Radiography and MRI. Radiography and computed

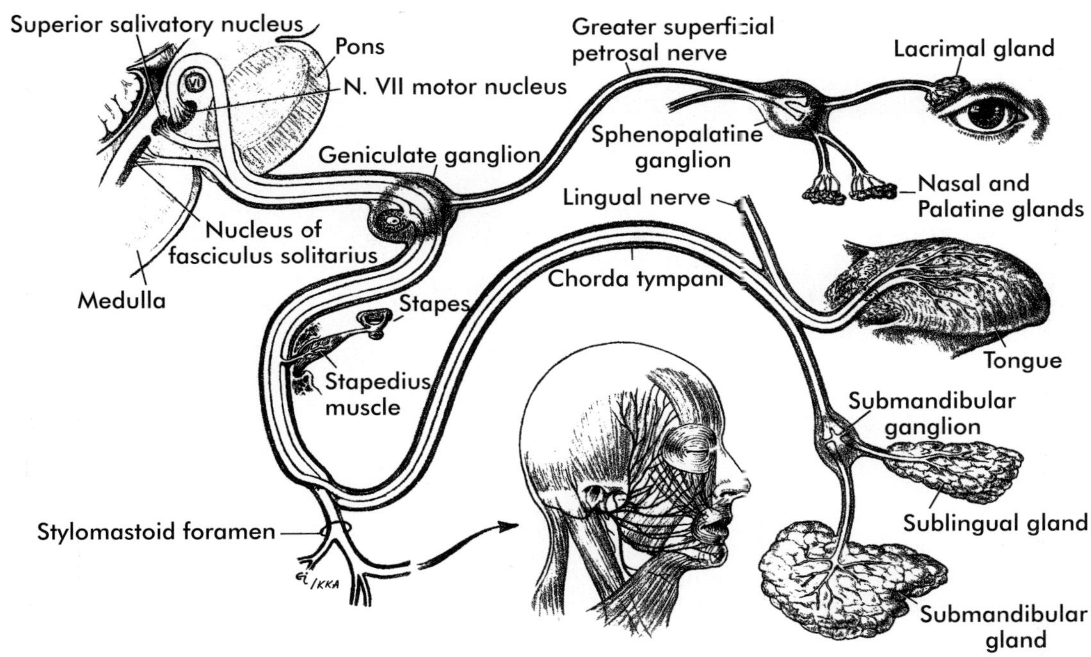

FIG 21-4
Drawing showing the anatomic and physiologic functions of the facial nerve used in topographic diagnosis. (Reproduced by permission of the editor and publisher from Adour KK: Facial nerve testing and evaluation. In House JW, O'Connor AF, editors. *Handbook of Neurotological Diagnosis.* New York, 1987, Marcel Dekker.)

tomography are not needed for assessment of Bell's palsy and Ramsay Hunt syndrome (herpes zoster cephalicus), which represent 90% of all cases of facial paralysis.[21] Computed tomography scanning has been replaced by MRI, which is safe, noninvasive, uses nonionizing radiation, and has superior soft tissue contrast. MRI produces unique high-resolution images using radio waves, magnetic fields, and computer processing. The technique provides exquisite anatomic definition and also distinguishes subtle biochemical changes. Assessment by MRI is preferable when a soft-tissue or inflammatory lesion is suspected.

Treatment

Natural course of Antoni's palsy. Familiarity with the natural course of the disease is a necessary part of therapy for Antoni's palsy. The more knowledge you have of the disease, the more confidence you have in your treatment and the more reassurance you can offer the patient.

The ratio of male to female patients is about equal; however, among persons age 10 to 19 years, the condition is twice as common in girls. Whereas after age 40 years, it is 1.5 times more common in men. This distribution suggests a relation to menarche and menopause. The rate of occurrence in menstruating women is highest during the first menstrual day; secondary peaks of incidence are seen on the eleventh through seventeenth day of the cycle and are probably related to ovulation. The frequency of Antoni's palsy in pregnant women is 45 in 100,000 births. Per year of exposure, pregnant women are 3.3 times more likely to develop Antoni's palsy than nonpregnant women in the same age group. The palsy is statistically more likely to occur during the third trimester or immediate postpartum period.[68]

The left and right sides of the face are equally affected and less than 1% of cases are bilateral.[14] The recurrence rate is about 10% and can be ipsilateral or contralateral.[118] Persons with one recurrence are more likely to have a third recurrence, and 50% of those with a third recurrence will probably have a fourth recurrence. One third of those with recurrence are likely to have an abnormal glucose tolerance test but not necessarily clinical diabetes. But, diabetic persons are 4.5 times more likely to get Antoni's palsy.[5,8]

A positive family history of Antoni's palsy is noted in about 10% of all patients. The annual incidence of Antoni's palsy is about 20 per 100,000, but age-corrected figures show an increased incidence in each decade of life, reaching 30 to 35 per 100,000 after age 60 years.[14]

Corticosteroids. In 1993, Austin et al,[30] in a double-blind prospective study, confirmed the finding that treatment of Bell's palsy patients with prednisone significantly reduces the number with electrical denervation.[3,136,137,139] Corticosteroids per se are considered excellent treatment for a viral, inflammatory autoimmune disease. Prednisone dramatically relieves the pain of Bell's palsy so that analgesics are usually not necessary.[2,3] For adults, a total of 1 mg per kilogram of body weight daily (1 mg/kg/day) is suggested, taken in divided doses morning and evening. The patient should be seen on the fifth or sixth day after onset of the paralysis. If the paralysis remains incomplete (Type I), the dose of prednisone is tapered to zero during the next 5 days. If the paralysis is complete (Type II), the 1 mg/kg/day dose should be continued for 10 more days and tapered to zero during the next 5 days (total, 21 days). Prednisone is discontinued after day 21, even though return of facial function cannot be expected until 3 to 6 weeks after onset of paralysis. Prednisone should never be stopped abruptly because rebound inflammation can lead to further denervation. Because Ramsay Hunt syndrome is more severe and has late neural degeneration, prednisone should be continued at a 1 mg/kg/day dose for 14 days and then tapered during the next week.[20,21,23,24]

When the classic distribution of otic vesicles (Ramsay Hunt syndrome) is absent, diagnosis of herpes zoster facial paralysis is dependent on results of complement fixation tests weeks into the course of disease. Presence of severe pain is a general indicator of poor prognosis, and such pain may represent a forme fruste of herpes zoster, or the zoster-like form of Bell's palsy.[26] Therefore, presence of severe pain is an indication for treating patients with the dose schedule advised for herpes zoster.

Acyclovir. Acyclovir alone and acyclovir with prednisone are becoming the preferred treatment of herpes zoster facial paralysis.[23] Although such treatment reduces pain and heals the vesicles, its effect on the facial nerve is unknown. The acyclovir can be given intravenously or orally. If oral treatment is elected, 800 mg every 5 hours is necessary because absorption from the gut is limited. When treating HSV-1 Antoni's palsy, 200 mg of acyclovir every 5 hours for 10 days is suggested (Adour KK, unpublished data, 1994). Once again, the effect of acyclovir *alone* on outcome has not been determined, and treatment with prednisone and acyclovir is advised.

Facial nerve decompression. The history of facial nerve decompression reflects lack of uniformity in selecting patients for surgery and in selecting areas for decompression.[19] From 1932 to the 1950s, decompression of the distal 1 cm (⅜ inch) of the facial nerve at the stylomastoid foramen was proposed, but no consensus on timing of surgery was reached.[32,43,82,84] In 1939, decompression for the entire vertical segment was suggested by Morris.[108] In the 1940s and 1950s, decompression of the vertical and pyramidal segments within 12 weeks of onset of paralysis was advocated when the reaction of degeneration was present.[75] In the 1960s, the iter chordae posterius was thought to be the most constricting area, and chorda tympani neurectomy for "internal" facial nerve decompression was instituted.[36,96] And, finally, in the late 1970s and early 1980s, decompression of the meatal and labyrinthine segments only through a middle cranial fossa approach was advocated[60] (Fig. 21-5).

The transmastoid total facial nerve decompression pro-

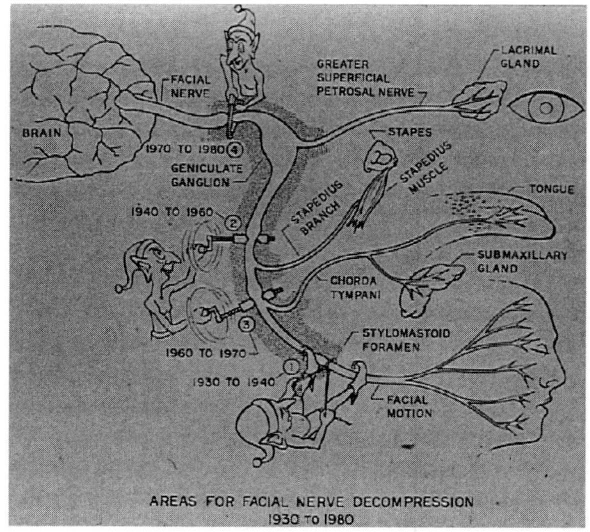

FIG 21-5
Schematic drawing depicting the previously perceived areas most likely to cause compression in Bell's palsy used as the basis for illustrating the history of facial nerve decompression. (Reproduced by permission of the special issue editor and publisher from Adour KK: Medical management of idiopathic [Bell's] palsy. *Otolaryngol Clin North Am* 24:663-673, 1991.)

posed by May[99] as treatment for Bell's palsy has been invalidated, and May no longer performs decompression surgery.

All decompression surgery is based on lack of understanding that Antoni's palsy is a viral demyelinating disease which is longitudinal, not perpendicular, to the facial canal and that surgery cannot possibly help a viral disease (Fig. 21-6).

Eye care. Protecting the eye from foreign bodies and drying is paramount. Dark glasses must be worn during the day, artificial tears instilled at the slightest evidence of drying, and a bland eye ointment used before sleep. Taping the eye closed is not recommended, but early exposure keratitis may require patching or, rarely, tarsorrhaphy.

Physiotherapy. Just as fewer clinicians are offering facial nerve decompression, fewer are offering electrical stimulation of paralyzed muscles. Physiotherapy has been suggested as valuable for maintaining patient morale. Cost to the community and to the patient of daily visits to the hospital for electrotherapy does not seem justified.[110] An accurate diagnosis and a reliable estimate of prognosis, with careful explanation and reassurance, can give full confidence to the patient. Further, experimental research has shown that electrical stimulation of a denervated muscle retards ingrowth of neurofibrils to the motor endplates. Therefore, electrotherapy may be detrimental and is not advised.

Prognosis

Making a reliable prognosis in early stages of facial paralysis is difficult. Electrodiagnostic testing attempts to pre-

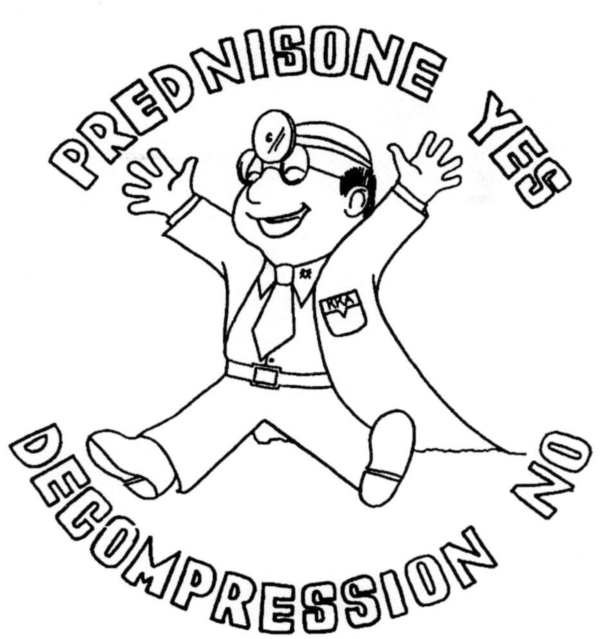

FIG 21-6
Prednisone Yes—Decompression No.

dict prognosis by determining the physiologic extent of nerve damage.[45,114,123,138] However, results of available electrical tests (nerve excitability, facial nerve latency, evoked and volitional electromyography, and strength duration determination) show abnormality from days to weeks after degeneration. In the case of a severed nerve, nerve excitability, facial nerve latency, and ENOG results are normal for 72 hours.[48,49,63] All stimulatory nerve test results reflect what has occurred 3 days earlier, and volitional electromyography results do not become abnormal for 2 to 3 weeks.[121,134,135] Moreover, once stimulatory electrical test results become abnormal, they remain abnormal and cannot be used to monitor regeneration and reinnervation.[133] In cases in which regeneration is expected, electrical test results are good prognostic indicators but differ in interpretation on the basis of the bias of various authors.

The findings from all electrical testing must be correlated with the clinical and pathologic process causing paralysis.[127,133] In general, test results are useful only during the first weeks of disease. Because degree of regeneration is related to degree and rate of denervation, serial electrical tests are performed. If denervation has progressed from minimal to severe degeneration in 7 to 10 days, a greater and earlier return of volitional muscle motion can be expected in these patients than in those who have progression from minimal to severe denervation in 3 to 4 days.[17,124]

If test results indicate equal muscle response on both sides of the face, the patient can be expected to have complete return of facial function in 3 to 6 weeks without complications of faulty nerve regeneration. The most common complications of faulty nerve regeneration are contracture,

TABLE 21-1
Method for computing average MST results

Branch tested	Visual muscle response	Numeric score
Forehead	Minimal Decrease	3
Eye	Moderate Decrease	2
Mouth	Severe decrease	1
Averaged score (3 + 2 + 1 ÷ 3)		2

synkinesis (associated facial motion), and facial spasms (tics). An uncommon complication is gustatory tearing ("crocodile tears").

Maximal stimulation test. Because reliability of minimal NET results was challenged, a modification called maximal stimulation test (MST) was developed and has become the most accepted.[87,124] The observer is placed so as to see both sides of the face simultaneously. The stimulating probe is applied to the nerve branch at that intensity which produces a just visible muscle twitch. When the first contraction is observed, the area is explored to find the most sensitive point—that which displays the maximal amount of muscle motion. The current is then increased 1 to 2 mAmp above this threshold to obtain maximal nerve excitability stimulation. Test results are expressed as the difference in facial muscle movement when comparing the affected side of the face with the normal side; those results are recorded as equal or decreased movement. Additionally, when muscle response to maximal nerve excitability stimulation is decreased, the observer notes whether this decrease response on the affected side is minimal, moderate, or severe compared with the nonaffected side. The findings equate very well with the degree of denervation. No response indicates complete denervation of the nerve branch being tested.

We prospectively compared the ability of ENOG, facial nerve latency, and MST to predict prognosis in 150 patients with facial paralysis.[124] The degree of neural degeneration is not always equal in every branch of the facial nerve. Therefore, to refine statistical analysis and more accurately reflect the status of the entire peripheral nerve branch system, we devised a modified method of reporting MST results similar to that used for electromyographic reporting. Electromyographic technicians report the estimated degree of muscle action potentials (known as interference patterns) on a scale of 0 to 4, with 0 being no muscle action pattern and 4 being a normal response. For MST reporting, 4 is assigned to equal muscle reponse on both sides of the face; 3 is assigned to minimally decreased, 2 to moderately decreased, and 1 to severely decreased response compared with the response of the same branches on the unaffected side. We can now compute an average MST for the entire face. An example of such a computation is shown in Table 21-1.

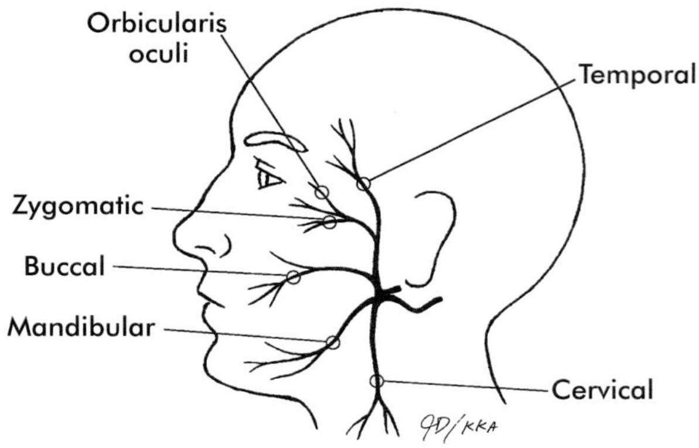

FIG 21-7
Schematic drawing depicting the location of the facial nerve branches to be stimulated when performing maximal stimulation tests (MST). (Courtesy Juan Domingo.)

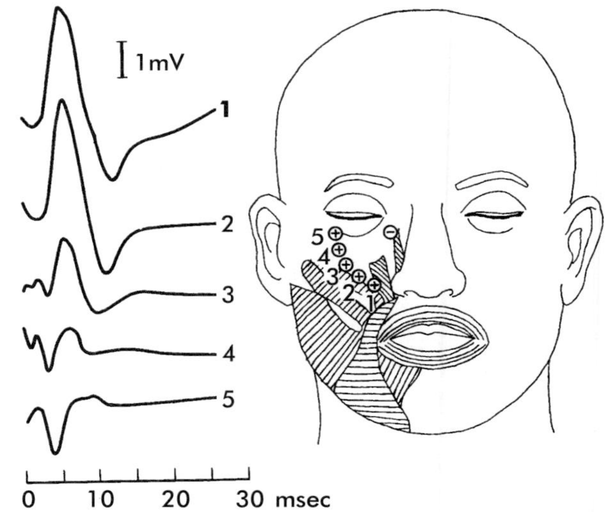

FIG 21-8
Schematic drawing showing the variations in compound muscle action potential when the recording electrode is moved as little as 1 cm in any direction. (Reproduced by permission of the publisher from Adour KK, Sheldon MI, Kahn ZM: Maximal nerve excitability testing versus neuromyography: prognostic value in patients with facial paralysis. *Laryngoscope* 90:1540-1547, 1980.)

TABLE 21-2
Prediction of recovery based on averaged MST scores

MST scores	% Recovery	Time (weeks)	Sequelae (severity*)
4	100	3-6	None
3-3.9	75-100	4-8	Minimal
2-2.9	75	6-12	Moderate
1-1.9	50-75	8-12	Moderate/severe
0-.9	<50	12+	Severe

*Contracture with synkinesis.

This hypothetical patient suffered a "moderately" degenerated facial nerve, and recovery would be delayed and followed by sequelae. A score of ≤2.7 is 94% accurate in predicting incomplete final recovery with midface contracture with synkinesis (Table 21-2).

Although facial nerve excitability testing is a simple procedure, determining location of the peripheral branches requires experience. The branch to the frontal muscle is usually found about 1 cm lateral to the eye; the branch to the orbicular muscle of the eye is stimulated at the lateral border of the orbit. Location of the branch to the orbicular muscle of the mouth varies the most of all 3 branches but is usually just anterior to the notch where the facial artery traverses the mandible. The stimulating probe may need to be moved to determine point of maximal response as the facial nerve can branch in many directions beyond the stylomastoid foramen (Fig. 21-7).

Electroneurography versus maximal stimulation testing. ENOG not only permits study of muscle excitability and state of muscle fibers but also provides useful information regarding conduction properties of nerve fibers. ENOG is the basis for determining conduction time, or latency (expressed in milliseconds), and motor nerve conduction, or velocity (expressed in meters/second). When testing the facial nerve, distance between stimulation and recording electrodes is only 10 to 12 cm, and tradition has established that facial nerve latency is preferable to conduction velocity as a measure of nerve function.

The stimulating electrode is placed over the nerve trunk at the stylomastoid foramen; the surface recording electrode is placed over the muscle group to be tested. The nerve is stimulated with a supramaximal stimulus. Functional status of the nerve is assessed by comparing amplitude of the compound muscle action potentials on both sides of the face.* The interval between nerve stimulation and start of muscle potential—facial nerve latency—can be accurately measured and is an acceptable indication of nerve function. This method is considered an improvement of MST. Instead of visual estimate, muscle action potential is recorded.

ENOG testing has yet to be standardized.[62,120,124,130] The test-retest result variability between both sides of the face and between tests on different days ranged as high as 50% with an average difference of 20%. This level of variability is in agreement with our research findings (Fig. 21-8).

MST has the disadvantage of relying on a visual endpoint, and ENOG has the advantage of possessing a recorded and often reproducible endpoint. However, ENOG has the disadvantage of reliance on stimulating the nerve trunk. Because the facial nerve trunk is deep in the stylomastoid foramen, an increased stimulus level is required which often triggers a reaction in the masseter muscle, the

*References 46, 56, 61, 71, 72, 80, 138.

"trigeminal nerve artifact." Moreover, ENOG findings are interpreted on the basis of muscle reaction in only one part of the face. If the upper division of the facial nerve is cut, ENOG would record a compound muscle action potential equal to that of the other side. MST, which records individual peripheral branches, would accurately show abnormal absent muscle response.[16,25] Because an electrical impulse can stimulate only neuropraxic fibers, none of the tests distinguish between axonotmesis and neurotmesis or second- and third-degree nerve injury. The recorded compound muscle action potential from a nerve with 25% of its fibers neuropraxic is the same, regardless of the degree of injury to the remaining fibers.

Comment. All stimulatory electrical facial nerve test results become abnormal 3 days after neural degeneration has taken place. The ostensible goal of facial nerve decompression is to prevent neural degeneration. Therefore, using any stimulatory electrical test results to predict need for possible surgery is an anathema. Even though instrumentation is elaborate and recordings impressive, it is still apparent that ENOG cannot be considered sufficiently sensitive to select Antoni's palsy patients for surgery. The sources of error are considerable: (1) electrode placement, (2) skin impedance, (3) masseter muscle artifact, (4) patient tolerance, (5) equipment variability, (6) lack of standardization, (7) inter-test results variance, (8) interside results variance, (9) lack of understanding that Bell's palsy is a viral disease which causes longitudinal, not perpendicular, damage to the intratemporal facial nerve. Surgery cannot possibly help to cure a viral disease.[2,11,88,115]

Conclusions

The term Bell's palsy should be discarded in favor of Antoni's palsy or mononeuritis multiplex to reflect the true nature of the disease: a viral inflammatory autoimmune disease probably resulting from HSV-1 reactivation in the ganglia of the head and neck. The diagnosis is not one of exclusion, and the clinician is capable of establishing a positive diagnosis to begin treatment. Treatment should include corticosteroid and acyclovir. MST is a simple, inexpensive method of predicting prognosis,[87] and topographic diagnosis is completely unreliable and unnecessary. Radiography and MRI are not necessary. Facial nerve decompression and electrotherapy are probably detrimental[2,115] to recovery and are not recommended.

PART III—PRESENT STATUS OF ELECTRICAL TESTS FOR BELL'S PALSY

To better understand the present status of electrical tests for Bell's palsy, a short historic background is appropriate, beginning with the demise of *minimal* NET in 1971 and 1972. At that time, the Hilger 2 and 2R percutaneous nerve stimulator replaced the previous model, which did not have a linear output and required using a mathematic conversion factor to determine true output of the stimulating electrode. The amperage necessary to obtain a just visible muscle twitch by stimulating the nerve trunk was obtained on both the paralyzed and nonparalyzed side. A difference of 2.0 to 3.5 mAmp was considered clinically significant, and surgical facial nerve decompression was recommended when the difference reached 3.5 mAmp.

From 1970 through 1972, Yanagihara and Kishimoto,[152] May,[95-97] and Adour[16] simultaneously became disenchanted with the results of minimal nerve excitability tests. Yanagihara and Kishimoto[152] compared the prognostic value of stimulatory electromyography using needle recording electrodes and minimal NET in facial paralysis. They stated that stimulatory electromyography is superior to minimal NET in determining the true neurophysiologic state of the nerve. May[95] and Adour et al[16] chose MST and abandoned minimal NET.

Since the 1950s, neurologists had used facial nerve conduction tests utilizing a surface recording electrode to determine facial nerve latency as a prognostic tool in patients with facial paralysis. In 1972, Esslen,[56] using a similar technique, advocated measurement of the compound summation muscle action potential under the surface recording electrode as a more accurate indicator of neurophysiologic status of the facial nerve and superior to stimulation electromyography, which uses a needle electrode to record individual rather than compound action potentials. He called the test electroneurography, which has received greater acceptance than the term electroneuronography suggested by Fisch[59] (both abbreviated as ENOG).

In 1980, Adour et al[16] noted that ENOG is a multichain event which includes nerve conduction, transmission time at the neuromuscular junction, and conduction time in the muscle and that this technique is properly called neuromyography (this term did not gain popularity).

Although ENOG became popular, we have not located any articles concerning its reliability published before 1977. Adour et al[16] compared ENOG with MST and concluded that the high rate of fluctuation observed with ENOG indicates the need to further assess test/retest result reliability and to standardize normal values. ENOG is a less accurate measure of the state of the facial nerve than is MST, and selecting patients for facial nerve surgery on the basis of ENOG results would be hazardous.

Three years later, Hughes et al[72] again noted universal lack of understanding, lack of normative and experimental data, and lack of control variables for ENOG. In their prospective study, they also concluded that: "Despite careful controls, test-retest variability can significantly influence ENOG measurements." Whereas Fisch and Esslen[58] advocated changing position of the stimulating and recording electrodes (optimized lead placement) (Fig. 21-9) to obtain maximum compound summation muscle action potential as the endpoint for comparison between both sides of the face, Hughes et al[7] concluded: "Repeated and averaged measures on a given patient will increase the precision of

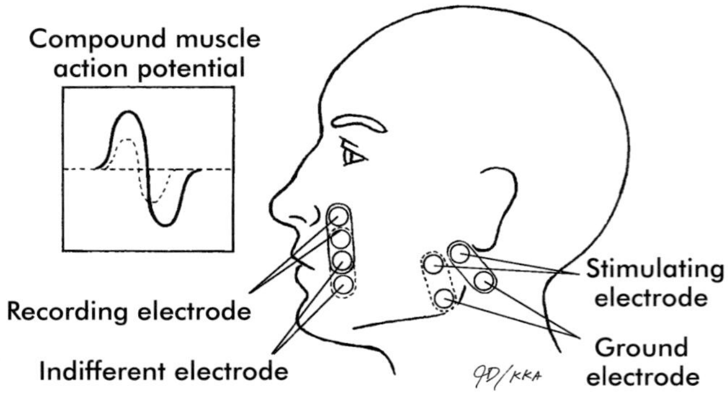

FIG 21-9
Electroneurography (ENOG): Schematic drawing showing the optimized lead placement of stimulating and recording electrodes and depicting the possible variation in size of the compound muscle potentials. (Courtesy Juan Domingo.)

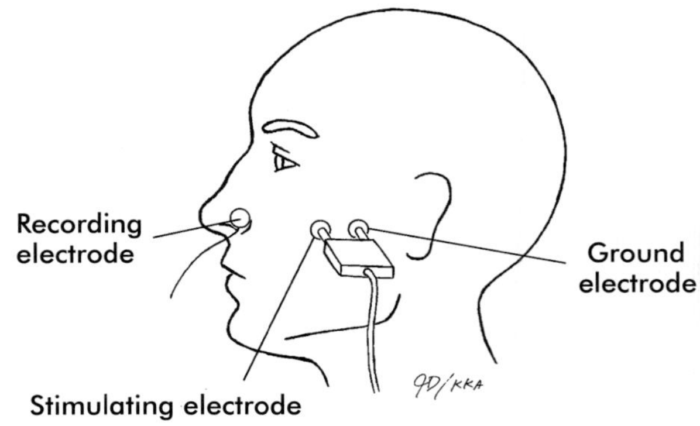

FIG 21-11
Electroneurography (ENOG): Schematic drawing showing the lead placement of stimulating and recording electrodes suggested by May who prefers the term "evoked electromyography." (Courtesy Juan Domingo.)

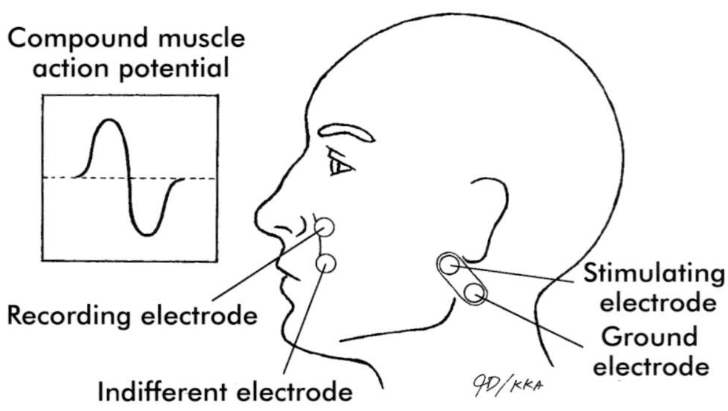

FIG 21-10
Electroneurography (ENOG):Schematic drawing showing the standardized lead placement of stimulating and recording electrodes and depicting a compound muscle action potential. (Courtesy Juan Domingo.)

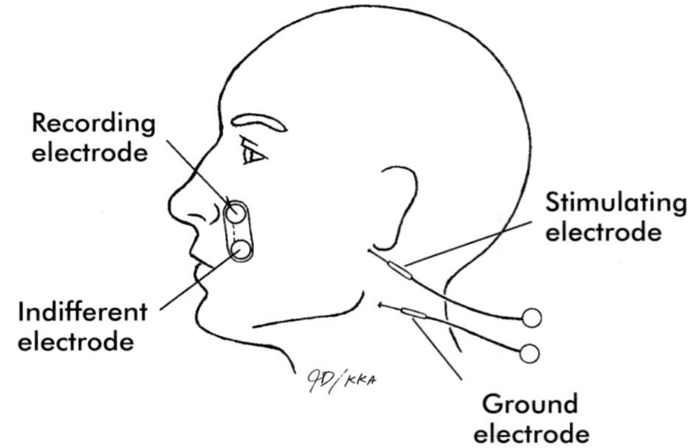

FIG 21-12
Electroneurography (ENOG): Schematic drawing showing the placement of the recording electrode and the insertion of the needle stimulating electrodes suggested by Kobayashi. (Courtesy Juan Domingo.)

ENOG." They also suggested standardized lead placement of the recording electrode (Fig. 21-10).

By 1983, ENOG testing was not standardized, and May et al,[100] prospectively studying normal subjects and patients with acute facial palsy, found the test-retest result variability between both sides of the face and between tests on different days ranged as high as 50% with an average difference of 20%, which was in agreement with our 1977 research results.

May et al[100,101] preferred the term "evoked electromyography" instead of "electroneurography." Gantz et al[61] felt this preference was inappropriate because electromyography, in neurologic terms, refers to the use of needle electrodes (Fig. 21-11).

In 1985, Kartush et al[46,80] conducted a clinical and experimental study to determine reasons for inaccuracy of ENOG in some patients. In contrast to May[100] and Hughes et al,[72] Kartush et al[80] advised optimized lead placement and still found an intertest result variance of 18%. When comparing interside variance, the optimized lead placement difference was 10% compared with 21% for the standardized lead placement. Kartush et al[80] further commented that a supramaximal level of stimulation was less often achieved with standardized lead placement because of pain or masseter muscle artifact.

In 1988, Kobayashi et al[83] reemphasized the disadvantages of surface-stimulating electrodes: placement of electrodes; electrical characteristics of the skin which may vary with temperature, moisture, thickness of the soft tissue covering the nerve; and patient tolerance to pain. They devised a needle-stimulating electrode inserted subcutaneously to a depth of about 1 cm (Fig. 21-12).

As would be expected, the threshold for nerve excitability testing using surface electrodes ranged from 30 to 160 mV, whereas the needle electrode had a range of 2 to 70 mV. Some patients without response to nerve excitability testing when conventional surface electrodes were used made a complete recovery. However, the needle method produced more effective stimulation of the nerve in these patients. Kobayashi et al[83] stated that by using the needle stimulation electrode, "We believe that unnecessary risk of early decompression surgery for Bell's palsy or Hunt's syndrome can be avoided."

In 1988, Raslan et al[120] performed a statistical study of ENOG test error. Using optimized lead placement, the test error was 18% compared with a test error of 20% using standardized lead placement; they also found that unconventionally small recording electrodes (3 to 7 mm) produced up to 4% less error.

Neurodiagnostic tests

Neurodiagnostic tests are used not only to determine the site of the lesion producing the paralysis but also to evaluate the physiologic extent of nerve damage, to predict prognosis, and to determine treatment.*

Because reliability of the tests has been challenged and newer forms of x-ray imaging and MRI have been developed, traditional testing has been modified, and electrical tests are considered the best prognosis and physiologic evaluation.

Nerve injury

Interpretation of electrical test results is necessary to understand types of nerve damage. The most useful classification is Sunderland's[133] 5 degrees of injury expressed in terms of damage to the endoneurium, perineurium, and epineurium. The 5 degrees of injury are of increasing severity according to effect of injury and not cause of injury. The older classifications which used neurapraxia, axonotmesis, and neurotmesis are not sufficiently precise but are in common usage.[127]

Again, I emphasize that these are pathologic classifications, and electrical test results are prognostic, not diagnostic, tests.

Methods of electrical testing

All electrical tests mentioned, except electromyography, are performed percutaneously. Most electrical tests are comparative, using the normal side as a control for the abnormal side. Because neural degeneration is often neither acute nor complete, a single examination is not sufficient: reexamination days or weeks later is necessary.†

Nerve excitability tests

The minimal NET requires simple percutaneous stimulation of the facial nerve at the stylomastoid foramen while raising the intensity of a short-duration current to the threshold at which a just visible muscle contraction is observed. Both the affected and the unaffected side are then stimulated and the two compared.

Because the reliability of minimal nerve excitability testing was challenged, a modification called the MST was developed (see Part Two).

*References 46, 70, 92, 101, 102, 114, 138.

†References 27, 28, 45, 70, 87.

Electromyography

The term electromyography refers in general medical usage to volitional electromyography, differentiated from ENOG. The muscle action potentials produced by stimulating the nerve differ somewhat from those produced by voluntary effort. Muscle action potentials produced by voluntary effort are associated with a graded response which varies according to strength of effort.

A needle electrode is placed into the muscle to be tested, and the signal is monitored visually and audiographically on an oscilloscope. When muscle denervation has been present for 2 to 3 weeks, the muscle begins to fibrillate so that the needle electrode records fibrillation potentials, a sign of denervation. At a later stage, if recovery has begun, reinnervation potentials can be recorded.

Strength duration curve

Determining the strength duration curve is tedious and somewhat painful, and is not widely used. Briefly, this curve depicts the relation between amplitude and duration of a stimulating impulse at the threshold for muscle response. If denervation has occurred, a stronger than normal stimulus is needed to activate the muscle, and the shape of the strength duration curve is thus changed.

Interpretation of electrical tests

In the surgical management of facial paralysis, stimulatory electrical test results are often used to select patients for treatment, and these test results must be fully understood to make the best decision. In the nonsurgical management of facial paralysis, these test results are used primarily to predict prognosis. Each test has limitations, and all test results show abnormality days to weeks after degeneration. Minimal and maximal nerve excitability tests both have the disadvantage of relying on a visual endpoint.

Because stimulatory electrical test results remain abnormal even when volitional facial muscle action has returned, electromyography may be of prognostic value in the regenerative period, but this is late in the entire course of the disease. During reinnervation, when there is visible facial muscle motion, obtaining an electromyogram is superfluous. If the nerve has been severed, regeneration cannot be expected unless repair is instituted. Even then, stimulatory electrical test results are of no benefit because they cannot monitor regeneration. For the three most common causes of facial paralysis (cranial polyneuritis, temporal bone fracture, and acute otitis media), which account for 95% of all cases in which the facial nerve is intact, regeneration can be expected and is predictable.

History repeats itself. In 1940 to 1950, when facial nerve decompression for Bell's palsy was in vogue (according to Adour and Diamond[19]), Sullivan and Smith[132] noted that they would identify the nerve at the stylomastoid foramen, directly stimulate the nerve, and, if there was any muscle response, cancel decompression. If surgery is considered on the basis of electrical test results, we advocate the use of Kobayashi's technique of needle stimulation of the facial nerve.

REFERENCES

1. Abramsky O, Webb C, Teitelbaum D, Arnon R: Cellular immune response to peripheral nerve basic protein in idiopathic facial paralysis (Bell's palsy). *J Neurol Sci* 26:13-20, 1975.
2. Adour KK, Swanson PJ Jr: Facial paralysis in 403 consecutive patients: emphasis on treatment response in patients with Bell's palsy, *Trans Am Acad Ophthalmol Otolaryngol* 75:1284-1301, 1971.
3. Adour KK, Wingerd J, Bell DN, Manning JJ, Hurley JP: Prednisone treatment for idiopathic facial paralysis. (Bell's palsy). *N Engl J Med* 287:1268-1272, 1972.
4. Adour KK, Doty HE: Electronystagmographic comparison of acute idiopathic and herpes zoster facial paralysis. *Laryngoscope* 83:2029-2034, 1973.
5. Adour KK, Bell DN, Wingerd J: Bell's palsy: dilemma of diabetes mellitus. *Arch Otolaryngol* 99:114-117, 1974.
6. Adour KK, Wingerd J: Nonepidemic incidence of idiopathic facial paralysis: seasonal distribution of 419 cases in three years. *JAMA* 227:653-654, 1974.
7. Adour KK, Wingerd J: Idiopathic facial paralysis (Bell's palsy): factors affecting severity and outcome in 446 patients. *Neurology* 24:1112-1116, 1974.
8. Adour KK, Wingerd J, Doty HE: Prevalence of concurrent diabetes mellitus and idiopathic facial paralysis (Bell's palsy). *Diabetes* 24:449-451, 1975.
9. Adour KK, Bell DN, Hilsinger RL Jr: Herpes simplex virus in idiopathic facial paralysis (Bell's palsy). *JAMA* 233:527-530, 1975.
10. Adour KK: Bell's palsy: a complete expression of acute benign cranial polyneuritis. *Prim Care* 2:717-733, 1975.
11. Adour KK: The bell tolls for decompression? *N Engl J Med* 292:748-750, 1975. (editorial.)
12. Adour KK: Cranial polyneuritis and Bell's palsy. *Arch Otolaryngol* 102:262-264, 1976.
13. Adour KK, Boyajian JA, Kahn ZM, Schneider GS: Surgical and nonsurgical management of facial paralysis following closed head injury. *Laryngoscope* 87:380-390, 1977.
14. Adour KK, Byl FM, Hilsinger RL Jr, et al: The true nature of Bell's palsy: analysis of 1,000 consecutive patients. *Laryngoscope* 88:787-801, 1978.
15. Adour KK, Hilsinger RL Jr, Byl FM: Herpes simplex polyganglionitis. *Otolaryngol Head Neck Surg* 88:270-274, 1980.
16. Adour KK, Sheldon MI, Kahn ZM: Maximal nerve excitability testing versus neuromyography: prognostic value in patients with facial paralysis. *Laryngoscope* 90:1540-1547, 1980.
17. Adour KK: Medical management of Antoni's palsy (Acute infectious polyneuritis cerebralis acusticofacialis). In Shambaugh GE, Shea JJ, editors: *Proceedings of the Sixth Shambaugh International Workshop on Otomicrosurgery and Third Shea Fluctuant Hearing Loss Symposium, March 2-7, 1980, Chicago, Illinois,* Huntsville, Alabama, 1981, Strode.
18. Adour KK: Current concepts in neurology: diagnosis and management of facial paralysis. *N Engl J Med* 307:348-351, 1982.
19. Adour KK, Diamond C: Decompression of the facial nerve in Bell's palsy: a historical review. *Otolaryngol Head Neck Surg* 90:453-460, 1982.
20. Adour KK, Hetzler DG: Current medical treatment for facial palsy. *Am J Otol* 5:499-502, 1984.
21. Adour KK, Hilsinger RL Jr, Callan EJ: Facial paralysis and Bell's palsy: a protocol for differential diagnosis. *Am J Otol Suppl*:68-73, 1985.
22. Adour K: Nonsurgical management and intervention in disorders of the facial nerve. In Alberti PW, Ruben RJ, editors: *Otologic medicine and surgery,* vol 2. New York, 1988, Churchill Livingstone.
23. Adour KK: Acute facial paralysis method of Kedar Karim Adour, M.D. In Rakel RE, editor. *Conn's Current Therapy,* Philadelphia, 1991, Saunders.
24. Adour KK: Medical management of idiopathic (Bell's) palsy. *Otolaryngol Clin North Am* 24:663-673, 1991.
25. Adour KK: Facial nerve electrical testing. In Jackler RK, Brackmann DE, editors: *Neurotology.* St. Louis, 1993, Mosby–Year Book.
26. Adour KK: Otological complications of herpes zoster. *Ann Neurol* 35:S62-64, 1994.
27. Alford BR, Jerger JF, Coats AC, Peterson CR, Weber SC: Neurophysiology of facial nerve testing. *Arch Otolaryngol* 97:214-219, 1973.
28. Alford BR: Electrodiagnostic studies in facial paralysis. *Arch Otolaryngol* 85:259-264, 1967.
29. Antoni N: Herpes Zoster med Forlamning. *Hygiea* 81:340-353, 1919.
30. Austin JR, Peskind SP, Austin SG, Rice DH: Idiopathic facial nerve paralysis: a randomized double blind controlled study of placebo versus prednisone. *Laryngoscope* 103:1326-1333, 1993.
31. Aviel A, Ostfeld E, Burstein R, et al: Peripheral blood T and B lymphocyte subpopulations in Bell's palsy. *Ann Otol Rhinol Laryngol* 92(2 Pt 1):187-191, 1983.
32. Ballance C, Duel AB: The operative treatment of facial palsy: by the introduction of nerve grafts into the fallopian canal and by other intratemporal methods. *Arch Otolaryngol* 15:1-70, 1932.
33. Baringer JR, Swoveland P: Persistent herpes simplex virus infection in rabbit trigeminal ganglia. *Lab Invest* 30:230-240, 1974.
34. Bell C: On the nerves; giving an account of some experiments on their structure and functions, which lead to a new arrangement of the system. *Philos Trans R Soc Lond,* 111:398-424, 1821.
35. Blackley B, Friedmann I, Wright I: Herpes zoster auris associated with facial nerve palsy and auditory nerve symptoms: a case report with histopathological findings. *Acta Otolaryngol (Stockh)* 63:533-550, 1967.
36. Blatt IM, Freeman JA: Bell's palsy. 3. Further observations on the pathogenesis of Bell's palsy and the results of chorda tympani neurectomy. *Trans Am Acad Ophthalmol Otolaryngol* 73:420-438, 1969.
37. Blunt MJ: The possible role of vascular changes in the aetiology of Bell's palsy. *J Laryngol Otol* 70:701-713, 1956.
38. Blunt MJ: Neurovascular considerations in Bell's palsy. *Med J Aust* 49:74-77, 1962.
39. Bumm P, Schlimok G: Lymphozytensubpopulationen- und HLA-DR-Bestimmungen bei Erkrankungen des Innenohres und Bellschen Paresen (Lymphocyte subpopulations and HLA-DR determinations of diseases of the inner ear and Bell's palsy). *HNO* 34:525-527, 1986.
40. Bumm P, Schlimok G: The results of immunological regulation and immunogenetics in Bell's palsy. In Castro D, editor: *Proceedings of the Sixth International Symposium on the Facial Nerve. Rio de Janeiro, Brazil, October 2-5, 1988,* Amsterdam, 1989, Kugler & Ghedini.
41. Byl FM, Adour KK: Auditory symptoms associated with herpes zoster or idiopathic facial paralysis. *Laryngoscope* 97:372-379, 1977.
42. Campbell EDR: A simple prognostic test in facial palsy. *J Laryngol Otol* 77:462-466, 1963.
43. Cawthorne T: The pathology and surgical treatment of Bell's palsy. *Proc R Soc Med* 44:565-572, 1951.
44. Citron D III, Adour KK: Acoustic reflex and loudness discomfort in acute facial paralysis. *Arch Otolaryngol* 104:303-306, 1978.
45. Coker NJ, Fordice JO, Moore S: Correlation of the nerve excitability test and electroneurography in acute facial paralysis. *Am J Otol* 13:127-133, 1992.
46. Cramer HB, Kartush JM: Testing facial nerve function. *Otolaryngol Clin North Am* 24:555-570, 1991.
47. Dalton GA: Bell's palsy: Some problems of prognosis and treatment. *Br Med J* 1:1765-1770, 1960.

48. Denny-Brown D, Brenner C: Paralysis of nerve induced by direct pressure and by tourniquet. *Arch Neurol Psychiatry* 51:1-26, 1944.
49. Denny-Brown D, Brenner C: Lesion in peripheral nerve resulting from compression by spring clip. *Arch Neurol Psychiatry* 52:1-19, 1944.
50. Devriese PP: Experimental facial nerve decompression in the cat. *Arch Otolaryngol* 95:350-355, 1972.
51. Devriese PP, Schumacher T, Scheide A, et al: Incidence, prognosis and recovery in Bell's palsy: a survey of about 1000 patients (1974-1983). *Clin Otolaryngol* 15:15-27, 1990.
52. Djupesland G, Berdal P, Johannessen TA, Degre M, Stein R, Skrede S: Viral infection as a cause of acute peripheral facial palsy. *Arch Otolaryngol* 102:403-406, 1976.
53. Djupesland G, Degre M, Stien R, Skrede S: Acute peripheral facial palsy: part of a cranial polyneuropathy? *Arch Otolaryngol* 103:641-644, 1977.
54. Duchenne GBA: *De l'électrisation localisée et de son application à la pathologie et à la thérapeutique,* ed 3. Paris, 1872, Baillière. (Cited by Campbell EDR, Hickey RP, Nixon KK, Richardson ST: Value of nerve-excitability measurements in prognosis of facial palsy. *Br Med J* 2:7-10, 1962.)
55. Edström S, Hanner P, Andersen O, et al: Elevated levels of myelin basic protein in CSF in relation to auditory brainstem responses in Bell's palsy. *Acta Otolaryngol (Stockh)* 103(3-4):198-203, 1987.
56. Esslen E: Electrodiagnosis of facial palsy. In Miehlke A, editor: *Surgery of the Facial Nerve,* ed 2. Philadelphia, 1973, Saunders.
57. Esslen E: *The acute facial palsies: investigations on the localization and pathogenesis of meato-labyrinthine facial palsies,* New York, 1977, Springer-Verlag.
58. Fisch U, Esslen E: Total intratemporal exposure of the facial nerve: pathologic findings in Bell's palsy. *Arch Otolaryngol* 95:335-341, 1972.
59. Fisch U: Maximal nerve excitability testing vs electroneuronography. *Arch Otolaryngol* 106:352-357, 1980.
60. Fisch U: Surgery for Bell's palsy. *Arch Otolaryngol* 107:1-11, 1981.
61. Gantz BJ, Gmuer AA, Holliday M, Fisch U: Electroneurographic evaluation of the facial nerve: method and technical problems. *Ann Otol Rhinol Laryngol* 93(4 Pt 1):394-398, 1984.
62. Gavilan J, Gavilan C, Sarria MJ: Facial electroneurography: results on normal humans. *J Laryngol Otol* 99:1085-1088, 1985.
63. Gilliat RW, Taylor JC: Electrical changes following section of the facial nerve. *Proc R Soc Med* 52:1080-1083, 1959.
64. Greer JA, Cody DT, Lambert EH, Weiland LH: Experimental facial nerve paralysis: influence of decompression. *Ann Otol Rhinol Laryngol* 83:582-595, 1974.
65. Hanner P, Andersen O, Frisen L, et al: Clinical observations of effects on central nervous system in patients with acute facial palsy, *Arch Otolaryngol Head Neck Surg* 113:516-520, 1987.
66. Hilger JA: The nature of Bell's palsy. *Laryngoscope* 59:228-235, 1949.
67. Hilger JA: Facial nerve stimulator. *Trans Am Acad Ophthalmol Otolaryngol* 68:74-76, 1964.
68. Hilsinger RL Jr, Adour KK, Doty HE: Idiopathic facial paralysis, pregnancy, and the menstrual cycle. *Ann Otol Rhinol Laryngol* 84:433-442, 1975.
69. House WF: Surgical exposure of the internal auditory canal and its contents through the middle, cranial fossa. *Laryngoscope* 71:1363-1385, 1961.
70. House JW, O'Connor AF, editors: *Handbook of neurotological diagnosis.* New York, 1987, Marcel Dekker.
71. Hughes GB, Josey AF, Glasscock ME, et al: Clinical electroneurography: statistical analysis of controlled measures in twenty-two normal subjects. *Laryngoscope* 91:1834-1836, 1981.
72. Hughes GB, Nodar RH, Williams GW: Analysis of test-retest variability in facial electroneurography. *Otolaryngol Head Neck Surg* 91:290-293, 1983.
73. Hughes GB: Prognostic tests in acute facial palsy. *Am J Otol* 10:304-311, 1989.
74. Hunt JR: On herpetic inflammations of the geniculate ganglion: a new syndrome and its complications. *J Nerv Ment Dis* 34:73-96, 1907.
75. Jongkees LBW: Treatment of Bell's palsy. *Neurology* 7:697-702, 1957.
76. Jongkees LBW: Bell's palsy: a surgical emergency? *Arch Otolaryngol* 81:497-501, 1965.
77. Jongkees LBW: The timing of surgery in intratemporal facial paralysis. *Laryngoscope* 79:1557-1561, 1969.
78. Jonsson L, Sjoberg O, Thomander L: Depression of T cells in Bell's palsy, *Ann Otol Rhinol Laryngol* 97(2 Pt 1):138-141. 1988.
79. Jonsson L, Alm G, Thomander L: Elevated serum interferon levels in patients with Bell's palsy. *Otolaryngol Head Neck Surg* 115:37-40, 1989.
80. Kartush JM, Lilly DJ, Kemink JL: Facial electroneurography: clinical and experimental investigations. *Otolaryngol Head Neck Surg* 93:516-523, 1985.
81. Kerbavaz RJ, Hilsinger RL Jr, Adour KK: The facial paralysis prognostic index. *Otolaryngol Head Neck Surg* 9:284-289, 1983.
82. Kettel K: *Peripheral facial palsy: pathology and surgery.* Springfield, Ill., 1959, Charles C Thomas.
83. Kobayashi T, Kudo Y, Chow M-J: Nerve excitability test using fine needle electrodes, *Acta Otolaryngol Suppl (Stockh)* 446:64-69, 1988.
84. Lathrop FD. The treatment of Bell's palsy. *Lahey Clin Bull* 8:45-48, 1952.
85. Laumans EPJ: Nerve excitability tests in facial paralysis. *Arch Otolaryngol* 81:478-488, 1965.
86. Lewis ML Jr: A variation in technique of facial nerve decompression. *Laryngoscope* 66:1451-1463, 1956.
87. Lewis BI, Adour KK, Kahn JM, Lewis AJ: Hilger facial nerve stimulator: a 25-year update. *Laryngoscope* 101(1 Pt 1):71-74, 1991.
88. Liston SL, Kleid MS: Histopathology of Bell's palsy. *Laryngoscope* 99:23-26, 1989.
89. Magielski JE, Blatt IM: Submaxillary salivary flow: a test of chorda tympani nerve function as an aid in diagnosis and prognosis of facial nerve paralysis. *Laryngoscope* 68:1770-1789, 1958.
90. Manos-Pujol M, Buendia E, Mestre M, et al: Cellular immunity abnormalities in patients with recurrent Bell's palsy, *Clin Otolaryngol* 12:283-287, 1987.
91. Markby DP: Lyme disease facial palsy: differentiation from Bell's palsy. *Br Med J* 299:605-606, 1989.
92. Marsh MA, Coker NJ: Surgical decompression of idiopathic facial palsy. *Otolaryngol Clin North Am* 24:675-689, 1991.
93. Martin RC: Intratemporal suture of the facial nerve. *Arch Otolaryngol* 13:259-264, 1931.
94. Matsumoto Y, Yanagihara N, Sadamoto M: Gd-DTPA-enhanced MR imaging in peripheral facial palsy. *Facial Nerve Res Jpn* 11:93-96, 1991.
95. May M, Harvey JE, Marovitz WF, Stroud M: The prognostic accuracy of the maximum stimulation test compared with that of the nerve excitability test in Bell's palsy. *Laryngoscope* 81:931-938, 1971.
96. May M, Hawkins CD: Bell's palsy: results of surgery; salivation test versus nerve excitability test as a basis of treatment. *Laryngoscope* 82:1337-1348, 1972.
97. May M: Nerve excitability test in facial palsy: limitations on its use, based on a study of 130 cases. *Laryngoscope* 82:2122-2128, 1972.
98. May M: Bell's palsy: progressive ascending paralysis, therapeutic implications. *Laryngoscope* 88(1 Pt 1):61-72, 1978.
99. May M: Total facial nerve exploration: transmastoid, extralabyrinthine, and subtemporal indications and results. *Laryngoscope* 89:906-917, 1979.
100. May M, Klein SR, Blumenthal F: Evoked electromyography and idiopathic facial paralysis. *Otolaryngol Head Neck Surg* 91:678-685, 1983.
101. May M, Blumenthal F, Klein SR: Acute Bell's palsy: prognostic

value of evoked electromyography, maximal stimulation and other electrical tests. *Am J Otol* 5:1-7, 1983.

102. May M, Klein SB: Differential diagnosis of facial nerve palsy. *Otolaryngol Clin North Am* 24:613-645, 1991.
103. McCormick DP: Herpes-simplex virus as cause of Bell's palsy. *Lancet* 1:937-939, 1972.
104. McGovern FH, Konigsmark BW, Sydnor JB: An immunological concept for Bell's palsy: experimental study. *Laryngoscope* 82:1594-1601, 1972.
105. Metz O: The acoustic impedance measured on normal and pathological ears: orientating studies on the applicability of impedance measurement in otological diagnosis. *Acta Otolaryngol Suppl (Stockh)* 63:1-254, 1946.
106. Meurman OH: Endaural tympanic approach to the facial nerve. *Acta Otolaryngol* 49:495-498, 1958.
107. Morris WM: Surgical treatment of Bell's palsy. *Lancet* 1:429-431, 1938.
108. Morris WM: Surgical treatment of facial paralysis: a review of 46 cases. *Lancet* 2:558-561, 1939.
109. Morris WM: Surgical treatment of Bell's palsy. *Neurology* 7:697-702, 1957.
110. Mosforth J, Taverner D: Physiotherapy for Bell's palsy. *Br Med J* 2:675-677, 1958.
111. Nahmias AJ, Roizman B: Infection with herpes-simplex viruses 1, 2, and 3. *N Engl J Med* 289:781-789, 1973.
112. Nakamura Y, Yanagihara N: Neutralization antibody to herpes simplex virus type 1 in Bell's palsy. *Ann Otol Rhinol Laryngol* 137*(suppl)*:18-21, 1988.
113. Ney KW: Facial paralysis and the surgical repair of the facial nerve. *Laryngoscope* 32:327-347, 1922.
114. Olsen PZ: Prediction of recovery in Bell's palsy. *Acta Neurol Scand Suppl* 61:1-121, 1975.
115. Olson NR, Goin DW, Nichols RD, Makim B: Adverse effects of facial nerve decompression for Bell's palsy. *Trans Am Acad Ophthalmol Otolaryngol* 77:ORL67-71, 1973.
116. Park HW, Watkins Al: Facial paralysis: analysis of 500 cases. *Arch Phys Med* 30:749-762, 1949.
117. Peitersen E: The natural history of Bell's palsy. *Am J Otol* 4:107-111, 1982.
118. Pitts DB, Adour KK, Hilsinger RL Jr: Recurrent Bell's palsy: analysis of 140 patients. *Laryngoscope* 98:535-540, 1988.
119. Proctor B, Corgill DA, Proud G: The pathology of Bell's palsy. *Trans Am Acad Ophthalmol Otolaryngol* 82:70-80, 1976.
120. Raslan WF, Wiet R, Zealear DL: A statistical study of EnoG test error. *Laryngoscope* 98:891-893, 1988.
121. Richardson AT, Wynn Parry CB: The theory and practice of electrodiagnosis. *Ann Phys Med* 4:3-16, 1957.
122. Robillard RB, Hilsinger RL Jr, Adour KK: Ramsay Hunt facial paralysis: clinical analysis of 185 patients. *Otolaryngol Head Neck Surg* 95:292-297, 1986.
123. Rosenhall U, Edstrom S, Hanner P, et al: Auditory brain stem response abnormalities in patients with Bell's palsy. *Otolaryngol Head Neck Surg* 91:412-416, 1983.
124. Ruboyianes JM, Adour KK, Santos DQ, Von Doersten PG: The maximal stimulation and facial nerve conduction latency tests: predicting the outcome of Bell's palsy. *Laryngoscope* 104(Suppl 61):1-6, 1994.
125. Safman BL: Bilateral pathology in Bell's palsy. *Arch Otolaryngol* 93:55-57, 1971.
126. Sandstedt P, Hyden D, Odkvist L: Bell's palsy: part of a polyneuropathy? *Acta Neurol Scand* 64:66-73, 1981.
127. Seddon HJ: Three types of nerve injury. *Brain* 66:237-288, 1943.
128. Shambaugh GE Jr: *Surgery of the ear.* Philadelphia, 1959, Saunders.
129. Shiotani M, Yuda Y, Wakasugi B: Comparison of prognoses in Bell's palsy, Ramsay Hunt syndrome and zoster sine herpete. *Facial Nerve Res Jpn* 11:207-210, 1991.
130. Smith IM, Murray JAM, Prescott RJ, Barr-Hamilton R: Facial electroneurography: standardization of electrode position. *Arch Otolaryngol Head Neck Surg* 114:322-325, 1988.
131. Sugita T, Murakami S, Hirata Y, Fujiwara Y, Yanagihara N: Experimental facial nerve paralysis induced by herpes simplex virus. *Facial Nerve Res Jpn* 11:52, 1991.
132. Sullivan JA, Smith JB: The otological concept of Bell's palsy and its treatment. *Ann Otol Rhinol Laryngol* 59:1148-1170, 1950.
133. Sunderland S: *Nerves and nerve injuries,* ed 2. Edinburgh, 1978, Churchill Livingstone.
134. Taverner D: Bell's palsy: a clinical and electromyographic study. *Brain* 78:209-235, 1955.
135. Taverner D: Electrodiagnosis in facial palsy. *Arch Otolaryngol* 81:470-477, 1965.
136. Taverner D: Surgery versus conservative treatment in peripheral facial palsies: round table discussion. (Jongkees LBW, moderator). *Arch Otolaryngol* 81:532-546, 1965.
137. Taverner D, Cohen SB, Hutchinson BC: Comparison of corticotrophin and prednisolone in treatment of idiopathic facial paralysis (Bell's palsy). *Br Med J* 4:20-22, 1971.
138. Thomander L, Stålberg E: Electroneurography in the prognostication of Bell's palsy. *Acta Otolaryngol (Stockh)* 92:221-237, 1981.
139. Thomas MH: Treatment of Bell's palsy with cortisone and other measures. *Neurology (Minneap)* 5:882-886, 1955.
140. Tickle TG: Nerve graft operation for facial paralysis. In Symposium: Deep infections of the neck. *Laryngoscope* 49:475-481, 1939.
141. Tien R, Dillon WP, Jackler RK: Contrast-enhanced MR imaging of the facial nerve in 11 patients with Bell's palsy. *Am J Neuroradiol* 11:735-741, 1990.
142. Tonning FM: The reliability of level-diagnostic examinations in acute, peripheral facial palsy. *Acta Otolaryngol (Stockh)* 84(5-6):414-415, 1977.
143. Tschiassny K: The site of the facial nerve lesion in cases of Ramsey Hunt syndrome. *Ann Otol Rhinol Laryngol* 55:152-174, 1946.
144. Tschiassny K: Eight syndromes of facial paralysis and their significance in locating the lesion. *Ann Otol Rhinol Laryngol* 62:677-693, 1953.
145. Tumarkin IA: Some aspects of the problem of facial paralysis. *Proc R Soc Med* 29:1685-1691, 1936.
146. Tumarkin IA: The pathology and surgical treatment of Bell's palsy. *Proc R Soc Med* 44:565-572, 1951.
147. Tzadik A, Babin RW, Ryu JH: Hypotension-induced neurapraxia in the cat facial nerve. *Otolaryngol Head Neck Surg* 90:163-167, 1982.
148. Ushiro K, Yanagida M, Iwano T, Hosoda Y: Gd-DTPA enhanced MRI in patients with Ramsay Hunt syndrome. *Facial Nerve Res Jpn* 11:133-138, 1991.
149. Vahlne A, Edström S, Arstila P, Beran M, Ejnell H, Nylén O, et al: Bell's palsy and herpes simplex virus. *Arch Otolaryngol* 107:79-81, 1981.
150. Warren KG, Brown SM, Wroblewska A, et al: Isolation of latent herpes simplex virus from the superior cervical and vagus ganglions of human beings. *N Engl J Med* 298:1068-1069, 1979.
151. Wayman DM, Pham HN, Byl FM, Adour KK: Audiological manifestations of Ramsay Hunt syndrome. *J Laryngol Otol* 104:104-108, 1990.
152. Yanagihara N, Kishimoto M: Electrodiagnosis in facial palsy. *Arch Otolaryngol* 95:376-382, 1972.
153. Yanagihara N: Etiology and pathophysiology of Bell's palsy. *Ann Otol Rhinol Laryngol Suppl,* 137, 1988.

22

Evaluation of the Dizzy Patient

Dennis I. Bojrab, M.D.,* Joel A. Goebel, M.D., F.A.C.S., and Charles W. Stockwell, Ph.D.

Although many technologic advances have become readily available to the practicing otolaryngologist, an accurate and thorough clinical history and physical examination remains the most important part of the evaluation of the patient that complains of dizziness. A specific diagnosis can be reached in the majority of patients with dizziness with a careful bedside evaluation. This chapter is dedicated to the understanding of the clinical approach to the dizzy patient. The good clinician must have a methodic approach to obtaining the clinical history and physical examination. The complete physical examination is based on a thorough knowledge of the relevant anatomy and pathophysiology of the vestibular system and its central projections. Understanding the vestibular evaluation by electronystagmography, rotation chair testing, posturrography, and head shake testing is demonstrated from a practical standpoint. (Medication, rehabilitation, and surgical treatment of the dizzy patient with emphasis on specific disease entities and case management presentations are presented in the sequel course.)

DEFINITIONS

Dizziness is a nonspecific term that describes a sensation of altered orientation in space. Because vestibular, visual, and proprioceptive signals provide the main source of information about the position of the head and body in space, damage to any of these afferent systems can lead to a complaint of dizziness. Changes in the brain centers that integrate these orienting signals can also result in the sensation of dizziness (see box on p 266).

Types of dizziness

Vertigo. Vertigo is a sensation of movement, of either self or of the environment. The illusion is that of rotation, linear displacement, or tilt. This perception is distinct from self motion during natural locomotion; vertigo is linked to impaired perception of a stationary environment. It is the mismatch between the actual multisensory inputs and the expected pattern of sensory stimulation with the head stationary that causes vertigo. The nature of the vertigo may distinguish between disturbance of the semicircular canals, which sense angular rotations, and the otoliths, which sense linear movements or tilts of the head. Thus, rotational vertigo connotes disturbance of the semicircular canals or their central projections. Sensations of body tilt, levitation, or lateropulsion imply otolithic disturbance or central projections.

The afferent nerves from the semicircular canals and otoliths of each labyrinth maintain a balanced tonic rate of firing into the vestibular nuclei. Asymmetric involvement of this baseline activity anywhere in the peripheral and central vestibular pathways leads to an illusion of movement. For example, damage to a semicircular canal or its afferent nerve produces a sensation of angular rotation in the plane of that canal similar to the sensation experienced during physiologic stimulation. Lesions of all canals and otoliths of one labyrinth become injured, a sensation of rotation in the plane determined by the balance of afferent signals from the contralateral labyrinth (usually the horizontal plane, since the vertical canals and otoliths signals partially cancel out).

The direction of the patients vertiginous illusions is often uncertain. This is because the vestibular sense indicates self-rotation in one direction, but the eye movements (slow phases of vestibular nystagmus) cause visual image movements that, when self referred, denote self-rotation to the opposite side. It is therefore worthwhile to evaluate the vestibular sense alone by asking specifically about the perceived direction of self-rotation with the eyes closed, thus eliminating any possible confounding visual stimuli. On the other hand, with the eyes open, one should ask about the

*Send reprints and questions: Dennis I Bojrab, M.D., EAR Consultants of Michigan Assistant Clinical Professor, Wayne State University, 3535 West 13 Mile Road, Suite 444, Royal Oak, Michigan, 48075

Classification of Dizziness

Dizziness is the term used to describe any of a variety of sensations that produce spacial disorientation

Vertigo	Disequilibrium
Oscillopsia	Lightheadedness
Visual distortion	Multisensory
Physiologic	Psychophysiologic

direction of image motion from which one can deduce the direction of the nystagmus (slow-phase direction is opposite to image motion). Another factor that may confuse the interpretation of acute vestibular symptoms is that compensatory vestibulospinal reactions may cause a sensation of falling toward the side of the lesion.

Central verses peripheral causes of vertigo are often difficult to differentiate. The same sensation can result from such diverse locations as the inner ear, the deep paravertebral stretch receptors of the neck, the visual-vestibular interactions centers in the brain stem and the cerebellum, or in the subjective sensation pathways of the thalamus or cortex. Distinction between peripheral and central causes of vertigo can frequently be made based on other features in the history. For instance, peripheral causes of vertigo are often associated with severe nausea and possibly vomiting and mild imbalance, occasionally with hearing loss, tinnitus, aural fullness, or otalgia. Recovery is relatively rapid. Central causes of vertigo causes less nausea and greater imbalance, rarely with hearing problems. Compensation is slow, and there may be the presence of other neurologic symptoms of headache, cranial neuropathy, or confusion.

Disequilibrium. Patients may use the term of dizziness to describe a sensation of imbalance or disequilibrium that occurs when they are standing or walking that is unrelated to an abnormal head sensation. Imbalance is common with acute unilateral peripheral vestibular lesions, but it is transient and invariably associated with subjective vertigo. The symptom of disequilibrium represents the normal pattern of compensation after an acute vestibular loss pattern and can last weeks to months, depending on the severity of the injury. The imbalance due to loss of vestibulospinal and proprioceptive function is typically worse in the dark when the patient is unable to use vision to compensate for the loss. Patients with cerebellar lesions show little change in the balance with and without vision (Romberg test). Disequilibrium may be the presenting symptom of lesions involving the motor centers of the basal ganglia, and frontal lobes such as with Parkinson's disease, hydrocephalus, and the multiple lacunar infarct syndrome.

Presyncopal lightheadedness. This is a sensation of impending faint. It is often associated with a sensation of unsteadiness or falling. This results from pancerebral ischemia and is not a sign of impending stroke or focal occlusive cerebrovascular disease. This symptom has been experienced by all of us by rapidly standing from a supine or sitting position. This may be secondary to *orthostatic hypotension* from acute or chronic blood volume loss, antihypertensive drugs, autonomic dysfunction, antidepressants, and major tranquilizers. Decreased cardiac output from arrythmia, valvular heart disease, or heart failure are other causes of lightheadedness. *Vasovagal attacks* may occur with such emotions as fear and anxiety. Symptoms include lightheadedness, giddiness, nausea, and an abdominal sinking sensation. Parasympathetic hyperactivity may elicit piloerection, sweating, slowing of the heart rate, and diminished sympathetic tone leading to vasodilation. *Hyperventilation* syndrome is a common cause of lightheadedness found in young adults.

Ocular dizziness. This is the sensation that many people have experienced when they first wear glasses. The description is that of disorientation and headache. The dizziness most frequently accompanies correction of astigmatism but also occurs after a change in magnification. This sensation may occur in patients who undergo lens implant after cataract removal to correct severe visual loss. Dizziness may also be a result from an imbalance in the extraocular muscles. Oscillopsia is the optic illusion that stationary objects are moving back and forth or up and down. When brought on or accentuated by head movement, it is usually of vestibular origin and reflects an inappropriate vestibulo-ocular reflex (VOR) gain or phase. Vision becomes blurred so that fine print on grocery items can only be detected if the patient stands still in the store aisle. It is usually a sign of vestibular, brain stem, or cerebellar involvement. Rarely it may be secondary to a lesion in the visual association areas in the cortex. In the acute phase of loss of labyrinthine function, the inadequate VOR results in movements of visual images on the retina with every head movement; this causes oscillopsia and impaired vision. Patients with partial bilateral vestibular loss tend to show preferential sparing of the VOR for high-frequency stimuli.

Multisensory dizziness. Occasionally, one can trace dizziness to disease involving multiple sensory systems, especially in the elderly and in patients with systemic disorders such as diabetes mellitus. This condition may be found in the diabetic patient with peripheral neuropathy (decreasing proprioceptive cues), retinal disease (decreasing visual acuity), and vestibular dysfunction.

Physiologic dizziness. Physiologic dizziness refers to a group of phenomena that occur in normal subjects with physiologic stimulation of the vestibular, visual, or somatosensory systems. It typically results from a mismatch in sensory signals, resulting in a feeling of disorientation, imbalance, and vegetation symptoms. Motion sickness, space sickness, height vertigo, and Mal de Barquement syndrome are examples of physiologic dizziness.

Psychophysiologic dizziness. A wide range of dizzy sensations are associated with psychiatric illness. Feelings

Dizziness Questionnaire

1. Patient's description	To write out description		
2. Medical description	"Spinning in circles, world spinning around you, spinning in head, falling or pulling to one side, etc."		
3. Typify dizzy spell	When was the first occurrence		
	Continuous or in spells, how long, and how often		
	Related to head or body positions	Yes	No
	Occurs when laying down or rolling over in bed	Yes	No
	Nausea associated with spells	Yes	No
	Fullness or ringing of ears associated with spells	Yes	No
	Hearing loss associated with spells	Yes	No
	Recent ear drainage or pain in the ear	Yes	No
	Are you better when lying still during a spell	Yes	No
	Trouble walking in the dark	Yes	No
	Weakness after eating	Yes	No
	Dizzy after standing up suddenly	Yes	No
	Dizziness related to menstrual cycle	Yes	No
	Dizziness after exertion	Yes	No
4. Other sensations	Fainting	Yes	No
	Headaches	Yes	No
	Double or blurred vision	Yes	No
	Numbness in the face or extremities	Yes	No
	Weakness or clumsiness in arms or legs	Yes	No
	Slurred speech or difficulty swallowing	Yes	No
	Tingling around your mouth	Yes	No
	Spots before your eyes	Yes	No
	Jerking or trembling of extremities	Yes	No
	Confusion or memory loss	Yes	No
5. Hearing	Hearing loss in one ear	R	L B
	Ringing in one ear or both	R	L B
	Change of hearing with dizziness	Yes	No
	Previous ear surgeries	Yes	No
	Exposure to loud noises	Yes	No
	Family history of deafness	Yes	No
6. Past medical history	Allergies	Medications, foods, or inhalants	
	Medications	Especially for hypertension, diabetes, thyroid, asthma, seizures, sleep, nerve pills, dizziness, nonprescription drugs	
	Surgeries	Ear, endocrine, brain, other	
	Social history	Smoking, drinking, stress	

of dissociation, as though one has left one's own body, are common. Patients use the term of floating or swimming. They may report a feeling of imbalance (commonly a rocking or falling sensation) or even spinning inside the head. These sensations may be confused with vertigo, except that they are not associated with an illusion of movement of the environment or with nystagmus. This dizziness may be constant or occur in attacks frequently associated with symptoms of anxiety. Commonly associated somatic complaints include a sensation of tension headache, heart palpitations, gastric distress, urinary frequency, backache, or a general feeling of weakness. Common examples of this type of disorder are panic attacks, agoraphobia, and acute and chronic anxiety.

HISTORY

Vertigo is a frightening and potentially debilitating disease. Treatment of the disorder begins with reassurance to the patient of the availability and the interest of the physician. A complete history should include a description of the nature of the dizziness, time course, precipitating factors, and associated symptoms. A patient questionnaire is helpful in allowing the patient to organize thoughts. This is given to the patient prior to the initial physician-patient encounter. The questionnaire is organized into segments to augment the clinical history (see box above). The initial task of the clinician is to obtain a description of what the patient means by dizziness. Patients should be encouraged to use their own words to describe the sensation and how

Duration of Common Causes of Vertigo

Seconds	Benign positional vertigo
	Posttraumatic labyrinthine dysfunction
Minutes	Vertebrobasilar insufficiency
	Migraine attacks with or without headache
Hours	Meniere's syndrome
Days-weeks	Vestibular neuritis
	Acute toxic or traumatic labyrinthine injury
	Labyrinthine infarction

this sensation interferes with their daily activities. In the authors' experience, less than half of patients complaining of dizziness actually have vertigo. Because the diagnostic evaluation and management differ markedly depending on the category of dizziness, it is critical that the examining physician determine the type of dizziness before proceeding with exhaustive diagnostic studies.

The time course of vertigo is helpful in determining the type of lesion present. Continuous dizziness without fluctuation for long periods of time is not typical of vestibular disorders. (See box above).

Episodes lasting for seconds suggest the diagnosis of benign positional vertigo. During the acute phase patients may report a nonspecific feeling of disorientation and imbalance along with nausea and vomiting that lasts for minutes to hours. The vertigo is often short in duration and quite severe, with a more persistent nonspecific dizziness lasting for hours to days. Some patients with posttraumatic labyrinthine injuries may experience brief spells of vertigo, lasting for seconds, that may occur spontaneously or with certain head or body movements. An episode of vertigo lasting for minutes suggests a transient vascular ischemic attack such as that experienced in patients with transient ischemia within the basilar vertebral circulation and for migraine attacks with or without headache. With a typical bout of Ménière's syndrome, the vertigo may occur abruptly or crescendo over minutes and remain severe for one or two hours. The symptoms usual include disorientation or imbalance for hours to occasionally days. Vestibular neuritis, toxic labyrinthitis, labyrinthine trauma, infarction of the labyrinth, or any lesion that produces acute and permanent damage to the inner ear or vestibular nerve produce vertigo, disorientation, and disequilibrium that lasts for days to weeks. Even with a complete unilateral loss of vestibular function, the vertigo will gradually resolve as central compensation occurs.

Associated symptoms are usually presents with vertigo of vestibular lesions. Autonomic symptoms such as sweating, pallor, and nausea with or without vomiting. Typically, the autonomic symptoms are more pronounced when the vertigo has a peripheral origin, although there are frequent exceptions to this dictum. This is due to the numerous interconnecting pathways between brain stem vestibular and autonomic centers which accounts for this close association of vestibular and autonomic symptoms. The site of lesion determines the symptoms that accompany vertigo (see box above).

Associated Symptoms and Site of Lesion

- Inner ear
  - Hearing loss
  - Tinnitus
  - Aural pressure
  - Otalgia
  - Drop attacks (rarely)
- IAC* and C-P angle†
  - Hearing loss
  - Tinnitus
  - Facial numbness or weakness
- Brain stem
  - Facial numbness or weakness
  - Diplopia
  - Dysarthria
  - Extremity incoordination, weakness, or numbness
  - Drop attacks
- Cerebellum
  - Imbalance
  - Incoordination
- Temporal or occipital lobes
  - Visual, olfactory, or gustatory hallucinations
  - Visual field loss

*IAC = internal auditory canal.
†CPA = cerebelopontine angle.

Precipitating factors are important in the clinical history and may determine the illness. Rapid head movements commonly induce vertigo because they accentuate any imbalance within the vestibular pathways. Positional vertigo is commonly induced by turning over in bed, sitting up from a lying position, extending the neck to look up, or bending over and straightening up. Even after compensation has occurred, head movements or change in position can lead to a brief sensation of vertigo and disorientation. In a patient with an hypofunctioning labyrinth, movement toward the side of lesion is generally more troublesome because of the lack of usual stimulation of the vestibulocular or vestibulospinal reflexes. Patients with a perilymphatic fistula develop brief episodes of vertigo precipitated by changes in the middle ear pressure. The pressure change in the middle ear is transferred directly to the inner ear through the fistula. In patients with Ménière's syndrome or disease, patients may occasionally experience transient vertigo with pressure changes in the middle ear or with loud noises (Tulio's phenomenon). This may occur because of adhesions between the stapedius footplate and the membranous labyrinth with sudden movement of the stapes.

Predisposing factors should be investigated in the past medical history. The patient's general health prior to the onset of dizziness should be carefully investigated. Patients with an acute severe vertigo attack suggestive of a peripheral vestibular loss pattern may have a viral neurolabyrinthitis with a history of previous upper respiratory tract infection. Chronic middle ear or mastoid infections may lead to bacterial or serous labyrinthinitis. Patients with bacterial meningitis may develop a bacterial labyrinthitis through the direct cerebrospinal fluid and perilymph connections.

Patients with Ménière's syndrome may have ingested a high salt load, allergic stimulant, or another substance triggering endolymphatic hydrops. Some systemic disorders such as vasculitis, endocarditis, or septicemia may incur damage to the vestibular system by damage to vestibular system that causes acute interference with its blood supply. Other chronic systemic illnesses such as diabetes mellitus, atherosclerotic vascular disease, syphilis (congenital or acquired) may cause a vestibular system injury. Viral illnesses (rubella, mumps, rubeola) that damage the inner ear in utero, infancy, or childhood may initially cause only symptoms of hearing loss which may be followed years later by episodic vertigo. The deafened ear may be the focus of so-called delayed endolymphatic hydrops years later (frequently the third or fourth decade of life).

A careful drug history is important when evaluating any patient with dizziness. Ototoxic drugs such as the aminoglycosides and salicylates occasionally may cause vertigo but more typically an unsteadiness or oscillopsia from bilateral symmetrical vestibular endorgan damage. Antihypertensive medications may produce lightheadedness secondary to postural hypotension. Anticoagulants can be associated with an acute inner ear hemorrhage. Alcohol and phenytoin produce acute reversible disequilibrium from cerebellar dysfunction. Positional vertigo and nystagmus commonly occur with acute alcohol intoxication. Sedative drugs (antihistamines, benzodiazepines, or barbiturates) cause a nonspecific dizziness typically described as giddiness or cloudiness presumably secondary to diffuse depression of the central sensory integration.

Family history may be of help, especially in those patients with a family history of migraine, Ménière's syndrome, otosclerosis, neurofibromatosis, and spinocerebellar degeneration.

Head injury commonly damages the delicate labyrinthine membranes with or without associated temporal bone fracture. Labyrinthine trauma may result in a single prolonged episode of vertigo, positional vertigo, or sudden bursts of vertigo episodically or associated with head or body movements. Surgery in or about the ear may result in trauma to the delicate membranes of the labyrinth.

PHYSICAL EXAMINATION

The critical areas in the examination of the patient with dizziness are summarized in Table 22-1. They include a general thorough examination to include vital signs, head and neck, ear, otoneurologic, cranial nerves, and cerebellar function. The vital signs are to include respiration rate, heart rate, and blood pressure. If the patient has complaints of presyncopal lightheadedness, it is beneficial to hyperventilate the patient to see if the symptoms are reproduced. Also, lightheadedness may be associated with body position changes that cause fluctuations in blood pressure, therefore a fluctuation of heart rate or blood pressure may be of significance when standing up quickly after sitting or lying down. The head and neck includes a good otolaryngologic examination. Auscultation for bruits in the neck is included. Heart murmurs may also be of significance.

TABLE 22-1
Critical areas in the physical examination of the patient with dizziness

Vital signs	Head and neck
Ear	Otoneurologic
Cranial nerves	Cerebellar

The external ear is examined for signs of obstruction, swelling, otorrhea, or skin lesions such as vesicles that may indicate herpes zoster oticus. The ear is examined for signs of previous surgery. Next an otoscope or microscope is used to examine the tympanic membrane to search for retraction pockets, cholesteatoma, middle ear fluid, or middle ear masses such as vascular lesions (glomus tumors or aberrant carotid artery). Movement of the tympanic membrane is performed with pneumotoscopy to check for middle ear fluid. Hearing testing for estimating loudness sensitivity and for differentiating between a conductive and a sensorineural hearing loss is performed with tuning forks. The Rinne test is performed with first a 512 Hz fork. If the test is negative (bone conduction louder than air conduction), indicating a conductive hearing loss, the test is repeated with the 1024 Hz fork to assess the degree of loss. If the test is still negative, the patient has at least a moderate conductive loss. If the test is positive (air conduction louder than bone conduction), hearing is tested with a higher tuning fork to check for a high-frequency sensorineural hearing loss. The Weber test is performed as a check for lateralization to either the conductive hearing loss ear or for the ear with the sensorineural hearing loss.

The otoneurologic examination is performed with particular attention to the fistula test, vestibulo-ocular reflexes, and the vestibulospinal reflexes. The fistula test is performed by transiently increasing and decreasing the pressure in the external ear canal. Pressure is maintained for 20 seconds. Added pressure may be administered by instructing the patient to hold the nose and swallow to essentially perform the Valsalva maneuver. A positive fistula sign is a transient burst of nystagmus and vertigo. This occurs in patients with a labyrinthine fistula, and the nystagmus may be in the direction toward or away from the tested ear. Some patients may experience symptoms of nausea or dizziness without frank nystagmus, and this may be of clinical significance. Patients with Meniere's syndrome may in fact have adhesions between the stapedius footplate and the membranous labyrinth, and sudden movement of the stapes produces vestibular symptoms.

If the patient wears glasses, he/she is allowed to wear glasses during the examination. The eyes are examined in the primary position for any nystagmus. The examiner places his two thumbs approximately 60° apart at least 3 ft from the patient and the patient is to simply fixate from thumb to thumb several times to determine overshoot or undershoot nystagmus. Then pursuit is checked by following the examiner's thumb in the horizontal and vertical planes, then divergence and convergence is checked. If any of this is abnormal, these maneuvers are repeated.

Following this, a Snellen wall chart is used and the patient undergoes passive then active head shake tests, at which time the head shakes for approximately 20 seconds. The eyes are left open and the patient is asked if the chart blurs. Remember, that an intact vestibular ocular reflex should keep the image fairly still. The patient should be able to read within three lines on the chart. If the chart cannot be read within three lines of the initial still head reading, the test is considered a positive test for oscillopsia or vestibular asymmetry (see head shake nystagmus).

Further tests of the vestibulo-ocular reflex include head shake nystagmus, positioning and positional testing, and caloric testing. The head shake test is performed with Frenzel glasses, and the head is tilted roughly at 30° downward to place the lateral canal in the horizontal plane. The head is then passively vigorously rotated in the horizontal plane for 20 seconds. The eyes are then examined with the backlit Frenzel glasses for any nystagmus. Patients with a compensated vestibular imbalance due to either peripheral or central lesions may develop a transient spontaneous nystagmus after vigorous head shaking. Spontaneous nystagmus after head shaking is abnormal, indicating an imbalance within the vestibulo-ocular pathways.

Positional testing is an important part of the vestibular examination, particularly in patients who complain of vertigo with change in head position. A distinction should be made between paroxysmal nystagmus induced by rapidly placing the patient in specific head-hanging positions and nystagmus that persists while the patient is held in a static position.

The most useful procedure is to rapidly bring the patient to a supine, head-handing position, with the head turned to the right, left, or center. With the patient sitting, the head is turned toward one shoulder. The examiner stands in front of the patient and grasps the head bitemporally. Having informed the patient of the nature of the test, the head, neck, and trunk are briskly moved to a head-hanging position (Hallpike maneuver) about 30° below the horizontal. Note the eye movements in primary position and on left and right gaze. After about 45 seconds, return the patient to the primary position and observe the eye movements again. Repeat the whole procedure with the head rotated toward the other shoulder and, finally, with the head directed straight back. Transient nystagmus induced by these maneuvers is usually diagnostic of benign paroxysmal positional vertigo.

Testing for nystagmus with static changes in head position (e.g., with the subject lying supine, head turned to the right or the left) is less useful since some normal subjects show a horizontal nystagmus (with respect to their heads) in this position in darkness. In some subjects, this horizontal nystagmus occurs with the head turned right or left (direction fixed), but in others it changes direction with lateral head turn (direction changing) such that it is either always beating toward the earth (geotropic) or always beating away from the earth (ageotropic or apogeotropic). Geotropic and ageotropic nystagmus probably represent the effects of changing otolithic inputs but may be encountered with either peripheral or central vestibular lesions. Findings that point to a pathologic process causing positional nystagmus include nystagmus with large slow-phase velocity, persistence during visual fixation, nystagmus present with more than one head position, and purely vertical or torsional nystagmus. These tests are best performed with the patient wearing Frenzel goggles.

The caloric test uses a nonphysiologic stimulus to induce endolymphatic flow in the horizontal semicircular canal and thus horizontal nystagmus by creating a temperature gradient from one side of the canal to the other. Because of its availability, iced water (approximately 0° C) is usually used for bedside testing. A major advantage over rotatory testing is that caloric testing allows selective stimulation of one labyrinth at a time. It is usually performed with the patient in the supine position, head tilted 30° up, placing the horizontal canal in the vertical plane. To avoid inadequate stimulation, 10 ml of iced water should be used. After infusion of the water into the external canal (with as little as 0.2 ml), the endolymph circulates because of the difference in specific gravity on the two sides of the canal. This induces a brief burst of nystagmus (1 to 2 min in duration), with slow phase toward and fast phase away from the side of stimulation. In a comatose patient only a slow tonic deviation toward the side of stimulation is observed. In normal subjects the duration and speed of induced nystagmus varies greatly depending on the size of the external canal, the thickness of the temporal bone, the circulation to the temporal bone, and the subject's ability to use fixation to suppress the nystagmus. In any given subject, however, the responses tend to be symmetric. Greater than 20% asymmetry in nystagmus duration is usually abnormal.

Physical examination signs of vestibulo ocular reflex (VOR) dysfunction

During the physical examination of the dizzy patient, certain findings are highly suggestive of peripheral labyrinthine dysfunction. These key signs include: (1) spontaneous nystagmus, (2) post-headshake nystagmus, (3) paroxysmal positioning nystagmus, (4) refixation saccades, and (5) impaired dynamic visual acuity.

Spontaneous nystagmus. Spontaneous nystagmus of peripheral vestibular origin is the result of static asymmetry in eighth nerve input to the brain stem between the intact and the impaired labyrinth. The nystagmus is seen best in the dark (recorded by electro-oculography) or behind Frenzel's glasses to inhibit fixation. By definition, this nystagmus is seen in the sitting position with no provocation. The nystagmus increases in intensity while the patient gazes in the direction of the fast component. Most authors feel that the slow-component velocity of a significant spontaneous nystagmus is >5 to 7 deg/s. Spontaneous nystagmus usually denotes a recent onset of injury since the static asymmetry is modified by CNS input rather quickly.

Post-headshake nystagmus. In certain patients with peripheral disease and no spontaneous nystagmus, a 20 to 30 second headshake at 2 Hz produces a post-headshake nystagmus which usually beats (fast phase) toward the stronger ear. This reaction is thought to occur due to the asymmetric input during head rotations toward versus away from the intact ear (stronger signals with ipsilateral rotations) and the storage of this input within the brain stem and ultimate discharge immediately following the maneuver. Although not all post-headshake nystagmus is due to peripheral disease, the presence of this sign in conjunction with a history suggestive of labyrinthine dysfunction is quite helpful to strengthen the case for inner ear dysfunction.

Paroxysmal positioning nystagmus. The finding of a horizontal-rotary nystagmus (horizontal component ageotropic) during the Hallpike maneuver is diagnostic of benign paroxysmal positioning nystagmus. The characteristic latency, fatigue and habituation of the nystagmus are noted and the disease is nearly always localized to the downmost ear. No further workup is indicated at this point if the nystagmus is typical in all the above-mentioned features and hearing is symmetric on audiometry.

Refixation saccades. In high-velocity head movements, the VOR is the predominant (if not sole) mechanism for maintaining visual fixation. If the VOR is deficient, the eye travels with the head during rotation and then relocates the intended target with a compensatory saccade. This can be seen in the office easily by either keen observation of the pupillary landmarks or ophthalmoscopy of retinal vessels during impulsive head movements with attempted fixation. When seen in one direction only, the presence of refixation saccades implies VOR dysfunction on the ipsilateral side to the head turn. This may be the only localizing sign on examination. When bidirectional, refixation saccades imply bilateral VOR dysfunction (e.g., ototoxicity, trauma, aging).

Dynamic visual acuity. In a related fashion to refixation saccades, impairment of visual acuity during head movement implies impairment of VOR function. Another way to document this is the so-called dynamic visual acuity test. Have the patient read the lowest line on an eye chart with the head still and then repeat the task 30 seconds later with the head in motion above 2 Hz. If visual acuity degrades more than three lines, VOR function is considered significantly impaired. Changes in dynamic visual acuity almost certainly imply bilateral VOR dysfunction.

As a general rule, bedside tests of vestibulospinal function lack specificity and sensitivity. It is difficult to distinguish vestibular signs from those resulting from lesions of the proprioceptive and cerebellar pathways. Furthermore, an acute vestibulospinal imbalance is rapidly compensated for so that a chronic lesion may be undetectable even when the tests are performed with the patient's eyes closed. "Past pointing" refers to a reactive deviation of the extremities caused by an imbalance in the vestibular system. The test is performed by having the patient place his extended index finger on that of the examiner, close his eyes, raise the extended arm and index finger to a vertical position, and attempt to return his index finger to the examiner's. Consistent deviation to one side is termed "past pointing." As with all tests of vestibulospinal function, extralabyrinthine influences should be eliminated as much as possible by having the patient seated, with eyes closed and arms and index fingers extended throughout the test. The standard finger-to-nose test does not identify past pointing since joint and muscle proprioceptive signs permit accurate localization even when vestibular function is lost. Patients with acute peripheral vestibular damage past point toward the side of loss, but compensation rapidly corrects the past pointing and can even produce a drift to the other side.

For the Romberg test the patient stands with feet together, arms folded against the chest, and eyes closed. Patients with acute unilateral labyrinthine lesions sway and fall toward the damaged side. Like the past pointing test, however, the Romberg test is not a good indicator of chronic unilateral vestibular impairment, and sometimes the patient will fall toward the intact side. The sharpened Romberg test is often a more sensitive indicator of vestibular impairment. For this test the patient stands with feet aligned in the tandem heel-to-toe position with eyes closed and arms folded against the chest. Normal subjects can stand in this position for 30 seconds, whereas patients with unilateral or bilateral vestibular impairment can rarely sustain the position.

When performed with the patient's eyes open, tandem walking or heel-to-toe walking is usually a test of cerebellar function since vision compensates for chronic vestibular and proprioceptive deficits. Acute vestibular lesions, however, may impair tandem walking with the patient's eyes open. Tandem walking with the patient's eyes closed provides a good test of vestibular function as long as cerebellar and proprioceptive function are intact. As with other tests of vestibulospinal function, however, the direction of falling in patients with chronic lesions is not a reliable indicator of the side of the lesion. So-called stepping or

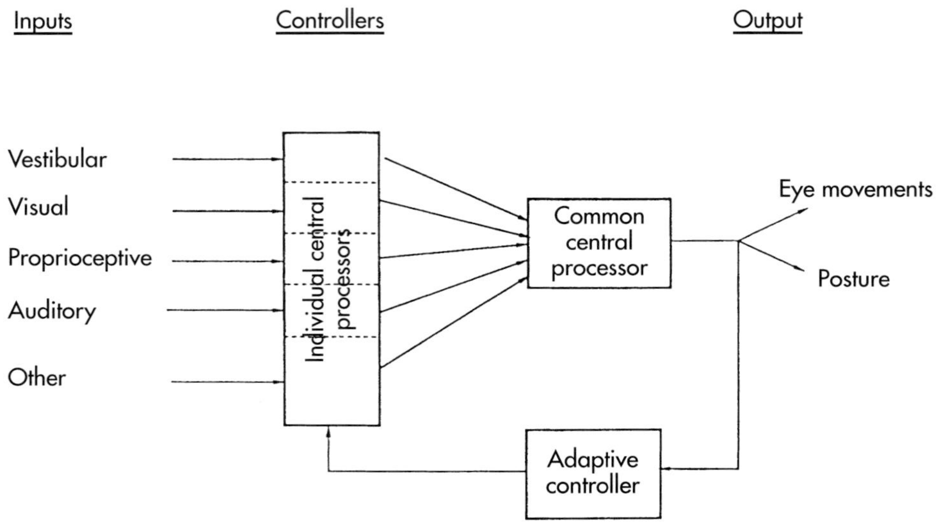

FIG 22-1
Integrative nature of oculomotor and posture control. (Reprinted with permission: Baloh, RW, Honrubia, V: Clinical Neurophysiology of the Vestibular System. Philadelphia, 1990, FA Davis.)

TABLE 22-2
Otoneurologic exam

Ear	Appearance, pressure test, tuning fork
Eyes	Ocular motility, pursuit, convergence and divergence pathologic nystagmus
VOR*	Frenzel glasses used Head shake, positional, and calorics
VSR†	Romberg, Fukuda, Tandem, past ponting

*Vestibulo-ocular reflex.
†Vestibulospinal tract reflex.

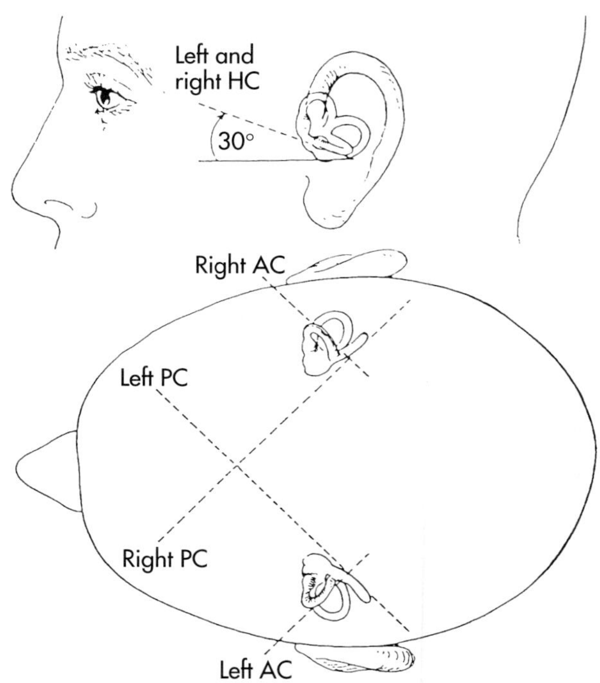

FIG 22-2
Bilateral orientation of the semicircular canals and otic capsule within the human temporal bones. (Reprinted with permission: Baloh, RW, Honrubia, V: Clinical Neurophysiology of the Vestibular System. Philadelphia, 1990, FA Davis.)

marching tests have the same limitations as the tandem walking test (see Table 22-2).

APPLIED ANATOMY AND PHYSIOLOGY

Maintenance of visual and postural control is a complex process involving: (1) multiple sensory inputs, (2) central integration and selection of orientationally correct inputs, (3) execution of proper motor commands, and (4) feedback. The prime inputs for these tasks come through the visual, vestibular, and somatosensory and proprioceptive pathways (Fig. 22-1). Fortunately, visual stability and posture control can be maintained with as little as one correct sensory input, although, under ideal circumstances, all sensory systems deliver overlapping orientationally correct information. Therefore, in order to evaluate and treat dizziness and imbalance, the examiner must understand each sensory input and its integration within the CNS into a usable motor command.

The vestibular labyrinth and central connections

Semicircular canal anatomy and physiology. The otic capsule (the hardest bone in the body) houses the three semicircular canals, utricle, and saccule within the paired temporal bones in the human skull (Fig. 22-2). The semicircular canals are arranged at approximate right angles to each other and each canal is coplanar with its partner on the other side. The paired horizontal (lateral) canals are actually tipped 30° backward off the yaw axis. The superior (anterior) canal on one side is roughly coplanar with the

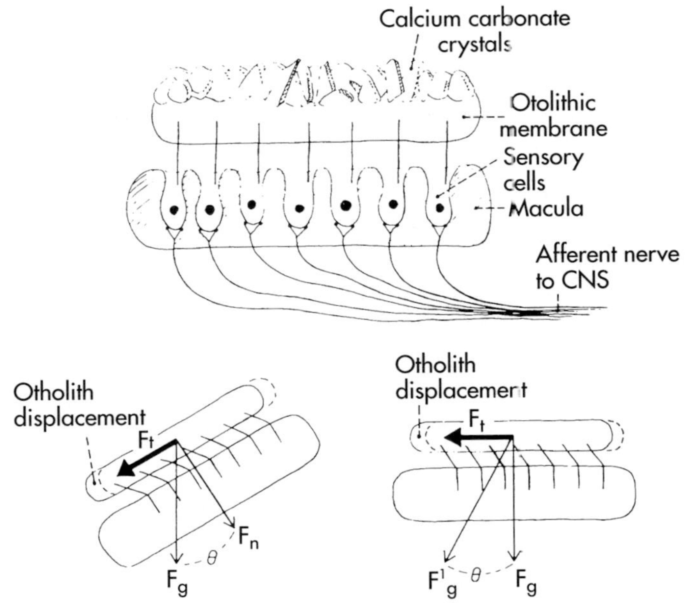

FIG 22-3
Hair cell structure and electrical activity following mechanical stimulation of the stereocilia and kinocilium. (Reprinted with permission: Leigh, RJ, Zee, D: The Neurology of Eye Movements, Philadelphia, 1991, FA Davis.)

posterior canal on the opposite side. Hence, with any head motion in space, endolymph movement occurs in at least two canals—most head movements trigger all six canals. Due to the bilateral representation, it is also apparent that one can function quite well on one labyrinth for almost any head movement.

The sensory transducer in each semicircular canal—the hair cell—is located in a dilated portion of the endolymphatic space termed the ampulla. In the ampulla, the hair cells are imbedded in a supporting mound of tissue called the crista ampullaris. Attached to the long (kinocilia) and short (stereocila) projections from the apex of the hair cell is a sail-like structure called the cupula. The hair cells in each canal are oriented in a consistent polarity such that cu-pular deflection prompted by endolymph movement causes either depolarization (stereocilia bend toward kinocilium) or hyperpolarization (stereocilia bend away from kinocilium) (Fig. 22-3). In the horizontal canals, movement of the cupula toward the utricular recess (utriculopetal) causes increased firing; in the vertical canals, movement away from the utricle (utriculofugal) produces increased neural activity.

The combination of bilateral endorgan coupling and hair cell orientation is the basis for the "push-pull" mechanism of the labyrinth to any angular acceleration of the head. In the absence of motion, the hair cell has a resting firing rate of about 90 spikes/second. Head rotation in the yaw plane, for example, increases the firing rate in the ipsilateral ear (utriculopetal flow) and decreases the firing rate in the contralateral ear (utriculofugal flow). The overall effect is a magnification of the difference in firing rates between the two end organs which is sent to the vestibular nuclei and interpreted as movement in the direction of the higher firing rate. If one ear is nonfunctional, the other ear can still sense motion to both sides, but the "push-pull" amplification is lost. Moreover, an inherent bias is present such that yaw rotations trigger a greater change in the ipsilateral ear (from 90 to 500 spikes/second) than the contralateral ear (from 90 to 0 spikes/second). Hence, certain high acceleration head movements toward a damaged ear can result in a less than perfect neural response.

Signals from the semicircular canals are carried by the superior (serving horizontal and anterior canals) and inferior (serving the posterior canal) divisions of the vestibular nerve medially to the brain stem. The vestibular and cochlear nerves run with the facial nerve together within the internal auditory canal to the brain stem. From there, most of the semicircular canal afferents synapse in the medial and superior vestibular nuclei. A second neuron leaves the nuclei on both sides of the brain stem to synapse within the appropriate ocular motor nucleus. The final neuron in this three neuron arc runs from the ocular motor nuclei to the appropriate eye muscle. This three neuron arc is termed the vestibuloocular reflex (VOR) (Fig. 22-4). Its main function is to cause conjugate equal and opposite eye movement to any angular head movement within the frequency range 0.1 to 10 Hz. Such neural activity preserves visual acuity during head movement by creating equal and opposite eye movement, thus minimizing retinal slip. Damage to the VOR produces retinal slip and decreased visual acuity with head motion termed oscillopsia.

Otolith organ anatomy and physiology. The utricle and saccule lie within the vestibule of the labyrinth at roughly 90° to one another. The utricle is vertically oriented within the elliptical recess and the saccule horizon-

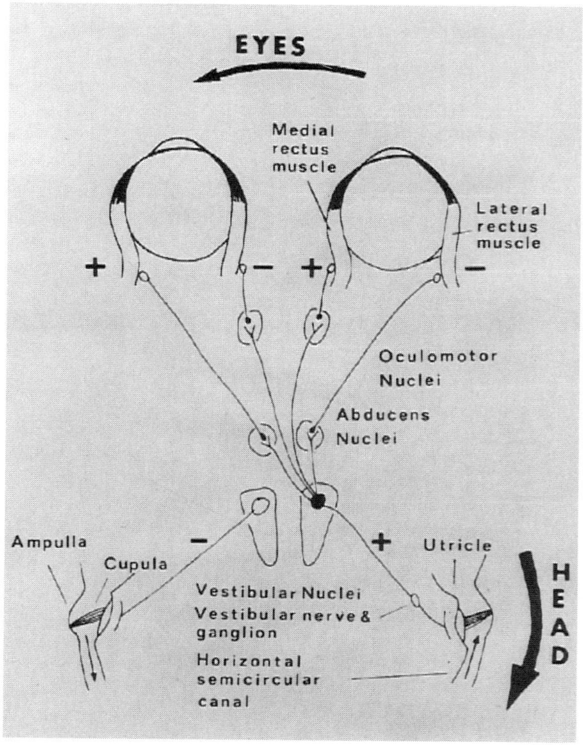

FIG 22-4
The vestibulo-ocular reflex (VOR). Head rotation to the right causes excitation of the right lateral canal receptors and inhibition of the left lateral canal receptors. This is carried to the brain stem by the eighth cranial nerve nuclei (neuron 1). Second-order neurons send projections ipsilaterally and contralaterally up the brain stem to the ocular motor nuclei (neuron 2). Third-order neurons leave the nuclei to synapse on the appropriate eye muscle groups to cause conjugate eye deviation to the left.

tally oriented within the spherical recess. The hair cells are found within the maculi of each otolith organ with the cilia imbedded into a calcified proteinaceous membrane (Fig. 22-5). The kinocilium of each hair cell faces a line called the striola, thus imparting a complex polarity to both otolith organs. Changes in orientation to gravity or linear acceleration produces a shift in the otolithic membrane, ciliary deflection, and increased neural activity.

Otolithic afferent activity is carried via the superior (utricle) and inferior (saccule) vestibular nerves to the brain stem. These fibers synapse primarily within the lateral or inferior vestibular nuclei. Descending fibers from these nuclei form the medial and lateral vestibulospinal tracts which innervate the antigravity muscles of the neck, spine, and lower extremities. Hence, the vestibulospinal reflex (VSR) carries information regarding body orientation in space and changes in linear velocity to the body musculature for the appropriate compensatory response to perturbations. It is important to note that vestibulospinal activity is combined with segmental spinal reflexes generated by tendon stretch receptors to produce the best response to changes in both body position and the support surface conditions.

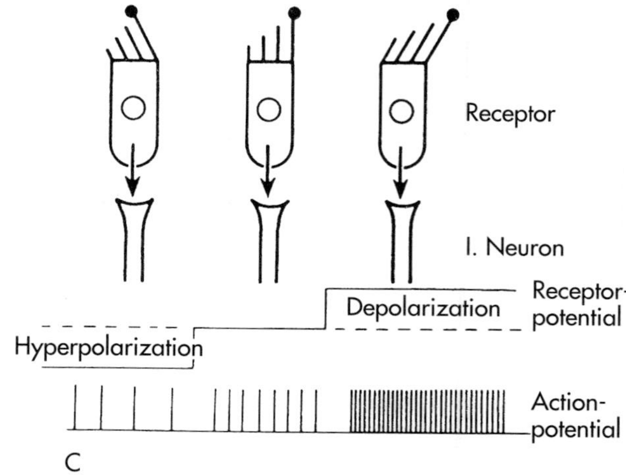

FIG 22-5
Diagramatic representation of the otolithic membrane. **A,** Anatomic features of the macula. **B,** Effects of head tilt on the otolithic membrane. **C,** Effects of linear acceleration on the otolithic membrane. (Reprinted with permission: Baloh, RW, Honrubia, V: Clinical Neurophysiology of the Vestibular System. Philadelphia, 1990, FA Davis.)

Ocular motor systems—anatomy and physiology. There are three important ocular movement systems which interact with the vestibular input (1) saccadic, (2) smooth pursuit, and (3) optokinetic.

The saccadic system generates eye movements which are rapid, conjugate, and accurate to change gaze from one stationary target to another. The origin of this activity is within the frontal eye fields (each lobe generating contralateral deviations). From there the signal reaches the midbrain (vertical saccades) and pons (horizontal saccades) where certain populations of cells are activated to move the eye to the new target (burst cells) and keep the eye on the new target (tonic cells). The cerebellum plays a key role in modulating the accuracy of saccadic movements. In addition, the fast phase of nystagmus (vestibular, optikinetic, or gaze evoked) is produced by the brain stem components of this system.

The smooth pursuit system allows for ocular tracking of small, discrete, slowly moving objects within the visual field. Foveal vision is required, and the retinal stimulation is processed within the occipital cortex, forwarded to the caudal brain stem (associated with the vestibular nuclei), and from there the signal reaches the ocular nuclei and eye muscles for conjugate movement. Decline in this system comes from age, medication, visual acuity, inattention, and CNS lesions of the brain stem, cerebellum and occipital-parietal junction (for ipsilateral pursuit).

The optokinetic system is closely related to smooth pursuit and receives its visual input from perifoveal and peripheral retinal receptors in order to sense motion in the visual environment. The resulting nystagmus is a combination of an involuntary pursuit of repetitive images (slow phase) followed by a saccade to recenter the eyes (fast phase). The main purpose of this visual system is to augment the low-frequency vestibular information during slow, sustained head rotations to produce adequate visual image stability. Lesions of smooth pursuit often affect optokinetic responses as well.

These three systems interact constantly with the vestibular reflexes to modulate visual input consistent with the task at hand. At lower frequencies of motion, the visual-mechanisms dominate. With faster head accelerations, however, the automatic VOR inputs are the primary stabilizers of gaze. Hence, over a wide frequency and velocity range, the visual and vestibular inputs combine to assure visual world stability.

Dizzy patients are evaluated by three vestibular function tests—(1) electronystagmography, (2) rotation test, and (3) posturography.

Electronystagmography (ENG). ENG has been used to examine the eye movements of dizzy patients for more than 30 years. It essentially replicates the physical examination of eye movements and has approximately the same clinical utility as such an examination, but it offers certain advantages—it provides the rigor of a prescribed test protocol, it provides quantification and well-defined normal limits, and it provides documentation in medicolegal and workers' compensation cases. Moreover, the most important ENG test—the caloric test—cannot be done as accurately without the precise stimulus control and response quantification provided by ENG. On the other hand, ENG suffers certain disadvantages—it is insensitive to torsional eye movements, it does not reliably register eye position, and, in some patients, the background noise obscures small eye movements—although an experienced examiner can overcome these disadvantages by direct observation of the patient's eyes with and without Frenzel's lenses.

The standard ENG test battery consists of the following tests: (1) the saccade test, in which horizontal voluntary saccades are evaluated, (2) the spontaneous nystagmus test, in which the patient is evaluated for nystagmus or other gaze-holding disorders with the eyes in various positions of gaze, (3) the positional nystagmus test, in which the patient is evaluated for nystagmus with his head in various positions, (4) the caloric vestibular test, in which the patient is evaluated for a loss of sensitivity of one or both labyrinths to caloric stimulation, (5) the optokinetic nystagmus test, in which nystagmus responses to horizontal optokinetic stimuli are evaluated, (6) the oscillating tracking test, in which horizontal ocular tracking is evaluated, (7) the Hallpike maneuver, in which the patient is evaluated for paroxysmal positional and other types of nystagmus following a brisk movement from the sitting to head-hanging position, and (8) the head shaking test, in which the patient is evaluated for vestibular asymmetry. In addition, an ice water caloric test is performed whenever the caloric vestibular test fails to provoke any response from a given labyrinth, and a pressure test is performed when the physician wishes to know if a given labyrinth is sensitive to pressure in the external ear canal.

For decades, eye movements were recorded on strip-chart recorders until the first computerized ENG system was introduced in 1985. The tests are performed in the same way, but computerized ENG permits quantitative analyses of test data that simply are not feasible to do by hand.

Three examples are given below.

The results of a computerized saccade test are shown in Fig. 22-6. The patient was asked to follow a visual target that jumped back and forth in an unpredictable sequence under computer control. The sequence consisted of 80 target jumps (40 to the right and 40 to the left) with amplitudes ranging from 5° to 25°. A segment of the eye position tracing, with stimulus position superimposed, is shown in the upper left panel. After testing, the computer eliminated invalid data, then calculated three values—peak velocity, accuracy, and latency—for each saccade and plotted these values in graphic form. The test revealed that this patient has slow saccades, an abnormality that is associated with lesions in the basal ganglia, cerebellum, or peripheral oculomotor nerves or muscles.

The results of a computerized tracking test are shown in Fig. 22-7. The patient was asked to follow a visual target moving back and forth following a sinusoidal waveform at frequencies from 0.2 to 0.7 Hz under computer control. A segment of the eye position tracing, with stimulus position superimposed, is shown in the upper panel. After testing, the computer eliminated invalid data, then deleted interpolated saccades, differentiated the eye position signal, calculated the gain of eye velocity with respect to target velocity, and plotted these values in graphic form. This patient has defective pursuit, which indicates a CNS lesion.

The results of a computerized caloric test is shown in Fig. 22-8. The computer calculated slow-phase eye velocity for the entire response and plotted these values in graphic form. It then automatically determined peak response intensity for each of the four responses and calculated unilateral weakness. This patient has a 39% unilateral weakness in the right ear, which indicates a lesion of the right labyrinth or vestibular nerve.

Rotation test. Rotation testing has been done in various ways in the past, but the type of test used most widely today is the slow harmonic acceleration test. The patient is seated in a chair in complete darkness with the head firmly restrained so that it exactly follows chair motion and positioned so that the horizontal semicircular canals are in the plane of rotation. The patient undergoes sinusoidal oscillation about a vertical axis at various frequencies from 0.01 Hz to 0.64 Hz. The patient's nystagmus is recorded by the same method used in ENG.

After testing, the computer differentiates the eye position signal and removes the fast phases of nystagmus, yielding slow-phase eye velocity. Then the computer compares the head velocity and slow-phase eye velocity signals and, for each test frequency, calculates three response indices—phase, gain, and asymmetry.

An example of a rotation test result is shown in Fig. 22-9. The patient has a right peripheral vestibular lesion and

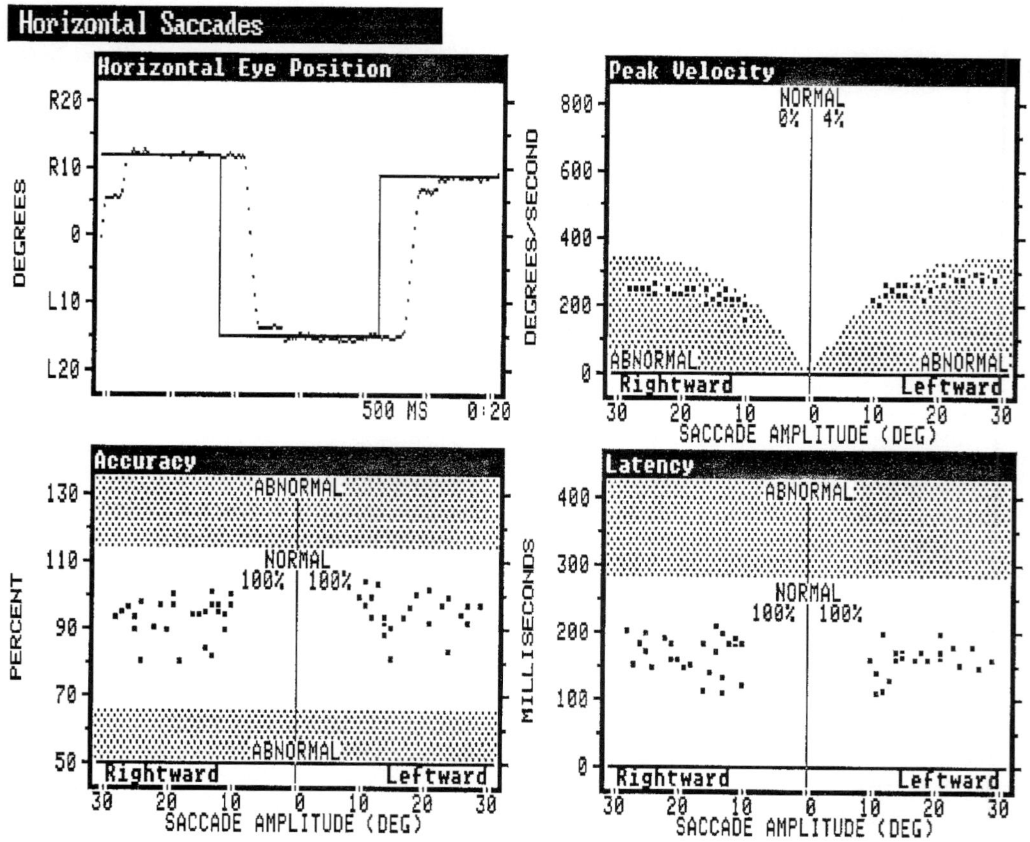

FIG 22-6
Results of a computerized saccade test in a patient with slow saccades. *Upper left,* horizontal eye position *(dotted line)* and target position *(solid line),* with upward deflection denoting rightward movement. *Upper right,* peak saccadic velocity. *Lower left,* saccadic accuracy. *Lower right,* saccadic latency. Shaded areas denote the abnormal range.

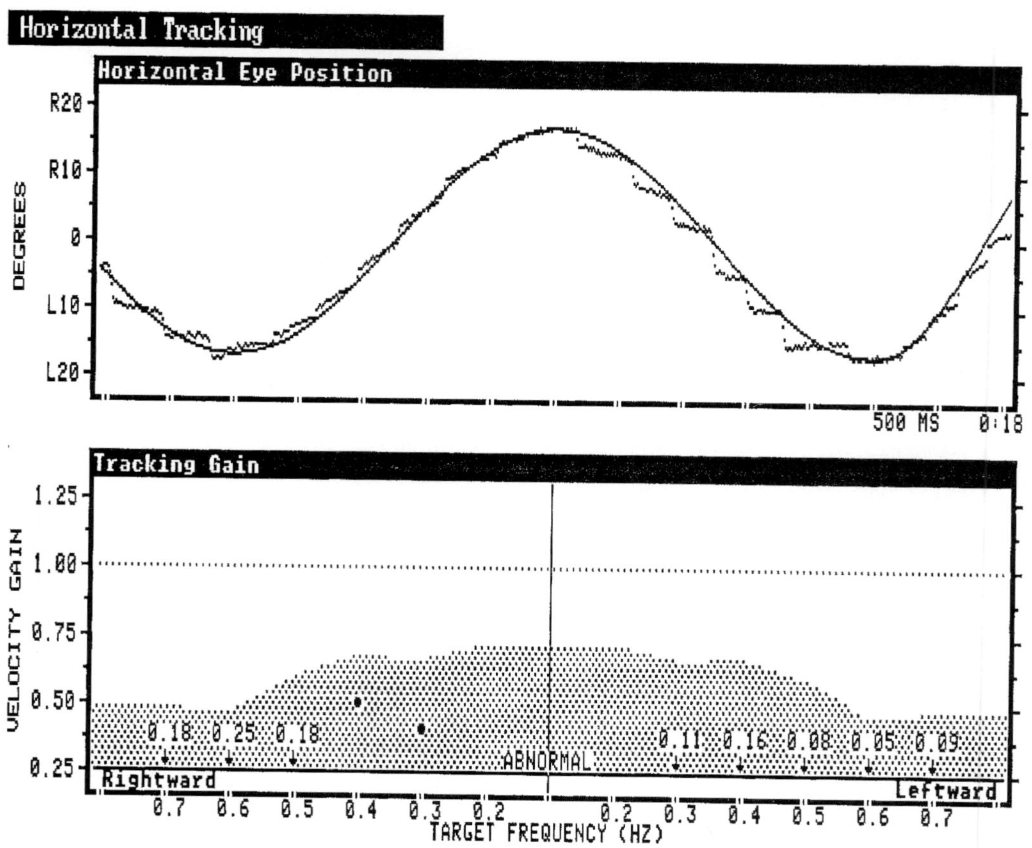

FIG 22-7
Results of a computerized tracking test in a patient with defective pursuit. *Top,* horizontal eye position *(dotted line)* and target position *(solid line),* with upward deflection denoting rightward movement. *Bottom,* gain of peak eye velocity *re* target velocity. Shaded areas denote the abnormal range.

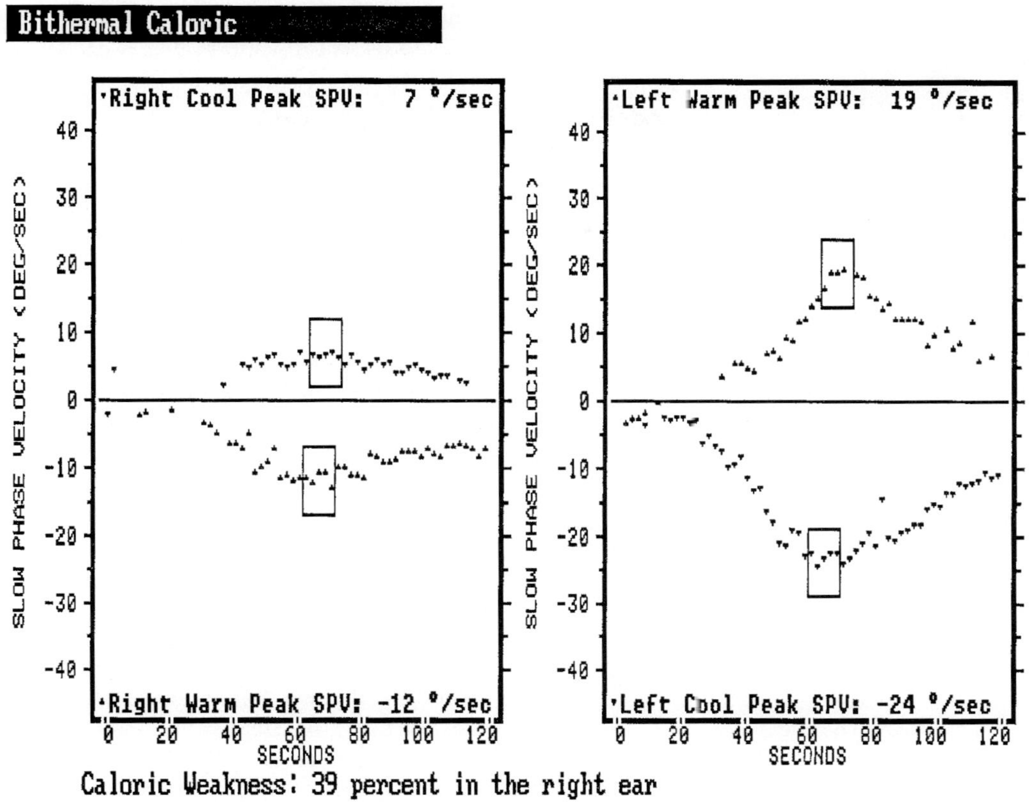

FIG 22-8
Results of a computerized caloric test in a patient with a right caloric weakness. Slow-phase eye velocity is on the vertical axis, with positive values denoting rightward velocities. Time is on the horizontal axis.

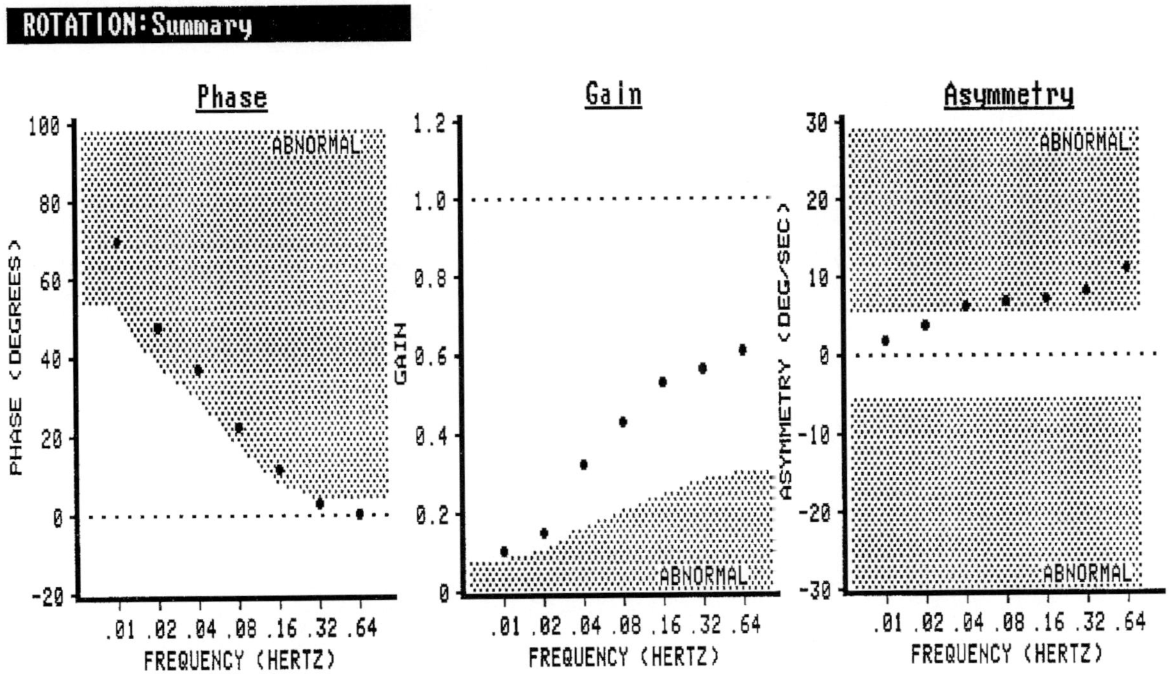

FIG 22-9
Results of a rotation test in a patient with a right peripheral vestibular lesion. The eye velocity signal is inverted during analysis, so that a phase of zero indicates eye velocity exactly opposite head velocity. Shaded areas denote the abnormal range.

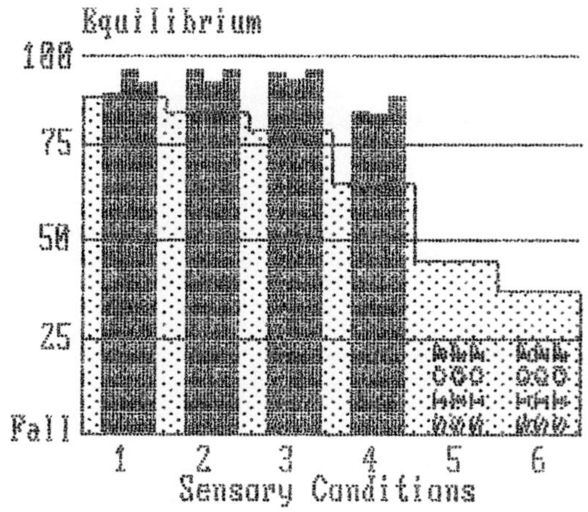

FIG 22-10
Results of a posturography test in a patient with total bilateral loss of vestibular function. Higher scores indicate less body sway. *"STOP"* indicates that the patient fell before completing the trial. Numbers at bottom of chart indicate test condition, as follows: condition 1, both the supporting surface and visual scene are fixed; condition 2, the supporting surface is fixed and the patient's eyes are closed; condition 3, the supporting surface is fixed and the visual scene is tilted in proportion to the angle of body sway; condition 4, the supporting scene is tilted in proportion to the angle of body sway and the visual scene is fixed; condition 5, the supporting surface is tilted in proportion to the angle of body sway and the patient's eyes are closed; condition 6, both the supporting surface and visual scene are tilted in proportion to the angle of body sway. Shaded areas denote the abnormal range.

shows two abnormalities. First, he has progressively greater-than-normal phase leads at the lower test frequencies, which is presumed to reflect a loss of velocity storage that is normally provided by the central vestibular system to enhance the low-frequency response of the vestibulo-ocular system. Second, he shows a rightward asymmetry at the higher frequencies—that is, nystagmus with rightward slow phases is stronger than nystagmus with leftward slow phases. This abnormality is presumed to be due to saturation of inhibitory responses of the intact labyrinth during rotation toward the side of the lesion.

Posturography. Posturography is based upon a computerized testing device, called Equitest, manufactured by Neurocom International, Inc., of Portland, Oregon. This device consists of a platform that is capable of moving back and forth and of tilting in the pitch plane about an axis colinear with the patient's ankle joints. The patient stands facing a visual screen that is capable of tilting about the same axis as the platform. As the patient sways on the platform, a built-in force plate measures the changes in the position of his body's center of pressure. These data are transmitted to the computer, which calculates the angle of his body sway in the pitch plane.

Posturography consists of two tests—the sensory organization test and the movement coordination test. Of the two, the sensory organization test is the more interesting to those of us who examine dizzy patients, because it is designed primarily to test vestibular function. The patient's postural stability is tested under various conditions in which either visual or proprioceptive cues (or both) are denied.

An example of a posturography test result is shown in Fig. 22-10. The patient has suffered a total bilateral loss of vestibular function due to ototoxicity. He has normal postural stability when tested under conditions 1 through 4, when he had either correct visual or correct proprioceptive cues (or both), but marked instability on Conditions 5 and 6, when he was required to rely solely upon vestibular cues. Such an abnormality is not surprising in patients who, like this one, lack vestibular function, but we have also seen it in patients with acute unilateral peripheral vestibular lesions, which is surprising because those patients still receive input from the intact labyrinth. Apparently acute unilateral lesions cause suppression of vestibulospinal input. We have seen this abnormality only rarely in patients with chronic unilateral peripheral vestibular lesions.

SUGGESTED READING

Nashner, LM: Posturographic testing. In Jacobson et al, editors: *Handbook of Balance Function Testing*. St. Louis, 1993, Mosby–Year Book.

Stockwell CW: Vestibular function tests. In Paparella, et al, editors: *Otolaryngology*, ed 3. Philadelphia, 1991, WB Saunders Co.

Stockwell CW, Bojrab DI: Rotation testing. In Jacobson et al, editors: *Handbook of Balance Function Testing*. St. Louis, 1993, Mosby–Year Book.

23

Surgical and Medical Treatment of Otosclerosis

Jean-Bernard Causse, M.D., Robert Vincent, M.D., and Martine Michat M.D.

In our mind, the goal of surgical treatment of a fixed stapes is to restore a physiologic hearing through the best possible physiological vibration of the inner ear fluids thanks to an as effective as possible impedance transfer of the ossicular chain, a good enough acoustic impedance of a new annular ligament around the lower tip of the piston.

If the piston is placed directly into the footplate hole, (without interposition of a living tissue graft) there is more risk of excessive motion of the inner ear fluids. A piece of vein graft is recommended as it provides 0.2mm thickness of elastic fibers. The hair of the Corti hair cells (0.5 micron in diameter) and the membranes of the inner ear can only withstand very small motion of the fluids, smaller than mechanical ones. Acoustic trauma or barotrauma may damage the hearing more easily if a "shock absorber " has not been rebuilt around the lower tip of the piston.

Rebuilding the stapes reflex tendon has also been our goal.

A yearly audiogram is recommended. Testing the 2 Khz is advised in order to detect a deterioration of the hearing due to a damage of the hair of the Corti hair cells by the proteolytic enzymes spread by the otospongiotic foci. Sodium fluoride, in small doses ranging from 2 to 20 mg, neutralizes the proteolytic enzymes in the perilymph and decreases the osteoclasts activity. At a higher dose than 40 mg a day, sodium fluoride may rebuild fragile pseudo-haversian bone and obstruct the cochlea.

JEAN-BERNARD CAUSSE SURGICAL TECHNIQUE FOR OTOSCLEROSIS

Case selection

If the surgeon is not experienced, we advise to follow the American Academy Guidelines which are:

Hearing loss should be sufficient to really bother the patient. Other ear must have surgical confirmation of otosclerosis. Family history of otosclerosis should be known. Progressive hearing loss should exist for at least one year. Tinnitus or vertigo prior surgery should not be too severe.

If there is also previous stapedectomy with recent vertigo and progressive or fluctuating hearing loss in the operated ear, the nonexperienced surgeon should refer the patient to a more trained surgeon.

Surgery should be referred to a more experienced surgeon when the previous stapedectomy was performed with unimproved conductive hearing loss either early or late onset after surgery.

Physical examination should show absence of acute or chronic infection. Tympanic membrane should be intact on the side scheduled for surgery.

Air and bone pure tone audiogram for both ears should demonstrate:

- SRT > 30 dB
- Air/bone gap > 20 dB: average at 0.5 kH, 1.0 kH, and 2.0 kH (in the ear to be operated); may add 10 dB at 2.0 kH to allow for effect of Carhart notch
- In cases of profound hearing loss and bone testing not valid, provide rationale for diagnosis of otosclerosis.

SRT and discrimination should be performed on both ears as well as the tympanogram and acoustic reflex. If tympanogram shows a negative pressure or acoustic reflex shows stapedius reflex present or only an on-off effect, surgery should be postponed or referred to a more experienced surgeon.

A tuning fork is highly recommended and should be positive in two or three speech frequencies.

If the surgeon is actually experienced, case selection does not need to be restricted to large gaps only. Surgery is indicated even if the gap is smaller than 20dB, if bone vibration is obviously heard in the deafest ear.

A very small change in the pressure and mobility of the labyrinthine fluids can alter the bone conduction level a great deal. The hair of the Corti cells are geared to react to a molecular size level vibration of the cochlear canal fluids. Bone conduction drops in case of hydrops due to a Menière's syndrome. As soon as the fluid pressure is released, the hearing level is improved.

A lack of elasticity of the annular ligament of the stapes footplate causes a reduction in the vibration of the inner ear fluids and consequently of the hair of the Corti cells (Figs. 23-1 and 23-2).

The acoustic impedance transfer of the ossicular chain[4,5] should be restored as much as possible.

Acoustic impedance transfer is the ratio between the effective vibrating surface of the tympanic membrane and the effective vibrating surface of the stapes footplate (Fig. 23-3).

Too small fenestra in the footplate, such as one that is O.4 mm, will produce too much energy near the lower tip of the piston and not enough farther on in the cochlear canal.[25] The high-pitched frequencies localized in the first basal turn of the cochlea are good with a small fenestra, but the mid and low frequencies located in the apical remote part of the cochlea are poor if too small a fenestra has been used.

The acoustic impedance of the annular ligament of the stapes footplate should be restored as much as possible.

The acoustic impedance is how a material will resist to its vibration, when a sound vibration is applied to this material.

The otosclerotic foci cause the annular ligament of the stapes footplate to lose its elasticity:

$$Z = \sqrt{R^2 + \left(2\pi f \cdot M - \frac{S}{2\pi f}\right)^2}$$

Z = Acoustic impedance of the annular ligament
R = Resistance
M = Mass
S = Elasticity is the contrary
f = frequency

R* = *resistance *which acts as a kind of a shock absorber:* It protects the inner ear membranes and hair of Corti cells against acoustic trauma or barotrauma. If the resistance around the lower tip of the piston is not rebuilt, the threshold at which an acoustic trauma or barotrauma will be able to damage the inner ear is lowered.

An acoustic or barotrauma may more easily rupture the Reissner membrane, leading to no Na+ K+ exchange and thus a drop in the cochlear potentials. The hearing level becomes extremely poor.

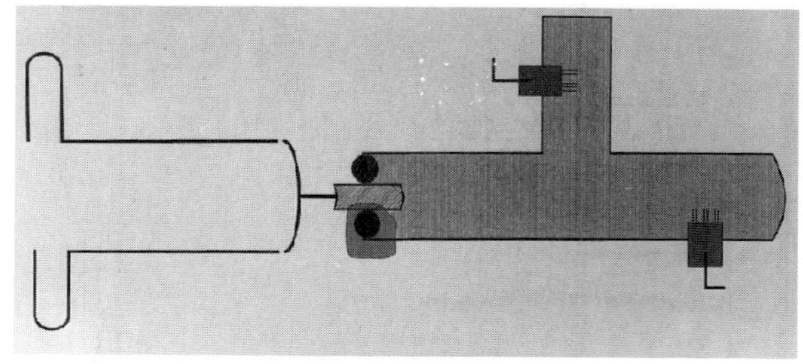

FIG 23-1
Schematisation of the effect of the fixation of the stapes on the vibration of the inner ear fluids.

Likewise, the attachments between the outer Corti hair cells and the membrana tectoria may rupture, leading to poor speech discrimination and tinnitus.

The annular ligament of the stapes footplate is a 0.2 mm^3 volume of elastic fibers.[1] We should interpose a living seal that will create around the lower tip of the piston the same volume of elastic fibers (Fig. 23-4).

Scuba diving and rough plane landings are no more dangerous if this technique has been used. A professional pilot or scubadiver may be able to keep his license if a videotape recording of the surgery proves that the resistance has been actually rebuilt around the lower tip of the piston.

M* = *Mass: The mass is multiplied by the frequency playing a role for high-pitched frequencies only.

A tiny bony spiculae helps making the long process of the incus act as a record player arm. Consequently, the long process of the incus should not be traumatized[29] during the joint separation for instance. The piston should be not too much heavier than the crura of the stapes.

***S* = *Elasticity*—**This is a kind of a trampoline helping the push-pull effect:

Elasticity is divided by frequency. It will play a role for mid and low frequencies, up to 3 kHz.

If the surgeon does not interpose a living tissue graft, the elasticity of the perilymphatic membrane only will not give an as good a push-pull effect as a normal annular ligament of the footplate, since the latter has many elastic fibers in the media layer as demonstrated by D. Lim.[1]

In this technique coupling the use of a piston and a piece of vein graft, the number of elastic fibers seen under microscope in the vein graft will be greater after two years than those found in a vein sample taken from the wrist of the patient on the same day.[6,7,28]

According to A Lopez and L. Juberthie, the elastic fibers are rebuilt from the fibroblasts (Fig. 23-5A and B).

Surgical technique

Many surgical techniques have been proposed so far. Two, more than others, are at the basis of the Jean-Bernard Causse technique.

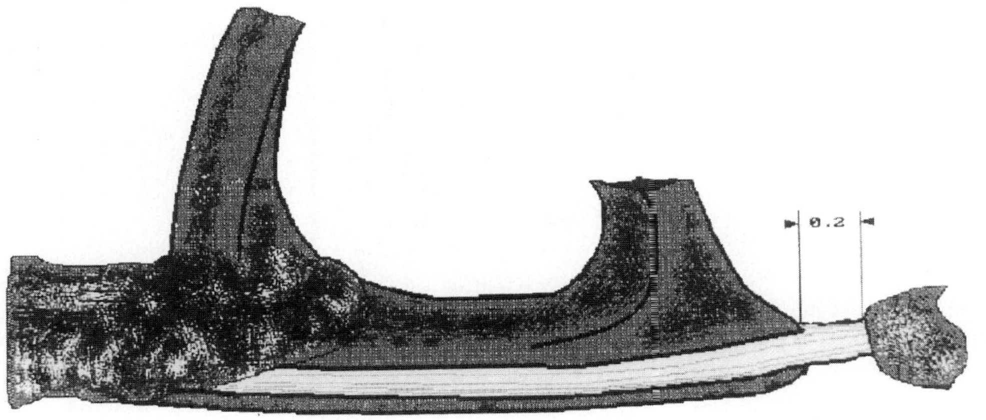

FIG 23-2
Increase of the ossicular chain impedance related to the lack of elasticity of the annular ligament invaded by the otosclerotic foci.

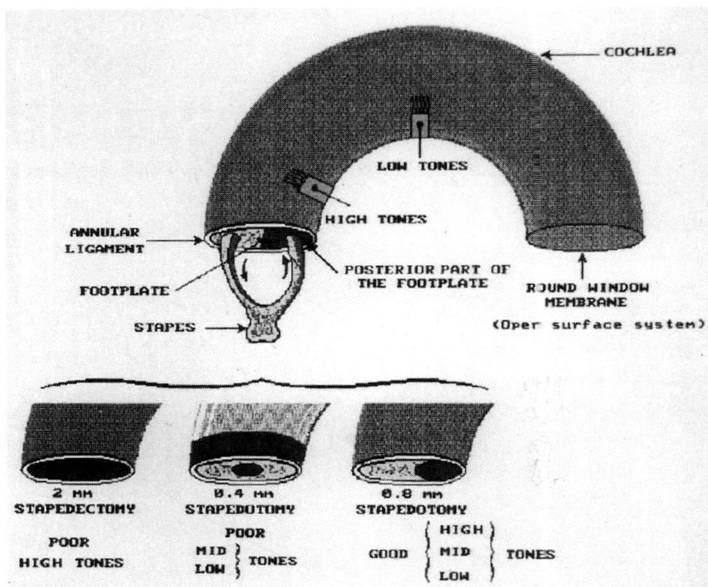

FIG 23-3
Total stapedectomy gives poor hearing for high tones and too small a fenestra gives poor hearing for low tones, whereas a transmission corresponding approximately to the posterior half of the footplate will create an acoustic vibration creating a better distribution of the vibration in the fluids along the cochlear canal.

The John Shea technique (1958) is more or less total stapedectomy with vein graft interposition and use of a polythene tube from the tip on the long process of the incus.[36]

The Jean René Causse technique (1962) combines two techniques of John Shea (that described above) and the use of the original Shea piston, resulting in a new more efficient technique, which he named Teflon-interposition.[8,38].

The Jean-Bernard Causse technique.[5,9-12] The posterior canal wall is removed with a curette to give a good exposure. The bone removal should not involve the superior aspect of the canal wall, as draping of the drum may occur postoperatively. Stagnating blood may form adhesions in the middle ear. The drum should rest as far as possible from the long process of the incus. Adhesions may retract, elevating the long process of the incus.

The stapes tendon is severed as near as possible of the posterior crus in order to be able to use this tendon for stapes tendon reconstruction at the end of the operation.

The crura are vaporized with an HGM Argon laser using the Gherini-Causse endootoprobe (beginning with the posterior crus).[13,23] Usually, the anterior crus is not visible, the fiber optic palpates the anterior crus before vaporizing it using a setting of 2 watts and O.5 seconds. Creation of the fenestra with the Argon laser : a round "rosette" is cre-

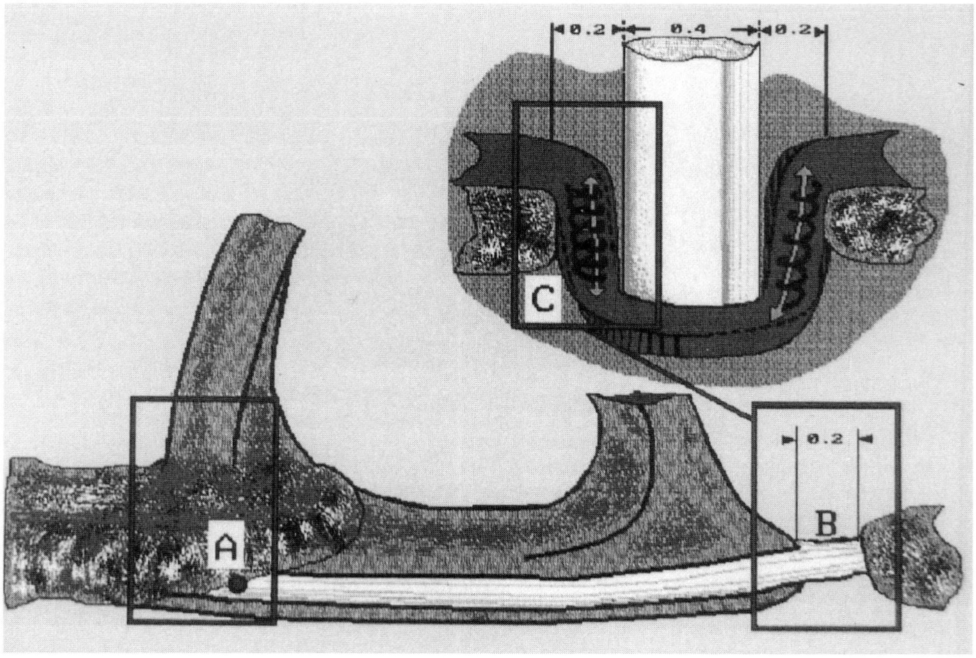

FIG 23-4
The new annular ligament, showed in *C,* has a volume and a structure comparable to the annular ligament of the stapes footplate, showed in *B.*

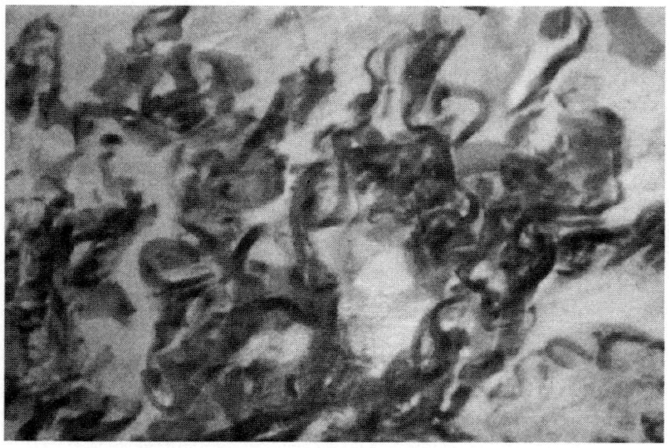

FIG 23-5, A
Old piece of vein graft—15 years—in a 63-year-old man. Histologic section. Elastic fibers colored with hydrochloric orcein.

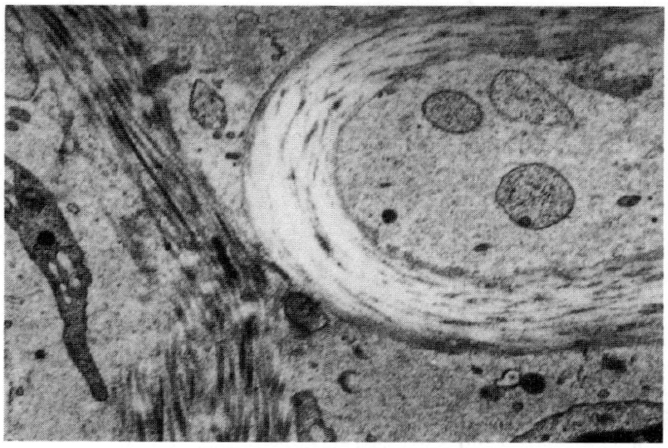

FIG 23-5, B
Old piece of vein graft—9 years—in a 42-year-old woman. Isolated elastic fiber. Ultrastructural aspect. Coloration with uranyle acetate-lead citrate.

ated in the stapes footplate with the Gherini-Causse endo-otoprobe. Settings of 1.2 watts and O.2 seconds pulse duration are used. Each laser impact site may or may not overlap the previous impact point until the shape and size of the "rosette" is complete (Fig. 23-6).

The power decreases immediately (200 μ only) thanks to the diffraction of the beam due to the fiber optic. The smoothing of the fenestra is then performed with the microdrill (Fig. 23-7). The Skeeter microdrill with a O.7 mm diamond bur removes the remaining bone and bone char and in addition smoothes the edges of the fenestra. The size of the fenestra is 0.8 mm.

A stapedotomy instead of a total stapedectomy will:

Avoid the spread of proteolytic enzymes into the vestibule: breaking the anterior otosclerotic foci may release proteolytic enzymes into the fluids. These enzymes may damage the membranes and Corti hair cells structure.

Avoid bleeding into the vestibule: breaking the anterior-foci may lead to such bleeding, as the foci are highly vascularized most of the time. The blood may float on the surface of the perilymph or penetrate into the vestibule leading to fibrous bands clogging of the cochlear canal.

Rebuild more resistance around the lower tip of the piston.

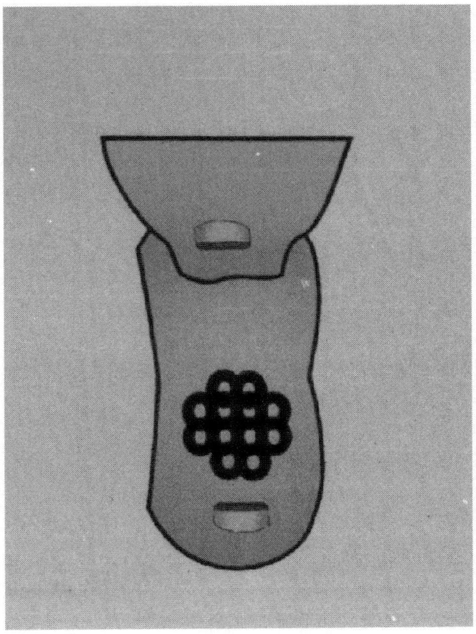

FIG 23-6
A rosette of spots determines the ulterior 0.8 mm stapedotomy.

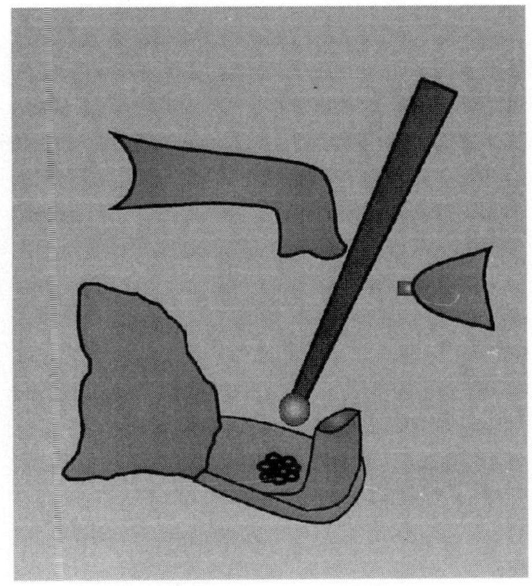

FIG 23-7
The Causse Skeeter Ototool abrading 0.8 mm of the footplate in the posterior half of the stapes footplate, approximately from one edge of the annular ligament to the other.

A piece of vein graft is placed in the oval fossa: A large piece of vein graft helps to prevent excessive motion and penetration of the piston into the vestibule. The piece of vein graft is placed adventitial "sticky" side down on the footplate (Fig. 23-8).

The piston is O.4 mm diameter. Thus the part of the vein graft sitting between the fenestra and the piston will be O.2 mm thick. The loop of the piston, being of Teflon, is soft on to the long process of the incus, as opposed to a wire loop. The position of the loop may be adjusted on the long process of the incus so that the piston shaft is perpendicular to the stapedotomy.

A cup piston with 0.4 mm shaft diameter is used when the long process of the incus is not long enough or when the second portion of the facial nerve is protruding too much in the oval fossa.

A stapes tendon reconstruction is performed:

To avoid penetration of the piston into the vestibule when the stapes tendon contracts, the tendon is severed as near as possible to the posterior crus at the beginning of the surgery, and at the end of the surgery it is attached to a Polycel platform (Xomed-Treace), in order to get the tendon at least perpendicular to the shaft of the piston. The tendon is glued to the Polycel platform, bridging the gap in between the Polycel and the tendon by a tiny drop of loose perivenous connective tissue. The amplitude of the acoustic reflex (impedancemetry is performed one year after surgery) shows a positive acoustic reflex back in 73% of the cases. The amplitude of the reflex will be less if the tendon is strictly perpendicular to the shaft of the piston (Fig. 23-9 to 23-14). Stapes tendon reconstruction is possible when a cup piston is used (Fig. 23-15).

Bending test: Proper placement of the piston is confirmed by the "bending test." A small pick is used to apply lateral pressure to the piston. If the piston bends slightly, the position is good. If the piston actually moves, it is not well seated in the stapedotomy fenestra.

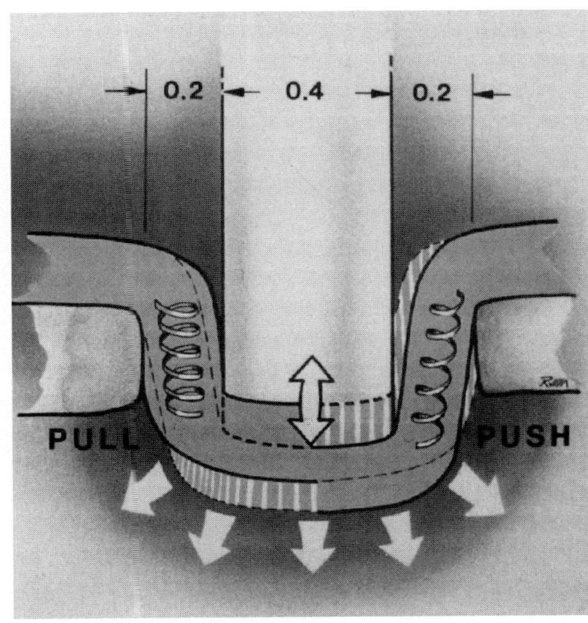

FIG 23-8
Resistance and elasticity around the lower tip of the piston are rebuilt thanks to the piece of vein graft.

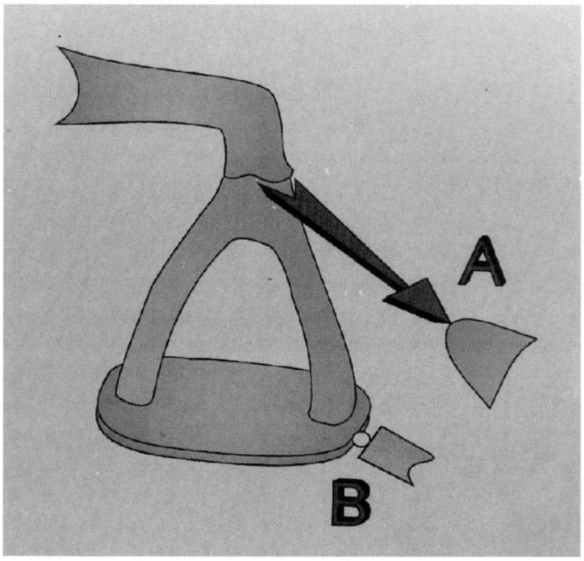

FIG 23-9
The stapes tendon force is backward and downward in order to allow the stapes footplate to be blocked on the edge of the oval fossa bony rim. **A,** Stapes tendon. **B,** Posterior annular ligament is higher and thinner than anterior annular ligament.

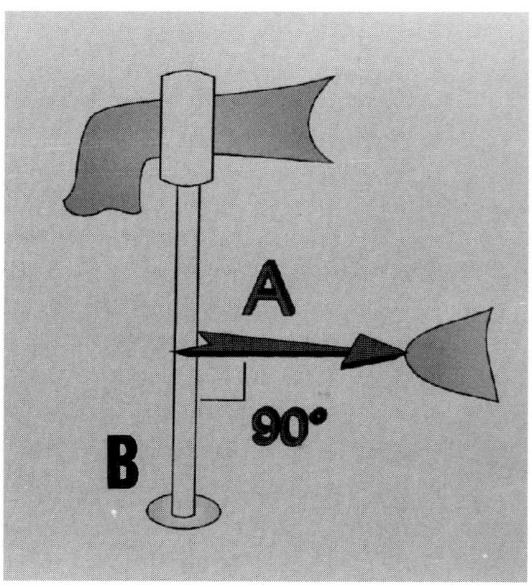

FIG 23-10
The tendon is placed perpendicular to the piston shaft, in order to pull the tendon and avoid the penetration of the piston into the vestibule when the tendon contracts. **A,** Polycel platform is placed on the shaft of the piston in order to get the tendon perpendicular to the piston. **B,** Shaft of the piston.

Middle ear inflation is advised after surgery for a few days: Such inflation is possible as the new annular ligament gives the system the same shock-absorber protection as an annular ligament of the stapes footplate. *Valsalva or Politzer maneuvers* prevent excessive penetration of the piston into the vestibule, due to tympanic membrane retraction, and helps to avoid adhesion formation in the middle ear postoperatively, due to blood stagnation.

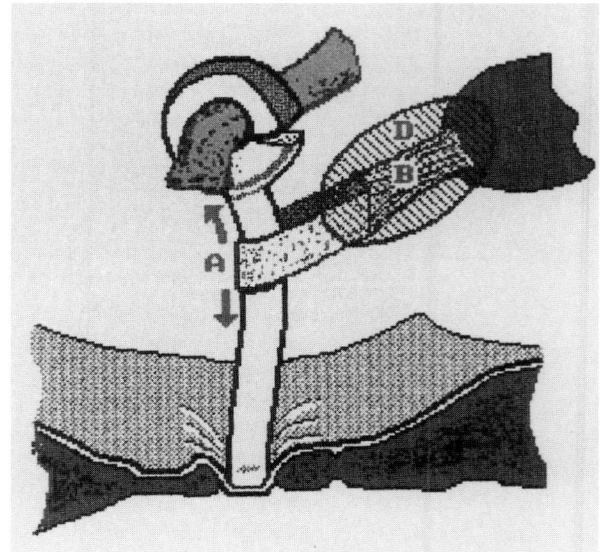

FIG 23-11
A, Causse Polycel device (Xomed-Treac). **B,** Stapes tendon. **C,** Pyramid of the stapes tendon. **D,** Fragment of connective tissue.

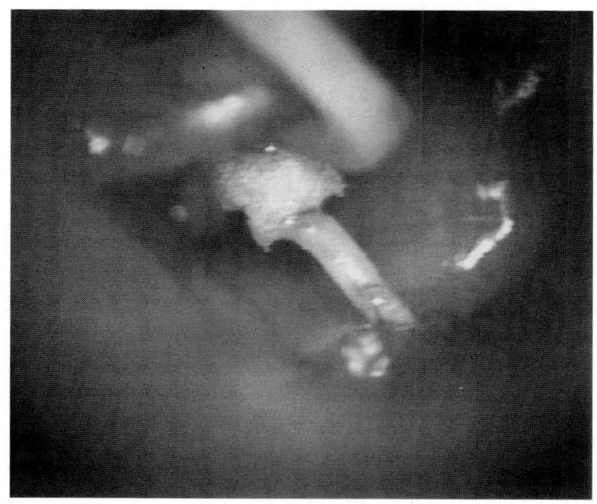

FIG 23-12
The tendon is glued to the Polycel platform.

RESULTS

The comparative results concerning these different techniques in otosclerosis surgery were studied one year after the operation. They are shown in Fig. 23-16. The statistics have been carried out by the Statistics Department of the Pierre FABRE Laboratories in Castres, France, on a series comprising 3.000 cases out of 54.000 cases corresponding to the total number of congenital ear defects operated on in our clinic.

According to these statistics, the removal of the whole

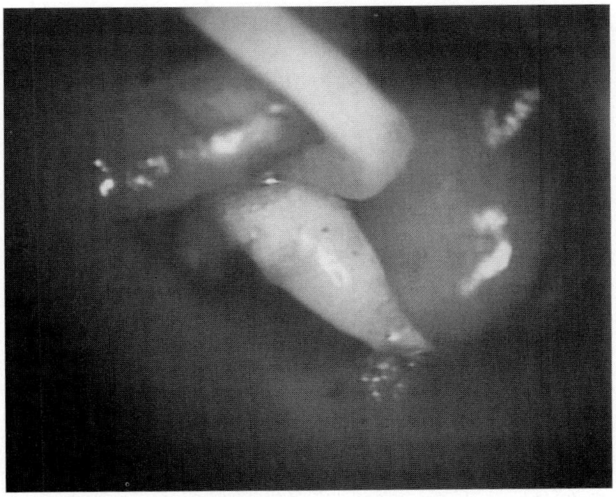

FIG 23-13
The tiny fragment of perivenous connective tissue ensures the adherence between the tendon and the Polycel, even if the tendon contracts.

stapes footplate gives poor high tones, and too small stapedotomy gives poor mid and low tones. The technique of reconstitution of good impedance transfer and good acoustic impedance of the annular ligament allows better vibration of the labyrinthine fluids on all the frequencies.

Dr. James Robinson (Gloucester, UK) carried out a statistical study relating to 125 patients, using a number of different techniques: total or partial platinectomy, interposition using vein graft and post crus of stapes, microfenestration using micro pick and hooks for fenestration (O.6 mm piston), O.65 mm microfenestration using a microdrill for fenestration (O.6 mm piston) and Causse technique. Airbone gap were measured using postoperative bone conduction and postoperative air conduction. His results are in the box on p. 287.

Results of Dr Christian Parahy with the JB Causse's technique[30]

Calculation of hearing results. The traditional way to report the results compares the preoperative bone conduction (preop BC) and the postoperative air conduction (postop AC) . Results showing an overclosure indicate the postop AC is above the preop BC. Closure is indicated when postop AC = preop BC. The preop BC does not show the real cochlear reserve and the improvement of the BC after surgery is due to a better pressure and mobility of the inner ear liquids in addition to a better impedance of the ossicular chain. These can explain the disappearance of the Carhart notch after surgery. Therefore, the results of these cases are reported comparing the best postop BC with the postop AC at 500 Hz, 1, 2, and 4 kHz. We do not talk about overclosure but about closure of gap only when the postop AC = postop BC. We include the 4 kHz in the calculation because of

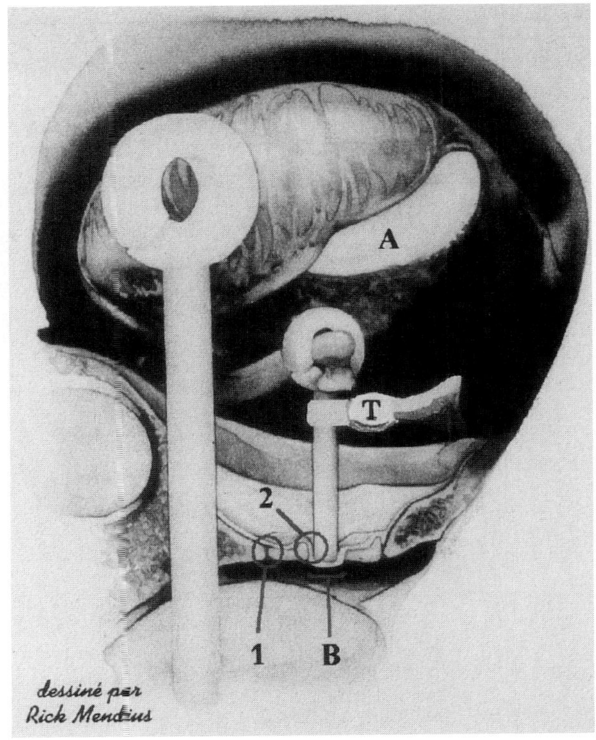

FIG 23-14
Technique of JB Causse using a ring teflon piston when the long process of the incus is long. A ring is preferable in order to get the piston perpendicular to the stapedotomy.

I = stapes tendon reconstruction (polycel platform)

A = vibrating eardrum surface

B = vibrating surface applied to the inner ear fluids

$\frac{B}{A} = \frac{1}{20}$ **at the posterior third of the footplate**

1 = annular ligament of the footplate (0.2 mm^2 of elastic fibers)

2 = part of piece of veingraft located between the piston and the footplate

1 = 2 { **same shock absorber effect (protects against acoustic trauma and baro trauma)**
same trampoline or spring effect (quantity and quality of hearing) }

its importance in speech discrimination and because it is improved in the small fenestra operation.

Comments on the results. Thanks to the surgical technique which reconstitutes the shape, dimension, and histologic structure of the annular ligament allowing the piston to exert a push-pull movement, vigorous inflation of the middle ear, and other treatments, the gap was closed to within 5 dB in 67% of the cases on the sixth postoperative day. The average bone conduction before surgery was 33.6 dB and increased to 20 dB after surgery. The improvement is possible by a perfect tension and better mobility of the inner ear liquids as well as good impedance of the chain. Both the middle ear and inner ear return to the normal ana-

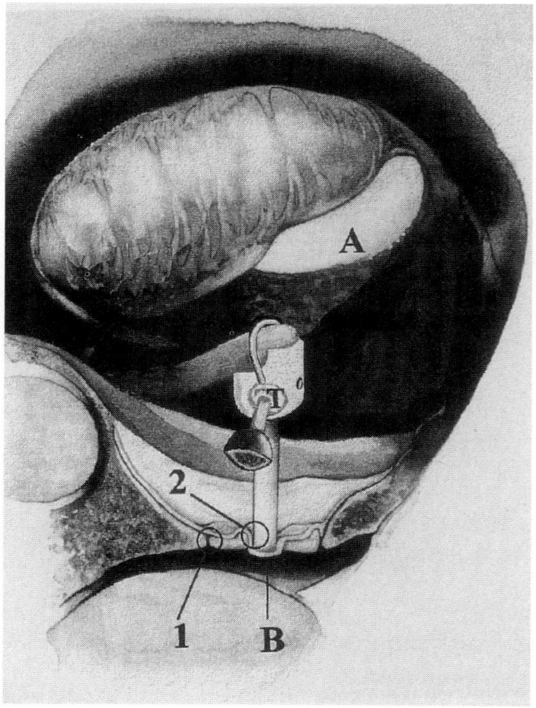

FIG 23-15
Technique of JB Causse using a cup piston when the long process of the incus is short or when the facial nerve is prolapsing. (+ legend same as that for Fig. 23-14)

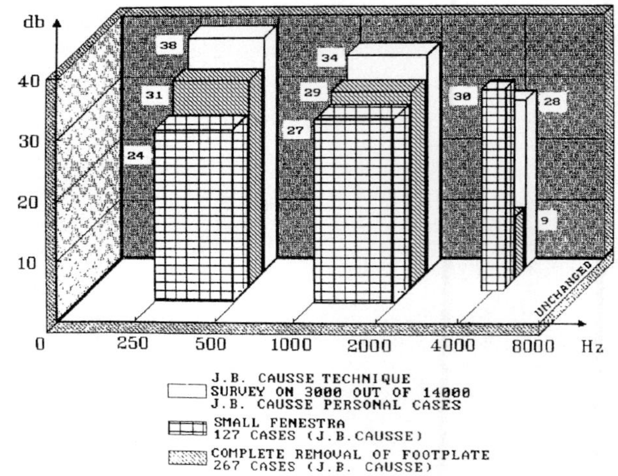

FIG 23-16
Comparison between preoperative and postoperative bone conduction (J.B. Causse cases). Number of dBs gained on the first postoperative year.

tomic and physiologic state. In the one-year follow-up audiograms done by other ENT specialists, the airbone gap stayed closed to within 5 dB in 64% of the cases, showing a good reliability of the technique. No dead ears were reported.

Preoperative dizziness was relieved in 19.5% of the patients, and 2.3% of the patients acquired light dizziness which disappeared completely after a few days. Preoperative tinnitus was relieved in 33% of the patients after surgery, mostly on the low frequencies because of a better tension of the inner ear liquids. The high-tone pitch often remained but at a lower intensity. With the improvement in hearing, patients no longer complained about tinnitus. The chorda tympani were cut, but never in both ears, in 5%.

MEDICAL TREATMENT FOR OTOSCLEROSIS

We will use the term otosclerosis when there is a gap on the audiogram showing a fixed stapes and the term otospongiosis when there is no gap and the stapes is not fixed. Family history of otosclerosis, progressive hearing loss on the mid frequencies, and foci suspected on CT scan are the main reasons for performing a hearing test and at least a pure tone audiogram once a year. If there is any sign of progressive deterioration on the mid frequencies, sodium fluoride as proposed by George Shambaugh[38] should be prescribed. If there is a progressive deterioration on the high-pitched frequencies, vascular drugs should be prescribed.

Two clinical proofs of the effectiveness of sodium fluoride

We administer sodium fluoride to combat the frequent progressive cochlear impairment that occurs in about 75% of all otospongiotic/otosclerotic cases, whether operated on or not, as a result of enzymatic action on the hair cells and on the bony cochlear duct which causes ligament distortion, atrophy of the stria vascularis, and hyalinization of the spiral ligament. Of course, the other causes of sensorineural hearing loss (SNHL), such as presbycusis, must first be excluded.

The optimum dosage is determined by the concept that sodium fluoride acts by its presence more than by weight, as any enzymogenesis inhibitor does. But a threshold must be achieved below which it does not act and above which its activity does not increase in proportion to the dose. The sodium fluoride action threshold stands around O.5 mg sodium fluoride/1 mg trypsin in vitro,[14] but this threshold is less accurate in vivo. Numerous clinical trials with various doses from 3 to 60 mg daily have shown that: first, small doses ranging from 2 to 10 mg daily are sufficient to act on pure cochlear otospongiosis, which is less active than stapedial fixation from the enzymatic point of view, and second, that in contrast, doses must be greater, about 20 mg daily for stapedial fixations with a cochlear component, in which extensive enzymatic activity is needed to produce both the bony rebuilding of the niche and the spreading of hydrolytic and proteolytic enzymes into the labyrinthine fluids. Larger doses of 60 mg daily did not appear to give any

Measurement of Airborne Gap using Postoperative Bone Conduction and Postoperative Air Conduction

Key:
(1) Total or partial
(2) Interposition
(3) Micro pick
(4) Micro drill without graft
(5) Micro drill with graft

Overclosure (500 Hz to 4 kHz)
(Average) (1) = 17 db
(2) = 10 dB (3) = 43 dB
(4) = 34 dB (5) = 36 dB

AC gain at 4 kHz
(Average) (1) = 6 db
(2) = 13 dB (3) = 16 dB
(4) = 17 dB (5) = 27 dB

AC improvement (500 Hz to 4 kHz)

AC 20 db or less:	(1) = 54%	
(2) = 57%	(3) = 82%	
(4) = 60%	(5) = 100%	
AC 30 db or less:	(1) = 23%	
(2) = 28%	(3) = 36%	
(4) = 40%	(5) = 69%	
Unchanged:	(1) = 19%	
(2) = 28%	(3) = 9%	
(4) = 0%	(5) = 0%	
Worse:	(1) = 4%	
(2) = 0%	(3) = 0%	
(4) = 7%	(5) = 0%	
Dead ear:	(1) = 4%	
(2) = 0%	(3) = 0%	
(4) = 0%	(5) = 0%	

Closure of airbone gap (500 Hz to 4 kHz)

Airbone gap 10 db or less:	(1) = 42%
(2) = 57%	(3) = 63%
(4) = 47%	(5) = 85%
Airbone gap 20 db or less:	(1) = 69%
(2) = 86%	(3) = 82%
(4) = 87%	(5) = 100%
Worse:	(1) = 19%
(2) = 0%	(3) = 18%
(4) = 7%	(5) = 0%
Dead ear:	(1) = 4%
(2) = 0%	(3) = 0%
(4) = 0%	(5) = 0%

Results of 100 Consecutive Cases of Stapes Surgery from January to June, 1988—Dr. Parahy

Average airbone gap preop:18 dB
Smallest: 5 dB
Largest: 37.5 dB
Average bone conduction:
Before surgery: 33.6 dB
After surgery: 20 dB
Airbone gap:
0 → 15 dB 67%
>5 dB 33%
One-year follow-up available in 77 cases:
0 → 5 dB 64%

No dead ear
Dizziness:
19.5% were relieved
2.3% acquired dizziness
0% disabling vertigo
Tinnitus:
33% were relieved
18.5% remain the same
3.5% acquired tinnitus
Chorda tympani cut in 5%

better results, because sodium fluoride has a double action according to the doses. Jowsey et al[24] have shown that sodium fluoride doses of 60 mg daily or more cause a pseudohaversian rebuilding resulting in the formation of a fragile new bone which may obstruct the cochlea, whereas daily doses of 45 mg or less do not increase bone formation and act on enzymatic activity only. For this reason, we always give our patients moderate doses of sodium fluoride, ranging from 2 to 20 mg daily, to stop cochlear deterioration without increasing stapedial fixation. We thus do not need to add vitamin D and calcium supplement to prevent the formation of abnormal bone.

On the basis of these data, we generally prescribe sodium fluoride as follows.

For adults we prescribe 20 mg daily, 5 days a week, for patients with advanced otospongiosis with a very active cochlear component and for those in whom smaller doses have not been effective, as well as before a stapedectomy to be performed on a patient showing an active Schwartze sign. This is continued for a short period of one year. For all operated patients with a progressive cochlear component, 20 mg is given daily for two years. The treatment will be resumed only if the yearly audiogram shows a deterioration of the hearing on the mid frequencies.

For children, we prescribe moderate doses (2 mg daily) to avoid possible stunting of growth due to premature calcification of the long bone matrix.[16,20]

Prevention currently relies first on the appearance on the audiogram of a Carhart notch at the 2 kHz frequency and more lately on the early detection of stapedial fixation by means of systematic testing for the "on-off effect," which

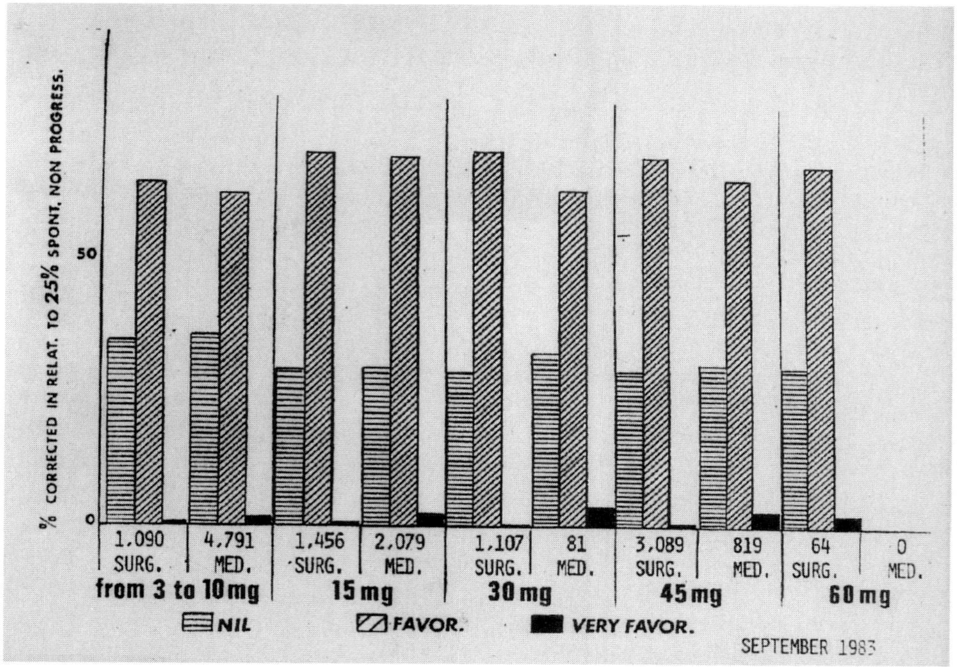

FIG 23-17
Percentages of functional results of NaF treatment in 14,576 surgical and medical cases.

TABLE 23-1
Sodium fluoride statistical data on 14,576 cases (Sept. 1983)

Doses of NaF (mg)	Surgical cases	Medical cases
3-10	1090	4791
15	1456	2079
30	1107	81
45	3089	819
60	64	—
TOTAL	6806	7770

is only a presumptive sign of an otosclerotic stapedial encroachment and must be confirmed by history, progression, or surgery and, second, on the early detection of cochlear involvement by repeated air conduction and bone conduction pure tone audiometry testing, and third, if the results show an otospongiotic involvement prevention requires immediate treatment with very small doses of sodium fluoride in young children.

The functional results of sodium fluoride therapy on the sensorineural component of mixed hearing losses of otospongiotic/otosclerotic origin, and/or on pure cochlear otospongiosis (presbycusis and other SNHLs excluded), garnered from our computerized data on patients with follow-ups ranging from 6 months to 15 years are favorable. However, "favorable results" means only arrest of cochlear deterioration in cases with a progressive cochlear component, because sodium fluoride acts only as a stabilization factor and thus cannot improve hearing, except in children. Moreover, a follow-up of at least 1 or 2 years is necessary for a sure approach to the problem, because otospongiotic disease generally develops in progressive steps separated by inactive periods due to spontaneous enzyme-antienzyme balance. For this reason, we have always corrected the functional results compared with control series, taking into account the 25% spontaneously nonprogressive otospongiosis operated or unoperated.

Our results are summarized in Table 23-1 and Fig. 23-17. Table I shows higher doses in surgical cases than in medical ones, as already reported. Fig. 23-17 proves that the various doses have been correctly established to slightly exceed the threshold of sodium fluoride action, since the percentages of favorable results in relation to different doses related to enzymatic activity are similar for medical cases (66.41%) and surgical ones (67.52%).

Fluoride action on vestibular function clearly appears. Patients generally show less vertigo after some months of sodium fluoride therapy, as well as less tinnitus for cochlear function. Moreover, we conducted a series of 224 comparative studies using the torsion swing test ENG recording, before and after sodium fluoride therapy on operated or unoperated otospongiotic patients.The more or less irritative type tracing, usual in otospongiotic patients, tends to become less irritative or even normal in almost 70% of operated ears and 60% of unoperated ears, compared with the control series, after 6 months or more of sodium fluoride therapy.

Linthicum et al[27] gave short-life radioactive strontium to patients undergoing stapedectomy. Histologic examination of the involved footplate from one side showed active vascular spongiotic changes and a low level of radioactive strontium. Sodium fluoride was then administered to the patient. When the second side was operated on, this footplate showed mature, inactive, sclerotic changes and a high level of radioactive strontium that had been taken up by the new bone formation.

Clinical studies of the effects of sodium fluoride on progressive sensorineural deterioration in large groups of patients operated on for fenestration or stapedectomy were reported in 1974 by Shambaugh and Causse.[17,35] Two thirds of 34 untreated control subjects showed further progression of the sensorineural hearing loss, while in one third of these subjects the hearing remained stable. In 80% of 575 patients treated with sodium fluoride in optimum dosage, the hearing remained stable, in 3% the hearing actually improved, and in 8% the hearing loss that had been arrested resumed when fluoride was halted. In 17%, the progression continued despite fluoride therapy. Thus, the medication was successful in more than 80% of treated patients. A similar study by Linthicum et al[27] showed the effect of sodium fluoride on otosclerosis activity.

Objective evidence of the favorable effect of fluorides on otospongiotic foci is afforded by comparative dosages of trypsin concentration in perilymph before and after sodium fluoride therapy in studies that we undertook with Uriel and Berges in 1980.[14] The results clearly show a constant and significant decrease in trypsin values, averaging 1 to 2 μg/ml after sodium fluoride therapy given over one year at moderate daily doses (15 to 45 mg a day). The clinical results of this study show that the trypsin level significantly decreases in about 66% of otosclerotic patients with moderate doses of sodium fluoride, compared with a control series.

Three double-blind, placebo-controlled studies have since been reported on small groups of patients elsewhere : two by Bretlau et al[2] in Denmark and another by Fisch[22] in Switzerland. Both authors verified the positive value of sodium fluoride in reducing progression of sensorineural hearing deterioration in stapedectomized patients.

Clinical

Double-blind placebo-controlled study on sodium fluoride treatment in otospongiosis. Bretlau et al[3] carried out this prospective study of 142 patients with clinical otospongiosis in the Ear, Nose, and Throat and Audiological Departments at Gentofte Hospital, to evaluate the effect of sodium fluoride treatment on otospongiosis. The diagnosis was based on audiometry, stapedial reflex tests, and x-ray examinations, and no patient underwent surgery during the observation period. Most of the patients had a mixed perceptive and conductive hearing loss: the remaining had a pure conductive or a pure perceptive hearing loss.

All patients agreed to participate in the double-blind, placebo-controlled trial testing the efficacy of medical treatment with sodium fluoride. They were assigned for each treatment group according to their odd or even birthdays. The active treatment consisted of 20 mg of sodium fluoride as enteric-coated tablets twice a day, 500 mg of calcium gluconate, and 400 units of vitamin D. The placebo treatment consisted of similar tablets without sodium fluoride but containing the same dose of calcium gluconate and vitamin D. Of the 142 patients, 47 were excluded before or during the investigation period, mostly due to different diseases or complications (4 kidney-bladder stones, 2 arthritis, 3 leukemia-metabolic disease, 4 dyspepsia, 6 eczema, 1 psychosis, 1 pregnancy). Seven patients moved away from the area and could not be reached: ten patients refused to join the investigation after the introduction: and 9 patients were treated only 3 to 6 months and therefore were excluded.

Ninety-five patients entered, went through the trial, and were controlled every third month in a 12- to 24-month period during the years 1978 to 1981. At each control the patients filled out a questionnaire in which they were asked about the daily intake of the medicine and if they had taken the medicine regularly. The subjective symptoms of change in hearing or vertigo and tinnitus were reported as well as side effects such as dyspepsia, nausea, eczema, obstipation, or diarrhea. A complete audiologic examination was performed including pure tone audiogram, SRT, and discrimination and stapedial reflex examinations. A polytomographic x-ray examination of the temporal bones together with a side view of the calcaneus bone was taken before treatment was started. Kidney function was tested by serum and urine analyses. Electrocochleography was done in several of the patients. The code was broken 24 months after the last patient had entered the trial.

Forty-three patients received the active treatment and 52 received the placebo medication. In the active group, 28 were women and 15 were men, and the corresponding figures in the placebo group were 32 women and 20 men. In the active group the ages ranged from 21 to 64 years, average 39.9 years: in the placebo group the average age was 39 years, ranging from 20 to 69 years.

Results. Subjectively, 3 patients (2 in the active group and 1 in the placebo group) experienced improved hearing during the trial; 11 reported reduced hearing (6 in the active and 5 in the placebo group), but the majority of the patients (35 active and 46 placebo) could not state any change in hearing. Regarding tinnitus, most of the patients indicated unchanged tinnitus or no tinnitus at all (41 active, 42 placebo), but 6 patients said that the tinnitus was improved and 6 found it worse. Five of these 6 in both situations were in the placebo group, but the difference was not significant. Sixteen patients complained of vertigo—5 in the active and 11 in the placebo group. This difference is not significant. The rest of the patients (38 active, 41 placebo) had no complaints of vertigo.

In the audiometric evaluation, a changed hearing was noted if the average threshold of 500 to 1,000 to 2,000 Hz improved 10 dB or more or deteriorated equally at the end

TABLE 23-2
Results of audiometric and speech reception—Treshold tests

	Audiometry (5---1000-2000 Hz)		SRT	
	A	P	A	P
Improved	1	3	1	1
Unchanged	39	36	37	36
Worse	3	13*	5	15+
TOTALS	43	52	43	52

$p < 0.025$ (2.5%)*
$p < 0.15$†

of the trial. In 4 patients, the hearing improved (1 in the active group and 3 in the placebo group), but in 16 patients a hearing loss was noted (3 in the active group and 13 in the placebo group, Table 23-2). This difference is significant ($p < 0.025$) using the χ^2 test. Using the SRT, the hearing loss deteriorated more in the placebo group, but this difference was not significant ($p < 0.15$).

The immune complex action of otospongiotic-otosclerotic disease is the subject of ongoing research, because otosclerosis may be an immune reaction of the enchondral otic capsule against the genetically determined cartilaginous remnants mainly located near the fissula ante fenestram as proposed by Jean-Bernard Causse.[38] TJ Yoo injected collagen II in rats animals models and claimed to have confirmed this.[37] Treatment could be directed toward antigen elimination, the manipulation of antibody response, the removal of circulating immune complexes, or the blocking of inflammatory mediators to inhibit the complement protein cascade that originates the destructive enzymatic process.

Sodium fluoride is an enzyme inhibitor

Studied trypsin and α_1-antitrypsin concentrations in the perilymph of surgically treated patients led to the conclusion that the basic mechanism of otospongiotic disease is a sudden reversal of the enzymatic equilibrium, the cochlear deterioration occuring when the normal balance is disrupted in favor of the tryptic activity.

The comparative studies undertaken by Jean-René Causse working with Uriel and Berges[14] in 1980 on trypsin, α_1-antitrypsin, and α_2-macroglobulin values in each of 811 samples of perilymph demonstrated that α_2-macroglobulin appears to have a synergic action with α_1-antitrypsin in the balance with trypsin. This is particularly important in otospongiotic disease, in which α_1-antitrypsin values are generally low. The interaction between α_1-antitrypsin and α_2-macroglobulin appears essential to the enzymatic mechanism in otospongiotic disease. The result of the breakdown of the normal equilibrium in favor of trypsin is an increase in trypsin values that damages the hair

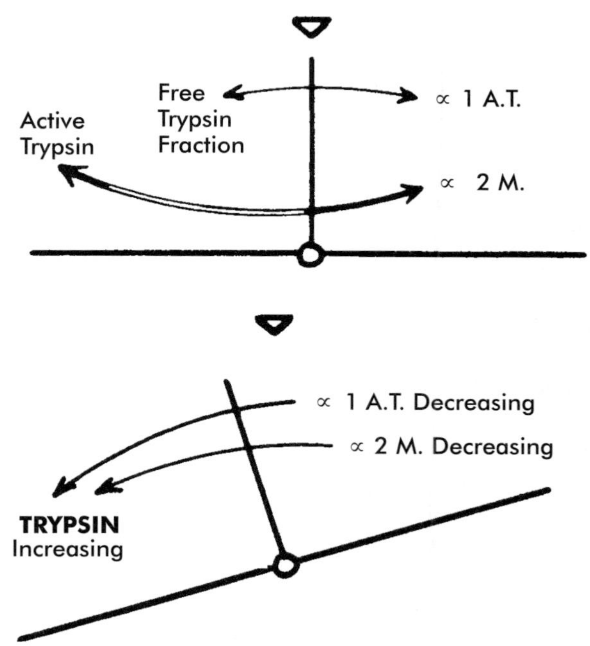

FIG 23-18
A and **B,** Balance with trypsin and rupture of equilibrium.

cells, leading to cochlear deterioration, and destroys the collagen fibrils during the first phase of bony lysis, resulting in the second pseudohaversian bony rebuilding phase (Fig. 23-18 *A,* and *B*).

The balance between trypsin and α_1-antitrypsin and other protease inhibitors is not the only mechanism involved in otospongiotic disease. Other enzymes, such as collagenase, α-chymotrypsin, phosphatasic acid, ribonuclease, lactate dehydrogenase, already found in the perilymph of otosclerotic patients, and cathepsin-B, recently studied by Ribari[34] in otosclerotic stapes, are also involved in active otospongiotic process. We are currently experimenting with collagenase, which plays a major role in the destruction of collagen tissues. In the past, we have found in vitro a synergic action between collagenase and α-chymotrypsin, similar to that recently found in vivo between α_2-macroglobulin and α_1-antitrypsin.

This enzymatic concept is quite similar to that proposed by Linthicum.[26] Linthicum and Parahy[31] stated that "otosclerosis" includes both otospongiosis and otosclerosis, and they statistically analyzed relationships between histologic and clinical data. They have found that ". . . active otospongiosis involving the endosteum is associated with hyalinization of the spiral ligament, atrophy of the stria vascularis and sensorineural hearing loss" and that ". . the most likely mode of action of sodium fluoride in halting the progression of hearing loss due to otospongiosis is to neutralize hydrolytic enzymes and inactivate the otospongiotic lesions," thus substantiating our belief. The only surprise is that they classify lesions as active otosclerosis, active otospongiosis, inactive otosclerosis, and inactive otospongiosis and emphasize that the absence of hyalinization adjacent to otosclerotic lesions suggests that these lesions were never otospongiotic. They conclude that otospongiotic and otosclerotic lesions can occur simultaneously and that otospongiosis does not necessarily precede otosclerosis, in contrast to the views that we have held so far.

In a relatively unexposed individual, about half of a single dose of fluoride is excreted in the urine within 24 hours. Steady static conditions develop after a regular daily intake of the same amounts for several months or even years.

The mechanism of sodium fluoride activity is an enzymatic action in the first phase of destruction. Experiments at many levels—in vitro, in vivo, on laboratory animals, and on human patients—from enzymatic, cytochemical, and anatomopathologic viewpoints[14] have proved that sodium fluoride can act directly on trypsin and other enzymes, which are inhibited in vitro in the proportion of O.5 mg sodium fluoride to 1 mg trypsin, and also that it reduces the levels of protease inhibitors, such as α_1-antitrypsin and α_2-macroglobulin. This overall reduction of enzymatic rates by inhibition favors the stabilization of the otospongiotic process. What occurs is a consequent arrest or slowing down of the cochlear deterioration which resulted from Corti cell alteration due to active proteases.

The atrophy of the stria vascularis and the hyalinization of the spiral ligament, explaining both pure cochlear otospongiosis and the sensorineural component of mixed hearing loss due to otospongiosis/otosclerosis,[15] are always found adjacent to active otospongiotic lesions. Sodium fluoride inactivates otospongiotic lesions by neutralizing hydrolytic and proteolytic enzymes. Linthicum and Parahy[31] believe that sodium fluoride slows down or halts the progression of otosclerotic hearing loss by neutralizing and inactivating the hydrolytic and proteolytic enzymes of otospongiotic foci, rather than by converting an active otospongiotic focus into an inactive otosclerotic one.

Diphosphonate has the reputation to be able to reduce the activity of the osteoclasts. Petrovic's work[32] demonstrated the effects of sodium fluoride on bone metabolism, reducing osteoclastic bone resorption as a major effect and at the same time promoting osteoblastic bone formation. In new bone, the fluoride ion replaces the hydroxy radical in hydroxyapatite; the resulting fluorapatite is harder, of better quality, and more resistant to bone resorption than hydroxyapatite.

Absorption and side effects of sodium fluoride therapy

Deka et al[21] investigated the intestinal absorption of sodium fluoride in human volunteers. They found that sodium fluoride in liquid preparation or in gelatin capsules provides the best absorption, but many patients suffer severe gastric distress. Enteric-coated sodium fluoride reduces the gastric irritation, but intestinal absorption is inconsistent and poor in some subjects.

Fluorosis is the most severe side effect in the treatment of generalized osteoporosis and it is an occupational hazard for workers exposed to fluorides in the aluminum industry. But we have never seen any case of confirmed fluorosis since the daily dose does not exceed 25mg.

In children, fluoride has a greater effect on bone because of increased bone turnover and the vascularity of young bones, so the dosage should be reduced relative to body weight.[19] Once-daily doses of 2 to 5 mg must be prescribed in order to avoid joint growth problems.

In case of intolerance of sodium fluoride, *diphosphonates* can take over from fluoride. Their mechanism of action could be due to a primary enzymatic inhibition, reducing the intensity of resorption phenomena and consequently promoting a stable secondary new bone formation.[3,18,33] Clinical trials showed a clear tendency toward stabilization of both conductive and sensorineural hearing loss following the regular use of EHDP for one year. But the five–year follow-up of our clinical comparative study of sodium fluoride and EHDP shows a poorer efficacy of EHDP in comparison with sodium fluoride. Diphosphonates appear to be only a relay therapy of fluorides.

CONCLUSION

Our experience leads us to our current opinion that it is necessary to perform an operation for stapes fixation considering:

With regard to the quality of hearing, the notion of impedance transfer of the ossicular chain, the notion of mass, as well as the quality of the system's elasticity, that is to say kind of a push-pull effect, replacing the annular ligament of the stapes footplate.

With regard to the safety of hearing, the resistance (or kind of shock absorber) of the system around the lower tip of the piston and, when possible, the reconstitution of the stapes tendon. Thus, the patient is allowed to scuba dive, fly, etc, even professionally.

The evolution of the vein graft in photonic and electronic microscopy and the comparative statistical results of the different surgical techniques replacing the fixed stapes have encouraged us to progress in this way.

Sodium fluoride therapy is second to none in our experience. Keeping the dose under 30 mg a day is essential to avoid a rebuilding of bone in the cochlea and still benefits both antienzyme and antiosteoclastic actions.

REFERENCES

1. Bolz EA, Lim DJ: Morphology of the stapediovestibular joint. *Acta Otol* 73:10-17 1972.
2. Bretlau P, Causse JR, Causse JB, et al: Otospongiosis and sodium fluoride: a blind experimental and clinical evaluation of the effect of sodium fluoride treatment in patients with otospongiosis. *Ann Otol Rhinol Laryngol* 94:103-107, 1985

3. Bretlau P, Hansen HG, Causse JR, Causse JB: Otospongiosis: morphologic and microchemical investigation after NaF-treatment. *Otolaryng Head Neck Surg* 89:646-650, 1981
4. Causse et al: Transfert d'impédance et impédance acoustique de l'oreille moyenne. Son intérêt dans la chirurgie des malformations d'oreille. LXXXVIIIè Cong 1993, *Congrès Annuel Français d'ORL,* Paris, Sept.30-Oct.3, 1991.
5. Causse JB, Gherini S, Lopez A, et al: Impedance transfer: acoustic impedance of the annular ligament and stapedial tendon reconstruction in otosclerosis surgery. *Am J Otol* 14:613-617, 1993
6. Causse JB, Causse JR, et al: The annular ligament of the stapes footplate: reconstitution of its function in otosclerosis and dysplasia surgery. International Workshop on Otosclerosis, Rome, April 25-27, 1989, XIV *World Congress of ORL, H&N Surgery,* Madrid, Sept. 10-15, 1989.
7. Causse J, Wiet RJ, Causse JR, Michat M: Le ligament annulaire de la platine de l'étrier: reconstitution de sa fonction dans la chirurgie de l'otospongiose et des dysplasies. *J Fr d'ORL,* 38:266-270, 1989.
8. Causse JR: Present problems in the surgery of otosclerosis. *J Laryngol Otol* 79:265-299, 1965.
9. Causse JB, Causse JR, Parahy CL : Stapedotomy technique and results. *Am J Otol* 6:68-71, 1985.
10. Causse JB: The twenty fine points of otosclerosis surgery— clinical vignette. *Am J Otol* 10:75-77, 1989.
11. Causse JB, Causse JR, Lopez A, et al: Subcophoses et otospongioses. Traitement médical et chirurgical. *Ann Otol Paris* 107:411-417, 1990.
12. Causse JB: Otosclerosis. The method of Jean-Bernard Causse. In Decker BC, editor: Current Therapy in Otolaryngology and Heah and Neck Surgery—4, 1990.
13. Causse JB, Gherini S, Horn K : Surgical treatment of stapes fixation by fiberoptic argon laser stapedotomy with reconstruction of the annular ligament *Otolaryngol Clin North Am* 26:395-416, 1993.
14. Causse JR, Uriel J, Berges J, et al : The enzymatic mechanism of the otospongiotic disease and NaF action on the enzymatic balance. *Am J Otol* 3:297-314, 1982.
15. Causse JR, Shambaugh GE, Chevance LG, Bretlau P: Cochlear otospongiosis: etiology, diagnosis and therapeutic implications. *Adv ORL* 22:43-56, 1977.
16. Causse JR, Shambaugh GE, Causse JB, Bretlau P: Enzymology of otospongiosis and NaF therapy. *Am J Otol* 1:206-213, 1980
17. Causse JR, Chevance LG, Shambaugh GE Jr: Clinical experience and experimental findings with sodium fluoride in otosclerosis (otospongiosis). *Ann Otol Rhinol Laryngol* 83:643-647, 1974
18. Causse JR, Causse JB: Clinical studies on fluoride in otospongiosis. *Am J Otol* 6:51-55, 1985
19. Causse JR, Causse JB: Otospongiosis as a genetic disease: early detection, medical management and prevention. *Am J Otol* 5:211-223, 1984.
20. Causse JR, Causse JB, Uriel J, Berges J, Shambaugh G, Bretlau P: Sodium fluoride therapy. *Am J Otol* 14:482-490, 1993
21. Deka RC, Kacker SK, Shambaugh GE Jr: Intestinal absorption of fluoride preparations. *Laryngoscope* 88:1918-1921,1978.
22. Fisch U: New dimensions in the management of otosclerosis. *Proceedings of the Thirteenth World Congress of Otolaryngology,*1985, pp 33-38.
23. Gherini S, Horn K, Causse JB, McArthur G: Fiberoptic Argon laser stapedotomy: Is it safe? *Am J Otol* 14:283-289, 1993
24. Jowsey J, Riggs L, Kelly P, Hoffman D: Effect of combined therapy with sodium fluoride, vitamin D and calcium in osteoporosis. *Am J Med* 53:43-49, 1972
25. Lesinski SG: Apical displacement of the traveling wave. Reprinted from the Transactions American Academy of Ophtalmology and Otolaryngology, Sept.-Oct., 1973.
26. Linthicum FH: Correlations of sensorineural hearing impairment and otosclerosis. *Ann ORL* 75:512-524, 1966.
27. Linthicum FH, House HP, Althaus SR: The effect of sodium fluoride on otosclerotic activity as determined by strontium-85. *Trans Am Otol Soc* 61:98, 1973.
28. Lopez A, Juberthie L, Olivier JC, et al: Survival and evolution of vein grafts in otosclerosis surgery: structural and ultrastructural evidence. *Am J Otol* 13:173-184, 1992
29. Marquet J: The incudo-mallear joint. *J Laryng and Otol* 95:543-565, 1981.
30. Parahy CL, Causse JB and Michat M: Stapes surgery—Minimizing the risks. Proceedings: 241-248, Ibiza, Spain, Sept. 10-15, 1989-1991, Kugler Pub.
31. Parahy CH, Linthicum FH: Otosclerosis. Relationship of spiral ligament hyalinization to sensorineural hearing loss. *Laryngoscope* 93:717-720, 1983
32. Petrovic A, Shambaugh GE Jr: Promotion of bone calcification by sodium fluoride: short-term experiments on newborn rats using tetracycline labeling. *Arch Otolaryngol* 83:104-112, 1966.
33. Petrovic A, Stutzmann J: Diphosphonates: a potential medication for evolutive otospongiosis. Proceedings of the Fourth Symposium CEMO. *Educ Med Hygiene* 84:275-282, 1988.
34. Ribari O, Sziklai I, Kiss JG, Sohar J: Cathepsin-B activity in otosclerosis. *Hun Arch ORL* 238:123-125, 1983
35. Shambaugh GE Jr, Causse JR: Ten years experience with fluoride in otosclerotic (otospongiotic) patients. *Ann Otol Rhinol Laryngol* 83:635, 1974.
36. Shea JJ: Fenestration of the oval window—*Annals ORL.* 67:932-951, 1958.
37. Yoo TJ, Tomoda K, Stuart JM, et al: Collagen-induced autoimmune neurosensory hearing loss, vestibular dysfunction and otosclerosis in rodents. Memphis, 1982, Dept of Medical University of Tennessee, Center for the Health Sciences and V.A. Medical Center.
38. Wiet JR, Causse JB, Shambaugh GE, Causse JR: Monograph on Otosclerosis. American Academy of Otology—Head and Neck Surgery Foundation, Inc., 1991.

24

Tinnitus: Evaluation and Treatment

John W. House, M.D. and M. Jennifer Derebery, M.D.

Tinnitus is a symptom and not a disease. Treatment cannot be based on one modality, and the evaluation is important to establish the etiology of this symptom. Goodhill put it well in 1953 when he said, "Any management which is based upon a single panacea for the treatment of a symptom and not a disease will result in failure."[7] In our practice, about 12% of the patients have a chief complaint of tinnitus. In most of these patients, the tinnitus is secondary to another otologic diagnosis, such as hearing loss. Fowler pointed out that 86% of patients with ear disease will have associated tinnitus.[6] About 5% of our patients who have tinnitus complain bitterly and are severely distracted by it. However, most patients are not particularly bothered by their tinnitus. Some are concerned that it may be a symptom of a more serious problem or that they may be going deaf. After an evaluation and explanation, they are usually satisfied. It is the 5% group of patients with severe tinnitus who present a management problem.

EVALUATION

All new patients at the House Ear Clinic undergo an initial audiogram, which includes air conduction, bone conduction, and speech audiometry. Following the audiogram, they are seen by the otologist who takes a history and performs the examination of the ears, nose, and throat. Depending on the situation, we may also do a brief neurologic examination emphasizing the cranial nerves. Further testing, if indicated, will be ordered. The management of the patient is based on the results of the audiogram, history, physical examination, and any further testing.

History

The patient is asked how long the tinnitus has been present, whether it was of sudden or gradual onset, and if it is constant or intermittent. We also must consider the possibility of objective tinnitus. Clues to this type of tinnitus include a pulsatile, rhythmic, or popping sound. A history of this type of tinnitus necessitates auscultation of the ear, head, mastoid, and neck for vascular bruits (box on p 294). In addition, if the patient describes a clicking sound and it is present at the time of the examination, the palate is inspected with mouth slightly opened. It is helpful to have the patient raise a finger when the click is heard. If the patient has palatal myoclonus, the palate will be seen contracting at the same time that the sound is experienced. Opening the mouth widely will stop the rhythmic contraction of the palate. The stapedial tendon and tensor tympani can also produce objective tinnitus.

Questions to assist in determining the severity of the tinnitus include: What time of day or night is it more bothersome? Is the patient aware of it constantly, just when it is quiet, or only when he or she thinks about it? One of the most important questions to ask is whether the tinnitus interferes with sleep. It is our experience that most patients with severe tinnitus have difficulty sleeping. Those patients who have difficulty sleeping are asked if they have trouble going to sleep or whether they awaken after a few hours of sleep and have difficulty going back to sleep. We find that most patients with severe tinnitus have problems staying asleep. Another common problem is difficulty concentrating during the day. Some patients may focus on the tinnitus to the extent that it interferes with daily activities or work. Patients are also asked if there is anything that seems to aggravate the tinnitus and if they are under stress or experiencing any depression. They may be asked if there was any precipitating event, such as trauma or a life crisis.

Physical examination

For the most part, the examination is not unique. The exception is when the history suggests a possible objective type of tinnitus. As mentioned earlier, auscultation is performed in these cases using a stethoscope and Toynby tube

Possible Vascular Causes of Objective Tinnitus

Venous

Chronic anemia
Pregnancy
Thyrotoxicosis
Intracranial hypertension
Large or exposed jugular bulb
Idiopathic venous tinnitus

Arterial

Fibromuscular dysplasia
Atherosclerosis
Styloid carotid compression
Petrous carotid aneurysm
Laterally displaced carotid
Persistent stapedial artery

Arteriovenous

Paraganglioma
Tympanicum
Jugulare
Other vascular tumors
Paget's disease of bone
Cerebral AV malformation
Dural AV fistula
Vertebral AV fistula

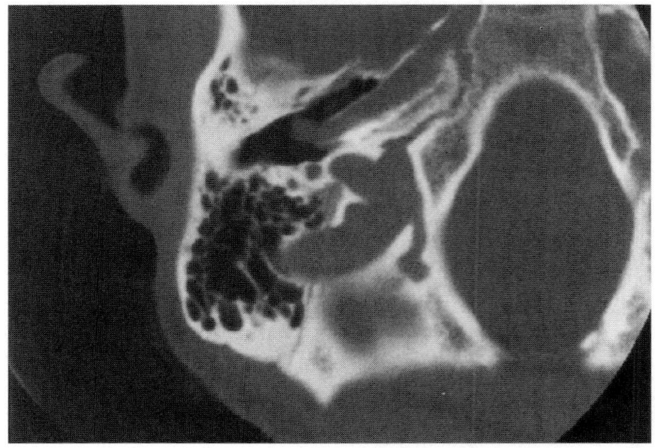

FIG 24-1
CT scan showing carotid artery in middle ear as associated with objective tinnitus. Reprinted with permission of House Ear Institute.

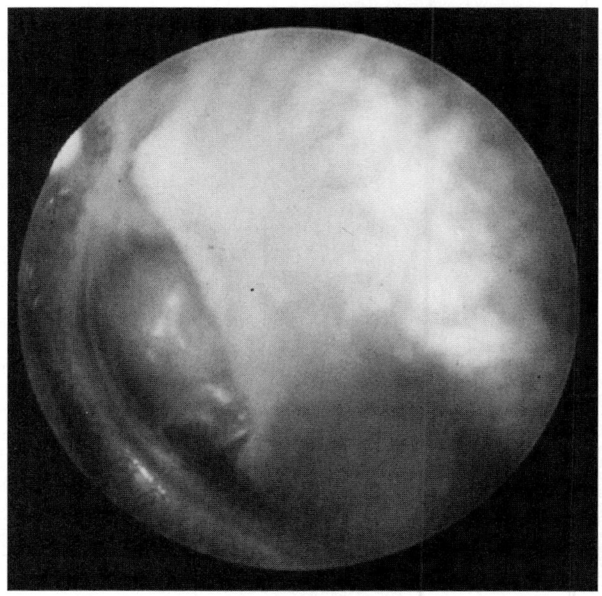

FIG 24-2
Photograph of tympanic membrane with exposed internal carotid artery in middle ear as cause of objective tinnitus. Reprinted with permission of House Ear Institute.

to listen in the patient's ear (Figs. 24-1 to 24-3). We routinely perform tuning fork examination (Weber and Renné) to confirm the audiometric findings.

Special testing

It is important to determine the etiology of this symptom and to rule out potentially serious pathology, such as an acoustic tumor. Of 1493 of our acoustic tumor patients, 9.5% presented with tinnitus as the chief complaint. We also want to rule out possible causes which would be associated with a progressive hearing loss. In some patients, allergy is a contributing factor. For this reason, an allergic history may be taken and allergy testing performed, if indicated.

When the symptom is unilateral or asymmetrical or if the audiogram is suggestive of a retrocochlear lesion (i.e., poor speech discrimination in one ear), further tests are ordered. Auditory brain stem response audiometry (ABR) is a good screening test for patients in whom we are minimally concerned regarding the presence of an acoustic neuroma. These include patients with asymmetric presbycusis and patients with normal audiograms and unilateral tinnitus. When the ABR test is positive, an MRI is ordered. Conversely, when the test is negative, it is still advisable to have the patient return in 6 months to one year to repeat the audiogram and be sure that there is not a progressive problem. If, at that time, there has been a change, further testing may be indicated. If the patient's history or audiometric tests are strongly suggestive of a retrocochlear lesion, an MRI with gadolinium is ordered. Other tests could include impedance audiometry and blood tests to rule out autoimmune disease or syphilis.

Management

The first step and the most important aspect of the management of patients with tinnitus is explanation of the problem to the patients. In most cases, this also includes strong reassurance that this is not a serious problem and that the patient will not go deaf. Many patients will be satisfied and are able to live with the tinnitus. They find that it fades into the background and that most of the time they are not aware of it.

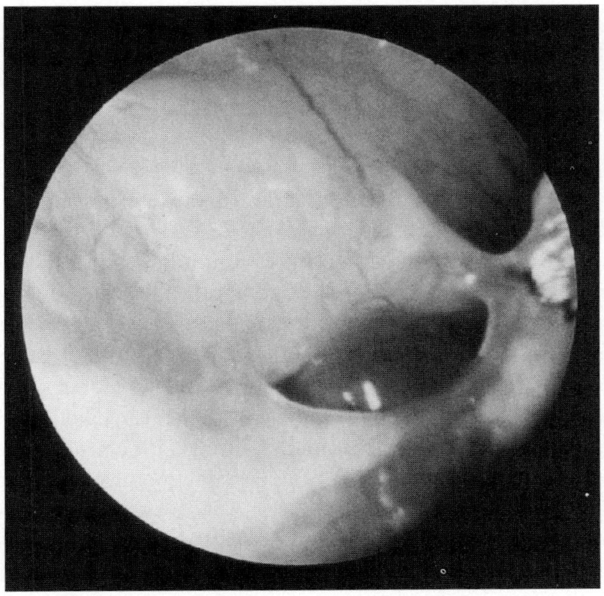

FIG 24-3
Photograph of dehiscent jugular bulb taken through tympanic membrane perforation. Reprinted with permission of House Ear Institute.

Medications

Intravenous Xylocaine will briefly relieve tinnitus in a significant number of patients. Emmett and Shea studied the effectiveness of tocainide hydrochloride, an oral analog of lidocaine, and reported some improvement; but side effects were too high to continue in most patients.[5] Subsequent studies have yielded similar results.

We have not had good results with other medications, including the anticonvulsants, vitamin therapy, vasodilators, or tranquilizers. Because our psychologic studies revealed that the majority of patients with severe tinnitus tend to be depressed, we often use antidepressants with good results. As previously mentioned, many of the patients have sleep disturbance. By using an antidepressant which has a sedative effect, the patient's sleep can be improved. We commonly use amitriptyline (Elavil) and, occasionally, a combination of antidepressant and sedative, such as Triavil.

There is evidence that a decrease in cochlear prostaglandins may play a role in the production of tinnitus. We performed a study to evaluate the effect of a synthetic prostaglandin E_1, Misoprostol on tinnitus.[3] Subjects were started on a regimen of placebo or 200 μg per day of Misoprostol. The dosage was increased every 5 days by 200 μg until a total dose of 800 μg per day was achieved. After one month of treatment, the placebo group was crossed over to the active drug phase. Eight (33%) of the 24 patients reported improvement during the active drug phase, while there were no placebo responders. Further study is needed before any conclusions can be drawn from this preliminary study. A different prostaglandin analog may need to be tried. The most abundant PGs in the cochlea of the guinea pig are PGI_2 and PGF_4, and an analog of one of these may be more appropriate for the treatment of tinnitus than a PGE_2.

TABLE 24-1
Use of a tinnitus masker in a series of 42 patients with tinnitus

Advised to try	27 (64%)
Rental trial	13 (31%)
Purchased masker	9 (17%)

TABLE 24-2
Use of a hearing aid in a series of 42 patients undergoing tinnitus masker evaluation

Advised to try	15 (36%)
Rental trial	14 (33%)
Wearing hearing aid	9 (21%)
Helps tinnitus	7 (175)

Masking and hearing aids

Vernon[13] first described the use of the tinnitus masker in 1977. We have been using maskers since he first described his experience. When we reviewed a series of 42 patients,[9] we found that only a small number of patients eventually purchased a masker and used it regularly (Table 24-1). Newer maskers allow adjustment of the masking sound and are also combined with hearing aids. We find that a few patients find these to be very helpful and give them some control over their tinnitus.

When a hearing loss is present, hearing aids can be of great help. It is not unusual to recommend a hearing aid in a patient with severe tinnitus who has a mild or unilateral hearing loss (Table 24-2). In these cases, the hearing aid is used to improve hearing but more importantly to mask the tinnitus with environmental sounds.

Biofeedback

In 1976, we first reported our results using biofeedback training in patients with severe tinnitus.[10] Biofeedback information from the frontalis muscle and skin temperature from the fingers was used to teach the patient relaxation techniques. When patients are able to do this and achieve a significant degree of relaxation, perception of the tinnitus is lessened greatly. In some cases in which stress is a major contributor to the tinnitus, we see the tinnitus disappear as the patient is able to relax and become more aware of bodily tensions. We have found that more than 70% of the patients with severe tinnitus had some improvement in symptoms. Depressed and anxious patients do best with this biofeedback, while severely disturbed patients have more disappointing results. We continue to refer selected tinnitus patients for biofeedback treatment with good results.

Surgery

Dandy[4] described sectioning the eighth nerve in 401 patients with Ménière's disease. He felt that 50% of the patients had improvement in the tinnitus. He stated that, "Tinnitus may or may not disappear after nerve section, and if it persists, it may or may not be improved.—No promise can be made concerning tinnitus, which a sensible person learns to disregard." When we looked at our experience with tinnitus in 500 patients undergoing translabyrinthine removal of acoustic tumors, we found that 40% felt it was better, 10% said it was the same, and 50% felt it was worse.[8] More recently, a questionnaire study of patients who had undergone acoustic tumor removal showed that those with preoperative tinnitus had some improvements in loudness, interference ratings, and frequency of occurrence, but rarely did tinnitus resolve entirely.[2] Thirty-seven percent felt the surgery made their tinnitus better, while 15% felt surgery made the tinnitus worse. In addition, 34% of those with no preoperative tinnitus felt the surgery made tinnitus worse (produced the symptom). When we carefully question a postoperative acoustic neuroma patient, most feel that the tinnitus is not altered by the removal of the tumor. This is despite the fact that the entire eighth nerve is removed with the tumor.

Even when stapedectomy closed the air bone-gap to within 10 db, only 37% of patients reported complete relief of their tinnitus (House HP: personal communication). An additional 39% reported improvement of the tinnitus, while 5% felt that it was worse. Microvascular decompression of the eighth nerve has also been proposed for the treatment of tinnitus.[11] Vascular compression of the eighth nerve would be a rare cause of tinnitus and the results of surgery would be unpredictable.

The effect of a cochlear implant in relieving tinnitus has been studied in profoundly deaf patients.[1] Of 90 patients who experienced tinnitus and completed a detailed postimplant tinnitus questionnaire, 53% stated that the cochlear implant made the tinnitus better, 36% felt that the tinnitus was unchanged by the implant, and 11% stated that the tinnitus was worse. There were reductions in the loudness of the tinnitus, the amount of interference, and the number of different sounds experienced. Interestingly, of those whose tinnitus was affected, 14% stated the implanted ear was affected, 52% indicated both ears, 13% indicated the other ear, and the remaining 22% could not localize the effect. Therefore, in at least some cases, the effect was most likely due to reduction of fatigue and stress. All of the patients in this study had received a cochlear implant for the purpose of hearing improvement. A small number of subjects have been implanted specifically for the indication of severe tinnitus.[12] In only one of five cases was the result considered a success.

From these studies and additional experience with other types of nerve sections it is apparent that, at this time, there is not an operation for tinnitus. We do not recommend surgery solely for the treatment of tinnitus.

SUMMARY

Tinnitus is a common symptom of ear disease and usually is not a major concern for patients. About 5% of our patients are driven to distraction by tinnitus. After an evaluation and examination, a thorough explanation is an important step in the management of these patients. Most of them are satisfied with the information and reassurance. Some patients will benefit from therapies such as biofeedback, tinnitus maskers, or, when appropriate, a hearing aid. Some medication such as antidepressants may be helpful. When surgery is indicated, some patients will report an improvement in tinnitus. This is especially true in otosclerosis surgery where hearing is improved. Transection of the auditory nerve in the removal of an acoustic neuroma does not necessarily eliminate tinnitus.

The key to all therapies for tinnitus is a complete evaluation, examination, and, above all, an explanation and reassurance.

REFERENCES

1. Berliner KI, Cunningham JK: Tinnitus suppression in cochlear implantation. In Hazell JWP, editor: *Tinnitus*. London, 1987, Churchill Livingstone.
2. Berliner KI, Shelton C, Hitselberger WE, Luxford WM: Acoustic tumors: effect of surgical removal on tinnitus, *Am J Otol* 13:13-17, 1992.
3. Briner W, House J, O'Leary M: Synthetic prostaglandin E1 misoprostol as a treatment for tinnitus. *Arch Otolaryngol Head Neck Surg* 119:652-654, 1994.
4. Dandy WE: Surgical treatment of Ménière's disease. *Surg Gynecol Obstet* 72:421-425, 1941.
5. Emmett JR, Sheat JJ: Treatment of tinnitus with tocainide hydrochloride. *Otolaryngol Head Neck Surg* 88:442-446, 1980.
6. Fowler EP: Head noises in normal and in disordered ears: significance, measurement, differentiation and treatment. *Arch Otolaryngol* 39:498-503, 1944.
7. Goodhill V: The management of tinnitus. *Laryngoscope* 60:422-50, 1950.
8. House JW, Brackmann DE: Tinnitus: Surgical management. *Ciba Found Symp* 85:204-216, 1981.
9. House JW, Johnson EW: Tinnitus: tinnitus masker and biofeedback training. *Trans Pac Coast Otoophthalmol Soc Annu Meet* 60:115-120, 1979.
10. House JW, Miller L, House PR: Severe tinnitus: treatment with biofeedback training (results in 41 cases). *Trans Am Acad Ophthalmol Otolaryngol* 84:697-703, 1977.
11. Moller MB, Moller AR, Jannetta PH, Jho HD: Vascular decompression surgery for severe tinnitus: selection criteria and results. *Laryngoscope* 103:421-427, 1993.
12. Thedinger B, House WF, Edgerton BJ: Cochlear implant for tinnitus: case reports. *Ann Otol Rhinol Laryngol* 94:10-13, 1985.
13. Vernon J: Attempts to relieve tinnitus. *J Am Audiol Soc* 2:124-131, 1977.

25

Immune Inner Ear Disease

Gordon B. Hughes, M.D. and Richard A. Moscicki, M.D.

Immune inner ear disease is a distinct clinical entity that characteristically produces bilateral, rapidly progressive sensorineural hearing loss. Unlike ototoxicity, trauma, and infection, which can produce profound hearing loss over hours or days, a presbycusis or noise-induced hearing loss, which occurs over years, immune-mediated hearing loss usually develops over weeks or months. Although sudden hearing loss can occur in one ear, loss is usually also rapidly progressive in the other ear. If only one ear is involved initially, the other ear often develops hearing loss within weeks or months. Sensorineural hearing loss can fluctuate or it can be profound. It can stabilize spontaneously if disease activity wanes or it can progress steadily without fluctuation. Typically the middle ear is normal, except in Wegener's granulomatosis, and there is no conductive component to the hearing loss.[5]

About 50% of patients complain of dizziness, usually lightheadedness if disease is early or ataxia if disease is advanced. Symptoms parallel hearing loss as activity waxes and wanes. True vertigo is rare but can occur, particularly with unilateral disease. Thus, dizziness is a nonspecific symptom.

The most common age group involved is 20 to 50 years at onset of symptoms. Many older patients can present with disease that, in retrospect, may have been present for many years. Disease can affect both sexes, but a female preponderance has been noted. Approximately 30% of patients will have evidence of a systemic immune disease such as rheumatoid arthritis, lupus erythematosus, or generalized vasculitis.

Immune-mediated inner ear disease should be suspected when a patient presents with unexplained, bilateral, rapidly progressive sensorineural hearing loss.

BACKGROUND

For decades researchers studied immune-mediated inner ear disease, however, it did not receive significant recognition until 1979, when McCabe[8] published his landmark paper, "Autoimmune Sensorineural Hearing Loss."

Mogi et al[10] (1982) and Harris[2] (1983) identified immunoglobulins within the inner ear. These consisted mainly of IgG, but also IgM and IgA. In a series of elegant studies, Harris et al[3] determined that the site of entry into the inner ear for immune inflammatory mediators was through the spiral modiolar vein adjacent to the tympanic lip.

In 1984 Arnold et al identified secretory IgA in the endolymphatic sac. In 1987, Takahashi and Harris[11] found proliferating immunocompetent cells and immunoglobulins within the sac. Tomiyama and Harris[12] confirmed the role of the sac in the efferent limb of immunity by observing decreased immunoglobulins in the inner ear following surgical ablation of the sac. Tomiyama and Harris[12] demonstrated the role of the sac in the afferent limb of immunity by selectively blocking the endolymphatic duct while preserving the sac. Such studies confirm that the endolymphatic sac plays a central role in immunoregulation of the inner ear and can participate in both afferent and efferent limbs of the immune response. Histologic endolymphatic hydrops has been noted in Cogan's syndrome and polyarteritis nodosa, as well as other systemic disorders. Furthermore, symptoms of idiopathic Ménière's disease are relatively common in patients with immune inner ear disease, suggesting that endolymphatic hydrops and related symptoms may be common manifestations of immune-mediated inner ear disease.

Thus, research has shown that the inner ear is immunocompetent and that systemic immune disease can produce immune-mediated inner ear disease. Still, our knowledge of inner ear immunology is poor, and the term "autoimmune inner ear disease" has been applied broadly to various immune-mediated disorders, including nonimmune indirect effects of systemic immune disease. Therefore, immune-mediated inner ear disease should be classified into primary (originating within the inner ear) and secondary (originating outside the inner ear).[5] Primary disease can be localized to the ear or generalized with systemic features. Secondary disease can produce direct effects on the inner ear (for example, Cogan's syndrome) or can produce indirect

Procedures for Collecting and Mailing Blood Specimens for LTT

Supplies

1. Three sterile green top (heparinized) vacutainers
2. Alcohol preps

Procedures

1. Draw blood into vacutainers and label tubes with patient's name, date, physician's name and "LTT-ear."
2. Please note on the vacutainer label whether the patient is allergic to Penicillin and/or Streptomycin.
3. Pack the vacutainers for shipping. Do not pack on ice. Avoid temperature extremes.
4. Blood must be delivered as soon as possible (no longer than 18 hours after being drawn). Mail by rapid carrier, overnight if necessary. Please do not ship on Fridays or the day preceding a holiday because the specimen cannot be processed on the weekend or holiday.
5. Label package: Human Blood, Deliver Immediately. Do Not Freeze.
6. Send to: The Cleveland Clinic Foundation, c/o Reference Laboratory, Laboratory Medicine Building, 9500 Euclid Ave., Cleveland, OH 44195. Do not mail samples directly to Dr. Hughes' office.

effects by alterations in circulation or biochemistry. Some of these effects remain theoretic and must be proved.

LABORATORY DIAGNOSIS

Immunologic laboratory tests may be specific for inner ear antigens, using homologous or heterologous inner ear membranes. Antigen-specific tests search for cellular or antibody immune reactivity and include the lymphocyte transformation test (LTT) and Western Blot immunoassay. [6] Other antigen-specific tests are used experimentally but not yet clinically. Antigen-nonspecific tests do not use inner ear tissue but search for indirect evidence of immune activity, for example, complement factor, rheumatoid factor, and erythrocyte sedimentation rate. Generally, antigen-specific assays are preferable as they provide more direct evidence of autoimmunity.

The lymphocyte transformation test assumes that circulating lymphocytes which have been sensitized to inner ear proteins will respond to the putative antigen(s) in vitro. When a previously sensitized lymphocyte receives a second similar antigen exposure, a proliferative response and release of lymphokines are identified as a positive laboratory test. Currently the Cleveland Clinic Foundation is the only laboratory to offer lymphocyte transformation testing. Procedures for collecting and mailing blood specimens for LTT are listed in box above.

Specificity of the LTT is 93%, but sensitivity is not known. It is estimated to be 50% to 80% if specimens are obtained when the patient's symptoms are acute and when the patient is not immunosuppressed. At the Cleveland Clinic Foundation, approximately 19% of LTT results are positive among those specimens mailed in by outside physicians. The predictive value of a positive LTT in a high-risk patient is estimated to be 56% to 73%. In the future, the authors hope to generate a panel of T lymphocyte clones that react to human inner ear proteins presented in associated with self human leukocyte antigen (HLA) determinants. The panel of T cell clones is developed by first identifying a group of patients with dramatic lymphocyte proliferation following exposure to inner ear homogenate. Subsequent purification through cloning should guarantee reactivity to inner ear antigen stimulation and further understanding of T cell reactivity in immune inner ear disease.

The Western blot immunoassay is used to identify serum antibodies that react with antigens of the inner ear.[9] The presence of such antibodies suggests specific immune pathogenesis of the sensorineural hearing loss in patients with idiopathic sensorineural hearing loss. The antigen extract is usually prepared from fresh bovine temporal bone specimens. The proteins present in the antigen extract are separated by electrophoresis and transferred onto membrane strips. Serum from patients is incubated with the separated antigen on the membrane. Unbound immunoglobulins are washed away, and the strips then are incubated with enzyme-linked antihuman IgG antibody. This reaction yields a band at the location of human antibody bound to bovine inner ear antigen.

Harris and Sharp[4] first described a positive band at 68 kiloDalten (kD) molecular weight in a patient with clinical features of immune inner ear disease. At the Massachussets Eye and Ear Infirmary, Western blot immunoassay identified antibodies to inner ear antigens in most patients with idiopathic bilateral progressive, sensorineural hearing loss and in all patients with Cogan's syndrome. The antibodies reacted with an antigen of 68 kD in about 60% of patients with idiopathic bilateral progressive sensorineural hearing loss. Only 2% of normal subjects and no patients with otosclerosis reacted to this antigen. In contrast, reactivity to other antigens was more common and did differentiate these groups well.

The relationship of the presence of such antibodies and the potential for response to treatment was studied. Patients were treated with prednisone 60 mg per day for 30 days; the doses were subsequently tapered. About 75% of the patients with antibody to the 68 kD inner ear antigen demonstrated improved hearing of greater than 10 dB on audiogram after one month of treatment. Of note, patients with Cogan's syndrome all demonstrated serum antibodies to the 55 kD but not the 68 kD antigen, yet all responded to corticosteroid therapy. Some patients with negative tests also responded to treatment. A correlation of antibody presence to activity of the disease in the patient was observed. Activity was defined as a progression of the hearing loss within 3 months of the assay. The test may, however, remain positive even after immunosuppressive medication is begun.

These studies demonstrate that inner ear disease responsive to corticosteroid is frequently associated with antibodies to inner ear antigens of 68 kD as detected by Western blot immunoassay. Unfortunately, this test is currently investigational. However, we anticipate it will be available for clinical use in the very near future.

Presently, the authors are evaluating and comparing the Western blot immunoassay and LTT in the same patient population. This comparison will be performed in a prospective trial in which response to therapy also will be evaluated.

MANAGEMENT

Very often, antigen-specific testing cannot be obtained, and antigen-nonspecific testing may be negative. Nevertheless, the patient with bilateral rapidly progressive sensorineural hearing loss should be given a treatment trial of corticosteroid. A beneficial response helps support a presumptive diagnosis of immune-mediated inner ear disease (primary or secondary), as proposed by McCabe[8] in 1979.

Cortisone

Corticosteroids are the mainstay of treatment. Unfortunately, the natural history of untreated disease is unknown. Because immune inner ear disease is one of the few forms of sensorineural hearing loss which responds to treatment and because preliminary results are encouraging, aggressive treatment should be considered in every case. Prednisone, 1 mg/kg/day, is continued for one month. This one month high-dose treatment is arbitrary; no study has determined what the minimal dose or length of treatment should be. However, some patients who will respond to steroids do so only after three or four weeks of treatment, and low-dose therapy may produce no benefit whatsoever or very short-term benefit at best.

The patient should be informed about side effects and risks of steroids. Relative contraindication may include pregnancy, glaucoma, hypertension, diabetes, tuberculosis, fungal infection, peptic ulcer disease, or any known "bone disease." Very often, however, medical prophylaxis for glaucoma, hypertension, inactive tuberculosis, and peptic ulcer disease will allow steroids to be given for the full course. Hypersensitivity to corticosteroid is rare. One additional rare but devastating risk is aseptic necrosis of the femoral head. This problem appears to be dose related but can be idiosyncratic and occur in any patient at any time. Total hip replacement may be required for complete rehabilitation. Patients should be warned of this risk.

With prednisone, effects of steroids can be noticed after approximately 4 hours, peak at 12 hours, then wane over the remaining 12 hours of the day. These effects include excitability, increased heart rate, flushing and sweating, increased urination, and increased appetite. They can be distracting but can be minimized by giving all of the medication at a single dose each morning.

After one month, an audiogram is repeated. A beneficial response supports the diagnosis of immune inner ear disease.

Steroids then are tapered down to the lowest dose required to maintain hearing. Steroids can be rapidly tapered to about 20 mg/day in the adult, then more slowly over several weeks. No study has determined ideal maintenance therapy. The authors recommend prednisone 10 mg daily or every other day initially for 3 to 6 months. Higher doses, or even high-dose repeat treatment for a second month, should be considered if hearing improves with treatment but falls again with tapering. Very often the patient learns to titrate the maintenance dose as disease activity waxes and wanes.

Cytotoxic drugs

The authors reserve cytotoxic drugs (cyclophosphamide in adults, methotrexate or azathioprine in children or young women) for patients with immune-mediated disease as second-line therapy. In diagnosed patients, lack of response to steroids, poor tolerance of steroids, or inability to withdraw from steroids are appropriate times to consider cytotoxic drug therapy. In contrast, McCabe[8] has suggested cyclophosphamide as part of initial therapy. Theoretically, such aggressive treatment would benefit some patients without waiting for steroids to fail. Also, it would be more appropriate than steroids alone for patients with granulomatus disorders such as Wegener's disease. At present, cytotoxic drugs are reserved for selected patients because the natural history of immune inner ear disease is not known, adverse effects of cytotoxic drugs are potentially more severe, and laboratory diagnosis does not allow a patient's disease to be divided into steroid vs cytotoxic treatment groups.

Plasmapheresis

Plasmapheresis has been examined by Luetje[7] who published detailed results of treatment in eight patients with average follow-up of 26 months. A significant difference was defined as greater than 10 dB pure tone average or 15% discrimination. Six patients had improved hearing that was previously stable in five and fluctuated mildly at menses in one. Four patients no longer required steroids or cytotoxic drugs. These preliminary results were very encouraging.

Unfortunately, plasmapheresis is expensive and inconvenient. Insurance companies must be petitioned to pay for this test which they often label as "experimental." Usually the procedure takes 3 hours and is repeated three times weekly for 2 weeks. In the authors' opinion, plasmapheresis should be reserved for well-documented cases of immune inner ear disease, with beneficial response to treatment, in whom steroid or cytotoxic drug side effects are severe. Plasmapheresis as adjuvant therapy may permit lower doses of medication with control of hearing. Unfortunately, plasmapheresis by itself will likely produce only transient improvement.

CONCLUSION

The diagnosis of immune-mediated inner ear disease should be considered when a patient has unexplained bilateral rapidly progressive sensorineural hearing loss. Even if laboratory testing is not possible or available, a treatment trial of high-dose steroids should be given for one full month. If there is no benefit, steroids can be tapered and stopped. If there is benefit, low-dose maintenance should be continued for 3 to 6 months. In this way, aggressive therapy helps as many patients as possible. Because immune-mediated inner ear disease is one of the few forms of sensorineural hearing loss that can benefit from medical therapy, a high index of suspicion and aggressive therapy should be the rule.

REFERENCES

1. Arnold W, Altermatt HJ, Gebbers JO: Demonstration of immunoglobulins (SIgA, IgG) in the human endolymphatic sac. *Laryngol Rhinol Otol*63:464, 1984.
2. Harris JP: Immunology of the inner ear: response of the inner ear to antigen challenge. *Otolaryngol Head Neck Surg* 91:17, 1983.
3. Harris JP, Fukuda S, Keithley EM: Spiral modiolar vein: its importance in inner ear inflammation. *Acta Otolaryngol* 110:356-357, 1990.
4. Harris JP, Sharp PA: Inner ear autoantibodies in patients with rapidly progressive sensorineural hearing loss. *Laryngoscope* 100:516, 1990.
5. Hughes GB, Barna BP, Calabrese LH, Koo A: Immunologic disorders of the inner ear. In Bailey BJ, editor: *Head and Neck Surgery—Otolaryngology*. Philadelphia, 1993, JB Lippincott. 1833-1842.
6. Hughes GB, Moscicki RA, Barna BP, San Martin JE: Laboratory diagnosis of immune inner ear disease. *Am J Otology* 15:198-202, 1994.
7. Luetje CM: Theoretical and practical implications for plasmapheresis in autoimmune inner ear disease. *Laryngoscope* 99:1137, 1989.
8. McCabe BF: Autoimmune sensorineural hearing loss. *Ann Otol Rhinol Laryngol* 88:585-589, 1979.
9. Moscicki RA, San Martin JE, Quintero CH, et al: Serum antibody to inner ear proteins in patients with progressive hearing loss. *JAMA* 272:611-616, 1994.
10. Mogi G, Lim D, Watanabe N: Immunologic study on the inner ear. Immunoglobulins in perilymph. *Arch Otolaryngol* 108:270, 1982.
11. Takahashi M, Harris JP: Analysis of immunocompetent cells following inner ear immunostimulation. *Laryngoscope* 98:1133, 1988.
12. Tomiyama S, Harris JP: Alteration of inner ear responses by endolymphatic duct obstruction. *Ann Otol Rhinol Laryngol* (In press.)

26

Otologic and Audiologic Evaluation of Infants and Young Children

Jane R. Madell, Ph.D., Judith S. Gravel, Ph.D., and Robert J. Ruben, M.D.

MEDICAL EVALUATION

Otolaryngic evaluation of the infant or child with a suspected communication disorder has five objectives. These are:

1. To *determine* the causes of the communication disorder.
2. To *carry out* the indicated intervention(s).
3. To *determine* which, if any, organ systems are involved.
4. To *monitor* the progression of the disorder(s).
5. To *evaluate* the effects of the interventions and access the *outcome*.

The determination of the cause(s) of the disorders and whether there are other organ systems involved is begun with a statement of the chief complaint then a review of systems followed by the detailing of the present illness. The review of systems is listed in box on page 302. The social history that must be obtained can be found in box on page 302. History of present illness is found in box on page 303. Features of the physical examination are found in box on page 304. The assessment of auditory function of other family members is in box on page 305. Hearing evaluation is covered in other sections of this paper.

There are other consultations and/or determination that may be required. These studies are obtained as a result of the information that has been discovered from the review of systems, present illness, physical examination, and audiologic and/or vestibular evaluations. They are found in box on page 306.

The completion of the evaluations are but one third of the function of the physician. There are two critical functions that the physician must undertake for and on behalf of the patient. These are to **communicate** the findings to the caretakers and to carry out **continued care** of the patient. Communication can be done by the means of a parent conference. This may be held at night to allow both parents to attend and to permit the staff to be free to spend uninterrupted time with the family. At this conference the staff discusses all of the findings and their implications. All of the health professionals who have participated in the evaluation and habilitation of the child should be at the conference. This will include those from audiology, habilitation, speech and language, genetics, pediatric neurology, and otolaryngology.

AUDIOLOGIC EVALUATION

Purpose of the audiologic evaluation

Audiologic evaluations may be performed for several reasons: to determine degree and type of hearing loss, to monitor middle ear status, to assess neurologic status, to assess auditory function (speech perception abilities), and to monitor progress of children with impaired hearing. To some extent, the purpose of the evaluation determines the type of testing that will be performed. For example, when seeking information about neurologic status, it will be necessary to include auditory brain stem testing in the evaluation. When seeking information about auditory function, it is necessary to perform a number of different speech perception tests at different intensities (normal and soft conversational levels) and under different test conditions (in quiet and in the presence of competing noise).

Early identification of hearing loss in children is critical. It has been well documented that even a mild hearing loss or a unilateral hearing loss can have a significant ef-

Review of Systems for Pediatric Otologic Evaluation

1. History of head trauma
   A. Temporal bone fracture
   B. Footplate dislocation
2. Ophthalmologic evaluation
   A. Deficiencies in visual acuity
      1. Additional sensory defects
      2. Correction needs
   B. Syndrome diagnosis
      1. Usher's
      2. Congenital rubella
      3. Others
3. Nose and paranasal sinuses
   A. History of infection, immune disorders
   B. Nasality
      1. Hearing-impaired children may be hypernasal
   C. Other syndromes
4. Mouth and pharynx
   A. Congenital abnormalities
      1. Cleft palate
      2. Submucosal cleft of palate
   B. Drooling
      1. Swallowing abnormalities
      2. Chewing abnormalities
   C. Infection, immune system
5. Larynx
   A. Hoarseness
   B. Other vocal qualities
6. Chest
7. Cardiac—congenital malformation
   A. Prolonged Q-T interval (Jervell and Lang-Neilson syndrome)
   B. VSDs with congenital rubella
   C. Other
8. Genitourinary tract
   A. All children with malformations of the pinna, external auditory canal, or the middle ear should have an ultrasonographic evaluation of the genitourinary system in the first few months of life
   B. Urine analysis
      1. Hematuria
      2. Proteinuria
   C. Enuresis
9. Endocrine system
   A. Goiter, patient and/or family
   B. Growth hormone deficiencies
10. Immune system
    A. Allergy
       1. Antibiotics or other medications
       2. Foods
       3. Hay fever
       4. Asthma
    B. Defects of the immune system
       1. HIV
       2. Other
11. Muscular and skeletal malformations
    A. Mouth
    B. Palate
    C. Limbs
12. Central nervous system
    A. Epilepsy
       1. Febrile convulsions
       2. Verbal auditory agnosia (VAA)
    B. Development
       1. Toilet trained
       2. Dresses self
       3. Feeds self
    C. Social development

Social History for Pediatric Otologic Evaluation

1. Place of birth
2. Occupation of parents
3. Type of "family"
   A. Both parents
   B. One parent
   C. Foster child
   D. Adopted
   E. Other

fect on speech and language development.[3,23,25] Early identification followed by enrollment in an early intervention program which includes the fitting of appropriate amplification, language therapy, and family counseling can reduce negative effects of hearing loss on language acquisition and have the additional benefit of reducing educational delays associated with hearing loss.

Screenings for infants frequently utilize electrophysiologic tests such as auditory brain stem response or otoacoustic emissions testing. Screenings for older children usually consist of behavioral tests such as play audiometry in which the child performs a motor act (placing a toy in a box) in response to the presentation of sound.

Diagnostic evaluations may consist of behavioral tests alone or include both behavioral and electrophysiologic tests depending on the purpose of the evaluation. Electrophysiologic tests assess the function of the auditory system but do not assess the infant's or child's ability to attend to or "tune in" to auditory stimuli. Behavioral assessments use observation of overt responses to calibrated sound stimuli and, therefore, can assess the ability of the child to attend to auditory stimuli. For this reason, behavioral testing should be a part of every audiologic evaluation. For infants,

Feature of the History of Present Illness for Pediatric Otologic Evaluation

4. Family history
   A. Genetic tree
      1. All members for two or more generations
      2. Note other family members affected with a communication disorder
         Any form of communication disorder, including presbycusis
         Brain tumors
   B. Consanguinity
   C. Geographic origin of the families
5. Prenatal factors
   A. Congenital infections
      1. Rubella
      2. Cytomegalovirus
      3. Other
   B. Abnormalities of pregnancy
      1. Diabetes
      2. Infertility
      3. Other
6. Perinatal factors
   A. Congenital infections
   B. Birth weight
   C. Neonatal intensive care unit (NICU)
   D. Ototoxic medications
   E. Kernicterus
   F. Head trauma
   G. Hearing status at birth
      1. Screening
      2. Caretakers evaluation
7. Developmental
   A. Changes in hearing
      1. Progressive loss
      2. Perilymphatic fistula
         Congenital/acquired
         Genetic/acquired
      3. Autoimmune disorders
   B. Changes in language—regression
      1. Hearing loss
      2. Language disorder
      3. Autism
   C. Motor development
      1. Perilymphatic fistula
      2. Meningitis
      3. Other
8. Early language milestone scale (ELM) (Coplan, 1993)
   A. Bench mark for language development
   B. Obtain in all patients from birth to 36 months of age (Ruben, 1991)
9. Review of other etiologies
   A. Sound trauma
      1. Fire crackers
      2. Guns
      3. Snowmobiles
      4. Rock concerts
   B. Physical trauma
      1. Temporal bone fracture
      2. Barotrauma
   C. Infections
      1. Meningitis
      2. Otitis media
      3. Labyrinthitis
   D. Ototoxicity
      1. Aminoglycosides
      2. Aspirin
      3. Other
10. Final question: "What have I not known to ask?"

behavioral testing (observation audiometry) relies on observation of changes in sucking, eye widening, or limb movement in response to presentation of an auditory stimulus. For slightly older infants and toddlers, the test protocol (visual reinforcement audiometry) uses a reinforced head turn in response to presentation of a sound stimulus. For older children the response consists of a motor act such as putting a block in a box or a ring on a ring stand in response to the presentation of a sound stimulus. The test protocol is selected based on the child's developmental and cognitive age. Infants who are developmentally or neurologically functioning below 6 months of age will be tested using observation audiometry. Children who are developmentally between 6 and 36 months will be tested using visual reinforcement audiometry. Children who are developmentally at or above 30 months will be tested using play audiometry. It is critical that the audiologist have an accurate picture of the developmental and neurologic status of the child to accurately select the appropriate test protocol.

Evaluating infants—birth to six months

Screening. Screening evaluations are recommended for all infants who are considered high risk for hearing loss.[17,18] Screening is recommended prior to hospital discharge but no later than 3 months of age. A list of high-risk factors is available in box on page 307. Virtually every infant in the NICU is high risk for hearing loss and should receive hearing screening. Many hospitals are developing hearing screening protocols to test high-risk infants. Screening protocols may include otoacoustic emissions and/or auditory brain stem response testing. Infants who fail the screening are rescreened prior to hospital discharge if possible and referred for diagnostic evaluation if they fail the second screening. The majority of infants identified with se-

Features of the Physical Examination for Pediatric Otologic Evaluation

1. The child
   A. Sit in the lap of the caretaker
   B. Relate to the child
   C. Do not hurt the child
      1. Crying will change the physical examination
      2. Probable need for subsequent examinations
2. Pinnae
   A. Direct observation
   B. Abnormalities associated with genitourinary malformations
3. External auditory canal
   A. Direct observation and otoscopy
   B. Abnormalities associated with genito urinary malformations
4. Cerumen
   A. Remove only:
      1. If the tympanic membrane is totally occluded and there is a need for information concerning the tympanic membrane
      2. May be causing a hearing loss
   B. Avoid instrumentation—use irrigation
5. Tympanic membrane
   A. Otoscope and/or microscope
      1. Make a drawing or record an image
      2. Microscope useful for:
         Congenital cholesteatoma
         Ossicular abnormalities
   B. Pneumotoscopy
      1. Diagnosis of otitis media with effusion (OME)
      2. Diagnosis of retraction and/or atelectasis
6. Head
   A. Direct observation, use of a measuring tape, palpation
   B. Closure of fontanelle—too early or too late
   C. Head size—too big or too small
   D. Shape of head—syndrome
7. Hair
   A. Direct observation
   B. White streak or lock of a few white hairs
8. Face
   A. Direct observation
   B. Symmetry face–size and function
      Paralysis or paresis
      Goldehar's
      Mobius
      Other
9. Eyes
   A. Direct observation
   B. Color of iris—heterochromia
   C. Conjunctivitis—autoimmune
   D. Spontaneous nystagmus—fistula or CNS abnormality
   E. Cataracts—congenital rubella
   F. Strabismus
10. Nose
   A. Direct observation
   B. Shape
   C. Fistula/cysts
   D. Intranasal
      Masses
      Discharge
      Epistasis
   E. Use of laryngeal mirror
      1. Patency of nares
      2. Quasiquantitative
   F. Speech—nose open—velopharyngeal competency
      1. "Susie's slippers"
      2. "Catch a fish"
   G. Speech—nose open and then gently closed
      1. Hyponasality or hypernasality
      2. Say the letter "M"
11. Mouth—palate and tongue
   A. Direct observation and palpation
   B. Mouth
      1. Drooling
      2. Masses
      3. Clefts
      4. Bifid uvula
      5. Tonsils
         Size
         Characteristics—erythema of the anterior pillars
      6. Palate
         Palpation of dorsal notching or dehiscence—occult submucosal cleft
         High arch
      7. Tongue
         Fasciculation—articulation deficiencies
         Asymmetry
   C. Larynx
      1. Auscultation with a small-diaphragm (1 cm diameter) stethoscope
      2. Examination with a flexible laryngoscope
         Record data
         Uses of topical anesthesia—can be carried out on almost all children older than 36 months
         Not to be undertaken when there is a question of airway compromise unless there is the ability to intubate and/or tracheotomize
         Examination of
            Oral pharynx
               Dorsal extension of tonsils
               Pharyngeal walls
            Larynx
            Hypopharynx
            Cricopharyngeus
12. Neck
   A. Direct observation
   B. Thyroid—goiter
      1. Pendred's disease
      2. Others
   C. Sinuses
   D. Cysts
   E. Palpation of the carotids
   F. Lymphadenopathy

Assessment of Auditory Function of Other Family Members for Pediatric Otologic Evaluation

1. Obtained in all families with
   A. Suspicion of genetic diseases
   B. No known cause of hearing loss
2. All members
   A. Especially important in younger siblings
   B. All subsequent siblings
3. Vestibular assessments
   A. Fistula test
      1. With all documented or suspected progressive sensory hearing losses
      2. Carried out as soon as possible
         Treatable cause of sensory loss
         Prevent further loss
         Possible prevention of meningitis
   B. Electronystagmography (ENG)
      1. Carried out in all with suspected sensory or neural losses
      2. Assessment includes
         Spontaneous
         Positional
         Optokinetic
         Rotary
         Caloric
      3. Information concerning CNS integrity
      4. Children with abnormal or absent vestibular responses may have motor delay
         Postmeningitis
         Fistula
         Not mental retardation

vere and profound sensorineural hearing loss are not identified by the high-risk register.[10,24,30,43] To accurately identify the majority of infants who have hearing loss at birth or early in infancy it would be necessary to screen in the well baby nursery in addition to the NICU. Certainly any infant for whom there is parent/caregiver concern about hearing should be considered at risk for hearing and be referred for audiologic evaluation.

Diagnostic evaluation. The diagnostic evaluation for an infant should consist of auditory brain stem response testing (ABR), otoacoustic emissions (OAE), behavioral observation to assess the infant's ability to attend and respond to auditory stimuli, acoustic emittance testing to assess middle ear function, and a report of parent/caregiver observations about the infant's response to sound. ABR testing should include frequency-specific testing to determine hearing levels at low and high frequencies and suprathreshold click-ABR to assess neurologic status. Otoacoustic emissions testing can be used to confirm other test results. Electrophysiologic tests such as ABR and OAE assess the auditory system but do not assess the infant's ability to attend to auditory stimuli. Behavioral evaluation using observation audiometry assesses the infant's ability to respond behaviorally to auditory stimuli. Research by Olsho et al,[28] Werner and Gillenwater,[48] and others has demonstrated that it is possible to reliably obtain hearing thresholds on infants as young as 2 weeks of age using an appropriate psychophysical method.

Sucking responses are the most reliable for obtaining threshold information,[19] while eye widening and limb movement are frequent responses to suprathreshold stimuli.[6,11,19,45,47] Reliable threshold information can be obtained best if infants are brought to the evaluation hungry. If they are to be bottle fed or use a pacifier they are placed in an infant seat in a position that permits the audiologist to get a good view of sucking activity. If they are to be nursed they are held in the mother's arms and, again, positioned so as to allow the audiologist to view the sucking. If the infant is being held, the mother must be cautioned not to move in response to sound since the mother's movement may cause the child to alter sucking behavior, confusing the determination of when a response is present. Ideally, the mother should be wearing ear protectors to reduce her ability to hear the stimuli and cue the infant.

After an initial period of feeding to get over the initial hunger, testing can be initiated. Stimuli may include pure tones, warble tones, noise bands, and speech stimuli. Testing is frequently conducted initially in soundfield, but all evaluations should include earphone testing to obtain ear-specific information. Timing of presentation of the stimuli is critical, since presentation of stimuli too close together may extinguish the response. To be certain that thresholds obtained with observation audiometry are reliable, a response should not be recorded until it has been obtained two to three times at the same intensity. In the hands of an experienced pediatric audiologist, behavioral testing is a reliable procedure capable of providing frequency-specific threshold information at multiple frequencies in a short period of time. Thus, threshold information obtained should be in agreement with the electrophysiologic test results but may be more extensive than the information that is obtained with electrophysiologic testing alone. In addition, observation audiometry can be used for evaluating function with amplification which cannot be obtained with electrophysiologic tests. However, observation audiometry has it's limits. It can be difficult to obtain reliable test results. Testing can be affected by the state of the infant, the infant's neurologic status, test stimuli, and the skill of the audiologist. Observation audiometry test results should be repeated at least once prior to finalizing a diagnosis and planning remediation.

Evaluating children 5 to 24 months

Visual reinforcement audiometry. The seminal studies of Wilson, Thompson, et al in the 1970s have served as the basis for incorporating the operant head-turn procedure

Other Consults for the Pediatric Otologic Evaluation

1. Ophthalmologic
   A. Who: all children with permanent or probable hearing loss
      1. Ophthalmologic signs
         Rubella
         Usher's syndrome
      2. Need for the optimization of sensory inputs
         Hearing impaired visually dependent
         Any additional defect has a greater effect than if it was the only defect
2. Pediatric neurology
   A. Who:
      1. Primary language disorders
      2. Cognitive disorders
      3. Seizures
      4. Developmental delay
   B. Children with developmental language delay and normal hearing—refer as soon as possible
      1. VAA
      2. Autism
      3. Developmental delay
3. Pediatric urology
   A. Who: those suspected or proven genitourinary abnormalities
4. Genetics
   A. Who:
      1. All with genetic history
         Autosomal
         X-linked
         Mitochondrial
      2. All who are syndromic
      3. All without an etiologic diagnosis
   B. Services
      1. Genetic diagnosis
      2. Genetic Counseling
         Prognosis
         Other siblings
      3. Chromosomal studies
      4. Linkage studies
5. Speech and language
   A. Who: all with communication disorders
      1. Hearing
      2. Voice
      3. Speech
      4. Language
   B. Baseline for language
      1. Direct the habilitation
      2. Evaluate the effects of the intervention-outcome
6. Imaging
   A. CAT
      1. Postmeningitis—monitor ossification for cochlear implantation
      2. Cochlear implant candidates
      3. Suspected bony labyrinth malformations
         Perilymphatic fistula
         CNS abnormalities
      4. External and middle ear malformations
         Obtain at time that surgical correction is considered
         Age 5 to 6 years
         There is an acceleration of new techniques, e.g., 3-D imaging, virtual reality, etc.
   B. MRI
      1. Who: infants and children suspected of neurological impairment von Recklinghausen II
      2. Possible in patients with suspected inflammation or allergic process of the membranous labyrinth
   C. Ultrasonography
      1. Who: suspected genitourinary malformations
      2. Who: swallowing disorders
7. Blood and serum determinations
   A. Autoimmune antibodies
      1. Who: patients with progressive losses
      2. When a perilymphatic fistula is felt to be unlikely
      3. Can occur
         In families
         In children with no other signs of autoimmune disease
      4. Immune profile
         Who:
            Postmeningitis
            Recurrent infections
         What:
            IgG, IgE, etc.
            WBC
            Phagocytic function
            Differential sedimentation rate
            HIV assay
      5. TORCH titters
         Who: as indicated from history and physical examination
         What:
            Toxoplasmosis
            Rubella
            Syphilis
            Cytomegalo virus
      6. Renal function
         Who: patients with suspected renal parenchymal disease
            Alport's syndrome
            Other
8. Urine analysis
   A. Who:
      1. Suspected or known real parenchymal disease
      2. Suspected or know genitourinary malformations
9. Electrocardiogram
   A. Who:
      1. Children suspected of having a cardiac abnormality
      2. Prolonged Q-T
      3. Congenital rubella
      4. Other
10. Medical records
    A. Who: patients with
       1. Unknown causes for communication disorders
       2. Suggestive pre- and perinatal histories
       3. What: review the records for
          Ototoxic medication
          Meningitis
          Other congenital function
          Anemia
          Anoxia
          Kernicterus

Indicators Associated with Sensorineural and/or Conductive Hearing Loss

A. Neonates (birth through age 28 days)
1. Family history of hereditary childhood sensorineural hearing loss
2. In uteroinfection, such as cytomegalovirus, rubella, syphilis, herpes, and toxoplasmosis
3. Craniofacial anomalies, including those with morphological abnormalities of the pinna and ear canal
4. Birth weight less than 1,500 grams (3.3 lb).
5. Hyperbilirubinemia at a serum level requiring exchange transfusion.
6. Ototoxic medications, including but not limited to the aminoglycosides, used in multiple courses or in combination with loop diuretics
7. Bacterial meningitis
8. Apgar scores of 0-4 at 1 minute or 0-6 at 5 minutes
9. Mechanical ventilation lasting 5 days or longer
10. Stigmata or other findings associated with a syndrome known to include a sensorineural and/or conductive hearing loss

B. Infants (age 29 days through 2 years) when certain health conditions develop that require rescreening.
1. Parent/caregiver concern regarding hearing, speech, language, and/or developmental delay
2. Bacterial meningitis and other infections associated with sensorineural hearing loss
3. Head trauma associated with loss of consciousness or skull fracture
4. Stigmata or other findings associated with a syndrome known to include a sensorineural and/or conductive hearing loss
5. Ototoxic medications, including but not limited to chemotherapeutic agents or aminoglycosides, used in multiple courses or in combination with loop diuretics
6. Recurrent or persistent otitis media with effusion for at least 3 months.

C. Infants (age 29 days through 3 years) who require periodic monitoring of hearing

Some newborns and infants may pass initial hearing screening but require periodic monitoring of hearing to detect delayed-onset sensorineural and/or conductive hearing loss. Infants with these indicators require hearing evaluation at least every 6 months until age 2 years, and at appropriate intervals thereafter.

Indicators associated with delayed onset sensorineural hearing loss include
1. Family history of hereditary childhood hearing loss
2. Inutero infection, such as cytomegalovirus, rubella, syphilis, herpes, or toxoplasmosis
3. Neurofibromatosis type II and neurodegenerative disorders

Indicators associated with conductive hearing loss include:

a. Recurrent or persistent otitis media with effusion
b. Anatomic deformities and other disorders that affect eustachian tube function
c. Neurodegenerative disorders

as the primary behavioral audiometric test procedure for infant assessment in the clinical setting. Visual reinforcement audiometry (VRA) has provided a means for the clinician to accurately and reliably determine threshold sensitivity in the vast majority (about 90%) of infants beginning at 5 to 6 months developmental age.[50,52]

Currently, there are various forms of VRA instrumentation and protocols that have been designed for logic system,[52] computer-mediated,[2,8,50] and manual[13,14] applications. The principles of VRA are fundamentally the same, however, across procedures. Briefly, a unidirectional head-turn response in the presence of a test signal is reinforced using a highly appealing animated and illuminated toy (the visual reinforcer). By initially pairing the test signal with the availability of the visual reinforcer, the infant's behavioral response is operantly conditioned. Reinforcement is contingent upon a "correct" response (a head turn only when a test stimulus is present). No reinforcement is provided for incorrect responding (turning when no stimulus is present).

The VRA procedure allows the clinician to obtain accurate adult-like thresholds from infants using frequency-specific signals.[52] Mean thresholds obtained from infants with normal hearing remain relatively invariant across a broad age range[52] and are only about 10 to 15 dB poorer than adult thresholds.[27] Test-retest reliability has also been shown to be excellent when early threshold estimates obtained with VRA are compared with thresholds obtained at older ages using play audiometry.[5,14] Behavioral thresholds obtained using VRA have also been shown to be in good agreement with those estimated using a frequency-specific ABR procedure.[39]

Ear-specific assessment. Ear-specific audiometric data are crucial to medical, surgical, and habilitative follow-up. Every attempt to acquire thresholds for each ear independently should be made. Standard earphones with a pediatric headband may be used successfully with the vast majority (≥ 80%) of infants between the ages of 6 months and 2 years.[16] Older toddlers (≥ 20 months) rather than younger babies (e.g., 6 to 18 months) usually resist earphone placement.[16]

Insert receivers offer significant advantages in the assessment of infants. The components (receiver/transducer, delivery tube, and ear insert) are lighter than the conventional earphone-headband assembly. Further, the risk of ear canal collapse or earphone misalignment are eliminated. Thresholds obtained from infants with sensorineural hearing loss using insert receivers better approximate real ear sound pressure levels. These values are useful in prescriptive amplification selection procedures. Finally, the use of insert receivers facilitates the use of noise masking when necessary.

VRA test equipment. Modifications of equipment necessary for VRA are usually inexpensive and will significantly enhance the effectiveness of the VRA procedure in the clinical setting. For example, multiple complex visual reinforcers housed in dark smoked-plexiglas units help to maintain the infant's motivation and attention during assessment.[13,32,33,34,46]

Recently, a commercially available PC-based VRA system (intelligent visual reinforcement audiometry, IVRA) has been developed. IVRA allows the clinician to conduct single examiner assessments using algorithms designed to be efficient and to document the reliability of the procedure (through the inclusion of control and probe trials). IVRA provides three protocols useful for screening and assessment purposes.[7,8,29,50,51] The Classification of Audiograms by Sequential Testing (CAST) screening and Optional Hearing Test Algorithm (OHTA) assessment procedures utilize innovative threshold search procedures based on Bayesian theory.

The advantages of computer-mediated VRA procedures are multiple. A single audiologist can complete bias-free threshold estimates. The inclusion of control and probe trials provides a means of quantifying the reliability of the threshold estimate and the degree of attention and motivation during assessment.[2,8] The inclusion and tracking of control (no stimulus) trial intervals during manual VRA threshold assessment can also provide the audiologist with an estimate of the reliability and validity of the test session. This can also be accomplished using a simple paper and pencil technique with one or two examiners.[14] The use of a second examiner, "blind" to the occurrence of a test trial, allows a bias-free assessment when using manual VRA. A naive assistant is the only reason to utilize two clinicians in the assessment of young children.[13,14]

VRA versus COR. VRA is often confused with another pediatric test procedure, conditioned orienting response (COR) audiometry. While both techniques incorporate the use of visual reinforcement for correct responding, they differ in methodology, intent, and information obtained.

In COR, two visual reinforcer displays are utilized—one located to the right, the other to the left side of the infant. The reinforcers are located on, or within close proximity to, soundfield speakers through which test stimuli are presented. The infant's task in the COR procedure is twofold: first, the infant must detect the presence of the test signal, and, second, in order to receive reinforcement, the baby must turn toward (localize) the sound source (right or left loudspeaker).

COR users suggest the technique provides qualitative information regarding localization ability. However, quantitative information regarding the specifics of any hearing loss (degree, configuration, and symmetry) cannot be accurately determined through soundfield COR testing alone. While COR may be qualitatively useful for examining localization accuracy, the traditional soundfield COR procedure is not recommended for use in a comprehensive audiologic assessment designed to determine ear-specific thresholds.

Evaluating children 24 to 30 months and older

Once children are cognitively and neurologically functioning at the 24 to 30 month level, they are able to cooperate for hearing testing. If screening tests are needed to determine hearing or middle ear status, the audiologist will usually use behavioral test protocols used for diagnostic testing but test at fewer frequencies. Children older than 30 months are tested using play audiometry. At this age children can be reliably taught to hold a toy up to their ears to "listen for the sound" and to put a block in a bucket or a ring on a ring stand after hearing the sound. An enthusiastic audiologist who frequently changes the toys used for the game will usually be able to get a reliable audiogram in a short period of time. Both air and bone conduction testing can be accomplished, which will provide information about degree and type of hearing loss. Acoustic emittance testing can easily be accomplished providing additional information about middle ear status.

Speech audiometry should be included in every evaluation to provide information about the child's ability to process auditory information. Even very young children can repeat words or point to pictures permitting a very thorough assessment of speech perception. (See speech audiometry below.) Auditory brain stem response testing can be performed if information about neurologic status of the child is needed or if there is some question about the reliability of the behavioral testing. Otoacoustic emissions testing is also used to provide confirmatory information and to give additional information about the status of the auditory system.

Evoked response measurements

Auditory brain stem response. The utility of the ABR in the pediatric assessment battery cannot be overstated. Very young infants and children whose developmental deficits preclude providing repeatable and valid threshold responses can now be assessed in a timely and reliable fashion. Not every child with hearing loss, however, requires an ABR. It is necessary only when the reliability of the behavioral assessment or the integrity of the auditory pathways to the level of the brain stem is in question.

The traditional click-ABR threshold estimation procedure provides only limited audiometric information. Because of its brief duration (100 us), the acoustic spectrum of the click is characteristically broad and essentially flat, with energy present in the 100 to 8000 Hz regions.[40] Thus, while general information regarding overall hearing sensitivity may be suggested by the click-ABR threshold, frequency-specific threshold information cannot be ascertained using the conventional click-ABR procedure alone.[31,38,41]

Inaccurate delineation of audiometric configuration may occur in children when only the click-ABR is utilized in assessment.[15,38] For example, infants with rising, trough-shaped ("cookie-bite"), and high-frequency (above 2000 Hz) hearing loss may exhibit normal click-ABR thresholds. Useable residual hearing may be present when no recordable click-ABR is obtained.[15] When only a click-ABR threshold is available, the clinician has insufficient information concerning the audiometric configuration to apply prescriptive amplification selection procedures.

Frequency-specific ABR: air and bone conducted. Frequency-specific ABR recording techniques are available that better predict audiometric configuration. Several approaches for obtaining frequency-specific thresholds have been suggested including the use of tone pips, tones having nonlinear gating functions ("Blackman" windows), derived responses (using click stimuli and various passbands of masking noise or tonal maskers) and tones in notched noise (see Stapells et al,[39] for a review). The tones in notched noise technique provides a valid estimate of behavioral hearing threshold in children, with correlations between behavioral and frequency-specific ABR thresholds better than 0.90.[39] It has been recommended that, at a minimum, threshold for 500-Hz tone pips be obtained in addition to the click-ABR threshold.[1].

The use of the bone-conducted ABR has allowed the differential diagnosis of sensorineural from conductive hearing loss and is particularly useful in the case of mixed deficits.[42]

Evoked otoacoustic emissions. Evoked otoacoustic emissions (EOAEs) are rapidly becoming part of the clinical assessment battery. Their obvious role in neonatal screening programs (NIH, 1993) has been documented.[49] Once again, however, it is important to consider the extent of the diagnostic information available through the use of the various EOAE procedures, such as transient OAE (TOAE) and distortion-product OAEs (DPOAE).[12,26] The benefits of this additional clinical tool have yet to be fully realized, particularly in the area of the differential diagnosis of hearing loss. Clinicians must interpret results obtained through EOAE as one component of the audiologic assessment process.

Acoustic emittance

Middle ear status must be assessed using acoustic emittance procedures (tympanometry and acoustic reflexes) at each audiologic assessment. This assessment is critical for the accurate interpretation of both behavioral and evoked response test procedures and to help verify the validity of degree-of-loss estimates.

Acoustic reflexes may be best elicited in infants with a 660 Hz probe frequency rather that the 220 Hz. The use of higher frequency probe frequencies for obtaining the tympanograms requires further examination. Regardless, it is clear that emittance procedures are invaluable and should be applied across the age range as part of the comprehensive audiologic assessment.[1]

The use of equivalent ear canal volume (Vec) is particularly useful in monitoring the viability of pressure-equalizing (PE) tubes in infants and toddlers. A recent report by Shanks et al[37] has provided normative data for clinicians for determining patency of PE tubes in young children. Obtaining Vec measures prior to myringotomy and tubes, however, provides a baseline for comparison of post-surgical PE tube evaluation.

An infant with sensorineural hearing loss should be monitored closely for middle ear involvement that could significantly exacerbate the degree of hearing loss. When the additional conductive hearing loss resulting from otitis media with effusion is imposed on the impaired sensory system, the difficulties impact on assessment, intervention, and follow-up.

Speech perception testing

Speech audiometry tests not only the subject's ability to know that a stimulus is present but also assesses the ability to identify and perceive what is said. Speech perception is a much more difficult task than threshold testing utilizing tones, noise bands, or speech stimuli. In addition to hearing the stimulus the child must have language and be able to process the stimuli. There are three different types of speech audiometry test protocols.

Speech awareness threshold (SAT). Speech awareness threshold (SAT) testing measures the softest level at which a child is aware of the presence of a speech stimulus. The task is the same as that is used for pure tone threshold testing (utilizing observation audiometry, visual reinforcement audiometry, or play audiometry), but the stimulus may consist of music, voice ("hello," or the child's name), or may be frequency specific and include low frequency ("bu"), mid-high frequency ("sh"), and high frequency ("s") speech stimuli.[21] The use of frequency-specific stimuli provides information that can be more easily compared with pure tone thresholds and provide information about how the infant may be expected to receive speech. Since understanding the stimulus is not required, an SAT can be obtained from neonates.

Speech reception threshold (SRT). Speech reception threshold testing assesses the softest level at which a child can identify speech stimuli. Testing is usually accomplished with pictures or objects representing spondee words (two syllable words with equal stress on both syllables). Older children may simply repeat the words presented by the examiner. The test protocol consists of familiarizing the child with the test stimuli to be certain that language comprehension is not a factor in test results. Presentation begins at an intensity level that is comfortably loud. Intensity is reduced to the point at which the child can correctly identify the words 50% of the time.[21] If the child is not familiar with the standard spondees, the tester may substitute pictures of familiar objects, Sesame Street characters, or body parts. The SRT should be in agreement with the pure tone average at 500, 1000 and 2000 Hz. If the audiogram is steeply sloping, the SRT may be closer to the best threshold than to the pure tone average.

Word recognition testing. Word recognition testing assesses the ability to correctly identify words that are presented at a comfortably loud level. Testing is usually accomplished at 40 dB above the SRT to be certain that the stimulus is comfortably loud. A word list of 25 or 50 words is used and the child is asked to repeat the words or point to pictures.[21] A percentage score is obtained. Picture pointing tests are available for children as young as 3 years of age.[9,35] A variety of word lists and picture pointing tests are available for children of different ages and with different vocabulary levels. Some have been specifically designed for assessing speech perception in children with severe and profound hearing loss.[21]

Describing auditory functioning. To fully assess a child's auditory functioning, it is necessary to test the child's word recognition abilities under different conditions.[21] In addition to testing at the standard level of 40 dB above threshold in each ear, a complete evaluation will assess the child's ability to understand speech in soundfield at a normal conversational level (50 dB) and at a soft conversational level (35 dB). In addition, testing should be accomplished in the presence of competing noise (four-talker babble) which is similar to what a child can expect to be exposed to at home or school.

Children who have borderline normal hearing (20 to 25 dB) thresholds can be expected to obtain a good word recognition score at 40 dB above threshold or at normal conversational level (50 dB) but will probably perform poorly at a soft conversational level (35 dB) and in the presence of competing noise. This means that they will have difficulty hearing in school or in a noisy home, and we can expect them to have academic difficulties. Auditory function at different levels and in the presence of noise needs to be considered as a factor in planning medical treatment, evaluating hearing aids, and determining if hearing aids or an FM system will be needed for school.

FOLLOW-UP EVALUATIONS

Otologic follow-up

Children with communication disorders require continued care. There are two essential aspects of this care. The first is the continued monitoring of the hearing function of the child. The primary disease may wax and wane, usually the latter. There will also be additional losses from OME which must be cared for. The second aspect of continued care is the continual assessment of the effectiveness of the interventions. The critical outcome is not hearing but the language of the child. This can be monitored periodically with the ELM[4,36] and, less frequently, with a complete language evaluation. Occasionally during the process of continued care, there will be new and/or additional information which can result in a change of diagnosis. The physician who undertakes the care of an infant or child with a communication disorder will be that child's physician for many years.

Audiologic follow-up

Children who are high risk for hearing loss should be followed audiologically on a regular basis. Infants who failed a hearing screening in the NICU should be followed until a complete frequency-specific audiologic evaluation with earphones (behavioral or electrophysiologic) can be accomplished which reveals normal hearing. This may require several re-evaluations at 3 month intervals. Children should return for re-evaluation after the development of speech and language to obtain speech perception testing, since the risk factors that cause hearing loss may also cause auditory processing disorders.

Children who are high risk for hearing loss because of family history need to be re-evaluated on a regular basis until past the age at which hearing loss has been identified in the family. While some hereditary hearing loss is present at birth, other children are born with normal hearing and loose hearing after birth, frequently in the first few months.[20,22] For this high-risk population, audiologic re-evaluation should be scheduled every 3 months until age two, every 6 months until age four, and annually or as needed after age four.

Children with identified hearing losses need to be followed audiologically to monitor changes in hearing and to monitor use of amplification. Evaluation should be scheduled every 3 months until age two, every 6 months until age five, and annually thereafter with amplification checks every 3 months. The purpose of audiologic followup testing for a child identified with impaired hearing is to monitor the progression of auditory development. At a minimum, testing should consist of air and bone conduction, emittance, and word recognition. A hearing-impaired child must be tested with and without amplification to monitor auditory development and progress.

Children who are otitis prone should be re-evaluated every 6 to 8 weeks as needed.[44]

CONCLUSION

In this paper we have attempted to demonstrate the importance of the collaborative effort of the otolaryngology-audiology team. We suggest that the comprehensive assessment and management of children with hearing loss is a critical factor in the success of the child and the family in dealing with the hearing loss and in managing progress. Good and continuous communication between these professionals insures optimal patient care.

REFERENCES

1. American Speech-Language-Hearing Association: Guidelines for the audiologic assessment of children from birth through 36 months of age. *ASHA* 33 (suppl 5):37-43, 1991.
2. Bernstein, RS, Gravel JS: A method for determining hearing sensitivity in infants: The interweaving staircase procedure (ISP). *J Am Acad Audiol* 1:138-145, 1990.
3. Bess F: The minimally hearing impaired child. *Ear and Hearing* 6:43-47, 1985.
4. Coplan J: *Early Language Milestone Scale, ed 2*. Pro-Ed, Austin, 1993, pp 1-95.
5. Diefendorf AO: Behavioral evaluation of hearing-impaired children. In Bess F, editor: *Hearing Impairment in Children.* Parkton, MD, 1988, York Press, pp 133-151.
6. Downs M, Sterrit G: A guide to newborn and infant hearing screening programs. *Arch Otolaryngol* 85:15-22, 1967.
7. Eilers RE, Ozdamar O, Steffins ML: Classification of audiograms by sequential testing: reliability and validity of an automated behavioral hearing screening algorithm. *J Am Acad Audiol* 4, 172-181, 1993.
8. Eilers RE, Widen JE, Urbano R, Hudson T, Gonzalez L: Optimization of automated hearing test algorithms: A comparison of data from simulations and young children. *Ear Hearing* 12:199-204, 1991.
9. Elliot LL, Katz D: *Development of a New Children's Test of Speech Discrimination.* St Louis, 1980, Auditec.
10. Elssman S, Matkin N, Sabo M: Identification of congenital sensorineural hearing impairment. *Hearing J* 40:13-17, 1987.
11. Gerber SE: Stimulus, response, and state variables in the testing of neonates. *Ear Hearing* 6:15-19, 1985.
12. Gorga MP, Neely ST, Bergman B, et al: Otoacoustic emissions from normal-hearing and hearing-impaired subjects: Distortion product responses. *J Acoust Soc Am* 93:2050-2060, 1993.
13. Gravel JS: Behavioral assessment of auditory function. *Semin Hearing* 10:216-228, 1989.
14. Gravel JS: Audiologic assessment of infants and toddlers. *ASHA Report 21,* 1992, pp. 55-62.
15. Gravel JS, Kurtzberg D, Stapells DR, et al: Case studies. *Semin Hearing.* 10:272-290, 1989.
16. Gravel JS, Trequina D: Experience with audiologic assessment of infants and toddlers. *Int J Pediatr Otorhinolaryngol* 23:59-71, 1992.
17. Joint Committee on Infant Hearing: 1990 position statement. *ASHA* 33(suppl 5):3-6, 1990.
18. Joint Committee on Infant Hearing (1994). *Audiology Today. ASHA,* 12:38-41, 1994.
19. Madell JR: Identification and treatment of very young children with hearing loss. *Infants Young Children* 1:20-30, 1994.
20. Madell JR: Progressive sensorineural hearing loss in young children: case reports. *Semin Hearing* 14:271-280, 1993.
21. Madell JR: Speech audiometry for children. In Gerber S, editor: *Handbook of Pediatric Audiology.* In press.
22. Madell JR, Sculerati N: Noncongenital hereditary hearing loss in children. *Arch Otolaryngol* 117:332-335, 1991.
23. Matkin N: Re-evaluating our approach to evaluation: demographics are changing—are we? In Bess F, editor: *Hearing Impairment in Children.* Parkton, MD, 1988, York Press, pp. 101-111.
24. Mauk GW, White KR, Mortensen LB, Behrens TR: The effectiveness of screening programs based on high-risk characteristics in early identification of hearing impairment. *Ear Hearing* 12:312-319, 1991.
25. Menyuk P: Effects of hearing loss on language acquisition in the babbling stage. In Jaffee BF, editor: *Hearing Loss in Children,* Baltimore, 1977, University Park Press, pp 621-629.
26. Norton SJ: Application of transient evoked otoacoustic emissions to pediatric populations. *Ear Hearing,* 14:64-73, 1993.
27. Nozza RJ, Wilson WR: Masked and unmasked puretone thresholds of infants and adults: development of auditory frequency selectivity and sensitivity. *J Speech Hearing Res* 27:613-622, 1984.
28. Olsho L, Koch E, Carter E, et al: Pure-tone sensitivity of human infants. *J Acoust Soc Am* 84:1316-1324, 1988.
29. Ozdamar O, Eilers R, Miskiel E, Widen J: Classification of audiograms by sequential testing using a dynamic Bayesian procedure. *J Acoust Soc Am* 88:2171-2179, 1990.
30. Pappas DG: A study of the high-risk registry for sensorineural hearing impairment. *Arch Otolaryngol-Head Neck Surg 91:*41-44, 1983.
31. Picton TW, Durieux-Smith A: Auditory evoked potentials in the assessment of hearing. *Neurol Clin* 6:791-808, 1988.
32. Primus M: Infant thresholds with enhanced attention to the signal in visual reinforcement audiometry. *J Speech Hearing Res* 31:480-484, 1988.
33. Primus M: Repeated infant thresholds in operant and nonoperant audiometric procedures. *Ear Hearing* 12:119-122, 1991.
34. Primus M, Thompson G: Response strength of young children in operant audiometry. *J Speech Hearing Res* 28:539-547, 1985.
35. Ross M, Lerman J: A picture identification test for hearing-impaired children. *J Speech Hearing Res* 13:44-53, 1970.
36. Ruben RJ: Language screening as a factor in the management of the pediatric otolaryngic patient. *Arch Otolaryngol Head Neck Surg* 117:1021-1025, 1991.
37. Shanks JE, Stelmachowicz PG, Beauchaine KL, Schulte L: Equivalent ear canal volumes in children pre- and post-tympanostomy tube insertion. *J Speech Hearing Res* 35:936-941, 1992.
38. Stapells D: Auditory brain stem response assessment of infants. *Semin Hearing* 10:252-261, 1989.
39. Stapells DR, Gravel JS, Martin B: ABR thresholds for tones in notched noise obtained from infants and young children with sensorineural hearing loss. *Assoc Res Otolaryngol: Abstracts of the Sixteenth Midwinter Meeting,* p. 59.
40. Stapells DR, Picton TW, Durieux-Smith A: Frequency specificity in evoked potential audiometry. In Jacobson J, editor: *The Auditory Brainstem Response,* ed 2. Allyn and Bacon, Boston.
41. Stapells DR, Picton TW, Smith A: Normal hearing thresholds for clicks. *J Acoust Soc Am,* 72:74-79, 1982.
42. Stapells DR, Ruben R: Auditory brain stem responses to bone-conducted tones in infants. *Annals of Otology, Rhinology, and Laryngology,* 98, 941-949.
43. Stein L, Clark S, Kraus N: The hearing-impaired infant: patterns of identification and habilitation. *Ear Hearing* 4:232-286, 1983.
44. Teele DW, Klein J, Rosner BA, Greater Boston Otitis Media Study Group: Otitis media with effusion during the first three years of life and development of speech and language. *Pediatrics* 74:282-287, 1984.
45. Thompson M, Thompson G: Responses of infants and young children as a function of auditory stimuli and test month. *J Speech Hearing Res* 15:699-707, 1972.
46. Thompson G, Thompson M, McCall A: Strategies for increasing response behavior of 1 and 2 year old children during visual reinforcement audiometry (VRA). *Ear Hearing* 13:236-240, 1992.
47. Thompson G, Weber B: Responses of infants and young children to behavior observation audiometry (BOA). *J Speech Hearing Dis* 4:140-147, 1974.
48. Werner L, Gillenwater J: Pure-tone sensitivity of 2 to 5 week old infants. *Infant Beh Develop* 13:355-375, 1990.
49. White KR, Vohr BR, Behrens TR: Universal newborn hearing screening using transient evoked otoacoustic emissions: results of the Rhode Island Hearing Assessment Project. *Semin Hearing* 14:18-29, 1993.
50. Widen JE: Behavioral screening of high-risk infants using visual reinforcement audiometry. *Semin Hearing.* 11:342-356, 1990.
51. Widen JE: Adding objectivity to infant behavioral audiometry. *Ear Hearing* 14:49-57, 1993.
52. Wilson WR, Thompson G: Behavioral audiometry. In Jerger J, editor: *Pediatric Audiology.* San Diego, 1984 College-Hill Press, pp 1-44.

27

Office Treatment of the Draining Ear

Jed A. Kwartler, M.D. and Clough Shelton, M.D.

THE PROBLEM

Office treatment of the patient with a chronically draining ear can be quite frustrating, both to the patient and the treating physician. Numerous factors, both intrinsic and extrinsic to the problem, block the attainment of a dry, safe, and hearing ear. These include failure to recognize underlying disease, such as cholesteatoma, pathologic synergy between aerobic and anaerobic bacteria that promote inhibition of phagocytosis, mucosal changes with subepithelial scarring and devascularization, poor drainage of inflammatory infiltrates, and lack of patient compliance with treatment. Some advocate that effective control of drainage with a low recidivism rate is unattainable and that the goal of office management is to prepare the ear for definitive surgery.[4,5,11] In contrast, others advocate the use of oral and intravenous antibiotic regimens to control drainage in suppurating ears without cholesteatoma.[7,12-14]

What types of ears drain? To come up with a treatment plan we define four groups: (1) ears with perforations, (2) ears with mastoid cavities, (3) ears with ventilation tubes, and (4) ears with problems limited to the canal.

PATIENT HISTORY

Our initial evaluation starts with a thorough history. What is the quality and pattern of the discharge? Is it serous, mucoid, or mucopurulent, and is it intermittent or constant? Is there a relationship between the drainage and upper respiratory tract infection (URI)? Has water gotten into the ear before the onset of drainage? Pain associated with a discharging ear is a serious symptom and may indicate an underlying osteitis or portend an impending neuro-otologic complication. Systemic conditions, particularly those that interfere with a normal immune response, are sought. Diabetes mellitus, autoimmune disorders requiring constant steroid use, anemia, malnutrition, and chronic dermatologic problems exemplify conditions that make treatment more difficult. Excessive manipulation of the ear by the patient can interfere with normal canal skin defense mechanisms. Q-tips, paper clips, bobby pins, and the like can seriously traumatize the canal skin or tympanic membrane setting up a vicious cycle of irritation and manipulation. Uncovering such behavior of which the patient may be unaware, is key to successful treatment. Hearing aid molds and ear plugs may also inflame the canal skin barrier. Their use is usually more obvious. Does the patient use any hair sprays, shampoos, or hair coloring? These may cause a contact dermatitis, easily treated by eliminating the offending chemical irritant. Has the patient used any ototopic medications containing neomycin or steroids? If so, for how long have drops been used? (Most patients referred from primary physicians will have been on a neomycin/cortisporin drop.) Has the patient taken any systemic antibiotics, either administered orally or intravenously? Associated symptoms of hearing loss, dizziness or vertigo, facial weakness, facial numbness, swallowing difficulty, and headache should serve as a red flag alerting the physician to a serious underlying problem, a "nonsafe" ear.

INITIAL EXAMINATION

The ears of all patients with drainage are examined under the microscope. Use of the microscope facilitates safer and more comfortable cleaning of the ear, as well as providing appropriate lighting and magnification to determine the extent of disease. A mental checklist of critical structural detail is used and all questions must be answered at the end of the examination.

Ears with perforations are divided into those with central perforations and those with marginal perforations. What

The authors wish to thank their teachers and colleagues at the House Ear Clinic for sharing many of the techniques and principles contained in this chapter. Dr. James Sheehy deserves special thanks for his superb teaching ability and willingness to instruct younger otologists in some of the "old-fashioned" but very useful techniques for managing the draining ear.

Instruction Card for Otitis Externa

Otitis externa

An infection of the ear canal (otitis externa) may be acute, subacute, or chronic. It may be due to a skin condition (dandruff, eczema), an allergy (to foods, inhalants, fungus, cosmetics, or jewelry), an irritation (from middle ear drainage or use of a hearing aid), or nervous tension (scratching the ear). In many cases a combination of these factors exists simultaneously. One problem may complicate or aggravate the other.

Regardless of the underlying cause, moisture and irritation (scratching) are usually responsible for keeping the problem active; both must be eliminated.

Under no circumstances should you allow water to enter the ear canal. When showering or washing the hair, place cotton or lambswool in the outer opening of the ear and cover the outside of this material with vaseline or use an ear plug.

It is natural to scratch your ear if it itches. Unfortunately, this rubbing or scratching aggravates the skin condition greatly, regardless of the underlying cause. A so-called vicious cycle of itch-scratch-itch occurs. Soon the ear opening and outer ear may become very sore. In most cases cleaning the ear with a Q-tip is only an excuse to scratch it and you must not do this unless your doctor specifically recommends using a Q-tip. Most treatment will be ineffective if you persist in scratching.

Treatment

1. Do not allow soap, water or peroxide to enter the ear canal.
2. Do not scratch or otherwise irritate your ear canal. Do not use Q-tips in the ear.
3. If you wear a hearing aid it is best that you leave it out of the involved ear as much as possible until the swelling or discharge subsides.
4. Your doctor will recommend medication to help the skin condition and decrease the itching. These medications may include ointments, medicated eardrops, alcohol eardrops or half-strength vinegar irrigations.
5. In certain cases allergy tests and injections may be indicated.

IF YOU HAVE ANY QUESTIONS ABOUT YOUR CONDITION PLEASE CALL OUR OFFICE.

Instruction Card for Draining Ear

Treatment of the draining ear

Your doctor will indicate the treatment he wishes you to use for your draining ear. This treatment may include cleaning of the ear and use of eardrops, powder, or half-strength vinegar irrigations.

It is important that you avoid getting soap or water into the ear. When showering or washing the hair, you may use ear plugs to prevent water from getting in the ear or you may place cotton or lambswool in the outer opening of the ear and cover the outside of the material with vaseline.

On rare occasions, the eardrops or powder may cause itching, burning, or increase in ear discharge. If these symptoms should develop after the first few applications of the medicine, please discontinue treatment and contact our office.

Discontinue all treatment to the ear 24 hours prior to your next visit to the doctor so that he may observe how much discharge, if any, has accumulated during this interval.

Cleaning the ear

If your doctor wishes you to clean your ear before treating it, you will be given a wire applicator and instructed in how to wrap it with cotton. Note that the cotton is tightly wound on the wire but is soft and fluffy on the end. Wash your hands before wrapping the cotton.

Use the hand opposite the ear to be cleaned, reach in back of the head and pull the ear up and back. This will straighten out the ear canal and make it easier to introduce the cotton-covered applicator. Gently insert the applicator as far as it will go and blot the ear (or mastoid cavity if you have had a mastoid or fenestration operation). Repeat this procedure with a fresh piece of cotton until the ear is dry.

Use of eardrops

If your doctor has instructed you to clean the ear before applying the eardrops, read the instructions above. With the head tipped well to the side, instill the prescribed number of drops. After five minutes, place a small piece of cotton loosely in the lower portion of the outer ear in such a way that it does not completely block the ear canal. This allows air to enter the ear canal. You may then resume normal activities. Change the cotton as necessary.

Use of antibiotic powders

If your doctor has instructed you to clean the ear before insufflating the antibiotic powders, read the section above on cleaning the ear.

Directions for use of the powder blower come with it. Review these before use.

The antibiotic powder capsules may be obtained locally or from Medical Square Pharmacy in Los Angeles (800-356-9440).

To use the powder blower remove the top of the powder capsule and insert the portion containing the powder in the chamber of the blower, *opened end toward the bulb*. Replace the small end of the plastic barrel of the blower.

To avoid having the powder fall into the bulb when not in use, keep the powder blower in an upright position (that is, with the tip downward). An empty drinking glass is a good container for storing the blower. Keep in a dry place to prevent caking of the powder. One capsule should last approximately one week.

If you have been instructed to clean your ear, insufflate one puff of the antibiotic powder into the ear canal after the cleaning procedure. Repeat the cleaning and powdering procedure in the morning and evening (or as directed). After there has been no evidence of discharge for three consecutive days, clean the ear only in the morning and do not insufflate powder unless the discharge reappears. If discharge does reappear, reinstitute cleaning and powdering the ear twice daily until the ear is dry again.

REFERENCES

1. Balkany T et al: A prospective study of infection following tympanostomy tube insertion. *Am J Otol* 4:288-291, 1983.
2. Braganza R et al: Closure of the soft palate for persistent otorrhea after placement of pressure equalization tubes in cleft palate infants. *Cleft Palate-Craniofac J* 28:305-307, 1991.
3. Brook I: Prevalence of beta-lactamase–producing bacteria in chronic suppurative otitis media. *Am J Dis of Child* 139:280-283, 1985.
4. Browning G et al: Controlled trial of medical treatment of active chronic otitis media. *Br Med J* 287:1024, 1983.
5. Browning GG et al: Medical Management of active chronic otitis media: a controlled study. *J Laryngol Otol* 102:491-495, 1988.
6. Cohen S et al: Otitic candidiasis in children: an evaluation of the problem and effectiveness of ketoconazole in 10 patients. *Ann Otol Rhinol Laryngol* 99:427-431, 1990.
7. Dagan R et al: Outpatient management of chronic suppurative otitis media without cholesteatoma in children. *Pediatr Infect Dis J* 11:542-546, 1992.
8. Fliss D et al: Aerobic bacteriology of chronic suppurative otitis media without cholesteatoma in children. *Ann Otol Rhinol Laryngol* 101:866-869, 1992.
9. Gates G et al: Delayed onset post-tympanostomy otorrhea. *Otolaryngol Head Neck Surg* 98:111-115, 1988.
10. Herzon JS: Tympanostomy tubes: infectious complications. *Arch Otolaryngol* 106:645-647, 1980.
11. Hussain S: Conservative treatment in the management of inflammatory aural polyp. *J Laryngol Otol* 106:313-315, 1992.
12. Kenna M et al: Medical management of chronic suppurative otitis media without cholesteatoma in children—update 1992. *Am J Otol* 14:469-473, 1993.
13. Lang R et al: Oral ciprofloxacin in the management of chronic suppurative otitis media without cholesteatoma in children: preliminary experience in 21 children. *Pediatr Infect Dis J* 11:925-929, 1992.
14. Lieberman A et al: Medical treatment of chronic suppurative otitis media without cholesteatoma in children—a two-year follow-up. *Int J Pediatr Otorhinolaryngol* 24:25-33, 1992.
15. Lundy L et al: Ototoxicity and ototopical medications: a survey of otolaryngologists. *Am J Otol* 14:141-146, 1993.
16. Mandel E et al: Acute otorrhea: bacteriology of a common complication of tympanostomy tubes. *Ann Otol Rhinol Laryngol* 103:713-718, 1994.
17. Merifeld D et al: Therapeutic management of chronic suppurative otitis media with otic drops. *Otolaryngol Head Neck Surgery* 109:77-82, 1993.
18. Morizono T: Toxicity of ototopical drugs: animal modeling. *Ann Otol Rhinol Laryngol* 99:42-45, 1990.
19. Podoshin L et al: Ototoxicity of ear drops in patients suffering from chronic otitis media. *J Laryngol Otol* 103:46-50, 1990.
20. Raju K et al: Reliability of conventional ear swabs in tubotympanic CSOM. *J Laryngol Otol* 102:460-462, 1990.
21. Schneider M: Bacteriology of otorrhea from tympanostomy tubes. *Arch Otolaryngol Head Neck Surg* 115:1225-1226, 1989.
22. Sheehy, JL: Surgery of Chronic Otitis Media. In English GM, (editor): *Otolaryngology.* Philadelphia, 1984, Harper and Row.
23. Wright C et al: Ototoxicity of otic drops applied to the middle ear in the chinchilla. *Am J Otolaryngol* 5:166-176, 1984.

28

Advanced Techniques in Tympanoplasty

Roger E. Wehrs, M.D. and David W. White, M.D.

HISTORICAL

In the early part of this century, ear surgery consisted of incision and drainage of the mastoid. There was no effort to save or restore the anatomy or to improve the hearing.

In the 1940s Lempert[2] introduced his endaural incision and mastoidectomy which was much more effective in eliminating disease and in exteriorizing cholesteatoma, preventing complications and fatalities. However these procedures changed the basic anatomy and function of the ear and did nothing to preserve or restore hearing.

The most widely performed procedure was the radical mastoidectomy, in which the mastoid was completely exteriorized, the eardrum and ossicles removed, and an effort made to obliterate the eustachian tube. Conservative otolaryngologists such as Shirley Barron[1] introduced the modified radical mastoidectomy for cases of attic cholesteatoma. These were used when the pars tensa was intact and the middle ear was sealed off. Tympanomeatal flaps were reflected back into the mastoid cavity. Hearing was preserved and sometimes improved by the tympanomeatal flap contacting the stapes and the structure providing some preservation or even increase of the patient's hearing.

In 1953 the term "tympanoplasty" was introduced by Horst Wullstein in Germany. The word "tympanoplasty" is quite descriptive as "tymp" refers to the eardrum and "plasty" refers to plastic surgery, therefore it is literally plastic surgery of the eardrum. For the first time a new concept was introduced into ear surgery, stressing not only the removal of the disease but also the preservation of as much of the normal anatomy and function of the ear as possible. It also recognized that the main function of the ear was to hear, and efforts were made to preserve or improve the hearing following the surgical procedures.

Wullstein soon introduced his 5 types of tympanoplasty with the different degrees of severity of disease.[10] Type I referred to a simple perforation of the tympanic membrane with an intact ossicular chain. In type II, there was a perforation with malleus present and erosion or absence of the incus, but usually an intact stapes. The graft was placed over the perforation with contact being made to the remaining incus and, hopefully, stapes. In type III, the malleus and incus had been destroyed by disease and the reconstruction carried directly to the stapes head. In type IV, the stapes superstructure was absent and the footplate was mobile. Here the graft had a cutout for the oval window so that there was sound protection for the round window, and hopefully the sound waves would go directly to the footplate. In type V there was absence of all ossicles and a fixed stapedial footplate. Here a fenestration was made in the horizontal semicircular canal in an effort to improve hearing. In the early Wullstein procedures, an elliptical piece of full-thickness skin was obtained from the postauricular sulcus. This was ingenious as the skin was thin, relatively hairless, easily available, and the defect closed with no cosmetic change at the end of the procedure. Unfortunately the full-thickness skin did not have the migratory characteristics of the canal skin and eardrum and would exfoliate with secondary infections and poor function. Occasionally the full-thickness skin would not survive but would act as a matrix to support the ingrowing canal skin, and in these ears excellent results were obtained.

The third stage of development was the intact wall tympanomastoidectomy.[4] This consisted of doing a mastoidectomy to remove the disease but preserving a thin bony barrier between the ear canal and the mastoid. Several significant improvements were accomplished. The eardrum would remain in an anatomical position rather than collapsing onto the horizontal semicircular canal, thus compromising the size of the middle ear. This also allowed normal mastoid air cells to be preserved with normal drainage beneath the bony wall into the middle ear and down the eustachian tube. It also provided for aeration of the mastoid as nature had intended. Due to the fact that there was no cavity to the outside, these ears healed much faster. There was no need for periodic cleaning of the mastoidectomy cavity. Elimination of the noncleaning cavity with its repeated infections and restriction on swimming and other activities was greeted with enthusiasm by the otological community. It seemed almost too good to be true and unfortunately it was.

With a large pneumatized mastoid and no cholesteatoma, the procedure lived up to all its expectations. However the enthusiasm spread to all cases of mastoidectomy including cholesteatoma. The surgeons, accustomed to doing surgery with only cursory attention to detail and removal of cholesteatoma, performed the intact wall mastoidectomy in the same manner as they had the modified radical and radical mastoidectomy procedures. The cholesteatoma left behind could no longer exfoliate to the outside as had been the case in the open cavities and therefore formed large cysts in the mastoidectomy cavity. Complications such as brain abscess or meningitis rarely developed, however the thin bony wall was soon eroded by the recurrent cholesteatoma. This was followed by infection and drainage. Occasionally cholesteatoma filled the ear canal. These early ears were revised, converting them back to an open cavity. Unfortunately these failures gave a bad name to the intact wall tympanoplasty and it was all but abandoned.

Compromise procedures were forthcoming. Among the more popular was the staging of tympanoplasty procedures.[3] The concept here was that following the initial procedure one would re-explore the ear in a few months to remove any residual cholesteatoma. An inducement to get the patient to return was to not do any ossicular reconstruction at the initial procedure so that the patient would not hear and be more apt to return for follow-up and the second stage. When cholesteatoma was found at the second stage, occasionally this was carried out further to third and fourth stage procedures.

Another compromise has been the use of the intact wall tympanoplasty for small cholesteatomas with large pneumatized mastoids and the canal wall down procedure for extensive cholesteatomas or contracted mastoids. This combined with staging of difficult cases was an acceptable answer for many surgeons.

PHYSIOLOGICAL TYMPANOMASTOIDECTOMY

To avoid the mistakes of the past and hopefully improve the results in the future, a technique of physiological tympanomastoidectomy has been developed. The goals here are to remove all disease and cholesteatoma and restore the middle ear and mastoid to normal anatomical configuration and function.

Let us review the normal anatomy and configuration of the middle ear and mastoid (Fig. 28-1). The cone-shaped tympanic membrane is situated at the medial end of the bony ear canal. The eardrum and ear canal are lined by a squamous epithelium which migrates to the outside with a self-cleaning action. The middle ear is aerated by the eustachian tube with continuation of the aeration into the honeycomb of the mastoid air cells. In reverse direction the mastoid air cells drain into the middle ear and down the eustachian tube. The middle ear space is maintained by the tympanic membrane being supported by the bony ear canal which provides space for the ossicular chain which converts air waves from the eardrum into fluid waves in the inner ear.

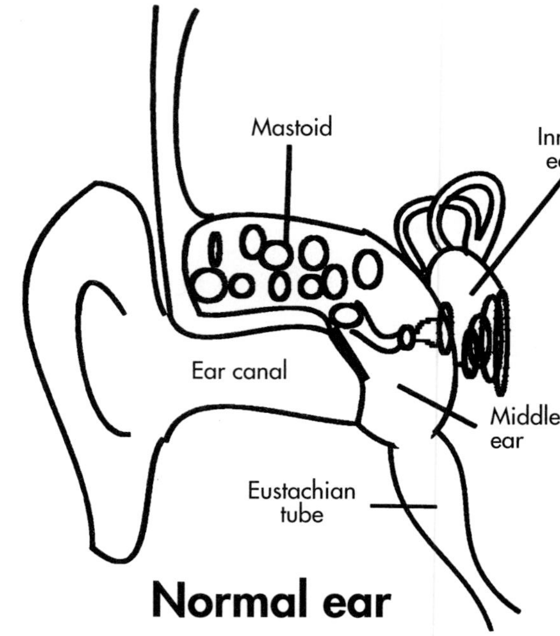

FIG 28-1
Normal anatomy of the middle ear and mastoid.

Now let us consider what happens when this bony barrier is removed (Fig. 28-2). The posterior superior part of the tympanic membrane has no support and collapses against the posterior middle ear and mastoid. The lever action and function of the ossicular chain is lost. The normal conduit from the middle ear to the mastoid is replaced by the collapsed tissues of the remaining eardrum and canal wall or graft. Air can no longer reach the mastoidectomy cavity. It can, of course, be aerated from the outside, however the drainage from the remaining air cells cannot reach the middle ear and is shunted to the outside where it softens and macerates the graft. The size of the middle ear is reduced. Loss of this reserve of air capacity forces the patient to equalize the pressure by swallowing or yawning much more often.

Now let us consider a physiological situation in which the posterior bony canal wall has been preserved or replaced with homograft knee cartilage (Fig. 28-3). Having the wall in place, the middle ear can be reconstructed to normal size. This is accomplished with the homograft tympanic membrane and malleus as a main building block. The ossicular reconstruction is carried out with the incus or incus stapes replacements of hydroxylapatite. Due to the fact that the

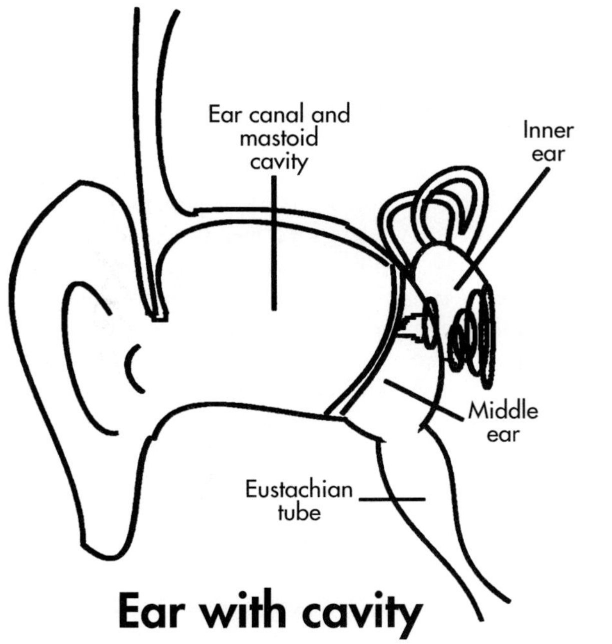

FIG 28-2
Altered anatomy of the middle ear and mastoid after removal of the bony posterior canal wall.

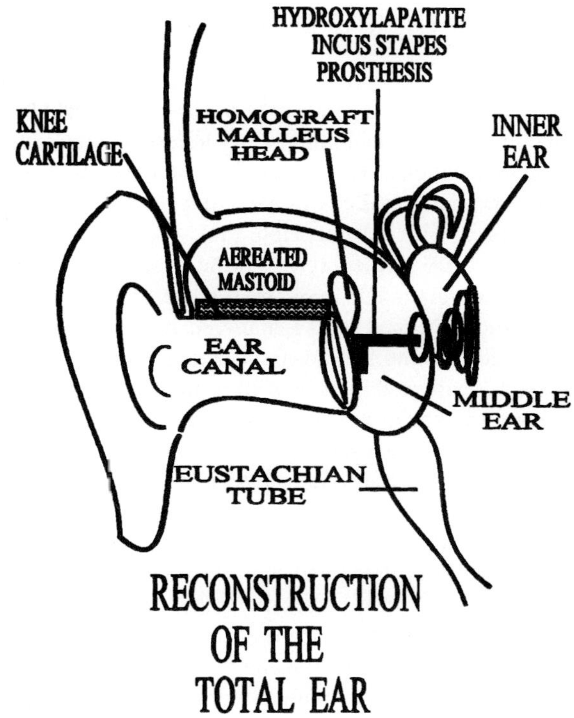

FIG 28-3
Restoration of the normal anatomy of the middle ear and mastoid with homograft knee cartilage, tympanic membrane, and incussta-pes prosthesis of hydroxylapatite.

conduit is once again established beneath the bony wall, the mastoid cavity which was a honeycomb of air cells is now one large air cell aerated from the middle ear. The remaining mastoid cells drain into the antrum and thus to the middle ear and eustachian tube. The external ear canal is of normal size and configuration and cleans itself by epithelial migration. In this technique, the middle ear and mastoid have once again been rebuilt to normal anatomical configuration and function.

PHILOSOPHY OF CANAL WALL UP OR CANAL WALL DOWN

The most important goal of using an open or closed technique is the complete and total removal of all disease. This is meticulous and time-consuming surgery, and without removal of all disease a good result will not be obtained. Most surgeons agree that it is better to preserve the bony canal wall if possible. Yet there is a difference in how to treat this structure. Surgeons who usually take the canal wall down want to create as small a cavity as possible so that it will epithelialize quickly and not drain. Therefore they begin the procedure with the thought in mind that if possible the canal wall will be preserved but they do not hesitate at all in taking it down. They therefore create a small cavity and soon find they do not have room to work and keep the canal wall up and so quickly concede that the wall cannot be preserved and take it down. Also some surgeons do not want to waste a lot of time preserving the canal wall, and then find that it cannot be preserved and they have to remove it.

Surgeons who usually leave the wall up make as large a cavity as possible so that there is better visualization and disease can be removed without sacrificing the bony wall. They do not hesitate to make a large cavity as they are going to have a closed cavity and the size does not matter. They are also willing to spend the extra time it takes to preserve the bony canal wall even if sometimes after spending an hour or more preserving it they find that in this case it does have to be removed. They figure the extra time spent in surgery preserving the wall is made up many times over by not having to clean a cavity in the office.

There are guidelines for preserving the canal wall. As previously stated, the first and most important goal is to make a large cavity, taper the edges so that one can have better visualization to remove the disease, and still keep the wall intact. Before removal of any cholesteatoma the cortex should be completely uncapped over the cholesteatoma, including the zygomatic portion. The dissection should be carried far enough forward over the zygomatic region to visualize the head of the malleus. When thinning the bony wall one should constantly check on both the canal as well as the mastoid side and avoid any drilling on the canal wall side. The incus and head of the malleus should be removed early as this will give much more room to adequately remove the cholesteatoma. In early removal of the incus the incudostapedial joint is separated as it is for stapedectomy. Following separation of the incudostapedial joint and elevation of the long process of the incus, it is best to go back to the mastoid cavity and separate the incudomalleolar joint with a right angle pick and remove the incus from the cavity side. At this time it is good to again go back to the canal side and elevate the skin and/or cholesteatoma from the neck of the malleus. The neck of the malleus is then cut with House Dieter malleus nippers and the head separated from the neck with a right angle pick. Again, one usually needs to go back to the cavity side to remove the malleus head with a right angle pick or forceps. The dural plate should also be thinned with a diamond burr until it is blue and translucent. One should avoid exposing the dura if at all possible. However, when drilling next to the dura one should use a large cutting burr or a diamond burr, as a small cutting burr will more easily perforate the dura.

Once the entire mastoid has been uncapped, the incus and malleus head removed, the cholesteatoma is accessible for removal. Before removal of the matrix, the cholesteatoma sac should be debulked and loose chunks and layers of cholesteatoma removed but the matrix preserved. Elevation of the matrix should begin at the most distal areas of the cholesteatoma ingrowth, usually at the antrum or tip of the mastoid. The matrix should be elevated with a blunt instrument. The matrix sac is kept intact if at all possible to avoid any residual cholesteatoma pockets. The sac is elevated from the bone and the cholesteatoma sac is always lifted from the bone with the blunt instrument, which is much better than pressing against the bone to elevate the sac as one can easily injure any underlying soft structures such as a fistula of the horizontal canal, dura, or facial nerve. The cholesteatoma should be followed into all cells usually elevating the mucosa as well. In an intact wall procedure it is important to remove all cholesteatoma from the undersurface of the preserved bony wall. This is done by working from both sides and keeping the sac intact. After removal one may use a mirror to view the undersurface of the wall and be sure that no cholesteatoma has been left behind. As the cholesteatoma is elevated toward the attic and middle ear, it becomes bulky. When it is no longer manageable the sac is cut across with a scissors, well away from the remaining attachments and the bulk is removed. In this way the sac is kept intact. The cholesteatoma is elevated from the bed of the addis ad antrum and over the Fallopian canal and up to the tensor tympani tendon and then under the bony wall to the middle ear. It is often necessary to open the facial recess widely with a diamond burr. After the cholesteatoma is freed from its bed it is reflected as far as possible into the middle ear, and then by turning attention to the canal side the cholesteatoma is picked up here and elevated into the middle ear and followed to its termination. Elevation here is similar to that used in the mastoid and consists of elevating an intact sac and then amputating the bulk and proceeding with the elevation until all the squamous ingrowth has been removed. Cholesteatoma removal is meticulous and time consuming and cannot be rushed. Often it is necessary to curette or burr down the bony annulus. Often the sac is adherent to the stapes and stapedial footplate or even the round window membrane. If one is to effect a cure every shred of cholesteatoma must be removed.

On occasion the dural plate is almost touching the superior bony ear canal and it is not possible to uncap the zygomatic mastoid portion. If the cholesteatoma cannot be removed by the above-described means then only that portion of the bony wall over the cholesteatoma is removed. Once the cholesteatoma has been completely removed, the defect in the bony canal wall is immediately reconstructed with homograft knee cartilage. This has the effect of creating an intact canal wall tympanoplasty. The advantage is that of removal of the obstructing bony portion of the wall so that the cholesteatoma can be removed under direct vision. Immediate reconstruction is much easier and more successful than reconstruction following a procedure where the wall had been completely removed. In the immediate reconstruction the facial ridge is high and intact as well as a zygomatic spur along the dural plate. With this support the cartilage button may be grooved to overlap the remaining bony wall which holds it securely in position. The new wall is covered with the facial graft and the tympanomeatal skin flaps replaced. Healing is usually rapid with a normal-appearing and functioning ear canal.

MIDDLE EAR RECONSTRUCTION

If the patient has a perforated eardrum and no cholesteatoma, the operative procedure is usually carried out through the ear canal by means of a canal skin type of tympanoplasty. In our practice we do a high percentage of revision cases from other surgeons. As the facial underlay graft has been widely used, it is important to have an effective and alternative surgery to revise these cases. I believe that the canal skin tympanoplasty meets these requirements.

The canal skin type of tympanoplasty is not new, as a matter of fact it is one of the older type of techniques, even predating the facial graft. Most procedures are carried out transmeatally through an ear speculum. The first incision is made just above the pars flaccida and is carried up the tympanosquamous suture line (Fig. 28-4). The second incision, a vertical one extends up the tympanomeatal suture line and outlines the vascular strip. The third incision is circumferential at the bony membranous junction and joins the two previously made incisions. By means of a round knife and with constant suction against the knife, the skin is elevated around the ear canal and down to the fibrous annulus. At this point one must be careful not to elevate the fibrous annulus from the bony annulus. The periosteum continues under the fibrous annulus into the middle ear. Therefore one must break through this periosteum in order to elevate the epithelial layer from the remaining drum remnant. Once a plane has been established it can easily be followed. However one must be careful not to leave any pockets of squamous epithelium behind. Once the proper plane has been

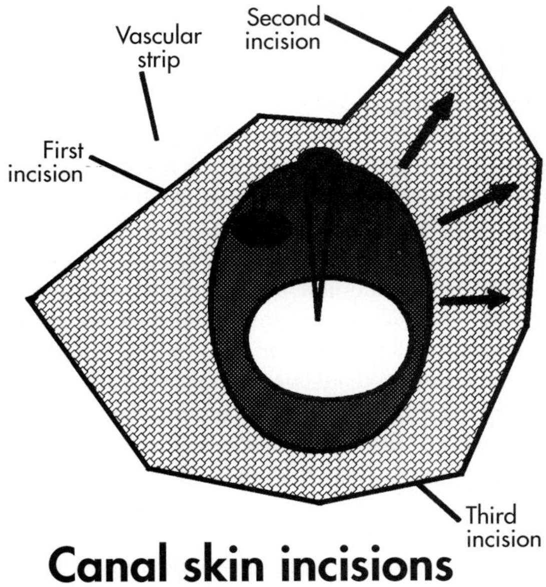

FIG 28-4
Incisions for removal of the canal skin graft.

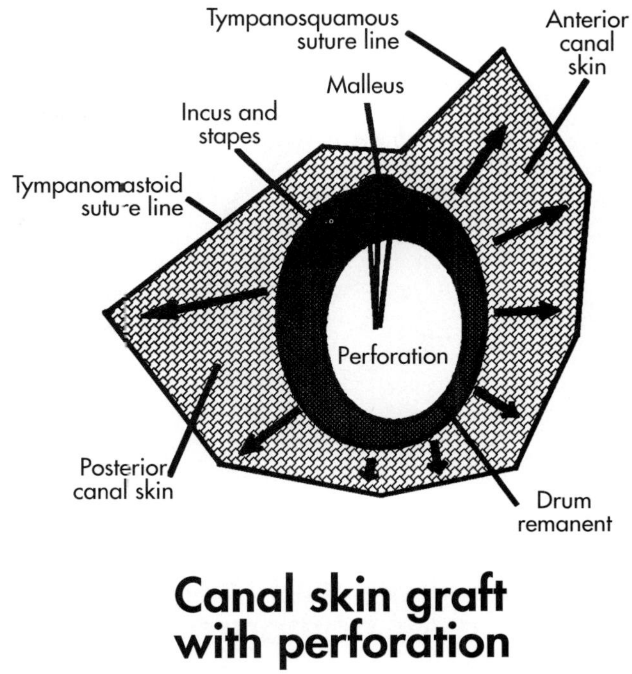

FIG 28-5
Diagrammatic representation of the canal skin graft removed as a cylinder.

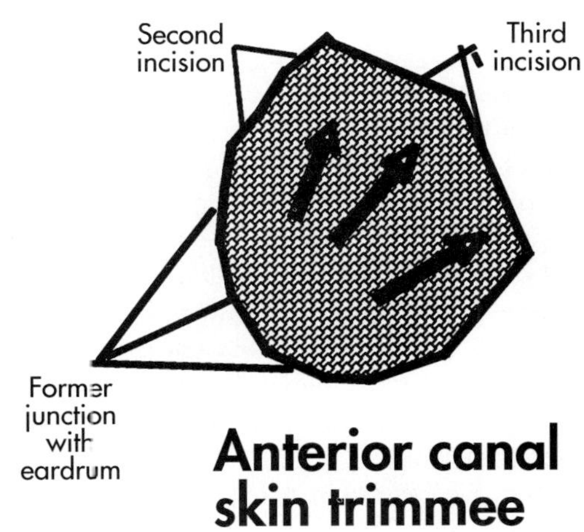

FIG 28-6
Canal skin graft trimmed. Note arrows match previous location of anterior canal skin.

found, the elevation proceeds easily and the canal skin is removed in continuity with the epithelial layer of the remaining eardrum. Occasionally there is squamous ingrowth around the margins of the perforations, and it is very important to follow this ingrowth beneath the eardrum, even removing parts of the drum if necessary, as any squamous epithelium left beneath the drum will cause recurrence of cholesteatoma with breakdown of the graft.

Another advantage of the canal skin type of tympanoplasty is that after its removal it gives access to remove any anterior bony overhang. Bony obstruction and failure to visualize the anterior annulus is in my experience one of the major causes for failure of an underlay fascial graft. The canal skin is elevated from the incision at the bony membranous junction over the bony overhang to the fibrous annulus. If the bony overhang is average and only moderate, the removal of the thickness of the canal skin often gives adequate visualization to remove the skin down to and from the fibrous annulus. If there is massive bony overhang it may be necessary to drill down some of the bony overhang with a diamond burr before the skin can be removed. All drilling on the anterior canal is performed with a diamond burr under constant irrigation. If the bone is heated by dry drilling it will not heal. This is especially true for our technique in which the anterior canal wall is left completely bare.

The canal skin comes out as a cylinder with a perforation at the bottom (Fig. 28-5). It is placed on a tongue blade and the skin area that had been over the pars flaccida is cut through with a knife and the epithelial layer of the drum is also trimmed to the area that had made up the fibrous annulus (Fig. 28-6). This allows the graft to lay flat and it becomes more rectangular in shape. The graft is turned 180° so that the thin area that composed the anterior canal skin now lies over the anterior ear drum (Fig. 28-7).

The canal skin is very thin and has no tendency to granulate or produce stenosis with obliteration of the anterior angle as happens with overlay tissue grafts. In the early 1960s, the senior author used the canal skin alone over the perforation. Although hearing results were good, the graft take rate was very poor at about 60%. It was found that if a homograft tympanic membrane or dural graft was put over

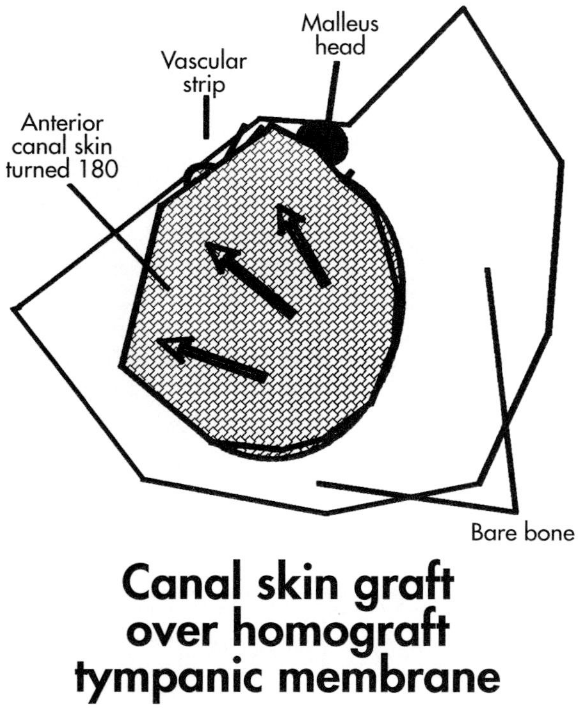

FIG 28-7
Canal skin graft in place. Note arrows and rotation.

the drum remnant and the canal skin placed over these structures, the graft take rate rose to 95% and there was still excellent preservation of the sharp anterior angle with good hearing results.[5] Homograft tympanic membranes must be preserved in 70% ethyl alcohol. If one uses a homograft which had been preserved in formalin or buffered formaldehyde, there appears to be a toxic reaction to the graft which produces granulation tissue, crusting, and delayed healing. Therefore I recommend that only tympanic membranes preserved in 70% ethyl alcohol be used with the canal skin technique.

Removal of the canal skin also gives good access to posterior superior canal. The bony scutum can be removed in a fashion similar to that used in stapedectomy. The chorda tympani nerve is preserved if possible. This gives good access to the ossicular chain and one can test for dehiscence or mobility. One of the most frequently seen defects is dehiscence of the long process of the incus. Usually the lenticular process of the incus is still attached to the stapes head, and if possible this should be removed as it often contains squamous epithelium. Also the reconstruction is easier to a normal capitulum than to one with the lenticular process attached. As a general rule the incus body is removed, as this gives better access for the reconstruction and opens aeration to the mastoid. The incudomalleolar joint is separated with a right angle pick and the incus body removed. The malleus is then checked for mobility and the mucosa elevated from the undersurface of manubrium of malleus in preparation for reconstruction.

The character of the middle ear mucosa is checked. If there is any squamous ingrowth, it must be followed to its termination and removed. There is often bare bone over the promontory after the removal of squamous ingrowth. Also the tip of the malleus may touch the mucosa or be buried in it. In this case the malleus tip is elevated and the adhesions severed. To prevent fixation of the malleus or bare areas, it is important to use silastic sheeting in the middle ear. Precut silastic inserts have been developed with the Xomed-Treace Company. The tympanoplasty silastic insert is used in conjunction with the canal skin tympanoplasty.[9] This silastic insert completely fills the inner ear with a cutout for the stapes or stapedial footplate and for the tensor tympani tendon. There is also a tongue which extends over the horizontal canal and into the first part of the mastoid antrum. Another insert called the mastoid silastic insert is used in conjunction with mastoidectomy. It does not have precut areas for the reconstruction as there are considerable variations of the anatomy in mastoid surgery. If the tip of the malleus touches the mucosa, a 4 × 6 mm insert is created and placed under the tip of the malleus.

As stated earlier special techniques are often needed for revision cases. The middle ear mucosa is often thick and scarred. Occasionally the underlay fascial grafts have blocked the mastoid antrum or posterior middle ear with resultant shunting of the mastoid flow to the outside. This keeps the ear wet and produces repeated infections. In revision cases in which cholesteatoma was elevated over bare bone, adhesions have formed because no silastic sheeting was placed in the middle ear. The technique here is to remove the canal skin and epithelial layer from the drum, following any squamous ingrowth over the graft into the middle ear to its termination. The scar tissue is elevated and dissected to normal appearing mucosa where it will be cut across and removed. There appear to be two areas that are vulnerable to obstruction by the fascia graft. This is the narrow area over the horizontal canal and Fallopian canal, especially with an intact ossicular chain. The other is beneath the manubrium of the malleus. Here the graft was placed under the manubrium of a malleus which almost touched the promontory. This scars in and effectively seals off the posterior middle ear so that any drainage cannot reach the eustachian tube and is trapped to the outside. This scar tissue and old graft must be dissected from the promontory and undersurface of the malleus. The anterior middle ear is usually found to have normal mucosa. Putting in the silastic insert will usually solve the problem with aeration of the posterior ear and mastoid. These silastic inserts completely fill the bony middle ear which is actually larger than the eardrum. This prevents them from rolling up or being displaced. The insert continues into the mouth of the eustachian tube and there is a tongue which extends into the

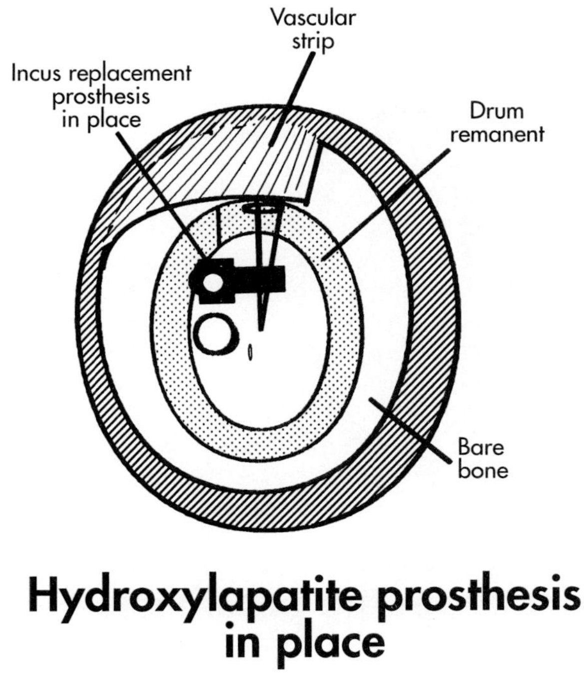

FIG 28-8
Hydroxylapatite incus replacement prosthesis in place over stapedial head and notch under malleus.

addis ad antrum. Sometimes the insert is too large for the middle ear and must be trimmed so that it will lie flat.

The next stage in the reconstruction of the middle ear is the ossicular reconstruction. This is usually performed with incus or incus-stapes replacement prostheses of hydroxylapatite.[6] However occasionally notched incudi sculptured from cadaver incudi are employed. When the stapes is intact and mobile, the incus replacement prosthesis is used. The hole through the prosthesis engages the head of the stapes and the notch in the body is placed beneath the manubrium of the malleus to stabilize the prosthesis in place (Fig. 28-8). The reconstruction begins with selection of the proper prosthesis. The short incus replacement in prosthesis is most frequently used, however, if the malleus appears high or anterior, an average or medium prosthesis may be selected. The prosthesis is placed in the middle ear with the cup near the stapes and the notch off the tip of the malleus. With a right angle pick in left hand, the malleus handle is elevated and, with gentle curve pick in the right hand, the prosthesis is slid up beneath the handle of the malleus to an upright and stable position. If the notch is loose on the malleus and the prosthesis tends to fall over, a larger prosthesis should be employed. It should fit snugly but not so tight as to depress the stapes. With a gentle curve pick the prosthesis is tested for motion at the stapes and there should be good motion of the footplate, stapedial tendon, or a round window reflex. One may pack the middle ear and prosthesis with gelfoam pledgets if desired.

When there is no stapes superstructure remaining but an intact and mobile footplate, an incus stapes replacement prosthesis is employed. Again the short prosthesis is the one most usually used, however, if the malleus appears high or further forward, then an average or medium prosthesis may be substituted. Prostheses come with a square shaft. It is advantageous to round this square shaft with a diamond burr to get a better fit on the footplate. These prostheses are put in place on the promontory with the shaft on the footplate and the notch off the tip of the malleus. The malleus handle is elevated with a right angle pick in left hand and with a gentle curve pick in the right hand. The prosthesis is slid up along the undersurface of the malleus to a stable and upright position. If the shaft does not remain on the footplate but tends to shift posteriorly, the shaft may be too long and it may be removed and shortened with a diamond burr. Again the prosthesis should fit snugly but no so tight as to crack or depress the footplate. Occasionally if the prosthesis seems slightly loose it can be reflected back toward the tip of the malleus and the natural spring of the malleus will hold it more securely in position. However, if it fits too loosely it should be removed and a longer prosthesis employed.

The next step is grafting of the perforation. If this is large a homograft tympanic membrane from which the homograft malleus had been removed is put in place over the patient's drum remnant. If the ossicular chain is intact and mobile it is important that the umbo of the homograft contact the tip of the patient's malleus to ensure good sound transmission. If reconstruction were done with the hydroxylapatite prosthesis, the drum contacts the prosthesis; but it is not so important that the umbo contact the malleus tip, as the hearing is by direct columellar pressure through the prosthesis (Fig. 28-9).

If the patient has an absent malleus or the manubrium has been badly eroded or involved in cholesteatoma, the head of the patient's malleus should be removed from the epitympanum. The reconstruction is then carried out with a homograft tympanic membrane with malleus. The head of the homograft malleus is then placed in the epitympanum where the patient's malleus head had been and it usually rests on the silastic tongue to prevent adhesions. Occasionally there is no room in the attic and the malleus head must be amputated in order for it to fit properly. Once the homograft tympanic membrane with malleus is in place, the posterior half of the eardrum is elevated anteriorly and the ossicular reconstruction carried out. The canal skin graft is now placed over the homograft tympanic membrane (Fig. 28-10). It has been trimmed and rotated 180° so that the thin portion which had been over the lower anterior bony wall now covers the anterior homograft tympanic membrane. It has been unfolded anteriorly inferiorly and touches but does not turn up anterior canal wall so as to create a sharp anterior angle. It does extend up the inferior and posterior canal walls usually about halfway to the previously made circumferential incision. Therefore, there is bare bone except along the vascular strip where the canal skin con-

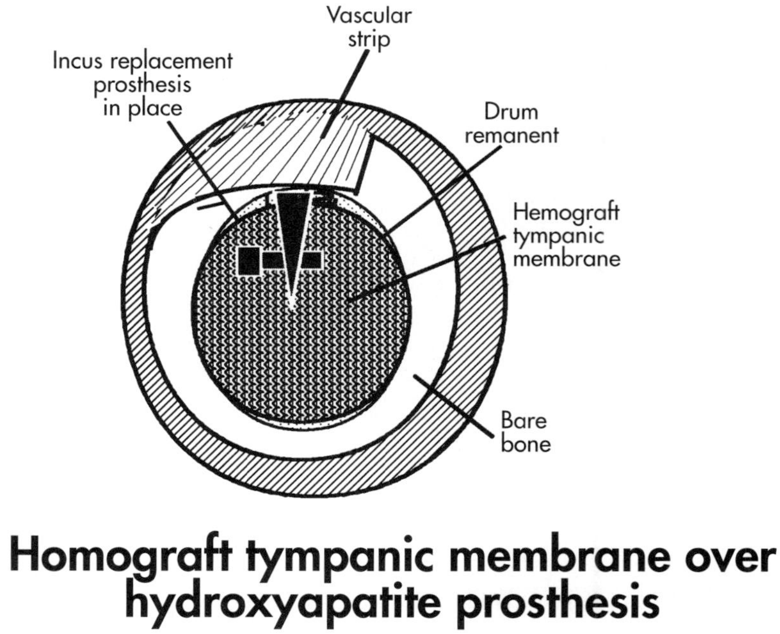

FIG 28-9
Homograft tympanic membrane in place over ossicular reconstruction.

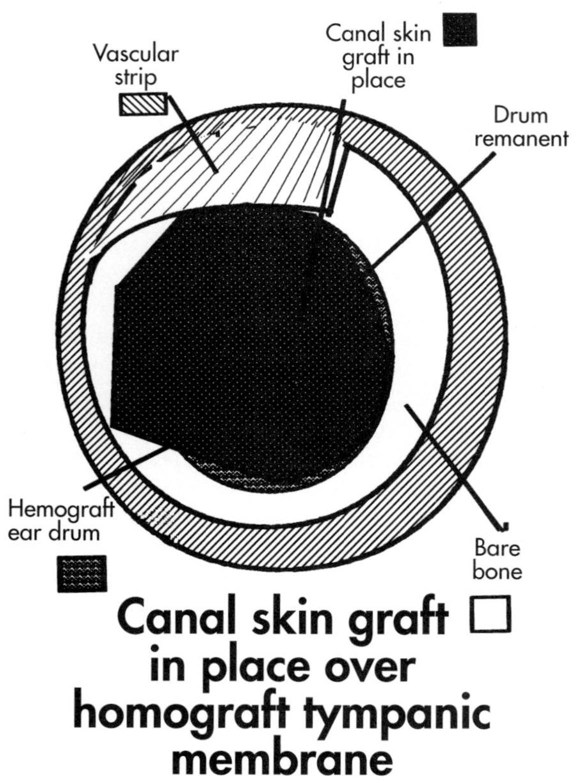

FIG 28-10
Canal skin graft in place. Note bare bone and contact to vascular strip.

tacts this structure. The entire anterior bony canal wall and half of the inferior wall is still bare bone. The graft is packed in place with formed drops of Gelfoam saturated in penicillin or Ansef antibiotic solution. Small pledgets are placed first in the anterior sulcus to secure the sharper angle and then larger ones to completely fill the ear canal. It is important to completely fill the ear canal and cover all the bare bone in order to keep it moist and ensure rapid epithelialization. A 3 to 4 cm strip of ¼ inch selvege edge gauze is placed in the external ear canal and a cotton ball is the final dressing. The gelfoam packing is removed in approximately 2 weeks along with the epithelial layer of the graft. It takes another 3 to 4 weeks for the skin to epithelialize over the bare bone. An audiogram is obtained at 6 weeks following the surgical procedure.

RECONSTRUCTION OF THE TOTAL EAR TO NORMAL ANATOMICAL CONFIGURATION AND FUNCTION

The final goal in reconstructive ear surgery is to have an ear which as nearly as possible resembles the normal ear in function and hearing.[7] Here we want to obtain a normal-appearing ear canal which cleans itself by epithelial migration so the patient can shower or swim. We hope to obtain an aerated mastoid with one large air cell rather than a honeycomb of air cells as nature planned. The mastoid can drain into the middle ear and down the eustachian tube and is also aerated in a reverse fashion. Another important goal is serviceable hearing.

To obtain these goals we preserve the bony ear canal or rebuild it with homograft knee cartilage. The tympanic membrane is reconstructed with fascia and homografts of the tympanic membrane, dura, or periosteum. The ossicular chain is reconstructed with the incus or incus-stapes prostheses of hydroxylapatite (see Fig. 28-3).

REVISION OF PREVIOUS CANAL WALL DOWN PROCEDURES

These are cases in which the patient has had previous surgery and has a remaining cavity. A patient usually seeks relief because of drainage from the ear, however in certain cases the loss of hearing is the principal concern. These ears are approached through a postauricular incision, subcutaneous flaps are elevated; if any fascia remains it is obtained for a graft. The periosteum over the temporal bone is then incised just posterior to the previously created mastoidectomy cavity. The lining of the cavity is then elevated toward the middle ear. Very often trapped cells filled with mucus will be encountered. Over these the skin of the cavity would be macerated and often granular. Also pockets of cholesteatoma may be encountered. These of course must be meticulously followed to their termination and removed. The dissection of the lining is carried forward over the facial ridge and horizontal canal to the middle ear. All normal mucosa in the mastoid as well as the middle ear is preserved. If the patient's malleus is present and not involved in disease it is preserved. After all disease and cholesteatoma have been removed the posterior canal wall will be constructed with homograft knee cartilage.

A template is made from the tin foil of the suture packet. It is cut with a scissors to approximate the defect in the canal wall. The template is then placed on the knee cartilage and it is cut around with a #15 Band Parker blade. The thin portion of the knee cartilage will overlap the facial ridge and horizontal canal and recreate a new posterior superior scutum. The interior and posterior edges of the cartilage are grooved with a sharp knife. The thin outer edge overlaps the bony facial ridge and the dural plate. The thicker inner layer goes to the mastoid tip and zygomatic portion of the temporal bone to support the wall in anatomical position. The finished cartilage wall should approximate the size and configuration of the normal bony canal wall.[8] When the knee cartilage wall has been modified to fit satisfactorily it is usually removed and placed in penicillin solution while the middle ear is reconstructed.

A Wehrs silastic mastoid insert manufactured by the Xomed Treace Company is then inserted from the mastoid cavity into the middle ear. A cutout is made for the stapes or oval window and the tensor tympani tendon if the patient's malleus is still present. If the patient has no malleus a homograft tympanic membrane with malleus is put in place. Again the head of the malleus is preserved if possible and placed in the previous epitympanum. It lays on the silastic sheeting. Ossicular reconstruction is next carried out with an incus or incus-stapes prosthesis as indicated. In the case of the homograft malleus the prosthesis actually helps to hold the malleus in anatomical position. The final reconstruction is carried out by replacing the knee cartilage wall. A facial graft or homograft dura extends up the posterior canal wall and over the cartilage. Skin flaps which had been elevated from the facial ridge and dural plate are reflected back over the fascia or dura. The new ear canal is packed with gelfoam pledgets saturated in antibiotic solution. The postauricular incision is closed in layers. A pressure-type mastoid dressing is applied.

EXAMPLE CASES

The following cases are used to present specific situations in which specialized techniques were used to perform tympanoplasty.

Case 1: Temporal bone fracture—ossicular discontinuity

History

This patient was a 15-year-old male injured in an automobile accident. He suffered abdominal and closed head injuries. No facial paralysis was reported. There were no complaints of vertigo and no history of cerebrospinal fluid otorrhea or rhinorrhea. The only otological complaint was hearing loss in the left ear.

Examination/audiometric evaluation

The external auditory canal on the right was normal, on the left there was a healing laceration of the canal but no evidence of CSF. At the time of the initial examination there was a hemotympanum present in the left middle ear. There was a disruption of the annulus in the posterior/superior quadrant of the left tympanic membrane. No abnormality was seen in the right ear. Rinne testing (512 Hz) was air conduction greater than bone in the right ear and bone conduction greater than air conduction in the left ear. The Weber lateralized to the left ear. Facial nerve function was normal.

Audiometric assessment demonstrated a mixed hearing loss with a discrimination score of 80% and a pure tone average (PTA) of 40 dB.

At follow-up in one month, the left hemotympanum had cleared. Both middle ear spaces were well aerated. The left incus was pressing laterally into the tympanic membrane.

Repeat audiometric assessment disclosed improvement in both the bone conduction and discrimination score. The conductive component persisted with a PTA of 35dB. Surgical exploration was planned.

Surgery

Working transcanal, a tympanomeatal flap was elevated. The flap was difficult to create due to the fracture line in the external auditory canal and at the bony annulus. The fibrous annulus was intact. The incus was avulsed from the malleus. The capitulum of the stapes was dislocated from the crura. The crura and footplate were intact and mobile. The annular ligament was intact. The incudostapedial joint was intact.

Repair was performed by removing the incus. The malleus was mobile. The ossicular chain was reconstructed with a Wehrs hydroxylapatite incus-stapes prosthesis. The shaft of the prosthesis was placed on the mobile footplate between the intact crura, and the notch was brought up beneath the malleus (Fig. 28-11).

A section of homograft dura was used to reinforce the posterior superior tympanic membrane at the site of the fracture. Postoperative course was uneventful.

Postoperative audiometric assessment shows closure of the air bone gap with a PTA of 16 dB and a discrimination score of 96%.

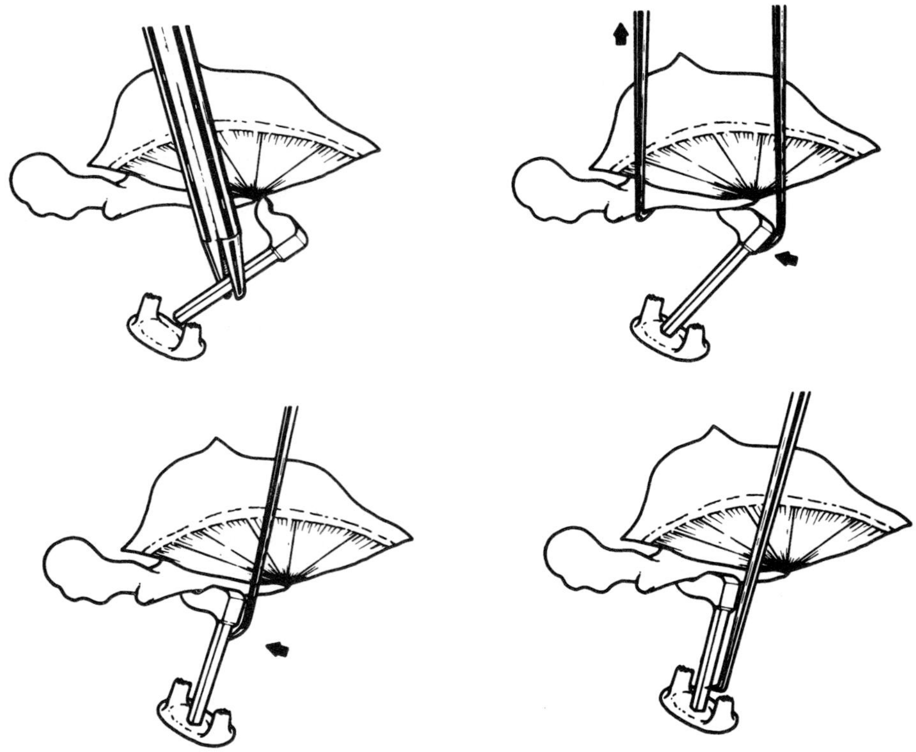

FIG 28-11
Placement of hydroxylapatite incus-stapes prosthesis from mobile footplate to malleus. (From Brochure on surgical technique, Wehrs hydroxylapatite incus-stapes repalcement prosthesis in middle ear surgery. Memphis, 1988, Richards Medical Co. With permission.)

Comment

The improvement in the bone conduction and discrimination score was felt to be due to a mild cochlear concussion which cleared between the time of the initial and follow-up examination. Temporal bone fracture can produce a variety of ossicular injuries. The disrupted incudomalleolar connection and the separation of the capitulum from the stapes necessitated a connection from the malleus to the mobile footplate. The surviving crura helped to support the shaft of the incus-stapes prosthesis.

Case 2: Persistent conductive hearing loss after stapedectomy

History

This patient was a 32-year-old female who had previously undergone a left stapedectomy elsewhere. There was no improvement in hearing postoperatively. The patient had experienced no infection or discharge from the ear. She had tolerated the stapedectomy well. There was no history of vertigo.

Examination/audiometric evaluation

Both tympanic membranes were intact and mobile. The middle ear was well aerated bilaterally. In the left ear, Rinne testing was bone conduction greater than air conduction.

Audiometric assessment disclosed a left conductive hearing loss, a PTA of 50 dB, and a discrimination score of 100%. Options of surgery or amplification were presented to the patient. The patient elected to proceed with revision stapedectomy.

Surgery

Working transcanal, a tympanomeatal flap was elevated. The malleus was found to be firmly fixed in the attic. The previously placed wire stapes prosthesis was removed from the incus, using a laser to free the prosthesis at the oval window. The incus was disarticulated from the fixed malleus and removed. Using the laser, the previously placed tissue graft was removed from the oval window. The oval window was sealed with a pressed fat graft harvested from the ear lobe. The malleus head was amputated at the neck, superior to the attachment of the tensor tympani tendon. Preserving the tendon helps to stabilize the malleus remnant. The ossicular chain was reconstructed with a Wehrs hydroxylapatite incus-stapes prosthesis. The shaft of the prosthesis was placed onto the fat graft over the oval window. The notch was brought up beneath the malleus remnant. A slightly longer prosthesis than usual was needed because the malleus remnant was no longer attached to the malleus head.

Postoperative audiometric assessment showed closure of the air bone gap with a PTA of 18 dB and a discrimination score of 100%.

Comment

Persistent conductive hearing loss after stapedectomy can result from many causes. In the illustrated case, a fixed malleus produced the conductive loss. Removal of the incus is necessary to complete the ossicular reconstruction. Removing the previous tissue seal at the oval window allows inspection of the oval window to ensure that there is no bony obstruction blocking conduction. Preserving the tensor tympani tendon not only stabilizes the malleus but helps to support the prosthesis.

Case 3: Soft tissue stenosis of the external auditory canal

History

This patient was a 35-year-old female with hearing loss in the left ear since childhood. The patient felt that the hearing had been steadily worsening during the past 5 years. There was no history of pain or discharge. A myringotomy with tube insertion had been performed on both ears as a child. Otherwise there was no history of ear surgery.

Examination/auditory assessment

On examination, the right ear canal, tympanic membrane, and middle ear were normal. The left ear canal was patent at the meatus but ended blindly in a soft tissue stenosis. No tympanic membrane could be seen. No ossicular landmarks were visible.

High-resolution computer tomography (CT) demonstrated a well-aerated middle ear with medial soft tissue stenosis of the external auditory canal.

Audiometric assessment disclosed a conductive loss in the left ear with a PTA of 40 dB and a discrimination score of 100%.

Surgery

A transcanal approach was used. Continuous facial monitoring was utilized in the event of abnormal middle ear anatomy. Using canal skin incisions, the stenotic tissue was dissected off of the tympanic membrane remnant. The posterior/central portion of the tympanic membrane was absent. The ossicular chain was malformed with only a fibrous band connecting the long process of the incus to the stapes capitulum. The malformed incus was removed and the malleus was mobile.

The ossicular chain was reconstructed using a Wehrs hydroxylapatite incus replacement prosthesis from the capitulum to the mobile malleus. The tympanic membrane was reconstructed with a sterile homograft tympanic membrane.

The stenotic ear canal skin was trimmed but was insufficient to cover the ear canal and tympanic membrane. The probable need for a split thickness skin graft was recognized preoperatively and the patient had been informed and prepared for the skin graft. A 3 × 4 cm split-thickness skin graft 10/1000 of an inch (0.25 mm) was harvested from the inner aspect of the left arm. This skin was used along with the canal skin to cover the ear canal and homograft tympanic membrane. The postoperative course was uneventful.

The postoperative audiometric assessment demonstrated marked improvement in the conductive loss with a PTA of 17 dB and a discrimination score of 96%.

Case 4: Tympanic membrane perforation with multiple ossicular fixation

History

This patient was a 6-year-old female with a history of a right tympanic membrane perforation. The patient had undergone a tympanoplasty which lateralized and then broke down producing an anterior perforation. There had been intermittent drainage from the right ear.

Examination/audiometric assessment

On examination, there was a lateralized tympanic membrane graft with an anterior perforation. The middle ear was dry with no evidence of cholesteatoma. Rinne testing was bone conduction greater than air conduction in the right ear. The left external canal, tympanic membrane, and middle ear were normal.

The audiometric assessment disclosed a large conductive component in the right with a PTA of 58 dB and a discrimination score of 96%.

Surgery

A canal skin tympanoplasty approach was used to repair the tympanic membrane. The lateralized fascia graft was removed. The patient had a total perforation of the tympanic membrane with only a thin rim of fibrous annulus remaining. On examination of the ossicular chain it appeared that both the incus and stapes were fixed. A staged procedure was planned. The tympanic membrane was reconstructed with a sterile homograft tympanic membrane which was covered with canal skin. The graft healed well, and, as would be expected, there was no improvement in hearing on audiometric assessment.

A series of counseling sessions were held with the parents during the postoperative period to discuss options of amplification or stapedectomy. To assist with evaluation, high-resolution computer tomography of the temporal bone was performed. There was no evidence of abnormal inner ear development, in particular a patent cochlear aqueduct. After considering all options and risks, the parents requested the second-stage surgery on the right ear.

At the second surgery, a tympanomeatal flap was elevated, raising the homograft tympanic membrane and fibrous annulus together. The middle ear was well aerated and free of infection. On palpation, the incus and stapes appeared to be fixed. The incudostapedial joint was separated, allowing independent inspection of the stapes and incus. Both were firmly fixed. A fat graft was harvested from the ear lobe and pressed to form a thin graft for the oval window. The incus was disarticulated from the malleus and removed. The malleus was mobile. The stapes superstructure was removed using a carbon dioxide laser and the central portion of the footplate was removed. The oval window was sealed with the thin fat graft. The ossicular chain was re-

inforced with temporalis fascia and homograft dura. The dura gave added support to the tympanic membrane. The ossicular chain was reconstructed with a Wehrs hydroxylapatite incus replacement prosthesis. The capitulum of the stapes was placed into the cup of the prosthesis and the notch was secured beneath the malleus. To ventilate the ear a Silverstein permanent aeration prosthesis was placed into the mastoid antrum.

The postoperative audiogram showed improvement of the conductive component of the hearing loss with a PTA of 30 dB and a discrimination score of 92%. Long-term follow-up has shown no recurrence of serous otitis media.

Comments

A combination of problems such as collapsed tympanic membrane, chronic serous effusion, and ossicular dislocation was treated in a single-stage surgery. The presence of a normal, mobile stapes facilitated a single-stage operation. A fixed stapes along with previous serous effusion may have prompted a staged repair with the first stage to restore a healthy, well-ventilated middle ear. The reconstruction of the attic was necessary to help stabilize the tympanic membrane and help prevent further collapse.

REFERENCES

1. Baron SH: Modified radical mastoidectomy. *Arch Otolaryngol* 49:280, 1949.
2. Lempert J: Improvement of hearing in cases of otosclerosis, new one stage surgical technique. *Arch Otolaryngol* 28:42, 1938.
3. Sheehy JL, Crabtree JA: Tympanoplasty: staging the operation. *Laryngoscope* 83:1594-1621, 1973.
4. Sheehy JL, Patterson ME: Intact canal wall tympanoplasty: a review of eight years experience. *Laryngoscope* 77:1502-42, 1967.
5. Wehrs RE: Homograft tympanic membrane after 12 years. *Ann Otol Rhin Laryngol* 91:533-537, 1982.
6. Wehrs RE: Ossicular reconstruction in revision ear surgery. *Oper Tech Otolaryngol* 3:51-54, 1992.
7. Wehrs RE: Reconstructive mastoidectomy with homograft knee cartilage. *Laryngoscope* 82:1177-1188, 1972.
8. Wehrs RE: Results of reconstructive mastoidectomy with homograft knee cartilage. *Laryngoscope* 88:1912, 1978.
9. Wehrs RE: Silicone sheeting in tympanoplasty. *Laryngoscope* 89:497-499, 1979.
10. Wullstein H: The restoration of function of the middle ear in chronic otitis media. *Ann Otol Rhin Laryngol* 65:1020, 1956.

Part Six

Pediatric

29

Pediatric Obstructive Sleep Apnea

Bruce R. Maddern, M.D., F.A.C.S., F.A.A.P.

Pediatric obstructive sleep apnea or obstructive sleep apnea syndrome (OSAS) is part of a clinical spectrum of obstructive sleep disorders in children. The significance of sleep-related respiratory obstruction in children is not completely understood. Many questions remain: "Is snoring alone clinically significant?" How much snoring or snoring with apnea is necessary to produce clinical features? What are the necessary criteria for the diagnosis of obstructive sleep apnea? When is therapy indicated, and what is appropriate therapy?

As the indications for adenotonsillectomy have evolved over the past 20 to 30 years, it is evident that airway obstruction is becoming more frequent an indication for adenotonsillectomy.[12,17] It has been argued also that the incidence of upper airway obstruction caused by adenotonsillar hypertrophy has increased.[9] This chapter will provide an overview of pediatric obstructive sleep apnea syndrome with specific information for the practicing otolaryngologist. Key differences between adults and children will be highlighted. Included are specific discussions of etiology, pathophysiology, and treatment options.

PATHOGENESIS

Obstructive sleep apnea is manifested by repeated episodes of decreased breathing of upper airway origin occurring during sleep. In obstructive sleep apnea, there is a decreased airway due to anatomic, neuromuscular, or other factors. To maintain adequate airflow through a diminished lumen, the patient must increase respiratory effort. This attempt to increase airflow requires increasing airway pressure. Because of the Bernoulli effect, increased intraluminal negative pressure, and a compliant airway structure, collapse of the airway and cessation of airflow results. Increasing negative airway pressures paradoxically causes further airway collapse and increased resistance to airflow.

Three physical parameters relate directly to the ease of airway collapse. They are compliance or elasticity of the soft tissues, spatial relationships, and anatomic narrowing of the available lumen. There are sleep-associated physiologic changes which lead to a decrease in muscle tone and support of the airway.

Peripheral and central neuromuscular regulation of respiratory function also contributes to the development of obstructive sleep disorders. There is a normal sleep cycle–related decrease in the activity of respiratory muscles such as the genioglossus and diaphragm. Obstructive apneas occur more frequently during these periods of decreased electromotor activity.[19]

During sleep, a repeating sequence of events occurs in which negative inspiratory pressure overcomes the ability of the airway to maintain patency, resulting in cessation of airflow. The cessation of airflow causes obvious physiologic changes, including acidosis, hypercapnia, and hypoxemia. Once sufficient changes in the partial pressure of oxygen (Po_2), the partial pressure of carbon dioxide (Pco_2), and the pH occur, central and peripheral chemoreceptors and baroreceptors are stimulated to cause arousal and awakening from sleep. This repeating cycle of sleep awakenings and restless sleep may occur many times in a night. This causes a repeating cycle of disordered sleep, along with chronic hypoxemia, acidosis, and hypercapnia. Certain clinical features and symptoms are directly related to these chronic pathophysiologic changes (Fig. 29-1).[2]

Long-standing obstructive sleep apnea may impair growth and development. Several studies have reported that poor performance in school and poor weight and height gains can be dramatically altered by therapy.[4,14,16] It is believed that, after the increased energy expenditure associated with breathing through a partially obstructed airway is removed, these children resume more normal growth and development.

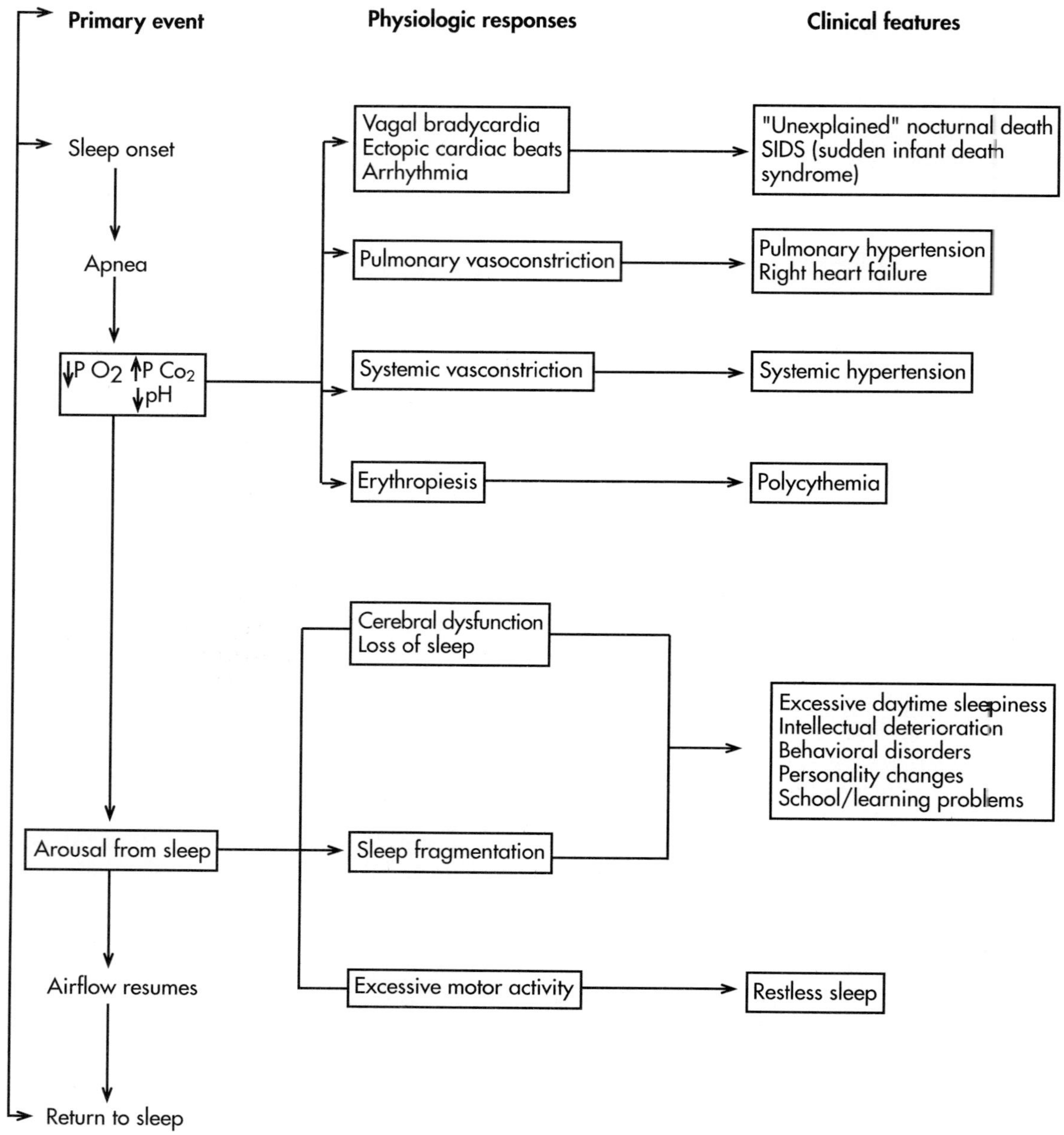

FIG 29-1

Clinical features and physiologic changes seen in obstructive sleep apnea. (Modified from Bradley TD, Phillipson EA: Pathogenesis of sleep apnea. *Med. Clin. North Am* 69:1169-1185, 1985.)

ETIOLOGY

Adenotonsillar hypertrophy is the most common cause of respiratory obstruction of upper airway origin during sleep in children. However, numerous other anatomic, congenital, neuromuscular, and miscellaneous causes are well documented (box on p 339). Any anatomic obstruction of the upper airway may potentially contribute to the development of obstructive sleep apnea. The site of obstruction and airway collapse is different for each patient. Other causes of airway obstruction, such as laryngotracheal abnormalities, may produce stridor and apnea, but they are not considered in this discussion.

Richardson et al,[22] using videofluoroscopy, demonstrated four mechanisms in the upper airway that contribute to obstruction during sleep: (1) collapse of the hypopharynx, (2) descent of the tonsil, (3) posterior tongue placement, and (4) occlusion of the velopharyngeal sphincter. These probably do not occur in isolation but may all contribute depending on each patient's anatomic and neuromuscular characteristics.

Pathologic Disorders of Upper Airway Obstruction Associated with Obstructive Sleep Apnea and Related Disorders

I. Anatomic

- A. Nasal
  1. Congenital nasal mass (glioma, encephalocoele)
  2. Anterior nares (fetal warfarin syndrome)
  3. Nasal septal hematoma
  4. Nasal polyposis
  5. Trauma—septal deviation
- B. Nasopharyngeal
  1. Choanal atresia/stenosis
  2. Choanal polyp
  3. CHARGE association
  4. Nasopharyngeal cyst
  5. Adenoid hypertrophy
  6. Cleft palate repair
  7. Velopharyngeal repair/stenosis
- C. Oropharyngeal
  1. Tonsillar hypertrophy
  2. Macroglossia
     - a. Down's syndrome
     - b. Acromegaly
     - c. Beckwith-Wiedemann syndrome
  3. Retrognathia, micrognathia
     - a. Pierre Robin sequence, Stickler's, Cornelia de Lange syndromes
     - b. Achondroplasia
- D. Laryngotracheal
  1. Laryngotracheomalacia
     - a. Subglottic stenosis
     - b. Vocal cord paresis
     - c. Vascular ring/sling
     - d. Glottic web
  2. Vallecular cyst
- E. Craniofacial syndromes
  1. Crouzon's
  2. Apert's
  3. Treacher Collins
  4. Down's

II. Neuromuscular

- A. Cerebral palsy
- B. Vocal cord paralysis
- C. Down's syndrome
- D. Myotrophic dystrophy
- E. Arnold-Chiari malformation
  1. Type I with Klippel-Feil syndrome
  2. Type II with spina bifida
- F. Syringomyelobulbia

III. Miscellaneous

- A. Congenital myxedema
- B. Prader-Willi syndrome (mental retardation, short stature, obesity, hypogonadic hypogonadism)
- C. Obesity
  1. Endogenous
  2. Exogenous
- D. Sickle cell disease
- E. Storage diseases (Hurler, Hunter, etc.)
- F. Chromosome disorders (trisomy 13, 18, 21)
- G. Fetal alcohol syndrome
- H. Allergic rhinitis

Anatomic

Nasal
Congenital nasal mass (glioma, encephalocoele)
Anterior nares (fetal warfarin syndrome)
Nasal septal hematoma
Nasal polyposis
Trauma—septal deviation
Nasopharyngeal
Choanal atresia/stenosis
Choanal polyp
CHARGE association
Nasopharyngeal cyst
Adenoid hypertrophy
Cleft palate repair
Velopharyngeal repair/stenosis
Oropharyngeal
Tonsillar hypertrophy
Macroglossia
Down's syndrome
Acromegaly
Beckwith-Wiedemann Syndrome
Retrognathia, micrognathia
Pierre Robin sequence, Stickler's, Cornelia de Lange syndromes
Achondroplasia
Laryngotracheal
Laryngotracheomalacia
Subglottic stenosis
Vocal cord paresis
Vascular ring/sling
Glottic web
Vallecular cyst
Craniofacial syndromes
Crouzon's
Apert's
Treacher Collins
Down's

Neuromuscular

Cerebral palsy
Vocal cord paralysis
Down's syndrome
Myotrophic dystrophy
Arnold-Chiari malformation
Type I with Klippel-Feil syndrome
Type II with spina bifida
Syringomyelobulbia

Miscellaneous

Congenital myxedema
Prader-Willi syndrome (mental retardation, short stature, obesity, hypogonadic hypogonadism)
Obesity
Endogenous
Exogenous
Sickle cell disease
Storage diseases (Hurler, Hunter, etc.)
Chromosome disorders (trisomy 13, 18, 21)
Fetal alcohol syndrome
Allergic rhinitis

Patients with craniofacial anomalies such as Crouzon's, Apert's, Treacher Collins, Pierre Robin's, and Cornelia de Lange syndromes will often have abnormalities of the upper airway. These patients will frequently have a history of snoring and disordered breathing during sleep. A broad range of phenotypic expression of the classic features for each syndrome is common. When evaluating these patients, the otolaryngologist should be suspicious of obstructive sleep apnea syndrome.

Down's syndrome patients are prone to obstructive sleep disorders. This is due to characteristic anatomic craniofacial features and, importantly, to neuromuscular control problems. These children have a small oro and nasopharynx along with a relative macroglossia. Poor gross motor and fine motor control of the velopharyngeal mechanism and tongue are common in these patients.[7]

Neuromuscular difficulties that contribute to airway obstruction are rare, however, decreased muscle tone regardless of etiology may potentially cause narrowing of the upper airway.

Iatrogenic causes of obstructive sleep disturbance are well documented. Repair of cleft palate and velopharyngeal flap surgery can obstruct an already compromised airway. Snoring and nasal obstruction are common postsurgical findings in these patients and warrant evaluation.

OBSTRUCTIVE SLEEP DISORDERS IN NEONATES/ YOUNG INFANTS

Neonates and young infants represent a special and increasing group of patients with obstructive sleep disorders. This is due in part to differences in respiratory physiologic responses exhibited by neonates.

Roloff and Aldrich[23] described several mechanisms in premature infants that are responsible. Central neuropathways which control ventilation are not completely developed and may lead to hypoventilation, central apnea, and periodic breathing. Physiologic responses to hypoxemia and hypercapnia are not fully developed due to chemoreceptor immaturity. Other neuromuscular control mechanisms, such as laryngeal abduction and diaphragmatic coordination, are incompletely developed.

Assessment techniques and treatment options in this group are different from those used in older children. History in neonates is largely observational, which makes reliability and interpretation of events difficult. Signs and symptoms in young infants with obstructive sleep disorders may include respiratory distress, stridor, cyanosis, feeding difficulties, pectus excavatum, and failure to thrive. These events are different and perhaps more severe than those seen in older children.

In young infants, an association between gastroesophageal reflux (GER) and apnea has been described. GER can cause airway occlusion by reflux of acid material directly into the glottis or secondary to central apnea by vagally mediated reflexes which inhibit respiration.[24] Considerable debate exists about causal relationships of GER and apnea. GER is common in all infants. Central nervous system disorders may also lead to GER and obstructive sleep apnea by separate mechanisms.

An association has been suggested between GER, apparent life-threatening event (ALTE), and obstructive apnea. Obstructive sleep apnea has been implicated in sudden infant death syndrome (SIDS). Autopsy studies have shown signs of upper airway obstruction in some patients.[1] Guilleminault et al[10] have documented five "near miss" SIDS cases, in which obstructive sleep apnea syndrome was subsequently identified.

DIAGNOSIS

Patients with snoring and obstructive sleep apnea may be classified according to the severity of symptoms and associated clinical features (box below). This suggested scheme takes into account signs, symptoms, and clinical

Classification of Obstructive Sleep Disorders and Related Disorders Based on Clinical Features and Symptoms

Primary snoring (alone)

Excessive oropharyngeal noise associated with sleep more prominent with inspiration
Respirations orderly and regular

Snoring with

Respiratory pattern changes
Irregular breathing cycle
Irregular breathing with short pauses (up to 5 seconds)

Snoring with

Breathing pauses up to 6 seconds
Periodic breathing (3 or more pauses of 3 seconds in a 20-second period)
Hypopnea (limitation of airflow)

Obstructive Sleep Apnea Syndrome

Obstructive apnea (cessation of airflow > 6 seconds)
- Airway obstruction
- Apnea, 20 to 30 episodes of obstructive type per evening (obstructive sleep apnea syndrome [OSAS])

Snoring with behavioral changes
- Hyperactivity, excessive daytime somnolence, aggression, depression
- Deteriorating school performance due to poor attentiveness, behavior changes, or hypersomnolence

Obstructive apnea with major clinical features
- Poor growth and development
- Heart failure
- Cor pulmonale
- Hypertension (other primary causes of hypertension ruled out)
- Hypoxemia with sleep

features to help aid the clinician in determining the severity of obstructive sleep disorders. Treatment options can then be outlined.

In the evaluation of obstructive sleep disorders, the assistance of pediatric subspecialists from pulmonary medicine, neonatology, radiology, and neurology is often valuable. A team approach in management, especially in complex cases, is recommended.

HISTORY

Several symptoms and complaints, which can be either daytime or nocturnal, occur with regularity in obstructive sleep apnea syndrome (box below). Snoring, mostly inspiratory in character, is a cardinal finding. The history often reveals a chronic and gradually worsening condition, which suggests upper airway obstruction during sleep. Parents will describe frank apnea with gasping for air following an episode of obstruction in their child.

Other complaints include frequent awakenings, restless sleep, diaphoresis, and night terrors. Diaphoresis is a result of the hypercapnia and secondary vasodilatation that occurs with obstructive sleep apnea.

In obtaining a nighttime history from parents about their child, it is important to determine chronicity, association with upper respiratory infections, character of the respiratory noise, and any other associations one would elicit from a complete history. Because of sleep dynamics, observations of sleep behavior should be taken at intervals throughout the sleep cycle, not merely from the first five minutes of active sleep, which is what parents frequently report.

Symptoms and Features Often Found in Obstructive Sleep Apnea Syndrome

Nocturnal	Daytime
Apnea	Mouth breathing
Snoring	Hypersomnolence (excessive daytime sleepiness)
Pauses with breathing at night	Poor school performance
Frequent awakenings from sleep, restless sleep	Abnormal daytime behavior
Nightmares	Aggression
Nocturnal enuresis	Hyperactivity
Nocturnal diaphoresis	Discipline problems
Cyanosis*	Short attention span
Near SIDS*	Morning headache
	Weight problem (failure to thrive or obesity)
	Frequent upper respiratory tract infections
	Chronic rhinorrhea
	Dysphagia
	School and learning problems
	Feeding difficulties*

*Neonatal/Infant.

Daytime complaints frequently include mouth breathing and behavior problems. Excessive daytime sleepiness or hypersomnolence may be interpreted in a young child as the normal need for a nap and makes this difficult to assess. In an older child this may indicate a poor nocturnal sleep pattern. Daytime hypersomnolence is a rare finding in children with OSAS.

Mouthbreathing is a frequent finding and often associated with a hyponasal speech quality. Both of these are due to the nasopharyngeal obstruction seen with adenoid hypertrophy.

The validity of clinical history in determining the diagnosis of obstructive sleep apnea syndrome has received extensive discussion. Brouilette[5] has suggested that thorough history and physical examination are adequate for the diagnosis to be made. Leach[13] and Loughlin[15] have fostered the idea that history alone is not sufficient because of the confusing nature of this disorder. They conclude that parents, as well as physicians, overestimate the severity of the disease and, therefore, other ancillary testing is required to confirm the diagnosis.

PHYSICAL EXAMINATION

Physical examination should include a complete otolaryngologic, head, and neck evaluation, with particular attention to potential sites of airway obstruction. Although pickwickian complex is one of the most well-known presentations of obstructive sleep apnea, it is not the most common clinical picture seen in children. Children with obstructive sleep apnea are more often slender and frequently lag in growth and development.[10] Observation should be made of any anatomic or functional limitations, as well as any anomalies suggestive of orofacial or craniofacial syndromes.

Oropharyngeal examination should assess pharyngeal dimensions, anatomy, and function. Neuromuscular assessment of velopharyngeal functions should be carefully assessed. Sphincter closure, appearance of Passavant's ridge, lateral and anteroposterior velar mobility, and gross and fine motor control of the tongue are all important determinations. Assessment should be made of pharyngeal dimensions, noting tonsil size and lingual anatomy.

Intranasal examination should include assessment of the nasal airway with particular attention to the nasal septum, nasal mucosa, and adenoids. A cervical and thoracic examination is necessary to rule out any processes that may contribute to or aggravate potential upper airway obstruction. A neuromuscular examination, including cranial nerves V, IX, X, XI, and XIII, is warranted to assess motor control and coordination of swallowing, phonation, and respiration.

When evaluating craniofacial dysmorphic patients, the otolaryngologist should be suspicious of airway problems and obstructive sleep disturbance. Specific abnormalities which should be considered in craniofacial syndromes are micrognathia, maxillary hypoplasia, choanal atresia/stenosis, cranial base anomalies, macroglossia, and pharyngeal hypotonia.

ANCILLARY STUDIES

Radiography

Soft tissue, lateral x-ray films are frequently ordered when one is suspicious of adenoid hypertrophy. However, these are two-dimensional airway and their usefulness has not been determined. Lateral and anteroposterior views of the head are included with a routine sinus radiography series. This may be a more cost effective choice in many of these patients and will provide more information. Assessment of overall craniofacial anatomy, airway dimensions, and adenotonsillar hypertrophy can easily be made. Sinus series radiography may be an important adjunct in evaluations, along with a complete history and examination.

Cephalometric study

Cephalometric studies are an accurate recording of bony landmarks; they provide precise dimensions but do not record soft tissue abnormalities, which are frequently the cause of airway difficulty. These studies are not part of the usual workup for OSAS but may be indicated in patients with craniofacial syndromes or suspected facial dysmorphia. This study is expensive and not all centers have the necessary equipment readily available.

Computed tomography

Computed tomographic (CT) scanning is an accurate and expensive method of recording bony and soft tissue landmarks but provides little information about functional problems. These studies may be indicated in complex cases.

Sleep tape audio-video recording

A frequently used, inexpensive study is the nighttime recording of sleep using an audiocassette tape recorder. This provides information regarding sleep sounds: snoring, pauses, apnea, and restlessness. Its disadvantages are background noise, necessity for parental compliance, and difficulty in distinguishing true apnea from depressed respiration or hypopnea. With new developments in video technology many families now have VHS or 8 mm recording for home use. A nighttime recording can be very helpful in visualizing sleep behavior and correlating sleep sounds.

Polysomnography

Polysomnography, or sleep study, is the gold standard for the diagnosis of sleep apnea and associated sleep disorders.

It consists of multiple physiologic and neurophysiologic simultaneous recordings of different variables, which include at least: (1) electroencephalogram (EEG), minimum two or three electrode placements, (2) electrocardiogram (ECG), (3) assessment of nasal and oral airflow by thermistors, (4) oxygen saturation monitoring, and (5) chest strain gauges or esophageal manometry to assess thoracic respiratory movements.

In addition, often the sleep study will include an electrooculogram to assess REM or NREM sleep stages, an electromyogram of the chin to assess muscle tone and activity, a recording of end-tidal P_{CO_2} by nasal sampling, and a videotape recording of sleep.

The sleep study can determine frequency, duration, type, and severity of apneic episodes. By monitoring oxygen saturation and P_{CO_2}, an assessment of physiologic changes associated with apnea can be made and the type of apnea, either central or obstructive (peripheral), can be determined. Apnea is defined as cessation of airflow for at least 10 seconds in adults and 6 seconds in children. Apnea has been observed in some patients with OSAS to last 70 seconds or more.[7]

Central apnea implies central nervous system dysfunction. The sleep study will demonstrate lack of respiratory movements, along with apneic episodes. This is an important distinction from obstructive apnea, in which respiratory movements continue despite the cessation of airflow, implying upper airway obstruction. The mixed pattern, which begins as central and then progresses to obstructive apnea, is frequently seen in OSAS and young children.

The disadvantages of polysomnography are that it is expensive and cumbersome to perform. It usually requires a one-night hospitalization and is better tolerated by adults than by children. The sleep study is not practical in the routine evaluation of the snoring child.

The sleep study is indicated when apnea is strongly suspected but history and physical examination findings are confusing. Often the neurologically impaired child is being assessed and there is a need to distinguish between central and obstructive apnea, as well as to determine the severity of OSAS before recommending appropriate therapy. Polysomnography is also indicated if one is considering tracheostomy in complex cases. Sleep study has many other uses in the evaluation of behavioral, psychiatric, and neurologic disorders.

Endoscopy

Flexible fiberoptic nasopharyngoscopy may provide useful anatomic and functional information. It can be performed in a clinical setting with minor coaxing and topical anesthesia. Newer, thinner fiberscopes make this especially useful in young children and neonates. Excellent visualization of static and dynamic components of the upper airway are possible and can greatly aid in the evaluation of all age patients for OSAS.

Rigid endoscopy is indicated in the patient with craniofacial abnormalities to determine nasopharyngeal, oropharyngeal, or supraglottic abnormalities and to rule out laryngotracheal problems. It may also be helpful in removing or correcting certain lesions that impinge on the upper airway.

THERAPY

Many different therapeutic options are available for the treatment of children with obstructive sleep disorders. A thorough understanding of each option and the risks versus

Therapeutic Options for Upper Airway Obstruction in Obstructive Sleep Apnea Syndrome and Related Disorders in Children

Removal of obstruction

Adenoidectomy
Tonsillectomy
Adenotonsillectomy
Uvulopalatopharyngoplasty (UPPP)
Middle partial glossectomy
Nasal surgery (septoplasty, polypectomy, etc.)

Bypass of obstruction

Nasopharyngeal airway
Tracheostomy

Positional manipulation of airway

Craniofacial surgery (midfacial, advancement)
Orthognathic surgery (e.g., maxillary or mandibular osteotomies)
Oral prosthesis (e.g., SNOAR)
Hyoidplasty

Medical (nonsurgical)

Medications—medroxyprogesterone, steroids, protriptyline, acetazolamide
Diet or weight reduction
Thyroid replacement (for congenital hypothyroidism)
Chemotherapy (Hodgkin's disease)
Nasal continuous positive airway pressure (CPAP)

benefits for each is necessary in order to treat these complicated patients.

Management decisions in obstructive sleep disorders can be surgical, medical, or airway position therapies. The clinician needs to take into account the exact etiology and severity of the problem in order to make an appropriate therapeutic choice. Anatomic craniofacial dysmorphism and patient compliance issues are important considerations.

Therapeutic choices vary according to the age of the patient. Young infants and neonates with obstructive sleep disorders may be amenable only to certain treatment options because of size and growth considerations. Conversely, teenagers may be effectively treated using the same paradigm as adults.

Surgery remains the mainstay of treatment in children. Newer nonsurgical choices have become more available but remain more useful in adults (box above).

Medical (nonsurgical) therapies

Nonsurgical options have included: (1) medications such as medroxyprogesterone, steroids, protriptyline, theophylline, and acetazolamide, (2) dietary measures or weight reduction, (3) nasal continuous positive airway pressure (CPAP), and (4) oral prosthetics (e.g., Snoar). These measures are useful in a specific few patients but remain largely ineffective in the treatment of the majority of children with sleep-related airway obstruction.[10,20]

Nasal continuous positive airway pressure is being used in children with increasing frequency. Advances in equipment and mask design have allowed young children and previously noncompliant patients greater ease in usage. Similar to adults, morbidly obese patients, those undergoing weight reduction, and surgical failures are the most successful users.[3,11] Long-term usage and patient compliance remain problems, but this technology is gaining wider acceptance in the treatment of children with obstructive sleep disorders.

Surgical therapy

Preoperative, operative, and postoperative management of patients with obstructive sleep apnea requires careful evaluation, an interdisciplinary team approach, and postoperative monitoring. These patients are frequently complex and need to be treated as such.

Preoperative evaluation should include chest radiograph, electrocardiogram, and anesthesia consultation in a patient with a confirmed diagnosis of OSAS. If cardiomegaly, right ventricular hypertrophy, or ECG abnormality are noted, cor pulmonale should be suspected and cardiology evaluation is warranted. Cerebral palsy, spastic diplegia, and static encephalopathy patients need preoperative assessment from a neurologist.

Surgery in complex craniofacial dysmorphic patients should be discussed well in advance with anesthesia colleagues. Decisions about airway management, anesthetic techniques, and postanesthesia care procedures need to be agreed to collaboratively prior to the procedure. This preoperative protocol ensures as safe a procedure as possible and encourages a team approach in management.

Surgical interventions are directed toward relieving the site of obstruction or bypassing the obstruction. Since adenotonsillar hypertrophy is by far the most common cause of obstructive sleep apnea, adenotonsillectomy is the most frequently performed procedure. This is very successful in relieving symptoms and correcting pathophysiologic changes due to OSAS.

Children with a compromised airway from anatomic or neuromuscular causes, such as Down's syndrome children, may be more susceptible to airway obstruction from even moderately enlarged adenoids or tonsils. Adenotonsillectomy may be definitive therapy in these borderline cases.[6] In addition, adenotonsillectomy may be appropriate initial management for complex or borderline cases before committing the patient and family to more long-term and invasive options such as tracheotomy.

Tracheotomy is an alternative to definitive correction of the obstructive lesion of the airway. This procedure bypasses the obstruction and can be a temporary solution used in combination with other future surgical reconstructive procedures. In complex craniofacial patients, this option may be especially helpful. Tracheotomy as a temporary solution is also used in conjunction with weight reduction therapy in morbidly obese patients.

In some patients, tracheotomy is a permanent treatment modality. This is appropriate in patients in whom other procedures have failed, multiply medically complex patients, and patients who refuse other treatment options.[10]

Uvulopalatopharyngoplasty (UPPP) has been popularized, especially for adults with OSAS.[8] This technique or a modification of it may be indicated in the child with redundant or poorly functioning pharyngeal soft tissues. UPPP has been used increasingly in children with severe mental handicaps, such as static encephalopathy and neuromuscular oromotor dysfunction. These patients have poor palatal control and redundant nonfunctional soft tissues. Simple removal of adenoids and tonsils in these patients may fail to relieve the obstruction and UPPP should be considered.[25] Conservative removal of soft tissue is warranted as postoperative velopharyngeal insufficiency may be especially detrimental in these patients.

Postoperative care of the patient with documented obstructive sleep apnea requires monitoring.[18] These children are at risk for postoperative edema, bleeding, and airway obstruction. Monitoring should include continuous oxygen saturation as well as ECG and respiratory rate.

It is recommended that adenotonsillectomy be performed as an inpatient or overnight monitored hospital stay.[21] Pulse oximetry and/or a cardiorespiratory monitoring aid in the immediate identification of respiratory compromise. Nursing staff must be aware that OSAS patients are not routine postoperative adenotonsillectomy patients. Humidification, oxygen support, and judicious use of narcotics are advocated.

SUGGESTED READING

Brouillette R, Hanson D, David R, et al: A diagnostic approach to suspected obstructive sleep apnea in children. *J Pediatr* 105:10-14, 1984. (The authors describe a clinically useful approach to the evaluation of snoring patients. A table of the signs and symptoms in OSAS based on an exhaustive statistical analysis is provided and could be quite useful to the clinician.)

Guilleminault C, Korobkin R, Winkle R: A review of 50 children with obstructive sleep apnea syndrome. *Lung* 159:275-287, 1981.

Koopman C, Moran W. Sleep apnea. *Oto Clinic NA* 23:571-575, 1990 (A complete reference on sleep disorders with well-written chapters on pathophysiology, polysomnography, and medical and surgical therapy is provided. The chapter on sleep apnea in children is an excellent review and is highly recommended.)

REFERENCES

1. Ariagno RL, Guilleminault C: Apnea during sleep in the pediatric patient. *Clin Chest Med* 6:679-690, 1985.
2. Bradley TD, Phillipson EA: Pathogenesis and pathophysiology of obstructive sleep apnea syndrome. *Med Clin North Am* 69:1169-1185, 1985.
3. Brooks LJ, Crooks RL, Sleeper GP: Compliance with nasal CPAP by children with obstructive sleep apnea. *Am Rev Resp Dis* 145:A556 1992 (abst).
4. Brouillette RT, Fernbach SK, Hunt CE: Obstructive sleep apnea in infants and children. *J Pediatr* 100:31-40, 1982.
5. Brouillette RT, Hanson D, David R, et al: A diagnostic approach to suspected obstructive apnea in children. *J Pediatr* 105:10-14, 1984.
6. Donaldson JD, Redmond WM: Surgical management of obstructive sleep apnea in children with Down Syndrome. *J Otolaryngol* 17:398-403, 1988.
7. Frank Y, Kravath RE, Pollack CP, et al: Obstructive sleep apnea and its therapy: clinical and polysomnographic manifestations. *Pediatrics* 71:737-742, 1983.
8. Fujita S, Conway W, Zorick F, et al: Surgical correction of anatomic abnormalities in OSAS: uvulopalatopharyngoplasty. *Otolaryngol Head Neck Surg* 89:923-934, 1981.
9. Grundfast KM, Wittich DJ: Adenotonsillar hypertrophy and upper airway obstruction in evolutionary perspective. *Laryngoscope* 92:650-656, 1982.
10. Guilleminault C, Korobkin R, Winkle R: A review of 50 children with obstructive sleep apnea syndrome. *Lung* 159:275, 1981.
11. Guilleminault C, Nino-Murcia G, Heldt G, et al: Alternative treatment to tracheostomy in obstructive sleep apnea syndrome: nasal continous positive airway pressure in young children. *Pediatrics* 78:797-802, 1986.
12. Kravath RE, Pollack CP, Borowiecki B: Hypoventilation during sleep in children who have lymphoid airway obstruction treated by nasopharyngeal tube and T and A. *Pediatrics* 59:865-871, 1977.
13. Leach J, Olson J, Hermann J, et al: Polysomnographic and clinical findings in children with obstructive sleep apnea. *Arch Otolaryngol* 118:741-744, 1992.
14. Lind MG, Lundell BPW: Tonsillar hyperplasia in children: a cause of obstructive sleep apneas, CO_2 retention, and retarded growth. *Arch Otolaryngol* 108:650-654, 1982.
15. Loughlin GM, Brouillette RT, Rosen C: Indications and standards for sleep studies in children. *Am Rev Respir Dis* 1994. (In preparation.)
16. Maddern BR, Reed HT, Ohene-Frempong K, Beckerman RC: Obstructive sleep apnea syndrome in sickle cell disease. *Ann Otol Rhinol Laryngol* 98:174-178, 1989.
17. Mangat D, Orr WC, Smith RO: Sleep apnea, hypersomnolence and upper airway obstruction secondary to adenotonsillar enlargement. *Arch Otolaryngol* 103:383-386, 1977.
18. McColley SA, April MM, Carroll JL, et al: Respiratory compromise after adenotonsillectomy in children with obstructive sleep apnea. *Arch Otolaryngol* 118:940-943, 1992.
19. Onal E, Lopata M, O'Connor T: Pathogenesis of Apneas in Hypersomnia-Sleep Apnea Syndrome. *Am Rev Respir Dis* 125:167-174, 1982.
20. Potsic WP, Pasquariello PS, Baranak CC, et al: Relief of upper airway obstruction by adenotonsillectomy. *Otolaryngol Head Neck Surg* 94:476-480, 1987.
21. Price SD, Hawkins DB, Kahlstrom EJ: Tonsil and adenoid surgery for airway obstruction: Perioperative respiratory morbidity. *ENT Journal* 72:526-531, 1993.
22. Richardson MA, Seid AB, Cotton RT, et al: Evaluation of tonsils and adenoids in sleep apnea syndrome. *Laryngoscope* 90:1106-1110, 1980.
23. Roloff DW, Aldrich MS: Sleep disorders and airway obstruction in newborns and infants. *Otolaryngol Clin North Am* 23:639-650, 1990.
24. See CS, Newman LJ, Berezin S, et al: Gastroesophageal reflux-induced hypoxemia in infants with apparent life-threatening event(s). *Am J Dis Child* 143:951-954, 1989.
25. Seid AB, Martin PJ, Pransky SM, Kearns DB: Surgical therapy of obstructive sleep apnea in children with severe mental insufficiency. *Laryngoscope* 100:507-510, 1990.

30

Head and Neck Masses in Children

Charles M. Myer III, M.D. and J. Paul Willging, M.D.

Head and neck masses in children may be classified into several categories, including congenital lesions, inflammatory diseases, noninflammatory benign lesions, benign neoplasms, and malignant neoplasms. This wide variety of pathologic processes makes it essential for a physician to develop an organized approach to such abnormalities when beginning a diagnostic evaluation. Rather than focus upon the nuances of therapy for many individual conditions, this manuscript offers an organized approach to guide the clinician in the evaluation of such abnormalities.

When evaluating a patient with a mass in the neck, it is essential to obtain as complete a history as possible. While congenital abnormalities may be present at birth or shortly thereafter, they may not present until later in life. Specifically, isolated branchial cysts often enlarge very slowly and may not become evident until the second or third decade of life. A thymic cyst or laryngocele should be differentiated from a branchial cyst. Computed tomography (CT) may confirm the origin of these anomalies which present more often just lateral to the midline in comparison to a branchial cyst. Surgical excision is the treatment of choice. Inflammatory diseases, in contrast, generally arise very rapidly and usually are associated with overlying erythema, edema, tenderness, and fever. Malignant and benign neoplasms are uncommon in the neonatal period and may not be accompanied by additional regional or systemic findings. Malignant neoplasms may be differentiated on occasion from benign lesions by their rapid growth, more indurated feel, and their frequent attachment to skin or surrounding tissues. If a mass undergoes enlargement associated with eating, inflammatory disease of the salivary glands should be suspected. Though there may be some generalized swelling at all times with an infected salivary gland, an increase in size is noted usually at the specific time of feeding. Other historic factors which should be obtained include any relationship to a preceding upper respiratory infection, rash, exposure to tuberculosis, travel, animal contact, or dental work.[4,7]

In children, there are several circumstances which deserve special consideration when taking a history. In newborn children, one should consider the possibility of neonatal sialadenitis when swelling develops over one of the salivary glands. Often seen in premature children, dehydration may be a factor, and broad-spectrum antimicrobial therapy along with adequate hydration is essential. This condition should be differentiated from facial cellulitis or a buccal space infection, both of which respond rapidly to antimicrobial therapy alone. Viral sialadenitis, especially mumps, is almost exclusively a disease of childhood. However, this should be differentiated from an acute parotitis of bacterial origin which may be recurrent in this age group. Whenever a child is diagnosed with an acute parotitis, the parents should be counseled that the disease process may be recurrent and chronic, often not ending until the child reaches adolescence. In addition, parents should be warned that the opposite gland may become involved also since at least one study has identified similar architectural changes in the clinically unaffected parotid gland as in the affected parotid gland. In adolescence, nutritional concerns may be associated with enlargement of the salivary glands. Malnutrition, including bulimia, obesity, and pica, all may be seen with enlargement of the salivary glands. Regardless of age group, salivary gland enlargement may follow administration of a general anesthetic and may result from either positive pressure ventilation through a mask or, when a mouth gag is used, compression of the submandibular ducts. Last, wind instrument players may find salivary gland enlargement due to pneumoparotitis, a condition in which air is forced into the salivary gland ductal system with resultant gland enlargement.[3]

As mentioned previously, the history of an animal scratch may be important in arriving at a diagnosis. When

Normal Cervical Masses
Mandible
Mastoid tip
Greater cornu of hyoid bone and thyroid cartilage
Lateral process of C-2
Lateral process of C-6
Styloid process

(From Myer III CM, Cotton RT: Lump in the neck. In Myer III CM, Cotton RT, eds: A practical approach to pediatric otolaryngology, Chicago, 1988, Year Book Medical Publishers.)

there has been a cat scratch, one must consider both cat scratch disease as well as toxoplasmosis. Toxoplasmosis must be considered also following raw meat ingestion. When posterior cervical adenopathy is noted, one should inquire about the possibility of a scalp infection.[5,8]

Once adequate historic information has been obtained, a complete physical examination of the patient should be performed with special emphasis given to the head and neck region. Many head and neck masses have their origin within the lymphatics of this region. Three functional units are usually considered: Waldeyer's ring, the cervical lymph nodes, and the transitional lymph nodes between these two areas. Waldeyer's ring is composed of the palatine tonsils, lingual tonsils, adenoids, and the adjacent submucosal lymphatic tissue. Both a superficial group of lymph nodes and deep group of lymph nodes compose the cervical chain. The superficial group drains the skin and muscles of the anterior part of the neck and passes through the superficial cervical fascia into the deep cervical nodes. The deep group is composed of medial and lateral compartments and lies medial to the superficial layer of the deep cervical fascia. Medially, there are prelaryngeal, prethyroid, pretracheal, and paratracheal lymph nodes. Laterally, nodes are found along the internal jugular vein, associated with the spinal accessory nerve, and within the supraclavicular fossa. Posterior triangle lymph nodes are part of this group and are located posterior to the sternocleidomastoid muscle. Transitional lymph nodes are found between the head and neck and include the submental nodes, submandibular nodes, parotid nodes, retroauricular nodes, occipital nodes, sublingual nodes, and retropharyngeal lymph nodes. They are located both superficial and deep to the superficial cervical fascia. Knowledge of the cervical lymphatics and the other normal cervical structures (box above) is crucial when formulating a differential diagnosis based on anatomical findings.[4]

Once a mass has been identified, specific characteristics should be noted in a checklist fashion, including size, surrounding edema, erythema, tenderness, and fluctuance. Making a drawing for the medical record may allow information to be communicated in an accurate manner. It should be remembered that the finding of lymph nodes in children

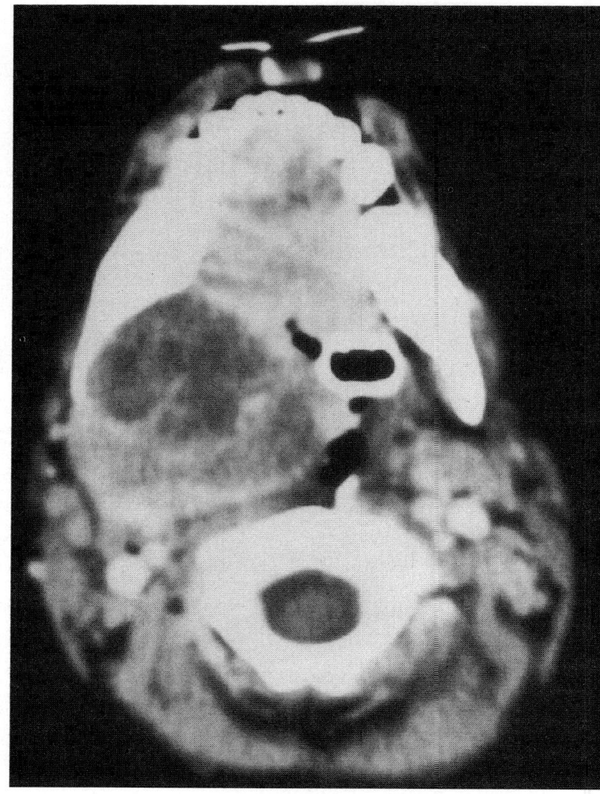

FIG 30-1
The right parapharyngeal mass as demonstrated on this CT was diagnosed as rhabdomyosarcoma following an incisional biopsy. The patient, a two year old female, presented with a cervical mass and obstructive sleep symptoms.

up to 2 cm in diameter is not uncommon, especially following an upper respiratory infection. The presence of multiple small lymph nodes bilaterally with such a history is generally of little concern. However, should there be a solitary lymph node or group of lymph nodes which is extremely hard, matted together, fixed to the skin, or demonstrating progressive enlargement without a history of associated respiratory infection, the concern regarding neoplasm becomes greater. Besides the cervical lymph nodes, one also must evaluate for the presence of generalized lymphadenopathy, hepatosplenomegaly, and fever, since cervical lymphadenopathy may be a reflection of a systemic condition. Head and neck regions which must be evaluated thoroughly as a possible primary site for infection include the ear, pharynx, tonsils, dental structures, scalp, and skin.[4,8]

Depending on patient age, one must consider the possibility of certain pathologic processes more strongly. Specifically, rhabdomyosarcoma is seen to peak in the head and neck region between 4 and 6 years of age as well as between 14 and 16 years of age (Figs. 30-1 and 30-2). Neuroblastoma is seen most commonly within the first several years of life. In contrast, Hodgkin's disease is seen more often in adolescents and adults, while non-Hodgkin's lymphoma is identified most commonly in children under

A

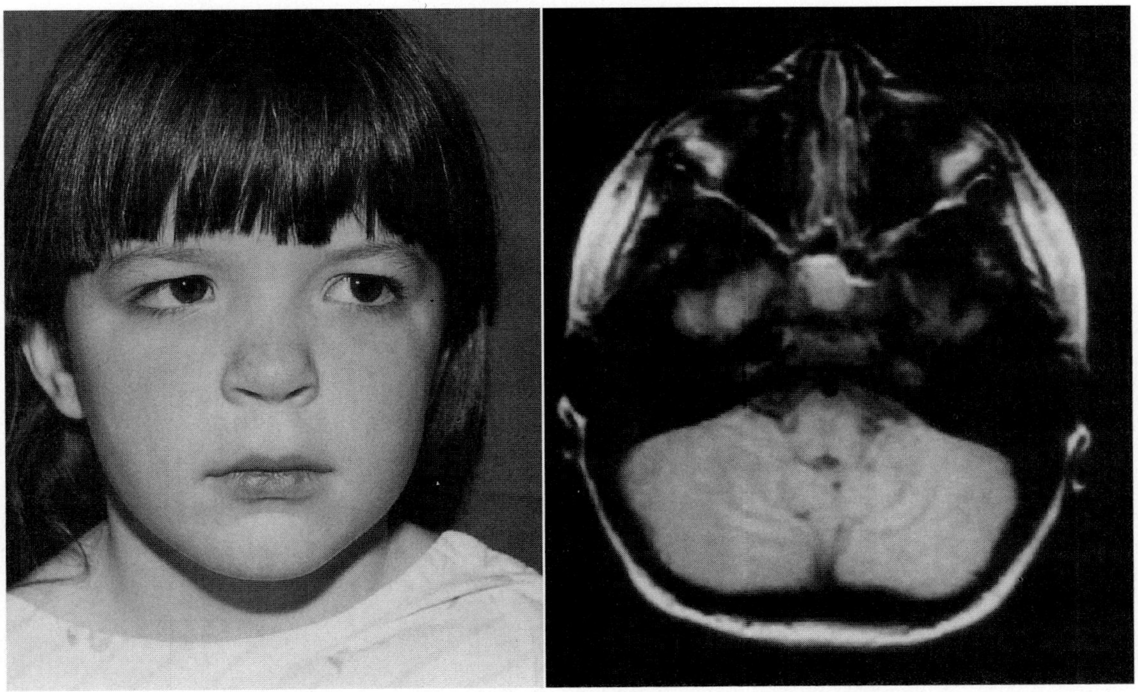

B

FIG 30-2
(A) A six year old female presented with a right lateral rectus palsy secondary to a mass within the right sphenoid sinus as demonstrated on the MRI **(B)**. Biopsy subsequently confirmed the diagnosis of rhabdomyosarcoma.

twelve years of age. In children under the age of two, Langerhans' cell histiocytosis is the most commonly diagnosed malignancy. It is usually the acute disseminated form, also known as Letterer-Siwe disease, and is almost universally fatal. The chronic disseminated form is seen in a slightly older age group (Hand-Schüller-Christian disease) and has a better prognosis with chemotherapy (Fig. 30-3). In adolescent patients, the chronic unifocal form (eosinophilic granuloma) is seen more often and therapy usually involves limited surgical resection or curettage and, in some patients, radiotherapy.[1,6]

An unusual systemic condition in which cervical lymphadenopathy is often a component is Kawasaki disease, also known as mucocutaneous lymph node syndrome. Other findings in this condition are a fever for five days or more, conjunctivitis, induration and erythema of the palms of the hands and soles of the feet with late desquamation, rash, and mucous membrane changes including red, cracked, and peeling lips or strawberry tongue. Late findings may involve coronary artery aneurysm formation and coronary thrombosis with myocardial infarction. Generalized lymphadenopathy is not part of this condition, though cervical lymphadenopathy is generally part of the disease complex. Antimicrobial therapy will not affect the cervical adenitis, but the adenopathy will respond to treatment of the overall disease process which usually involves intravenous infusion of gamma globulin in addition to daily aspirin.[5]

Laboratory and radiographic studies complement the history and physical examination of a child with a head and neck mass. As a baseline, a complete blood count with a differential should be obtained and may be indicative of inflammatory disease or, possibly, a blood dyscrasia. Depending on the other systemic findings, serum chemical profiles, a urinalysis, and an HIV test can be obtained. Before any biopsy procedure is performed, a chest x-ray should be performed. This is especially important when considering lymphoma, since mediastinal involvement can be very common with lymphomas in the pediatric population. Should there be metastatic disease to the mediastinum, it is imperative to have knowledge of this prior to administration of a general anesthetic, since loss of the airway can occur with a potentially disastrous outcome (Fig. 30-4). Serologic testing may be useful in the identification of viral infections (Epstein-Barr virus or cytomegalovirus), toxoplasmosis, tularemia, histoplasmosis, or syphilis. Though still relatively new, a serologic test for *Rochalimaea henselae* may be useful for the identification of this organism, which has been found recently to be the causative agent for cat scratch disease.[4,5]

Though cervical lymphadenitis in the United States due to *Mycobacterium tuberculosis* accounts for only about 10% of culture-proven mycobacterial infections, application of a Mantoux tuberculin test (5TU) should be a routine measure in children with persistent adenopathy. As noted in Table 30-1, there are characteristic differences of atypical and tuberculous mycobacterial adenitis which should assist the

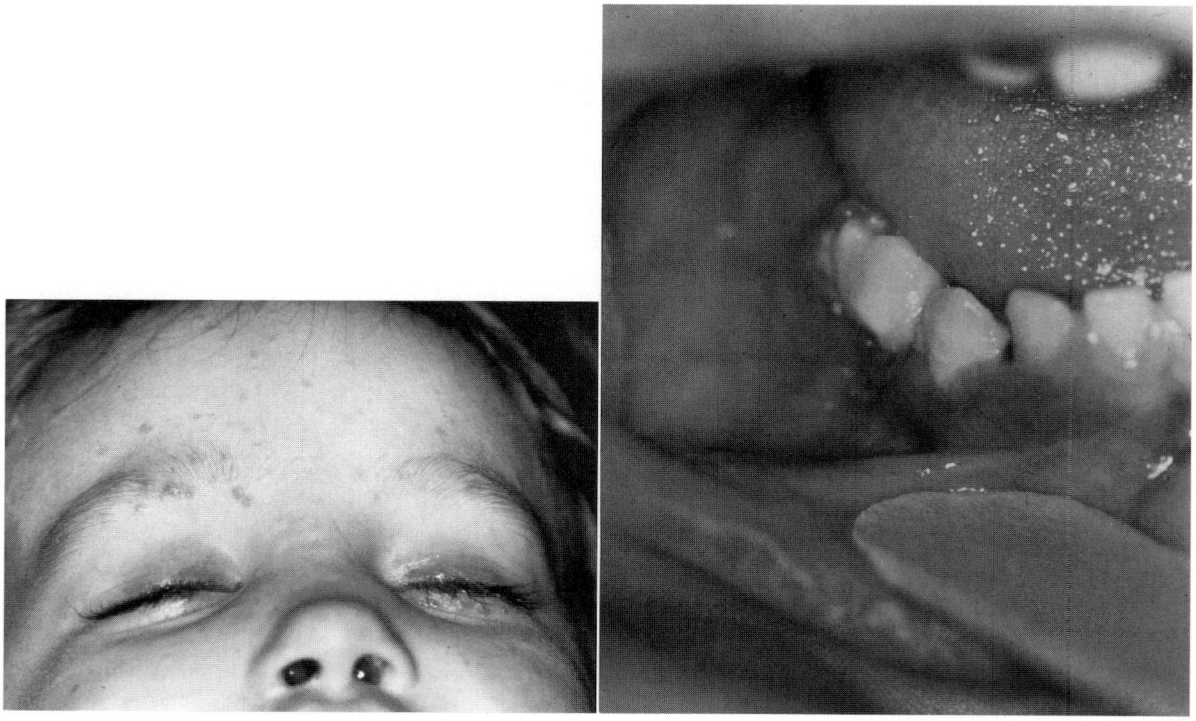

A

B

FIG 30-3
Child with Langerhans' Cell Histiocytosis who demonstrated papular rash typical of this process **(A)** and bleeding gums with loose teeth often seen with this condition **(B)**.

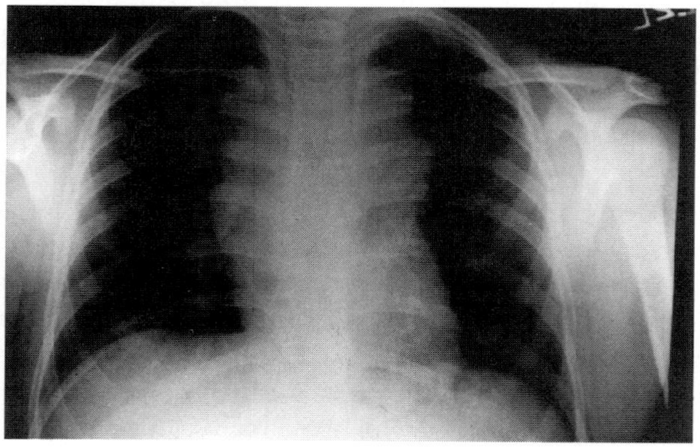

FIG 30-4
Anteroposterior chest radiograph demonstrating mediastinal widening in a child with biopsy-proven Hodgkin's disease.

TABLE 30-1
Comparative analysis of atypical and tuberculous mycobacterial adenitis

Factor	Atypical	Tuberculous
Age	Usually less than 5 years	Usually over 12 years
Site	Submandibular and jugulodigastric, frequently unilateral	Posterior triangle and supraclavicular
PPD* reactivity	Less than 10 mm	Greater than 10 mm
Chest x-ray	Frequently normal	Commonly abnormal
History of TB contact	No	Yes
Therapy	Surgical excision	Chemotherapy

From Myer CM III, Cotton RT: Lump in the neck. In Myer CM III, Cotton RT, editors: *A Practical Approach to Pediatric Otolaryngology*, Chicago, 1988, Year Book Medical Publishers, Inc., pp. 212-219. Used with permission.
*PPD = purified protein derivative.

clinician in differentiating these conditions. Consultation with a pediatric infectious disease expert may be appropriate when designing a chemotherapy course for the treatment of patients with *M. tuberculosis* and, on occasion, those with refractory atypical mycobacterial cervical adenitis following surgical therapy.[4]

Paranasal sinus radiographs may be beneficial when children present with loose teeth, epistaxis, or nasal obstruction associated with a cervical mass. Though the radiographic findings of sinusitis on plain films have a high rate of false positives and false negatives, the films may be helpful in demonstrating neoplasms or osteomyelitis. A lateral view of the nasopharynx allows evaluation of the retropharyngeal space as well as the cervical spine. Some of the conditions which may be identified on these films include juvenile nasal angiofibroma (bowing of the posterior wall

A

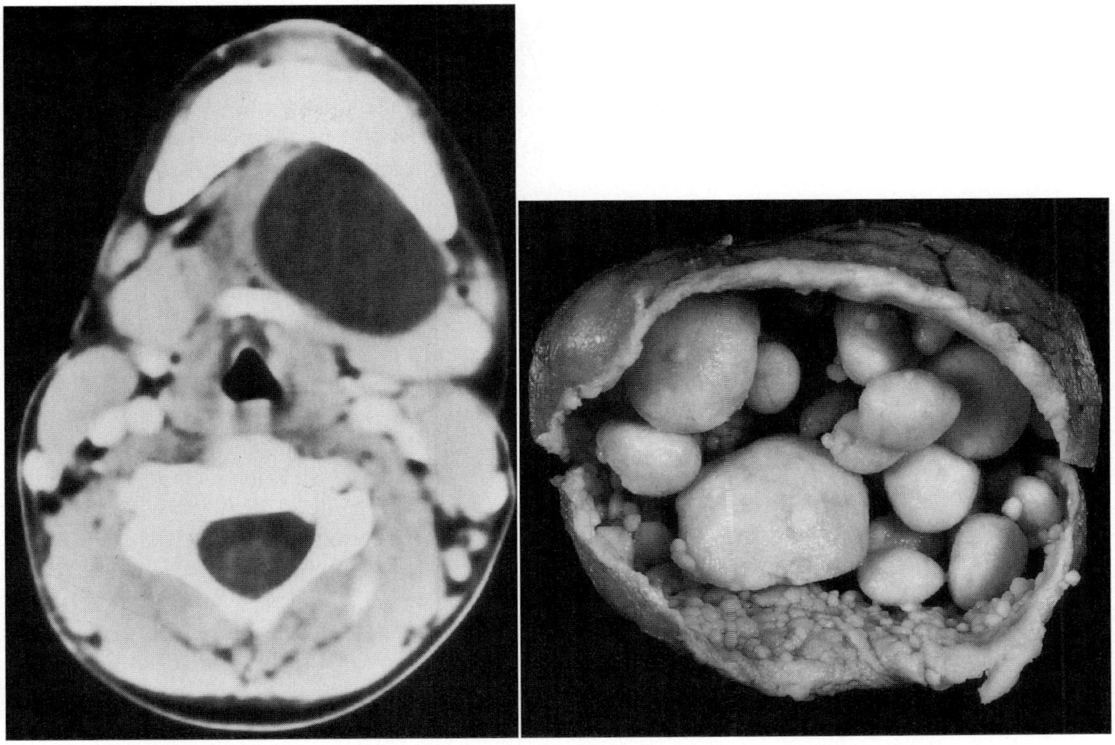

B

FIG 30-5
(A) Large submandibular mass of homogenous density on CT which proved to be a dermoid **(B)**.

of the maxillary sinus), Langerhans cell histiocytosis (solitary lytic lesion of bone, floating teeth), fibrous dysplasia (ground glass appearance of maxillary bone), and nasopharyngeal malignancy (bone destruction). When the enlarged cervical nodes are located in the supraclavicular region, one must consider the possibility of metastatic disease from a primary process located below the clavicles. Appropriate diagnostic tests may include any of the following: a barium esophagram, a barium enema, an intravenous pyelogram. When the mass is located anywhere from the base of tongue to the thyroid gland and is suspicious for a thyroglossal duct cyst, one may consider a thyroid scan or thyroid function tests, or both.[4]

Advanced imaging techniques such as CT and magnetic resonance imaging (MRI) may be appropriate in the assessment of head and neck masses. Consultation with a pediatric radiologist may allow one to obtain the most cost-effective study for the suspected pathology (Fig. 30-5). Though plain sialography is relatively limited in the assessment of salivary masses, a CT sialogram may be extremely beneficial in differentiating a mass lesion from an inflammatory condition.[4]

When prenatal ultrasonography identifies an anterior neck mass, consideration of teratomas, teratoid cysts, and lymphangiomas is most appropriate. Plans should be formulated to have a high-risk delivery team present at birth, including a pediatric surgeon, an anesthesiologist, an otolaryngologist, as well as a neonatologist. If the airway is obstructed, intubation or bronchoscopy should be performed without delay. If this is not possible, one might consider extracorporeal membrane oxygenation (ECMO) or a tracheotomy. Definitive therapy may proceed after the patient is stabilized and appropriate imaging studies obtained.

Fine needle aspiration (FNA) is an accepted diagnostic technique in the management of mass lesions of the head and neck in adults. The technique has not been used widely with pediatric patients, and its reliability is dependent on the experience and expertise of the cytopathologist performing the investigation. As noted in box on p 350, there are specific circumstances in which a needle aspirate may allow therapy to be directed more specifically. Whenever a neoplasm is suspected, failure to obtain a positive diagnosis with a needle aspirate should not deter one from performing an open biopsy procedure. If one is relatively certain that a mass is of inflammatory etiology, the needle aspirate may substantiate one's feelings and allow a more conservative approach to be taken. If, however, the aspirate is suspicious of a neoplasm or the mass has clinical activity more indicative of neoplasm, a biopsy should not be delayed.[2,4]

Malignancy should be considered more strongly and consideration of biopsy entertained at an earlier stage when there is persistent fever, weight loss, fixation of the mass to the skin or subcutaneous tissues, or supraclavicular adenopathy. Otherwise, biopsy may be most appropriate when there is progressive enlargement of the mass over a 2-week interval despite antimicrobial therapy, no change in size over a 6-week period, or failure to regress to what is considered normal size over a 3-month period, understanding that shotty adenopathy may be normal in all children.[1,7]

If a head and neck mass is felt to be of inflammatory etiology, antimicrobial therapy should be started empirically. Without identification of a primary source of infection, broad-spectrum therapy should be initiated and it should be effective against *Staphylococcus aureus* and group A beta-hemolytic streptococci. In very young children with periorbital inflammation, consideration should be given to *Hemophilus influenzae*. Anaerobic organisms must be considered when an odontogenic source is suspected. Several factors will influence the length of therapy with antimicrobial agents. As long as the mass responds to treatment, persistence with this method of therapy is appropriate. However, if the mass does not respond over some arbitrary time period (several weeks), alteration of therapy may be considered, especially if culture material has been obtained.[4]

If, however, no response is seen with prolonged antimicrobial therapy and the radiographic and laboratory studies

Cervical Lymphadenitis—Indications for Needle Aspiration

- Fever and toxicity requiring hospitalization
- Child less than 6 weeks of age
- Failure to improve with conservative management
- History suggestive of unusual pathogen
- Underlying altered immune status

From Myer CM III, Cotton RT: Lump in the neck. In Myer CM III, Cotton RT, editors: *A Practical Approach to Pediatric Otolaryngology,* Chicago, 1988, Year Book Medical Publishers, Inc., pp 212-219. Used with permission.

(From Myer III CM, Cotton RT: Lump in the Neck. In Myer III CM, Cotton RT, eds: *A practical approach to pediatric otolaryngology,* Chicago, 1988, Year Book Medical Publishers.)

A

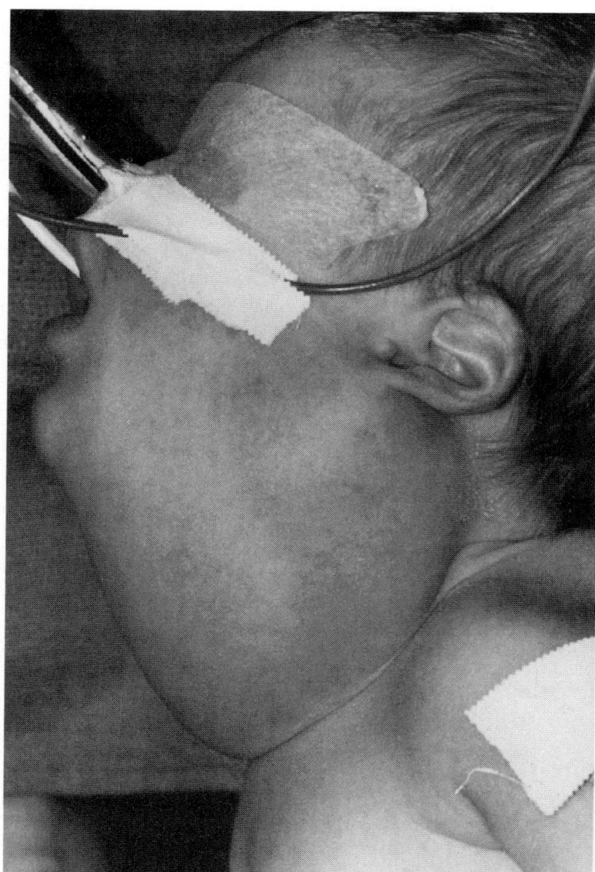

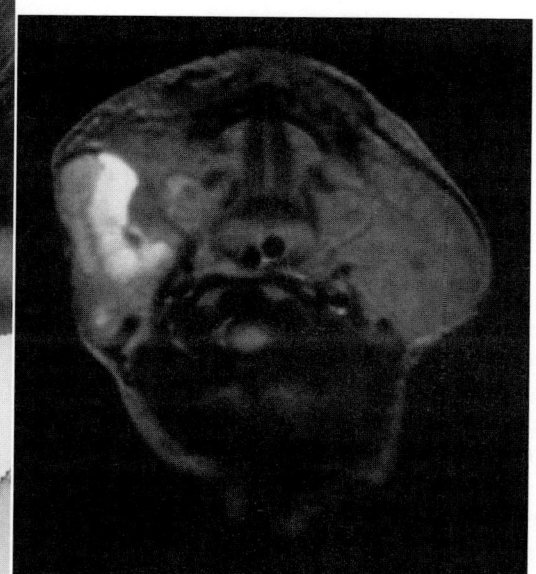

B

FIG 30-6
Newborn with large, compressible anterior neck mass clinically consistent with a vasoformative lesion **(A)** whose MRI scan **(B)** demonstrated components characteristic of both hemangioma and lymphangioma.

fail to establish a diagnosis, or both, an excisional biopsy should be performed to obtain material for culture and susceptibility studies and histologic examination. If a mass is extremely large and excisional biopsy is felt to be inappropriate, incisional biopsy is performed. Avoidance of excessive electrocautery around the specimen will minimize artifact. Similarly, cup forceps biopsy is to be avoided if possible to eliminate crush artifact. The specimen should be sent fresh or in isotonic saline to the pathologist who has been notified previously of the specimen and the clinical concerns of the surgeon. Appropriate cultures should be obtained if there is any consideration of an inflammatory etiology of the mass.[4,7]

One must remember that the minimum biopsy procedure for a parotid gland lesion is a lateral lobe parotidectomy and that complete submandibular gland excision is appropriate for a pathologic process in this region.[3] With some malignancies of the head and neck, including lymphomas, surgical therapy generally involves a biopsy procedure only. In rhabdomyosarcoma, unless the entire mass can be resected without compromising the function of normal structures, an incisional biopsy is an appropriate first step. Surgical salvage may play a role following chemotherapy or radiotherapy, or both. Posttransplant lymphoproliferative disease may be seen in immunocompromised patients following transplantation and is characterized by a discrete solid tumor or diffuse enlargement of lymphoid tissues. Following biopsy, reduction in immunosuppressive therapy usually will eliminate the abnormal tissue.[5] One must not forget the principles of evaluation of a metastatic lesion in the neck from an unknown primary, a condition seen more frequently in adults. In older pediatric patients, panendoscopy (direct laryngoscopy, bronchoscopy, esophagoscopy, nasopharyngoscopy) should be considered during the evaluation phase in order to rule out unrecognized primary lesions. Selective biopsies can be performed from the tongue base, nasopharynx, pyriform sinus, and tonsil. Additionally, bronchial washings for cytology and culture can be obtained. If a primary lesion is discovered, therapy of the cervical mass will be directed by the treatment necessary for the primary condition.[4]

Biopsy of the cervical mass should be deferred until evaluation of the remainder of the head and neck region has failed to uncover a primary lesion. Should biopsy be necessary, the incision should be planned so that it can be incorporated into an incision for a radical neck dissection at a later time. Therapy should be directed against the specific pathology identified at the time of biopsy. If squamous cell carcinoma is identified without a primary source, treatment should proceed in a fashion similar to that for the adult patient with the same condifion. If adenocarcinoma is identified, a primary source outside of the head and neck should be suspected, and patients generally have a poor outcome. Similarly, supraclavicular adenopathy often reflects metastatic disease from an intra-abdominal origin and often is associated with a poor outcome.[4]

Vasoformative lesions (hemangiomas, lymphangiomas, hemangiolymphangiomas) are found almost exclusively in children and are identified usually before the age of 2 years. Slow, progressive enlargement is common, but a rapid increase in size may be noted during periods of upper respiratory infection. In addition, hemangiomas often will demonstrate enlargement with exertion or dependency (Fig. 30-6). While lymphangiomas generally are soft, compressible, and relatively diffuse, hemangiomas may be more discrete and firm, especially when located within a muscle or the deep soft tissues. A lymphangioma may be more discrete and firm if it has been present for many years and has undergone morphologic alterations due to multiple infections with secondary scarring (Fig. 30-7). Cutaneous vascular changes may be indicative of hemangiomas which are diffuse and even infiltrative. CT and MRI can allow identification of the type of lesion and definite its extent.

The natural history of hemangiomas is resolution over a period of years, though surgical excision is appropriate when there is a diagnostic question, hemorrhage, repeated infections, airway compromise, high-output cardiac failure, or, rarely, significant cosmetic abnormality. Intravenous or oral steroids may be an appropriate initial alternative. Lymphangiomas rarely undergo spontaneous regression and should be managed surgically. The role of sclerosing agents and chemotherapy, though poorly defined, may be useful in unresectable lesions.

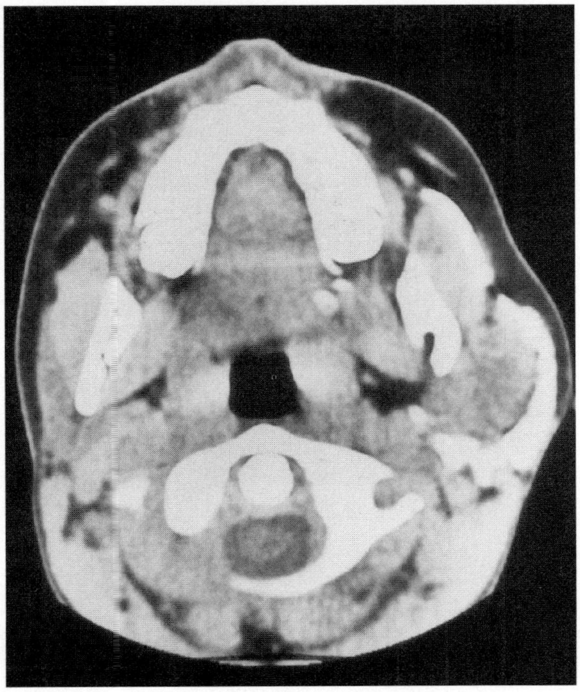

FIG 30-7
A CT sialogram demonstrating enlargement of the left parotid gland with the presence of contrast material extrinsic to the mass. Histopathology was consistent with a lymphangioma.

A relatively unique benign lesion in the pediatric population is the pilomatrixoma, or calcifying epithelioma of Malherbe. These are solitary masses located in the intradermal or subcutaneous soft tissues and represent hamartomas of hair follicle origin. They are of firm consistency and may be attached to the skin. Surgical excision is diagnostic and therapeutic.[4]

An algorithm is an effective method of approaching the diagnostic problem of a child with a mass in the neck. Fig. 30-8 is a schematic that details the appropriate studies necessary to develop such a differential diagnosis.[4]

REFERENCES

1. Bonilla JA, Healy GB: Management of malignant head and neck tumors in children. *Pediatr Clin North Am* 36:1443-1469, 1989.
2. Mobley DL, et al: Fine needle aspiration biopsy: application to pediatric head and neck masses. *Laryngoscope* 101:469-472.
3. Myer III CM: Salivary gland disease in children. In Johnson JT, et al, editors: *Instructional Courses,* vol 2, St. Louis, 1989, C.V. Mosby Co., pp 77-87.
4. Myer III CM, Cotton RT: Lump in the neck. In Myer III CM, Cotton RT, editors: *A Practical Approach to Pediatric Otolaryngology,* Chicago, 1988, Year Book Medical Publishers, Inc , pp 212-219.
5. Nuss RC, Cunningham MJ: Pediatric head and neck masses, cysts, sinuses, and tumors. *Curr Opin Otolaryngol Head Neck Surg* 1:153-160, 1993.
6. Robinson LD, et al: Head and neck malignancies in children: an age-incidence study. *Laryngoscope* 98:11-13, 1988.
7. Ward RF: Head and neck tumors in children. In Healy GB, editor: *Common Problems in Pediatric Otolaryngology,* Chicago, 1990, Year Book Medical Publishers, Inc., pp 349-355.
8. Wood II RP: Tumors and cysts of the neck. In Balkany TJ, Pashley NRT, editors: *Clinical Pediatric Otolaryngology,* St. Louis, 1986, C.V. Mosby Co., pp 427-430.

31

Surgical Treatment of Pediatric Airway Lesions

George H. Zalzal, M.D. and Robin T. Cotton, M.D., F.A.C.S., F.R.C.S.(C)

DIAGNOSIS OF PEDIATRIC AIRWAY LESIONS

Airway lesions in children can be life threatening, and stridor is often the initial symptom. As soon as a complete history and clinical examination are obtained, a treatment decision must be made quickly based on the nature and severity of the child's condition. Radiographic and endoscopic evaluations are key components in the workup of stridor,[30] with endoscopy providing the definitive diagnosis.[33]

Anterior-posterior and lateral plain films are very helpful in the evaluation of stridor. In an infant or very young child, it is essential that the neck be extended to prevent buckling of the posterior pharyngeal wall during inspiration and the misdiagnosis of a retropharyngeal swelling on the plain films. High kv voltage radiographs are especially useful, because the boundaries of air space and soft tissue are easily seen.

A barium swallow should be ordered for the evaluation of stridor in the presence of feeding difficulties such as aspiration, regurgitation, and reflux leading to cyanosis or if there is a suspicion of a vascular compression of the esophagus. A modified barium swallow should be performed in cooperation with a speech pathologist trained in the diagnosis of swallowing disorders if aspiration is significant. Appropriate liquid and solid food items are mixed with barium, allowing all phases of swallowing to be observed. The presence of a laryngotracheal-esophageal fistula or cleft should be apparent on a modified barium swallow.

Videofluoroscopy is an important tool for the study of structural and dynamic characteristics of the airway. It is particularly useful for the diagnosis of hypopharyngeal collapse, tracheomalacia, and foreign body aspiration. For instance, during inspiration the mediastinum always moves toward the side where the foreign body is located. Videofluoroscopy also can be performed while the child is sleeping to reveal dynamic airway collapse or other airway obstruction contributing to sleep apnea.

The detailed information available from modern imaging methods such as computed tomography (CT) and magnetic resonance imaging (MRI) is useful in some cases. However, sedation is usually necessary in young patients; and patient selection is important to avoid complications caused by further suppression of respiratory drive in infants already in respiratory distress. MRI is especially useful in the evaluation of vascular compressions and abnormalities.

Even the detailed images obtained with modern CT and MRI equipment are no substitute for endoscopic evaluation. Flexible fiberoptic endoscopes in a range of sizes have made it possible to examine the nasal cavities, hypopharynx, and larynx in the smallest infants. (Flexible fiberoptic endoscopy can be performed in the office with the proper administration of topical local anesthetic.)

Placed transnasally, a flexible fiberoptic endoscope provides a view of the airway superior to the subglottis and a view of the posterior oral cavity and pharynx during swallowing. By using colored foods and liquids of varying consistency, the mechanics of swallowing, particularly the time interval immediately after the swallow, can be observed from a vantage point above the valleculae and the larynx. Coordination disorders, excessive pooling of secretions, flooding of the laryngeal inlet, and aspiration may be seen during the examination. In some cases, this method of assessing swallowing function provides equivalent or better information than the modified barium swallow, and endoscopy has the additional benefit of not exposing the child to any radiation.[2,22]

Rigid endoscopy, although it requires the use of general anesthetic, affords the viewer an even more detailed view of the supraglottic region and also allows the examination to include the subglottic region and trachea down to the carina. Rigid endoscopy equipment also includes a variety of

Common Causes of Nasal Obstruction in Neonates

Most common	Less common
Septal deviation	Anterior nasal stenosis
Stuffy nose syndrome	Chlamydia trachomatis
Enlarged turbinates	Choanal atresia or stenosis
	Cystic fibrosis
	Diphtheria
	Drug-induced nasal obstruction
	Encephalocele
	Fetal alcohol syndrome
	Glioma
	Group A streptococus
	Hypothyroidism
	Infectious rhinitis
	Irritative obstruction
	Karagener's syndrome
	Nasal dermoid cyst
	Nasolacrimal duct cyst
	Nasopharyngeal stenosis
	Nasopharyngeal tumor
	Pertussis
	Rhinitis medicamentosa
	Septal hematoma
	Vascular malformation

instruments for treatment such as forceps for removing foreign bodies, obtaining biopsies, or removing excess tissue.[3] Endoscopic evaluation invariably yields a diagnosis.

PEDIATRIC RESPIRATORY DISTRESS

There is a wide variety of causes of pediatric respiratory distress involving any region of the airway from the nasal cavity down to the smallest bronchioles.[28,38] Because infants are predominantly nasal breathers at birth, they are particularly sensitive to nasal obstruction. The most common causes are listed in box above.

Disorders affecting the development of the oral cavity also may have an affect on airway patency. Micrognathia associated with Pierre Robin sequence contributes to stridor or airway obstruction while at the same time making intubation more difficult. Macroglossia can cause similar problems, and both conditions are seen frequently in conjunction with feeding disorders.

Obstruction of the larynx can have both dynamic and fixed components. The most common cause of laryngeal obstruction in infants is laryngomalacia, or collapse of the supraglottic structures of the larynx on inspiration. Laryngeal webs are usually located anteriorly, and they may be congenital or acquired following intubation trauma. Laryngeal papillomatosis and vocal fold paralysis may also contribute to airway obstruction at the level of the larynx. Subglottic hemangiomas and cysts can progress from nonobstructive to obstructive in a short time, therefore, they require careful and frequent monitoring.

Pediatric stridor may also be caused by tracheal pathology. Included are tracheomalacia, tracheal papillomatosis, complete tracheal rings, and vascular compressions. Tracheomalacia can be observed on a videofluoroscopic examination. Tracheal papillomatosis is less accessible than papillomatosis of the larynx, but for the most part this lesion is treated in the same manner. Complete tracheal rings represent a disturbance of cartilage development leading to what is sometimes called "stove pipe trachea." Vascular compression of the trachea can be caused by innominate artery, double aortic arch, or pulmonary sling.

Laryngeal incompetence is characterized by the frequent aspiration of foods and liquids. If the patient's history reveals a pattern of ingesting foreign bodies, a high index of suspicion should be maintained for the presence of a esophageal foreign body. Laryngeal cleft is a rare finding. The most severe cases include laryngotracheal-esophageal fistula. These malformations provide a conduit for gastric contents in the esophagus to spill into the larynx and trachea causing pulmonary disease.

ENDOSCOPIC LASER TREATMENT OF PEDIATRIC AIRWAY LESIONS

There are many kinds of lasers available to the pediatric otolaryngologist, including the CO_2, ND-YAG, ND-YAG-KTP, argon, tunable dye, krypton, helium-neon, and others. The two most commonly used for pediatric airway disorders are the CO_2 and the ND-YAG-KTP lasers. Laser therapy offers the advantages of nearly bloodless surgery and extreme accuracy.

A number of factors must be considered prior to using laser surgery in a pediatric airway. In general, children have a smaller oral cavity, the tongue is relatively larger, the larynx is more cephalad, and the plane of the glottis is not horizontal as that in the adult. Also, whereas the narrowest point in the adult airway is the glottis, the narrowest point in the pediatric airway is the subglottis bounded by the cricoid cartilage. Many pediatric patients have a small retrusive mandible that makes the larynx difficult to expose.

The small size of pediatric airways and the relative delicacy of pediatric tissues require much vigilance to avoid complications of laser surgery. It is especially important to avoid excess scatter of the laser beam when using the CO_2 laser in conjunction with the bronchoscope. It is also important that the depth of laser penetration be carefully controlled, and the configuration of the surgical wound that is created should never be circumferential, as this frequently leads to stenosis. Finally, the potential for the ignition of combustible materials by the combination of laser energy and high oxygen concentration is very significant. Endotracheal tubes, unless they are specifically made to resist laser energy, are extremely flammable. A laser induced airway fire is both terrifying for the surgeon and disastrous for the patient. In young children anesthetic techniques should be used that avoid an indwelling endotracheal tube during the use of the laser.

The CO_2 laser is well suited for treating intraoral and tongue base lesions, such as vallecular cysts, cystic hygromas, and lymphangiomas. The laser is used to open the cyst, the fluid contents are removed, and the entire cyst wall or lymphangioma is vaporized. Staged procedures may be necessary for treating lymphangiomas.

Laryngeal and subglottic cysts respond very well to simple unroofing by laser or the Bugbee electrode. The operative field usually remains bloodless, and the extreme accuracy of laser ablation allows the definitive cure of these lesions.

Papillomas are the most common benign neoplasm of the larynx, and the juvenile form of the disease is very unpredictable in its response to treatment and its tendency to spread. The papillomas themselves are wart-like in appearance and commonly involve the vocal cords and the anterior commissure. Here, as well as in the pharynx, oral cavity, or supraglottic area, they are readily accessible for treatment with the CO_2 laser. When used appropriately, the laser should vaporize only the abnormal tissue with little damage to adjacent normal tissue. The hemostatic properties inherent in laser surgery maintains a clear field of view. As mentioned, the final configuration of the surgical wound must be kept in mind to avoid supraglottic stenosis, fixation of the vocal folds, or other obstructive scar formation. The goal of laser management of papillomatosis is to maintain normal laryngeal function, not complete removal of the diseased tissue. The natural course of the disease is often complete resolution, so treatment must not compromise the long-term voice or airway result.

Papillomas in the cervical trachea in young children are accessible for laser treatment by using the subglottoscope, which is available in different lengths. In older children the use of the laser bronchoscope may be preferable.

Some endoscopic applications for laser surgery remain controversial. The appropriateness of laser for the division of laryngeal webs depends primarily upon the thickness of the web. Only webs that are uniformly thin in the vertical dimension are suitable for a laser procedure.[6] The tendency of the divided edges of the web to reapproximate contributes to a high recurrence rate. Scar tissue resulting from the division of a thicker web may cause greater obstruction than the web itself.

Subglottic hemangioma has a natural course ending in complete resolution and normal laryngeal function, so any intervention must maintain normal laryngeal function. Tracheostomy is used frequently to bypass the lesion until spontaneous resolution occurs, and efforts to avoid tracheostomy or expedite decannulation may be controversial. Isolated subglottic hemangiomas may be treated by CO_2 laser, provided the hemangioma does not incorporate the entire circumference of the airway. In that case, laser ablation will leave a circumferential surgical wound which will lead to subglottic stenosis.[16] Damage to the perichondrium of the cricoid cartilage must be avoided. Postoperative compression of the hemangioma by intubation and appropriate use of steroids will contribute to a successful procedure. Isolated subglottic hemangiomas that do not respond to laser treatment actually may be part of a large underlying tracheal or mediastinal hemangioma. Evaluation by CT or MRI is necessary to determine the extent of the hemangioma.

TABLE 31-1
Stenosis grades determined by endotracheal tube size

Classification (grade)	From	To
I	No obstruction	50% obstruction
II	51% obstruction	70% obstruction
III	71% obstruction	99% obstruction
IV	No detectable lumen	

The laser is very useful for the removal of granulation tissue but is indicated only in grade II lesions of mature subglottic stenosis (Table 31-1).[25] As in the other applications of endoscopic laser surgery, the potential for postoperative fixation or constricture of laryngeal structures is great, especially if the stenosis involves a significant portion of the airway vertically or circumferentially. In general, only very thin webs should be considered for laser therapy, and all other stenoses should be approached with an open laryngotracheal reconstruction procedure.[17]

PROCEDURES FOR THE TREATMENT OF LARYNGEAL SPHINCTER ABNORMALITIES

Vocal cord paralysis is the second most common cause of stridor in early infancy, and it is identified by flexible fiberoptic laryngoscopy. Unilateral paralysis rarely requires intervention, while bilateral involvement often requires tracheostomy for maintaining an adequate airway. In many cases of congenital idiopathic paralysis, spontaneous recovery of vocal cord function returns within 2 to 3 years but rarely after that. Surgical intervention is required to facilitate decannulation for patients in whom spontaneous resolution does not occur.

It is important to differentiate vocal cord paralysis from fixation prior to surgery, and this can be accomplished by electromyography under general anesthesia with direct laryngoscopic visualization.[35,36] If congenital paralysis is the diagnosis, the underlying cause should be thoroughly investigated, since vocal cord paralysis is frequently associated with central nervous system anomalies or cardiovascular disorders.

parison with certain death in children with severe long-segment stenosis. Although complete tracheal rings is a rare finding, additional research is needed to develop new techniques for handling this challenging problem.

REFERENCES

1. Barthez E, Rilliet F: *Traité clinique et pratique des maladies des enfants.* Paris, 1843, G. Bailliere.
2. Bastian RW: Videoendoscopic evaluation of patients with dysphagia: an adjunct to the modified barium swallow. *Otolaryngol Head Neck Surg* 104:329-350, 1991.
3. Benjamin B: Prolonged intubation injuries of the larynx: endoscopic diagnosis, classification, and treatment. *Ann Otol Rhinol Laryngol* 160:Supplement, 1993.
4. Bower CM, Choi SS, Cotton RT: Arytenoidectomy in children. *Ann Otol Rhinol Laryngol* 103:271-278, 1994.
5. Cotton RT: Management of subglottic stenosis in infancy and childhood. Review of a consecutive series of cases managed by surgical reconstruction. *Ann Otol Rhinol Laryngol* 87:649-657, 1978.
6. Cotton RT: Pediatric laryngotracheal reconstruction. *Oper Techniq Otolaryngol Head Neck Surg* 3(3):165-172, 1992.
7. Cotton RT: Prevention and management of subglottic stenosis in infants. *Pediatr Surg* 20:845-851, 1985.
8. Cotton RT: The problem of pediatric laryngotracheal stenosis: a clinical and experimental study on the efficacy of autogenous cartilaginous grafts placed between the vertically divided halves of the posterior lamina of the cricoid cartilage. *Laryngoscope* 101:Suppl 56, 1991.
9. Cotton RT, Evans JN: Laryngotracheal reconstruction in children. Five-year follow-up. *Ann Otol Rhinol Laryngol* 90:516-520, 1981.
10. Cotton RT, Gray SD, Miller RP: Update of the Cincinnati experience in pediatric laryngotracheal reconstruction. *Laryngoscope* 99:1111-1116, 1989.
11. Cotton RT, O'Connor DM: Evaluation of the airway for larygotracheal reconstruction. *Intl Anesth Clin* 30(4):93-98, 1992.
12. Cotton RT, Myer CM III, Bratcher GO, Fitton CM: Anterior cricoid split, 1977-1987. *Arch Otolaryngol Head Neck Surg* 114:1300-1302, 1988.
13. Cotton RT, Myer CM III, O'Connor DM: Innovations in pediatric laryngotracheal reconstruction. *J Pediatr Surg* 27(2):196-200, 1992.
14. Cotton RT, Schreiber JT: Management of laryngotracheoesophageal cleft. *Ann Otol Rhinol Laryngol,* 90(4):401-405, 1981.
15. Cotton RT, Seid AB: Management of the extubation problem in the premature child: anterior cricoid split as an alternative to tracheotomy. *Ann Otol Rhinol Laryngol* 89:508-511, 1980.
16. Cotton RT, Tewfik TL: Laryngeal stenosis following carbon dioxide laser in subglottic hemangioma. Report of three cases. *Ann Otol Rhinol Laryngol* 94:494-497, 1985.
17. Duncavage JA, Ossoff RH, Toohill RJ: Carbon dioxide laser management of laryngeal stenosis. *Ann Otol Rhinol Laryngol* 94:565-569, 1985.
18. Fearon B, Ellis D: The management of long-term airway problems in infants and children. *Ann Otol Rhinol Laryngol* 80:669-677, 1971.
19. Fearon B, Cotton RT: Surgical correction of subglottic stenosis of the larynx. Preliminary report of an experimental surgical technique. *Ann Otol Rhinol Laryngol* 81:508-513, 1972.
20. Holinger PH, Johnson KC, Schiller F. Congenital anomalies of the larynx. *Ann Otol Rhinol Laryngol* 63:581-606, 1954.
21. Iglauer S: Epiglottidectomy for the relief of congenital laryngeal stridor, with report of a case. *Laryngoscope* 32:56-59, 1922.
22. Langmore SE, Schatz K, Olson N: Endoscopic and videofluoroscopic evaluation of swallowing and aspiration. *Ann Otol Rhinol Laryngol* 100:678-681, 1991.
23. Myer CM III: Choanal atresia. In Gates GA, editor: *Current Therapy in Otolaryngology-Head and Neck Surgery.* Philadelphia, 1994, BC Decker, Mosby–Year Book.
24. Myer CM III, Holmes DK, Cotton RT, Jackson RK: Laryngeal and laryngotracheoesophageal clefts: role of early surgical repair. *Ann Otol Rhinol Laryngol* 99(2):98-104, 1990.
25. Myer CM III, Cotton RT, O'Connor DM: Proposed grading system for subglottic stenosis based on endotracheal tube sizes. *Ann Otol Rhinol Laryngol* 103 (4):319-323, 1994.
26. Narcy P, Contencin P, Viala P: Surgical treatment for laryngeal paralysis in infants and children. *Ann Otol Rhinol Laryngol* 99:124-128, 1990.
27. Narcy P, Bobin S, Contencin P, Le Pajolec C, Manach Y: Anomalies laryngies du nouveau-ne apropos de 687 observations. *Ann Otolaryngol Chir Cervicofac* 101:363-373, 1984.
28. Nowlin JH, Zalzal GH: The stridorous infant. *Ear Nose Throat J* 70:84-8, 1991.
29. Reardon TJ: Congenital laryngeal stridor. *Am J Med Sci* 134:242-252, 1907.
30. Schlesinger AE, Hernandez RJ: Radiographic imaging of airway obstruction in pediatrics. *Otolaryngol Clin N Am* 23(4):609-37, 1990.
31. Silver FM, Myer CM III, Cotton RT: Anterior cricoid split: update 1991. *Am J Otolaryngol* 12:343-346, 1991.
32. Smith GJ, Cooper DM: Laryngomalacia and inspiratory obstruction in later childhood. *Arch Dis Child* 56:345-349, 1981.
33. Tunkel DE, Zalzal GH: Stridor in infants and children: ambulatory evaluation and operative diagnosis. *Clin Pedictr* 31(1):48-55, 1992.
34. Variot G: Un cas de respiration stridoreuse des nouveau-nes avec autopsie. *Bull Mem Soc Med Hop Paris* 3:490-494, 1898.
35. Woo P, Arandia H: Intraoperative laryngeal electromyographic assessment of patients with immobile vocal fold. *Ann Otol Rhinol Laryngol* 101(10):799-806, 1992.
36. Zalzal GH: Posterior glottic fixation in children. *Ann Otol Rhinol Laryngol* 102(9):680-6, 1993.
37. Zalzal GH: Rib cartilage grafts for the treatment of posterior glottic and subglottic stenosis in children. *Ann Otol Rhinol Laryngol* 97(5 Pt 1):506-11, 1988.
38. Zalzal GH: Stridor and airway compromise. *Pediatr Clin N Am* 36:1389-402, 1989.
39. Zalzal GH: Stenting for pediatric laryngotracheal stenosis. *Ann Otol Rhinol Laryngol* 101:651-5, 1992.
40. Zalzal GH: Treatment of laryngotracheal stenosis with anterior and posterior cartilage grafts. A report of 41 children. *Arch Otolaryngol Head Neck Surg* 119:82-6, 1993.
41. Zalzal GH, Anon JB, Cotton RT: Epiglottoplasty for the treatment of laryngomalacia. *Ann Otol Rhinol Laryngol* 96(1):72-76, 1987.
42. Zalzal GH, Cotton RT: A new way of carving cartilage grafts to avoid prolapse into the tracheal lumen when used in subglottic reconstruction. *Laryngoscope* 96:1039, 1986.

Part Seven

Rhinology

32

Advanced Endoscopic Techniques

David W. Kennedy, M.D., Donald C. Lanza, M.D., F.A.C.S., and Eugenia M. Vining, M.D.

Although originally introduced for minimally invasive surgical therapy of inflammatory sinus disease, endoscopic endonasal surgery has been expanded to provide an alternative therapeutic modality for a variety of differing problems. Surgical procedures now performed in this manner include closure of cerebrospinal fluid (CSF) rhinorrhea,[9,14] orbital decompression,[7] dacryocystorhinostomy,[10] tumor surgery[14] and, more recently, optic nerve decompression and pituitary surgery. Performing these procedures endoscopically reduces morbidity by eliminating the necessity for external incisions and, at the same time, allows optimal visualization of the surgical site. For the experienced endoscopic surgeon such procedures are a natural extension of endoscopic surgery performed for inflammatory disease and, because the sinuses are typically not diseased in these cases, may be relatively easy to perform and less time consuming in severe cases of hypertrophic mucosal disease.

The aim of this presentation is to detail the key points in technique involved in several of the procedures and to discuss the advantages and disadvantages of the techniques relative to more traditional methods.

ENDOSCOPIC CLOSURE OF CEREBROSPINAL FLUID RHINORRHEA

The first extracranial repair of cerebrospinal fluid (CSF) rhinorrhea was reported in 1948 by Dohlman[2] using a naso-orbital incision. Chandler[1] advocated an external ethmoid incision, and, until recently, this has remained the procedure of choice for extracranial repair. Lehrer and Deutsch[8] recommended intranasal repair under the operating microscope. Endoscopic repair of CSF rhinorrhea during sinus surgery was first described by Wigand.[14] The technique as described below was first described by Mattox and Kennedy[9] and has now been utilized in a wide variety of patients with CSF rhinorrhea, meningoceles, and meningoencephaloceles.

Surgical technique

Prior to surgery, neurosurgical consultation is obtained in all cases. The surgery itself may be performed under local or general anesthesia. At the beginning of the surgery, a lumbar puncture is performed, and, if the defect is large or if the leak was spontaneous, a spinal drain may be placed. CSF (5 to 10 ml) is withdrawn and mixed with 0.2 ml of 5% fluorescein for injection (not topical) and slowly reinjected into the subarachnoid space. If a spinal drain is placed, it is clamped for the duration of the procedure. Although frequently not required, a blue light filter may be placed in the endoscopic light source to maximize the degree of fluorescence.

Endoscopic intranasal exposure of the skull base is then performed and the area of the defect carefully identified. Bony septae are meticulously removed to create a flat bed for the graft. If a meningocele or encephalocele is present, the neck is carefully isolated and it is cauterized bipolarly and transected. The remaining portion of the neck may then be inverted into the bony defect, and, if the defect is small, this may be sufficient to stop the gross leak. At least 5 mm of the mucosa around the defect is carefully removed in each direction, and the edges of the mucosa surrounding this area are elevated slightly.

A mucoperiosteal and mucoperichondrial graft is typically harvested from the septum of the opposite side of the nose, so that bleeding from the graft site does not interfere with visualization. If the defect is small, turbinate mucosa or mucosa from the floor of the nose can also be used. If the bony defect is large, some fascia or abdominal fat may be placed intracranially and the bony defect reconstructed with turbinate or septal bone or septal cartilage.

The mucoperiosteal graft is placed as a free graft over the bony defect with mucosa facing externally. The edges of the graft are tucked under the surrounding mucosa, and the graft is secured in place by packing the area with microfibrillar collagen. Fibrin glue may also be utilized. Gelfoam is then placed as further packing, and the remainder of the nose is packed with gauze or a Merocel sponge. If a spinal drain was placed it is opened at the end of the procedure and left in place for 72 hours. The nasal packing is removed at 4 to 7 days, and any remaining microfibrillar collagen is removed after about 3 to 4 weeks.

Comment

Endoscopic closure of CSF rhinorrhea allows excellent localization of the leak site when combined with intrathecal fluorescein. Although complications have been noted from the use of fluorescein, including status epilepticus, the risks appear to be minimal when utilized in the dose and manner recommended.[9] Utilization of a free graft rather than a pedicled graft helps to preserve nasal function and allows for better conformity of the graft to the recipient bed. It does not appear to affect graft viability. The donor site heals up well and is treated with the application of an antibiotic ointment postoperatively.

The authors have repaired a wide variety of different skull base lesions with this technique, including posttraumatic, iatrogenic, and spontaneous CSF rhinorrhea, meningoceles, and both frontal and temporal lobe encephaloceles. Only one failure to close a leak has occurred to date.

ENDOSCOPIC ORBITAL DECOMPRESSION

In 1911, Dollinger, using Kronlein's approach for access to the lateral orbit, performed a lateral orbital wall decompression for dysthyroid orbitopathy; however, the extent of decompression provided was minimal.[3] Sewall subsequently described a medial orbital wall decompression through an external ethmoidectomy approach.[12] Hirsch was the first to employ a Caldwell-Luc approach to obtain a decompression by removal of the orbital floor.[5] Walsh and Ogura extended this approach to include medial wall decompression, and this has subsequently become the most frequently utilized approach.[13] Endoscopic orbital decompression was described by Kennedy et al in 1990 and has subsequently been performed by a number of other surgeons with satisfactory results.[7]

Surgical technique

The patient is placed supine on the operating room table with the head slightly elevated. General anesthesia is provided through a right-angled endotracheal tube. Local vasoconstriction is obtained with topical cocaine and by injection of 1% xylocaine with 1 : 100,000 epinephrine. An intranasal endoscopic sphenoethmoidectomy is performed.[6] Care is taken to identify and skeletonize the medial orbital wall and the skull base. Posteriorly, the orbital apex and, when possible, the optic canal are identified. Anteriorly, the area of the frontal recess is opened. A very generous middle meatal antrostomy is then performed, creating an opening that extends anteriorly to the posterior margin of the nasolacrimal duct, inferiorly into the root of the inferior turbinate, and posteriorly to the posterior limit of the sinus. The infraorbital nerve is identified laterally within the sinus and defines the lateral limit for removal of the orbital floor.

At this point, the skeletonized medial orbital wall is gently removed with an angled spoon or fine Blakesly forceps. The orbital floor is removed with 70° or 110° Giraffe forceps while viewing the area with a 30° or 70° telescope. The inferior orbital wall may also be fractured inferiorly with a curved suction or a Kuhn angled spoon and removed. The medial and inferior orbital walls are removed to the orbital apex posteriorly. Anteriorly, it is essential to preserve the medial orbital wall in the region of the frontal recess if the possibility of stenosis and subsequent frontal sinus obstruction is to be avoided. Care is taken not to open the periobita during the bony removal as this would impair subsequent visualization.

Once meticulous resection of the bony orbital wall is complete, the periorbita is incised with a sickle knife in linear strokes from posterior to anterior. The initial incision is placed laterally within the maxillary sinus and is performed using a bent Beaver sickle knife. Successive incisions are performed medially within the maxillary sinus, so as not to obstruct the surgeon's view with the herniating intraorbital contents. Similar periosteal incisions are then made high on the medial orbital wall using a straight Beaver sickle knife or a No. 12 Bard Parker blade, and successive incisions are made inferiorly.

The immediate extent of decompression is assessed by gently palpating the orbit and endoscopically viewing the transmission of the palpations to the herniated orbital contents. At the end of the operation, a small piece of Gelfilm is placed in the middle meatus and a small Merocel sponge is placed in the nose. When maximum decompression is required, the endoscopic approach may be further augmented with a lateral orbital decompression performed at the same sitting.

Comment

Endoscopic orbital decompression has proved reliable for us, and recent presentations by other authors suggest that these results are being duplicated. An average of 4.5 to 5.0 mm of decompression can be expected, but the actual amount achieved is dependent on the amount of fibrosis and muscle hypertrophy present. Adding a lateral orbital decompression adds approximately 1 mm of additional decompression. As with other types of orbital decompression, diplopia may occur or worsen postoperatively, and the surgery is therefore usually reserved for patients with complications from exophthalmos.

Compared to the Walsh-Ogura technique, morbidity is

decreased while the total reduction of exophthalmos is similar. Decompression in the all important region of the orbital apex is maximized although inferior orbital decompression is less complete.

ENDOSCOPIC DACRYOCYSTORHINOSTOMY

Intranasal drainage of the lacrimal sac was originally described by West in 1911. However, at least in the United States, external dacryocystorhinostomy (DCR) has remained the most commonly performed procedure. In part it would appear that this may be due to the surgery being typically performed by ophthalmologists who are less familiar with intranasal surgical techniques. Endoscopic DCR provides excellent visualization for the surgery and enables concurrent sinusitis, a frequent cause of failure, to be accurately identified and removed. The use of endoscopes postoperatively allows both accurate visualization of the surgical site and debridement and removal of adhesions.

Surgical technique

The surgery can be readily performed under local anesthesia. We prefer to perform an infundibulotomy initially and then direct attention to the area of the nasolacrimal duct and sac anterior to the uncinate attachment. An inferiorly based mucosal flap is raised over the area immediately anterior and inferior to the anterior attachment of the middle turbinate and the mucosa is excised. The precise location of the lacrimal duct is most easily identified by placing a light pipe into the sac through the lacrimal canaliculus.

A diamond drill is used to widely remove the bone from the area of the sac and from the adjacent lacrimal duct. The sac is then incised vertically with a sickle knife at the junction of the anterior one third and posterior two thirds. Small horizontal incisions are made superiorly and inferiorly so that, when possible, flaps may be rotated anteriorly and posteriorly over the edges of the bone. Sufficient nasolacrimal duct should be opened inferiorly to ensure that there is not a second loculation of pus.

The light probe is now replaced with lacrimal probes and the area inspected to ensure that the common canaliculus is widely opened. Lacrimal stents are then placed, and the obturators are grasped intranasally and removed. The silastic stent is secured by tying intranasally. Attention is then redirected back to the area of the sac, and the flaps created from the sac mucosa are rotated outward over the bone and secured in place with a small amount of microfibrillar collagen or fibrin glue. Gelfilm is placed over the operative site and into the anterior middle meatus. The stents are left in place for 4 to 6 months.

Comment

Endoscopic visualization allows excellent identification of the operative site and avoids the morbidity associated with external DCR. It is our preference to remove the uncinate process during the operation to allow inspection of the infundibulum and to widen the posterior exposure of the sac. When, as is frequently the case in revision procedures, there is associated ethmoid sinusitis, this may be removed by performing and endoscopic ethmoidectomy. The use of a light probe makes identification of the sac easy, even in cases where it is severely fibrosed. Postoperatively the use of endoscopes allows for careful inspection of the surgical site and debridement of the area around the sac.

ENDOSCOPIC OPTIC NERVE DECOMPRESSION

The role of surgical decompression in traumatic visual loss remains controversial. Although megadose steroids remain the mainstay of treatment for this problem, variable success rates have been reported for return of vision with surgical optic nerve decompression.[4] Various routes have been proposed for extracranial decompression of the optic nerve. Our preference is for intranasal endoscopic decompression when surgical intervention is indicated.

Surgical technique

The surgery is performed under general anesthesia. After performing a complete endoscopic sphenoehthmoidectomy, the medial orbital wall is further skeletonized. The optic nerve is traced from the orbital apex through the lateral and superior aspects of the sphenoid sinus. If necessary some bone is removed from the orbital apex to aid in localizing nerve position. A diamond burr is then used to thin the bone of the orbital apex and optic canal. With smaller burrs, we attempt to skeletonize the nerve over greater than 180°. After the bone has been thinned, the eggshell thin remnants are removed with a curette. In selected cases, in which visual loss is complete, the sheath can be incised longitudinally with a disposable arachnoid knife. The patient is maintained on megadose steroids in the early postoperative period and these are then tapered.

Comment

At this time the role for surgical decompression of the optic nerve in traumatic visual loss remains unclear and further controlled studies are needed to identify the role for surgical intervention. However, the endoscopic approach provides excellent visualization with a minimum of morbidity and is probably the approach of choice when surgical intervention is indicated.

Discussion

For the experienced surgeon, endoscopes enable a minimally invasive approach to a wide variety of surgical problems. As instrumentation continues to improve, there is no doubt that a continually increasing number of procedures will become amenable to endoscopic intervention. Such surgery reduces morbidity by eliminating external incisions and, at the same time, allows optimal visualization of the surgical site. These procedures are a natural extension of endoscopic techniques performed for inflammatory disease and are not especially difficult for surgeons who have truly mastered the techniques of meticulous, atraumatic endoscopic surgery and who have an intimate knowledge of the anatomy of the area.

REFERENCES

1. Chandler JR: Traumatic Cerebrospinal Fluid Leakage. *Otolaryngol Clin North Am* 16:623-632, 1983.
2. Dohlman G: Spontaneous Cerebrospinal Fluid Rhinorrhea. *Acta Otolaryngol (Stockh)* 67(suppl):20-23, 1948.
3. Dollinger J: Die drickentlastlung der Augenhokle durch entfurnung der aussern Orbitalwand bei hochgradigen Exophthalmos und Koneskutwer hornhauterkronkung. *Dtsch Med Worhenschr* 37:1888-1890, 1911.
4. Girard BC, Bouzas EA, Lamas G, Soudant J: visual improvement after Transethmoid-sphenoid Decompression in Optic Nerve Injuries. *J Clin Neuro Ophthalmol* 12:142-148, 1992.
5. Hirsch, O.: Surgical Decompression of Exophthalmos. *Arch Otolaryngol* 51:325-331, 1950.
6. Kennedy DW: Functional Endoscopic Sinus Surgery: technique. *Arch Otolaryngol Head Neck Surg* 111:643-649, 1985.
7. Kennedy DW, Goodstein ML, Miller NR, Zinreich SJ: Endoscopic Transnasal Orbital Decompression. *Laryngoscope* 116:275-282, 1990.
8. Lehrer J and Leutsch H: Intranasal surgery for Cerebrospinal Fluid Rhinorrhea. *Mt Sinai J Med (NY)* 37:133-138, 1993.
9. Mattox DE, Kennedy DW: Endoscopic Management of Cerebrospinal Fluid Leaks and Cephaloceles. *Laryngoscope* 100:857-862, 1990.
10. Metson R: Endoscopic surgery for lacrimal obstruction. *Otolaryngol Head Neck Surg* 104:473-478, 1990.
11. Moseley JL, Carton CA, Stern WE: Spectrum of Complications in the Use of Intrathecal Fluorescein. *J Neurosurg* 48:765-767, 1978.
12. Sewell EC: Operative Control of Progressive Exophthalmos. *Arch Otolaryngol* 51:621-624, 1936.
13. Walsh TE, Ogura JH: Transantral Orbital Decompression for Malignant Exophthalmos. *Laryngoscope* 67:544-549, 1957.
14. Wigand ME: *Endoscopic Surgery of the Paranasal Sinuses and Anterior Skull Base.* New York, 1990, Thieme Medical Publishers, Inc.

Part Eight

Allergy

33

Otolaryngic Allergy

How To Do It—Update 1995

Hamilton S. Dixon, M.D. and Barbara J. Dixon, B.S.

This course gives the practicing otolaryngologist the necessary information for setting up an allergy department in his office, whether the otolaryngologist is a new practicing physician or has been in practice for many years and wishes to add allergy to his practice.

This course will explain the necessity of understanding and being able to perform skin endpoint titration (SET), even though the physician elects to mainly utilize some other form of IgE determination, such as the radioallergosorbent test (RAST). A step-by-step outline that follows the patient from the first office visit through testing by SET or RAST until treatment is in progress will be supplied.

THE PATIENT

Background

One method utilized in our allergy department is skin endpoint titration, as originally reported by Dr. Herbert J. Rinkel. Although the concept and technique is well established, widespread usage has begun only in the past 15 years.

Progressively stronger doses of a particular allergen or allergen group are injected intracutaneously, and, by watching the progressively larger wheal size, the endpoint of reaction is determined. The patient is then treated at this determined endpoint of reaction.

The concept of a starting therapeutic dose constitutes the main difference between the skin endpoint titration technique and that which is used by traditional allergists. Whereas the traditional allergist begins desensitization with an extremely dilute allergen (usually 1:100,000 or weaker) and gradually increases the strength hoping that eventually symptoms will be relieved, the therapeutic dose of the skin endpoint titration technique aims toward more immediate relief of symptoms as desensitization progresses.

Evaluation

History and physical examination. The patient's past medical history is *the* most important factor in determining the need for skin testing. As a matter of fact, in a very high percentage of cases, we could make our decision based almost totally on history if that history is adequate. Often, many important factors in the history are not obtained until a patient has been seen many times. Documenting specific symptoms is most helpful in determining whether skin testing is actually indicated and also in following the patient's progress in treatment. For example, we want to know how many times each day a person sniffs, blows, sneezes, coughs, etc. Initial screening histories may be obtained by trained medical assistants and questionnaires, but the physician must go into the details at some length in order to ascertain severity and put symptoms in proper perspective. Of utmost importance is a *continuing history* with each subsequent visit (Figs. 33-1 and 33-2.)

Examination. A complete ear, nose, and throat examination is done on every patient, including mirror exams of the nasopharynx, hypopharynx, and larynx, transillumination of the sinuses, and careful examination of the neck. Shrinkage of nasal membranes is often needed, and the skin should not be overlooked.

Cytogram—nasal cytology. A cytogram is performed on all patients with a suspicious allergic history and increased rhinorrhea. This is done by direct vision into the nose and the use of a Calgiswab to collect the secretions. Calgiswab is a calcium alginate swab on a malleable wire made by Spectrum Laboratories, Inc., 1100 Rankin Road, Houston, TX 77073 and comes in a sterile package. These secretions are carefully rolled over a glass slide and immediately sprayed with fixative or Aqua Net hair spray, regular hold, blue can. After the Wright-Geimsa stain has been

THE HAMILTON S. DIXON, M.D.
MEDICAL CENTER
3268 Martha Berry Highway, N.E.
Rome, Georgia 30165-9745

Referring ____________
Local M.D. ____________
Yellow pages ____________

Name ______________________ Age ________ Date ________
Present illness: ______________________

Past medical history: Bleeder Dia. Tbc. Ca. HBP
Ulcers Seizures Asthma CVR

Family history: Bleeder Dia. Tbc. Ca. HBP
Ulcers Seizures Asthma CVR

Ear:	Rt/Lt	Onset	Duration	Comments
Hearing loss				
Discharge				
Pain				
Fullness				
Tinnitus/roar				
Dizziness				
Itching				

Nasal:	Clear/ yellow	Duration	Seasonal	Perennial	Comments
drainage					
P.N.D.					
Blowing x's/day					

	x's/day	Duration	Seasonal	Perennial	Comments
Sniffing					
Sneezing					
Throat clearing					
Coughing dry/congestion					

Colds with yellow/green nasal drainage/12 months ______________
Antibiotics ______________
Nasal obstruction/itching ______________

	Days/week
Snore	
Mouth breather	
Waking with dry throat	
Waking tired	
Waking thirsty at night	
Eye symptoms	

Wheezing
Skin: Rash/ itching

FIG 33-1
Patient history.

EAR:

R L

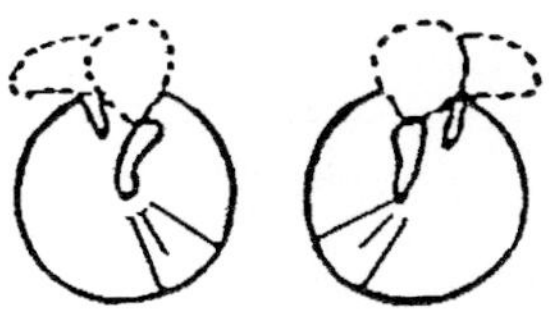

NOSE:

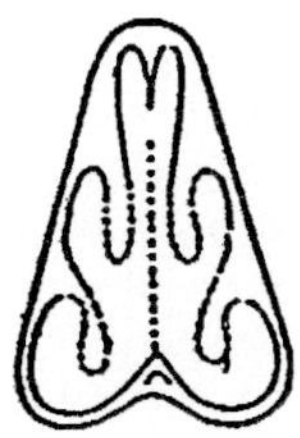

NASOPHARYNX:

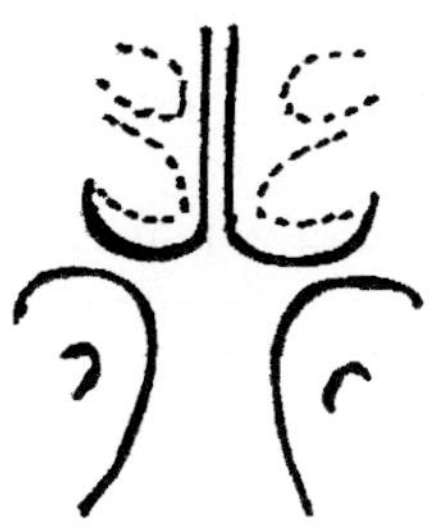

MOUTH:

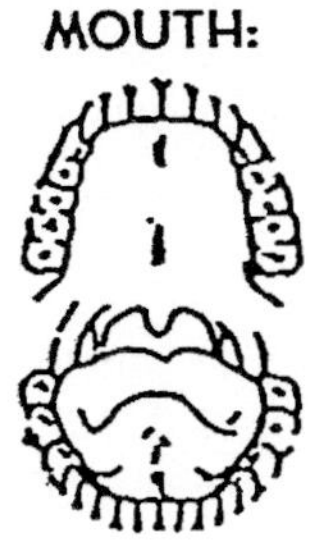

LARYNX:

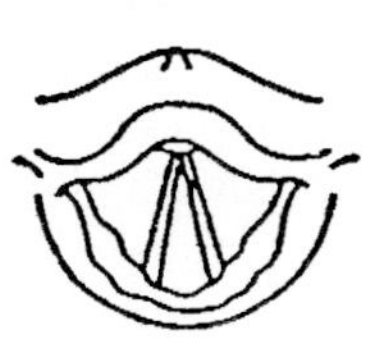

Throat:
Sore throat _______ with fever/12 months ________ Hoarseness ________
Dysphagia _______ Swelling/lump ______________ Choking __________

Headaches: Sinus/migraine/cervical	Type I	Type II
Location		
Frequency		
Duration		
Severity (scale of 1-10)		
Steady or pounding		
Medications used/effective		
Wake middle of night		
Unilateral tearing		

GI sxs Gas Belching Bloating Cramps
Nausea/vomiting Diarrhea Fatigue after meals Burning

Drug allergies: ______________
Surgeries/illness: ______________

Smokes/chews tobacco
Prescriptions:
Rx: OTC

Physical exam EARS: R | L | | L

	R	L		
Sinuses:	Frontal		Int. Ptg.	M.T.
	Antrum		Ext. Ptg.	Disch.
Nose:	M.M.	Disch.	TMJ	Weber
	Septum	Meati	Auricle	Rinne
			Canal	

Naso:	Turbs	Septum	Torus
	Adenoid	Disch.	Fossa
Oro:	Tonsil	Pharynx	Teeth
	Tongue	Palate	Gums
Hypo:	Lingual	Vallec	Ary.
	Epig.	Pyr.	Cords
Neck:	Nodes	Thyroid	Cerv. Sp.
	Sterno	Trap.	Post. Mm.

Skin: ______________

Diagnosis:

Disposition:

FIG 33-2
Patient history.

Nasal Cytoprofile

Allergy cells

Eosinophils
Goblet cells
Mast cells

Neutrophils

Infection cells

Bacteria
  Inside polys
  Outside polys
Virus effects
  Respiratory Epithelial clumping or tufting

Other cells

Squamous Cells
Lymphocytes
Monocytes

Comments

Patient name: ______________________ Date:______

Cytogram Procedure

1. Using a Calgiswab, draw it along the middle turbinate. Also, swing the Calgiswab up along the middle turbinate or roof of the nose.
2. Gently roll the secretion onto a clean glass slide. Don't rub, as this may damage some of the cells.
3. Immediately spray with Aqua-Net regular hold hair spray as a fixative or regular commercial fixative spray.
4. Allow to dry.
5. Flood slide with Wright-Giemsa stain and leave for 15 to 30 seconds.
6. Add hematologic buffer pH 6.5. A metallic precipitate will form. Leave this for 15 to 30 seconds.
7. Rinse slide thoroughly with distilled water. (Tap water is permissible if mineral content is not too high.)
8. Allow to dry or dry over an alcohol flame lamp, being careful not to hold in one spot and burn stain. A small inexpensive hair dryer works even better.
9. Add a few drops of immersion oil.
10. Examine under microscope with oil immersion lens.

completed, careful microscopic examination is accomplished.

Secretions representative of inhalant allergy usually contain many *eosinophils,* many goblet cells, and occasionally a few mast cells. In food allergy, one will see few to many goblet cells, a few eosinophils, and *many mast cells.*

Smears with predominantly neutrophils usually indicate infection–either bacterial or viral. In bacterial infections, *bacteria* will be present inside the neutrophils in acute infections or outside the polys in chronic infections (though both are usually present).

In viral infections, one will see many neutrophils accompanied by *viral-damaged respiratory epithelial cells.* Viral effects on these respiratory epithelial cells include progressive nuclear pyknosis, tufting, cell fragments with tufts separated from the nucleus, plus clumping of nuclear chromatin.

X-rays. The basic x-ray views of the sinuses are usually required. A Caldwell and a Waters View are done on the routine survey. If further problems are felt to be present in and around the sinus area, Stereo Rhese views can be done to pick up abnormalities in the sphenoid and ethmoid regions. Open-mouth sphenoid and lateral view of the sphenoid are also done in a complete sinus series. The base view is the best single view for the sphenoid. We especially look for thickening of the mucous membranes in any of the sinus areas, and the density seen is usually of diagnostic significance (see reference).

When routine plain films of sinuses are done on patients presently with allergies, 20% of these are found to have chronic sinus disease that were previously undetermined. It has been the experience of the author that clearing this problem up either medically or surgically before proceeding to allergy tests is the greater priority. Once the infection has been cleared, the patient will respond much better to immunotherapy. Since chronic sinusitis may be a relatively silent condition, thorough history and physical examination may not give any indication of its presence. Radiographic examination is safe, cost effective, and very diagnostic, even in small children.

Preparation of patient

Consultation. After the doctor has finished with his workup, the patient is escorted to the allergy department (or allergy nurse brought to patient). He is then given a *thorough* consultation concerning all the "hows, whys, whats, and how much."

It is of vital importance for the patient to understand, well ahead of testing time, exactly what is involved. He should be told of *basic* problems that could occur but not involved details. What causes allergy? What could be causing his allergy?

It is extremely important that the patient knows exactly how much money is involved for the test and first few weeks of treatment. Do not start working with a patient who will then have to stop in a few weeks because he cannot afford to continue shots. These are the "drop-outs" who ad-

RAST Patient Consult

Your doctor has suggested that allergy is probably a major cause of your problems. Therefore, a complete allergy workup and management program must be started for you.

The first step is to find out exactly what is causing your allergies. Some of the common causes are pollens (trees, grasses, and weeds) and inhalants such as house dust, mold, animal hair, feathers, and foods.

The method being used to test you is the Radio Allergo Sorbent Test method (RAST), developed to assist your physician in diagnosing allergic conditions.

After the laboratory blood testing has been completed, you will return, and your physician will explain to you which allergens are causing your problem. The nurse in the allergy department will then do two or three test wheals on your upper arm to determine that the mixture is the correct strength for your particular system.

We then begin your treatment. This consists of two shots per week for two to three weeks; then one shot per week for the first year. The status of your treatment will be determined and your injections may be moved to once every other week.

If food allergies are a part of your problems, you will be treated by omitting the food.

You must realize that if you use tobacco your allergy management will not be as successful as it could be if you were a nontobacco user. Therefore, every effort should be made to give up this habit before you become involved with allergy testing and treatment. Even if you are a nonsmoker, tobacco smoke in the home or office will affect treatment. Cigarettes should be kept out of the environment of an allergic patient.

Remember, allergy problems are inherited and therefore cannot be cured, only controlled. And this control will occasionally be interrupted by such occurrences as colds, infection, fatigue, nervous tension, and sudden temperature changes. These interruptions should not discourage you because they will usually be only temporary and your improvement will continue as usual.

The fee for your testing will be about ______. Insurance will be filed for you at your request. After your insurance company has paid, you will be responsible for the remainder of the bill. Your shots will cost ______. The first few weeks of your allergy treatment should be at our office, if at all possible. If you live out of town, you may take your medicine with you or to your family doctor after we have arrived at a maintenance dose of your treatment. But, of course, we prefer to give your treatment shots at our office.

If you have any questions regarding the testing, please feel free to call us.

vertise that your office is "expensive" and "does not help" (box above).

Scheduling. If allergy testing is just being set up, your office should be doing only pollen and inhalant testing. You should definitely not start any type of food testing at this point. In the beginning, you and your technician should test only one patient in the morning and one in the afternoon. Since your initial testing should begin on a no. 6 dilution, the test will naturally take longer. The relative inexperience of you and your technician will also slow you down. As you speed up your techniques, one technician can test two patients in the morning; thus, one test could be done at 9:00 and another at 10:30.

In our office, two technicians can, if necessary, do 16 tests a day—each technician testing two patients at 9:00, two at 10:30, two at 1:30, and two at 3:30; however, this could be done only if another nurse or technician is present for injection therapy and counseling. With the introduction and ease of RAST testing, this is usually no longer necessary to do.

Drugs. There are many widespread ideas as to what drugs affect allergy testing, how long drugs should be kept from a patient, and what drugs patients are allowed to continue before the test. We are reporting here to you strictly on experience. We have tried keeping a patient off a particular *antihistamine* one day, 3 days, and 5 days and have found that, to obtain what we consider an accurate skin test, that patient must be kept off a particular antihistamine at least 6 to 7 days. This also includes most "over the counter" medications, cough drops, nose sprays, some mouthwashes, cold tablets, and even aspirin combination drugs. We have proved this to ourselves by testing a patient on a particular day, finding negative results, and retesting that patient 6 days later to find a positive test. Some offices keep patients off a drug only 3 days and are successful.

Cortisone.—The patient should be kept off a long-acting cortisone at least 30 days, even longer if he has taken cortisone for a long period of time. Short-acting steroids do not require more than a 2-week wait.

Hismanal.—The patient should be kept off at least 30 days. This drug, as well as several other histamines, have a long life. Readers should refer to the PDR for information regarding specific antihistamines.

Tranquilizers and other depressant drugs.—Even though we have no strict rules, we try to keep the patient off these drugs for 24 to 48 hours, depending on the individual situation. Consideration is given to how long a patient has been on a particular drug.

At the end of the patient consult, an appointment is made for the patient to return. He is then given the "short" patient consult sheet on which we have written the test fee, injection costs, and appointment date for 2 weeks. The patient is instructed to *reread* the sheet before returning to the office.

THE TEST PREPARATION

Physical plant

Where to test. You will need: (1) a place to test, (2) a place to mix treatment and testing sets, and (3) a place to give injections

This can be, as in our office, separate rooms, or, as when we started, one tiny little room in which everything is done. Testing can be done in an examination room if one can be spared. If there is more than one physician in your office, an examination room can be used while one doctor is in surgery. You may also use a little corner of your lounge area or even the lab. All you need are two chairs and a table. This is not ideal, of course, but it is a start.

You *must* not test a patient if the doctor is not physically present in the office, i.e., not "across the street" in surgery.

Equipment. The equipment needed will probably be in your office already. If you do set up a separate room, there are several considerations:

1. If a location is available, a refrigerator *near* your department is excellent. We keep all the testing sets and patients' treatment sets in the refrigerator.
2. A large comfortable bar stool is ideal for the patient. A stool for the nurse should be one that will raise and lower easily.
3. Seating space should be available nearby for the family of the patient, preferably out of the room in which you are working.

Supplies

Below is a list of everything needed to begin allergy practice.

Exact allergens needed. You will need 30 cc of common, daily used allergens. Smaller amounts of more rarely used extracts will be needed, usually 10 cc at a time. (As your practice grows, you might find it necessary to have autogenous extracts made for you, such as Georgia's wood dust or Mobile's grain dust.) As soon as possible, extracts should be ordered on a yearly basis. The representative from the company of your choice will assist you in determining the amounts needed.

Other supplies.

1. 5 cc empty vials used for mixing individual patient treatment sets
2. 5 cc vials with 4 cc. phenolated albumin saline for mixing testing and treatment sets
3. 100 cc bottles bulk phenolated albumin saline

Most of the miscellaneous items are self explanatory. The new color-coded systems are great help in labeling bottles, especially for new offices.

In our office, we now use the B-D 27 G ½ inch regular bevel allergy pack for all skin testing and injections. We order the 26 G ⅜ inch intradermal bevel needle for mixing only. Both size needles are needed.

Tiered racks are more convenient but certainly not vital, for testing and treatment sets. The flat lucite or wooden ones will serve the same purpose.

Nearly all of these items can be ordered from your allergy company or purchased at your local medical equipment dealer or office supply store (box on p 373).

Mixing

Not enough importance can be placed on the need for an absolutely undisturbed time allotment for the preparation of testing sets, treatment sets, and individual patient's medication. This is a tedious and exacting responsibility and must be done with extreme care and caution (box on p. 374).

In our situation, no testing is done on Wednesday. On this day, two technicians prepare all the treatment sets, prepare mailouts, and update testing and treatment sets. This cannot be done in the hustle and bustle of a busy period of consultation, injections, and patient problems.

Computer records are checked, and allergy medicine will not be sent to a patient if he has not seen the doctor in 6 months. A reminder letter is sent so that an appointment can be made well ahead of time.

THE TEST

Method

The patient is here, sitting in the chair, ready to be tested. He is going to be sitting here for approximately 2 hours, as is the nurse; therefore, of prime importance is having both patient and nurse in a comfortable, pleasant atmosphere. For many years, we used an SMR chair; however, we now have a furniture store bar stool for the patient and a surgery stool for our use. The patient's arms and the testing equipment

Supplies Needed for Beginning Pollen and Inhalant Testing

Equipment

Chair for patient that can easily be turned—bar stool with arms works great!
Chair for technician
Shelves or portable cart for supplies
Trash can
Refrigerator

Antigen

10 to 30 cc vials of all allergens
Individual molds
Penicillium, Cladosporium, Halminthosporium, Aspergillus, Alternaria, Candida
Any other special area mixture
5 cc vial of:
Histamine phosphate (2.75 mg per 5 ml) (College Pharmacy, 1-800-748-2263)
Acetone-precipitated dust mix
House dust mites
Ragweed mix (giant)
2 to 3 individual weeds (for your area)
2 to 3 individual trees (for your area)
2 to 3 individual grasses (for your area)
Cat epithelium
Dog dander

Cytograms

Slides
Caligiswabs
Aqua Net regular hold spray
Bunsen burner or hair dryer
Wright-Giemsa stain
Buffer
Forceps
Microscope
Tray and slide holder

Vials

4 gross sterile 5 cc vials (size 5 to 22 small neck)—empty
2 gross 5 cc vials with 4 cc phenolated albumin saline
2 100 cc bottles bulk phenolated albumin saline
1 30 cc bottle 50% glycerine

Miscellaneous

2 × 2 gauze squares—2 packages of 200 (nonsterile)
Alcohol—4 bottles
Labels (white and various colors)
Wide Scotch tape
Cotton balls
Large three-ring notebook for treatment sheets
Printed testing and treatment sheets
2 cases B-D allergy trays for mixing (26G × ⅜ ")
2 cases B-D allergy trays for testing and treatment (27G × ½ inch)
2 tiered racks for test and treatment sets
Racks for patient's medicine—Wooden or Lucite
10 minute timer
Mailing bags or boxes
Metal trays for syringes
Metal containers for cotton balls

should be in easy reach of the nurse. Good lighting is essential. It is also essential that the nurses (as well as other employees in the allergy department) wear no scented cosmetics, hair sprays, or make up. Absolutely no smoking is allowed in our building.

1. Have the patient sign the consent for skin testing. This can be done at the same time of test scheduling or at the beginning of the test. This is especially necessary when seeing students or any patient who is not responsible for his own decisions.
2. Roll up the sleeve and clean both upper arms with alcohol; dry with a 2 × 2 gauze sponge.
3. Prepare patient's arm by initialing symbols for all allergens to be tested.
4. Follow the same procedure on the left arm for whatever allergens you decide best for your area.
5. From test rack, remove all the no. 6 bottles of each allergen mixture and place them within your reach.
6. Withdraw about 0.05 cc of the first allergen into the syringe (exact amount is *not* important).
7. Look at syringe and turn needle so that the bevel is toward you—it is important for you to *see* this bevel.
8. While holding skin taut, inject approximately 0.01 cc intradermally to make each wheal 4 mm in diameter.
9. Proceed with remaining allergens to be tested.
10. When all 4 mm wheals have been made for that particular dilution, set timer for *10 minutes* and wait. This is an excellent time for the nurse to delve further into the patient's past allergy history or possible food problems.

Mixing Test or Treatment Sets

1:20 concentrate—most pollen allergens
1:10 concentrate—most inhalant allergens, foods,
—special mixtures

	1:20 concentrate	1:10 concentrate
dilution no.1	4.00 cc. diluent 1.00 cc. allergen	4.00 cc. diluent * {.50 cc. additional} {diluent} .50 cc. allergen concentrate 5.00 cc. Total

From this point on, mix both identically

dilution no.2	4.00 cc.	diluent	4.00 cc
	1.00 cc.	no.1 dilution	1.00 cc
	5.00 cc		5.00 cc
dilution no.3	4.00 cc.	diluent	4.00 cc
	1.00 cc.	no.2 dilution	1.00 cc
	5.00 cc		5.00 cc
dilution no.4	4.00 cc.	diluent	4.00 cc
	1.00 cc.	no.3 dilution	1.00 cc
	5.00 cc		5.00 cc
dilution no.5	4.00 cc.	diluent	4.00 cc
	1.00 cc.	no.4 dilution	1.00 cc
	5.00 cc		5.00 cc
dilution no.6	4.00 cc.	diluent	4.00 cc
	1.00 cc.	no.5 dilution	1.00 cc
	5.00 cc		5.00 cc

This can be mixed to higher dilutions if needed.

For testing and treatment, phenolated albumin saline should be used as the diluent. The dilutions should be mixed to at least the no.6 dilution but can be mixed up to no.10 until you establish the toxicity of the allergen for your geographic area. This you will learn only after you have started your testing program.

The stability of the allergen is directly related to the degree of its dilution. The testing and treatment sets are valid up to 3 months, if mixed and diluted properly (no.5 and no.6 have to be remixed every two weeks).

*Other allergens, marked ______should be mixed as 1:50 dilutions (or simply as the 1:20 concentrates are mixed.)

11. At the end of 10 minutes, measure each wheal, record each result on the test sheet, and proceed to next stronger dilution.
12. The first dilution injected should result in a nonreacting (5 or 6 mm) wheal. *The first 7 mm wheal produced is a reaction but is not necessarily the endpoint.*
13. *When a 9 mm wheal is produced, the endpoint is the 7 mm wheal immediately preceding that 9 mm wheal. Stop the testing of each allergen as the endpoint is reached and record that endpoint on the test sheet.*
14. Proceed with the test until an endpoint has been reached on all allergens being tested.

Problems in testing

Routine. Various writers have elaborated on which allergens to test, on what dilution to start, and how to administer screening tests. Our method, essentially the *same* testing pattern for *all* patients, alleviates these decision. But more important, it also eliminates the possibility of missing an important allergic factor in the workup.

For example, if a patient shows symptoms of dust allergy and only tests for dust are ordered, then mold allergy could be overlooked, even though mold allergy could be an even more vital part of treatment than dust. The patient is usually unaware of which allergic problems exist in his area or in his particular environment.

For safety in doing skin endpoint titration, our office always begins testing all adults on the no. 6 dilutions for all allergens. Since children under 3 years old have not yet developed antibodies to pollens, they are initially tested for dusts, molds, and foods only. Pollens can be tested at a later time on an individual basis. Since children usually endpoint at stronger dilutions, we begin testing on the no. 4 dilution instead of no. 6.

There are also numerous screens one can utilize including:

1. Qualitative yes/no—one disc with 12 allergens per allergy group
2. Semiqualitative—a separate disc with mixture of all groups.
3. A serum dipstick test—with a separate test for inhalants and foods
4. Mini-screen—geographically relevant selected allergens

Our feeling, however, is that, if a thorough history and physical examination are taken, these tests are not critical. The RAST test, using either enzyme or isotope, can be used as a screen or can be used to base starting treatment.

Exceptions.

1. Children 3 years or under are usually tested only for inhalants and foods, and the skin test is started on a no.4 dilution. These children are tested for all pollens at a later time if they continue to have problems, especially if the mother reports added symptoms when they are exposed to grass, weeds, or trees in the spring or fall.

2. Patients with extremely high susceptibility, who know, from previous experience, that they become totally incapacitated during spring or fall pollen season are an exception. You may still begin testing on the no.6 (1:312,000 dilution). If *overreaction* occurs (a wheal 8 to 9 mm or longer), one may simply continue with a weaker, rather than a stronger, dilution to find the endpoint of reaction (or better called a "starting dose"). One may also choose to start only one or two allergens together, rather than the usual 8 to 10. If necessary, the test might be divided into several sessions.
3. Test variations—to repeat one of the most important concepts which we are trying to teach:

   When a 9 mm wheal is produced, the endpoint is the 7 mm wheal immediately preceding the 9 mm wheal. Stop the testing of each allergen as the endpoint of reaction is reached.

   However, now that we have stated an "absolute fact," let us consider the definite possibility that this "absolute" has variations.

   The procedure that has been taught over the years implies that when a test wheal is applied, a specific-sized wheal will *always* result after 10 minutes. This simply does *not* happen. As a matter of fact, it is much *more* infrequent to find the routine 5-7-9 patterns which we have all been taught.

   Therefore, we submit the following patterns, *not* as unusual or bizarre reactions but as various types of normal patterns you may possibly see:

Test Dilution no.	*6*	*5*	*4*	*3*	*2*	*1*	*EP*
Example 1	5	5	6	7	8	9	3
Example 2	5	5	5	6	8		3
Example 3	5	5	5	5	9		3
Example 4	5	7	7	7	9		3
Example 5	5	5	5	7	9		3

As you can see, here are at least five distinctly different whealing patterns, all showing an endpoint on the no.3 (or 1:2,500) dilution. We have seen these responses on five separate patients but also have seen these five different responses from individual allergens *on the same patient.*

Example 1

In this example, the no.6 and no.5 dilutions produced a 5 mm wheal. The no.4 dilution produced a 6 mm wheal. The no.3 dilution produced a 7 mm wheal. This 7 mm wheal is considered to be the first reactive wheal; that is, the first wheal which has grown at least 2 mm more than the initial 4 mm wheal which was injected. Following that, the no.2 dilution produced an 8 mm wheal. *The no.3 dilution with the 7 mm wheal is the endpoint.*

Example 2

Numbers 6, 5, and 4 dilutions produced 5 mm wheals. The no.3 dilution produced a 6 mm wheal. The no.2 dilution produced an 8 mm wheal. *Therefore, that no.3 is considered the EP, even though a 7 mm wheal was not produced.* Do not continue on to the no.1 dilution and do not attempt to treat on the no 2 dilution. Symptoms of overtreatment could be anticipated if a patient is treated on a dilution having an 8 mm wheal.

Example 3

In this situation, 5 mm wheals are produced on dilutions nos. 6, 5, 4, and 3. Dilution no.2 produced a 9 mm wheal. On reapplying dilution no.3, we found a wheal that is definitely *larger* than 6 mm, but smaller than 7 mm. It could be classed from 6.1 to 6.9 mm. We label it "6 slash 7" or 6/7. If that 6/7 is followed by a 8 or 9 mm wheal, it is the endpoint. If it is followed by a 7 mm wheal, it is not the endpoint. *The endpoint is the no.3 dilution.*

Example 4

Sometimes described as a "plateau," the no.6 dilution produced a 5 mm wheal. Nos. 5, 4, and 3 all produced 7 mm. Do not stop, however, until a progressive wheal after reacting 7 mm wheal is produced. When the no.2 dilution produced a 9 mm wheal, we knew the EP was the no.3 dilution; in this case, the third reactive wheal is produced.

Example 5

This is what is usually described as the "normal" whealing pattern. Dilution nos. 6, 5, and 4 produced 5 mm nonreacting wheals. The no.3 dilution produced a 7 mm wheal, followed by a 9 mm wheal on the no.2 dilution. *The endpoint is the no.3 dilution.*

Two other whealing patterns bear some discussion.

Test Dilution no.	*6*	*5*	*4*	*3*	*2*	*1*	*EP*
Example 6	5	5	6	7	15+		3
Example 7	5	5	7+	(9)			4

Example 6

Dilution nos. 6, 5, 4, and 3 were applied and showed a normal whealing pattern. When dilution no.2 was applied, a "flash" reaction occurred. (This "flash" reaction has been described as strictly a skin reaction and having no significance regarding the general allergic sensitivity of the patient. We have found, however, that it is the patient who is supersensitive who has this flash reaction. It is also the same patient who, after the testing is finished and the treatment started, seems to have problems adjusting to treatment and to dosages.) We have been taught to count back the number of dilutions which would normally give a 7 mm wheal. In this case, no.3 would give a 13 mm wheal; no.4–11 mm; no.5—9 mm; no.6—7 mm; and the no.7 dilution—5 mm wheal.

We have now found that this procedure usually accomplishes nothing. We almost always find the same type pattern repeated in the second test. A flash reaction almost always occurs again at exactly the same dilution.

Therefore, we have learned to back up (or move to the left to a weaker dilution) only *one* dilution. In almost all cases, this has neutralized the wheal. We must also be certain we have neutralized the symptoms the patient could possibly have developed.

Neutralizing is a well-established and clinically well understood phenomenon that is not well explained immunologically. Current theories include Trevino's work.

A skin test with a 4 mm intradermal wheal that grows to 15 mm or larger is called a "flash reaction," has pseudopods, considerable erythema, and provokes symptoms such as severe itching, runny nose, headaches, etc.

Neutralizing this large wheal is desirable since the large symptomatic wheal will disappear quickly and provoked symptoms will stop. Other alternatives to neutralization are the use of epinephrine, steroids, and antihistamines or simply waiting.

Neutralization, however, stops the allergic reaction and is far more satisfactory. This involves injecting a 5 times weaker dilution of the same allergen intradermally and waiting 10 minutes to see the response. If it is the correct neutralizing dose, the original large bound wheal will disappear and the new wheal will not grow. If the neutralizing dose is not correct, continue to administer 5 times weaker dilutions until symptoms disappear and the patient feels relieved. Testing is terminated at this point.

Example 7

We have called this reaction on the no.4 dilution a "7+" wheal. It is a skin reaction which we find is always followed by a 9 mm wheal. An experienced technician may *assume* this 9 mm wheal (which is in parentheses) and not proceed to the no.3 dilution. That "7+" is very red, more than normally raised, and usually erythematous. It frequently precedes a flash reaction; however, this testing procedure is to be used only after adequately experiencing whealing reactions.

Fig 33-3 shows a normal positive skin endpoint titration test.

Boxes on pp 378-379 and Fig. 33-4 explain the mixing of individual patient treatment vials.

Counseling

At the end of the test, the patient is told about positive findings and given a short information sheet which simply lists the allergic reactions but goes into no detail. No particular counseling is done at this time. The patient is told, however, that on the first return visit, an individual write-up of his particular case will be prepared and given to him. He is told to read the entire report carefully so that any questions he has can be answered. Patients rarely have questions if the case report is complete.

If the patient is tested by in vitro testing, blood will have been drawn previously, and when the patient returns, RAST test wheals will be done and the same type counseling instructions given.

Dosage schedule

Most patients will begin immunotherapy with a 0.05 cc dose of each vial of his individual treatment set. Injections will be given twice weekly (Monday and Thursday or Tuesday and Friday), increasing by 0.05 cc each injection. It does not work well to rely on the patient's judgment as to injections needed at the onset of treatment. The symptoms usually will not have changed enough during the first few weeks for the patient to be aware of whether or not an injection is necessary. Besides, if the patient is being tested and treated starting "out of season," there would be no symptoms.

After 0.25 cc is given (the fifth injection), the patient is instructed to wait one week, *if* his symptoms have not recurred. At this dosage, if the patient is receiving therapy outside our office, he is asked to call so we can follow his progress. He will then proceed with dosages as instructed.

Dosage then increases to 0.30 cc, 0.35 cc, 0.40 cc, 0.45 cc, and 0.50 cc of the treatment vials. After the patient has reached 0.50 cc and maintained that amount for at least two refills of his treatment vials, all "endpoints" or strengths are arbitrarily moved one dilution stronger. The dosage is dropped to 0.10 cc and increases to 0.50 cc again on this 5 times stronger dilution. (Fig. 33-5)

This "stronger dilution" concept involves moving the initial treatment dose, as tolerated, to the concentrates. While

Patient's Name Jane Dixon Date 5-24-90

Allergen	10	9	8	7	6	5	4	3	2	1	E.P. Dil.	Comments
Grasses												
Bermuda					5	5	6	(7)	9	→	3	
Fescue					5	(7)	9	→	→	→	5	
Weeds												
Ragweed					5	(7)	9	→	→	→	5	
Eng. Plantain					6	7	(7)	9	→	→	4	
Trees												
Oak					6	6	6	6	(7)	9→	2	
Elm					6	6	6	6/7	(7)	9→	2	
Molds												
Penicillium					5	5	5	(7)	9	→	3	
Cladosporium					5	(7)	9	→	→	→	5	
Aspergillus					5	5	(7)	9	→	→	4	
Candida					5	5	5	6	7	7	—	
Alternaria					5	5	5	5	(7)	9→	2	
Helminth.					5	5	6	6	7	7	—	
Epidermals												
Cat					5	5	7	7	7	7	—	
Dog					5	5	6	6	6	7	—	
Dust												
Farinae					5	(7)	9	→	→	→	5	
Pteronyssinus					5	5	5	5	7	7	—	
House dust mix				5	(7)	9	→	→	→	→	6	
Other												

FIG 33-3
Patient testing sheet.

the initial doses will often relieve symptoms, it has been shown that true "immunization" does not begin until the treatment doses are in the concentrates, no.1 or no.2 dilutions. This dose can be the "symptom-relieving dose" as well as the "maximum tolerated dose."

During the first year of therapy, at no point is the patient allowed to wait longer than one week for an injection.

Occasionally, a patient whose symptoms are controlled decides that he does not need to continue the injection therapy. After a year or more of therapy, he might take his-

Computing Individual Patient Treatment Sets

1. One treatment dose of any allergen is 0.50 cc of the endpoint dilution. This is an arbitrary figure, used first by Dr. Rinkle for ease of calculations, and an amount that, by trial and error, works well. (Dr. Rinkle, in his original articles, called it a "50X" dose, and that nomenclature remains in some older literature.)
2. When the endpoint dilution is determined, the volume is reduced to the lowest possible measurable quantity. This is done because an arm reaction is less likely with a smaller amount of allergen. This is simple to accomplish in our measuring methods since the SET technique makes each successive dilution change by multiples of 5.
3. Since it would be impractical to make only one treatment dose of an allergen, multiply by 10 the amount of allergen in one treatment dose. This yields 10 treatment doses of that individual allergen.
4. Since most patients are allergic to a number of pollens and inhalants, it is also not practical to give a separate injection for each allergen. Therefore, treatment doses of individual allergens are combined. A sufficient quantity of diluent is then added to those mixed allergens so that one combined treatment dose equals 0.50 cc, a number easy to add and multiply.
5. Multiplied by 10 doses, the amount mixed for a patient is 5.0 cc. This will yield 10 combined treatment doses of 0.50 cc each.
6. Patients may have more than one vial depending on the endpoint (or RAST class) and the number of positive findings. The allergens should be bottled (mixed together) depending on endpoint or RAST class rather than category or family. This allows for dosage increase on one vial, even if an arm reaction occurs with another vial. Vials are usually mixed with 1, 2, or 3 endpoints or RAST class in one vial and endpoints 4 and 5 in a second vial. In some cases, the allergens are even separated into three vials.

injections each month for a few months, then stop altogether. Suddenly, 2 or 3 months later (usually a change in season), when his symptoms recur, he returns, asking for treatment again.

If that patient has been on treatment for 10 to 12 months and returning symptoms are slight, therapy can be restarted by an experienced technician. The treatment should be restarted at 0.10 cc of each vial. If the patient gets symptomatic improvement, the next injection can be given in 3 to 5 days and can be 0.20 cc, followed by 0.30 cc in 8 to 10 days, then 0.40 cc or 0.50 cc in 10 to 14 days, or as needed. If, however, the patient returns and has had no injections for 6 months, the physician must see the patient before any therapy is reinstituted, and the dosage schedule must be followed as it was after the original testing.

If the original test was performed during a different season of the year, retesting might be warranted. If testing was done during the same season, one could conceivably start injections again on last year's endpoints, but with a warning to the patient of the possible need for retesting if response is not fairly rapid. Children must be retested every few years.

In children, retesting may be needed if the child has gone through puberty. In adults or children, immunotherapy may be stopped when the patient has been symptom free for 6-12 months. This usually occurs when treatment has been in progress for 3 to 4 years.

Records

Keeping allergy records, as well as chart records, is of vital importance in a therapy program. The technician must, at a moment's glance, be able to see: (1) how long the patient has been under treatment, (2) when any recheck was done, (3) any past local or systemic reactions, (4) the amount of the current treatment dose, and (5) when he last saw the doctor.

If he must first stop and look up the chart to go through reams of records for this information, overall efficiency will be limited. Therefore, a treatment sheet, in a loose-leaf notebook kept in the allergy department, is a simple answer.

The patient signs in at the front desk, receives a routing slip, goes directly to the allergy department, and hands the routing slip to the nurse. The nurse carefully checks the name on the slip and finds that patient's sheet, questions progress, records today's dose, gives the injection, records the charge, and the patient is quickly on his way.

THE FOLLOW-UP

Case records

The most important way to assure the "allegiance" of allergy patients is good follow-up. This begins with the patient's first injection as he is questioned about results of treatment, problems with injections, or any questions he might have. The drop-out rate in our allergy clinic is very low because of our continued attention and concern about the patient's problems and his treatment.

The nurse or technician who administers the injection is an extremely important part of the allergy team. He must not simply look at a schedule and administer a set dosage but, after intelligent questioning of the patient, make a decision as to whether to increase, decrease, stabilize, or in any other way change the treatment. This person also has the responsibility of deciding if a returning patient might

Instructions for Mixing Test or Treatment Sets

1. Arrange and label 5 cc bottles for each allergen you want in your testing set. The bottles contain 4 cc of phenolated albumin saline. Example: first group—ragweed. Label six bottles ragweed—nos. 1 to 6, and the date. Do this for all allergens to be included in the test.
2. Refer to our sheet no.10 labeled "Mixing Test or Treatment Set." There are two columns, one for 1:20 concentrates and one for 1:10 concentrates.
3. The left-hand column instructions are for mixing most pollen allergens which are 1:20 concentrates.
   For dilution no.1, use a 5 cc vial with 4.0 cc of premeasured phenolated albumin saline. To that 4.0 cc of saline, add 1.0 cc of the allergen concentrate. This gives a total volume of 5.0 cc in bottle no.1
   With bottle no.2 in readiness, withdraw 1.0 cc from bottle no.1. Inject this 1.0 cc into bottle no.2 and rinse syringe 5 to 6 times. With bottle no.3 in readiness, withdraw 1.0 cc from bottle no.2 and inject into bottle no.3. Continue with the same method to as high a dilution as you wish to mix (in most cases, a no.6 dilution).
4. The right-hand column instructions are for mixing most inhalant allergens, foods, and specials mixtures and are 1:10 concentrates.
   Begin with a 4.0 cc bottle of premeasured phenolated albumin saline. To this *add an addition 0.50 cc of albumin saline* from a separate bottle (usually from a 100 cc bottle included in your supplies list). The no.1 bottle now has 4.5 cc of albumin saline. To this add 0.50 cc of allergen concentrate. We now have a total volume of 5.0 cc of the no.1 mixture.
   With bottle no.2 in readiness, withdraw 1.0 cc from bottle no.1 and inject into bottle no.2, rinsing syringe 5 to 6 times. Repeat this procedure to bottle no.6 or as high as you wish to mix.
5. Testing and treatment sets are identical.
6. Dilution no.1 is the most used dilution, since it is used to make the remainder of the six dilutions. Therefore, one may exhaust this dilution more frequently. You may then, after allergy patient load has increased, wish to increase the amount of dilution no.1 mixed. This can easily be done by making a 10 cc bottle of no.1. It is possible to order premeasured 8 cc bottles of saline. To make a 10 cc bottle of 1:20 allergen, start with an 8 cc bottle of phenolated albumin saline. Add 2.0 cc of allergen concentrate for a total volume of 10 cc of no.1.
   For 1:10 allergens, add to the 8 cc bottle of diluent 1.0 cc of additional diluent and 1.0 cc. of allergen concentrate for a total volume of 10 cc. Remember, however, in proceeding to dilutions 2, 3, 4, etc. to add only 1.0 cc of allergen for each 4.0 cc of diluent for *both* 1:10 and 1:20 concentrates.
7. An important point to remember: the stability of the allergen is directly related to the amount of its dilution. The testing set is valid up to 3 months if kept refrigerated, but within the next 3-month period, the no.1 dilution is obviously more stable than no.2 to 6.

have a possible infection and need the doctor's attention, need any rechecking, any additional testing, or is simply having a flare-up of seasonal allergies, or allergic "overexposure."

The patient is instructed in the case history booklet to see the attending physician *every 6 months,* even though no problems exist at that time. Each patient must be assured that he has not been forgotten and simply left to the nurse or technicians for treatment. He is assured that his physician is available to him when needed.

Conversely, to assure the physician that he will not be besieged by allergy patients all day, an extremely important beginning of your allergy department is to find a person who is interested in learning absolutely everything he can about allergy. That person must not be saddled with x-ray, lab work, insurance, etc., but be given ample time to spend in the allergy department. As his knowledge increases through visits to other offices, allergy meetings, and reading current allergy literature, he will be able to take over the long "search and seek" sessions needed to analyze a particular allergy problem.

Instructions for out-of-town doctors

If the patient will not be returning to your office for treatment, arrangements must be made for follow-up injections with his local doctor or neighborhood nurse.

Many problems occur because doctors and nurses unfamiliar with TB syringes and measurements will mistake dosages. Therefore, not only do we show the patients the syringe used (plus supply these syringes along with the allergy medication), we include a picture of the syringe with dosages shown at the side. One might consider this an insult to a professional's intelligence, but, insults aside, the difference in 0.10 cc and 1.0 cc could cause problems in a highly allergic patient. These mistakes did happen in our area many times before we finally made our instructions so basic that a high schooler could understand them.

The dosage instructions are extremely simple and self

Name: Jane Dixon Date: 5/25/90

RAST-1 Endpoints		Bottle 1			Bottle 2			Bottle 3		
Bermuda	3	Ber 1	.02	.20cc	Fes. 3	.02	.20	Mite 3	.02	.20
Fescue	5	Oak c	.02	.20	Rag 3	.02	.20	Dust4	.02	.20
Ragweed	5	Elm c	.02	.20	Eng Pl.2	.02	.20			
Eng. Pl.	4	Pen. 1	.02	.20	Clad 3	.02	.20			
Oak	2	Alt. c	.01	.10	Asp. 2	.02	.20			
Elm	2									
Pen.	3									
Clad.	5									
Asp.	4									
Alt.	2									
Mite.	5									
House dust	6									
		Conc.	.09	.90	Conc.	.10	1.00	Conc.	.04	.40
		Dil.	.41	4.10	Dil.	.40	4.00	Dil.	.46	4.60
		TOTAL	.50	5.00	TOTAL	.50	5.00	TOTAL	.50	5.00

Comments: 5/25/90 Test Wheals 1- 7mm 2- 8mm 3-7 mm

5/28/90	-First Inj	.05cc	- no problems
5/31/90	-Second Inj.	.10cc	- "
6/4/90	3rd	.15cc	"
6/7	↓	.20cc	↓
6/11	etc.	.25cc	
6/14		.30cc	
6/18		.35cc	
6/25		.40cc	
7/2		.45cc	
7/9		.50cc	
7/16		.50cc	
7/23		.50cc	
8/6		.50cc	

FIG 33-4
Patient treatment sheet.

Name ______________________________ Vial # ______________
Date ______________

______ Test wheal Response after 10 minutes ______ mm.*
Most physicians choose to wait a 2-3 day period before beginning injections

______	1st dose	.05 cc. SQ	Wait 3-4 days
______	2nd dose	.10 cc. SQ	Wait 3-4 days
______	3rd dose	.15 cc. SQ	Wait 3-4 days
______	4th dose	.20 cc. SQ	Wait 3-4 days
______	5th dose call allergy department after this dose	.25 cc. SQ	Wait one (1) week-
______	6th dose	.30 cc. SQ	Wait one (1) week
______	7th dose	.35 cc. SQ	Wait one (1) week
______	8th dose	.40 cc. SQ	Wait one (1) week
______	9th dose	.45 cc. SQ	Wait one (1) week
______	Maintain at	.50 cc SQ	Wait one (1) week* *

* - See INSTRUCTIONS FOR VIAL TESTING

* * - When .50 cc. at RAST -1 is reached, the treatment sets can be mixed at RAST 0 (or 5 times stronger), and dosage starting at.10 cc. Injections are then increased at .05 cc. intervals. (You may back up to .05 cc. for the first dose of newly mixed bottle if you wish.)

ID — Intradermal SQ — Subcutaneous

Using a 27 gauge 1/2" TB syringe, remove the prescribed amount of allergen from each bottle. Your patient may have one, two, or three bottles of medication of the same dilution. Allergens are separated into different vials based on severity of allergy. If your patient receives more than one injection each time he comes in, it is important to keep track of which injection was given in which site. The reason for this is that in case a reaction occurs from one of the vials, you need to determine which vial is causing that reaction.

The injection is to be given in the fat in the back of the arm,approximately halfway between the elbow and the shoulder. It is never to be given in the muscle. The extract should be refrigerated. The only reaction there should ever be from these injections is a mild provocation of symptoms and/or redness of the arm (See RULES FOR LOCAL REACTIONS TO ALLERGY INJECTIONS).

FIG 33-5
Patient dosage schedule.

explanatory, but always make the patient understand that if any questions arise or any unusual reactions occur, he (or- the nurse or doctor's office) should feel free to call your office for advice (Fig. 33-6).

Mailouts

While some of our patients receive injections in our office, most of them, because of time or travel restrictions, are unable to come to the office. These patients receive their extracts by US Mail or UPS. A small fee is added to the bill to cover shipping charges.

It is the responsibility of the patient to request more treatment vials.

When the patient calls for treatment vials, if the technician sees that the patient has not been seen by his physician within the prescribed time period, a phone call is made or a post card sent reminding the patient to see the doctor. He is told that his treatment vial will be prepared when his

Patient's name: ____________________

Doctor: ____________________

Office phone number: ____________________

Special instructions: ____________________

____

____

____

HOW TO USE THE ALLERGY SYRINGE

1. Clean top of allergy medicine bottle with alcohol.
2. Twist and remove cap from syringe.
3. Insert needle into center of rubber stopper bottle and draw out medication as instructed.
4. Clean injection site with alcohol.
5. Give injection.
6. At a physician's office, drop needle into Sharps container. At home, replace cap on syringe, put used syringe into plastic bag, and dispose of them safely, or return them to our office for disposal.
7. This is a one (1) cc. needle. The first injection is 0.05 cc. (five-hundredths of one cc.), NOT 0.50 cc. Please read syringe and directions carefully.

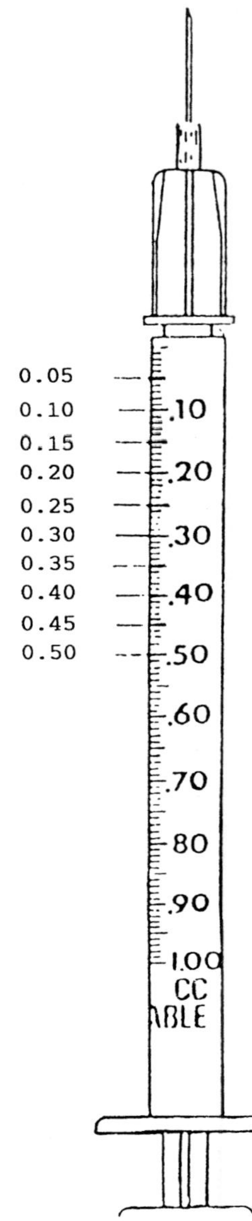

FIG 33-6
Syringe diagram.

physician has seen him again. After the initial 3-month visit, if the patient is totally asymptomatic, he need not see the doctor more than once every 6 months.

Need for food testing

After testing has been done and treatment is in progress, if we find that our patient is having only partial relief of symptoms, we begin to search for additional problems. We have found that these patients usually have food allergy.

In many instances, these problems relate to food allergy. So, while we continue to try to solve any pollen and inhalant problems, we start looking toward the possibility of food allergy as an added problem. Many times we know by history or by nasal cytoprofile that food allergy is possibly a problem (Fig. 33-7).

In any case, we always try first to "control" pollen and inhalant allergies, as well as start food elimination and rotation diets.

Date ____________________ Name ____

FOOD ALLERGY QUESTIONNAIRE

THIS QUESTIONNAIRE IS DESIGNED TO HELP DETERMINE IF SOME OF YOUR SYMPTOMS ARE RELATED TO DISTURBED BODY FUNCTIONS. PLEASE READ EACH QUESTION CAREFULLY; THEN ANSWER APPROPRIATELY.

	1. What foods do you crave or eat often? (Example: More than one glass of Coke, tea, or milk a day.) ____________________
	2. What foods do you dislike? Please list them. Do any foods make you sick? ____________________
1 2 3	3. Are you awakened between the hours of 1:00 a.m. and 5:00 a.m. with the following symptoms: Headache, dizziness, stomach cramps, bloating, or dry cough?
	4. Does any member of your family have hay fever, asthma, hives, chronic skin condition, migraine headache, dizziness, stomach cramps, bloating or dry cough? Which condition? Which family member? ____________________
Y N	5. During childhood, did you have any of the following: Eczema, hay fever, or asthma?
Y N	6. Were you told that you had feeding problems as a baby?
1 2 3	7. Do you have itching of the skin, palate, or roof of the mouth?
1 2 3	8. Do you notice swelling of the ankles, feet, hands, or face on arising in the morning?
1 2 3	9. After a full meal in the middle of the day, do you ever experience fatigue 2-3 hours later?
1 2 3	10. Do you eat snacks frequently between meals?
1 2 3	11. Do you have excessive chilling when a sudden change in temperature occurs?
1 2 3	12. Do you have migraine headaches?
1 2 3	13. Do you have pains in the back of the head?
1 2 3	14. Do you experience gas, bloating, abdominal distension, or cramps?
1 2 3	15. Have you noticed numbness of the face, arms, or legs at periodic intervals for no apparent cause?
1 2 3	16. Do you have drowsiness, headache, or bloating following the ingestion of a cocktail, glass of wine or beer?
Y N	17. Are you allergic to Penicillin?
Y N	18. Do you ever have any diarrhea, even mild or intermittently
Y N	19. Do you ever experience repeated symptoms on awaking in the morning such as headache? Can you make the the headache go away by eating or drinking any particular food such as coffee or Coke? What do you eat? ____________________

FIG 33-7
Food allergy questionnaire.

Y	N	20.	Are there any other reactions or problems you notice with any other particular food? If, so, please list. ____________
Y	N	21.	Are you aware of any symptoms occuring after meals that yoususpect may be due to a food allergy? If yes, please explain symptoms and any suspected foods: ____________ ____________
Y	N	22.	Have you experienced chronic cough?
Y	N		Is it a dry cough?
Y	N		Is it a productive cough?
Y	N		How many coughs in 24 hours on average?

1 = Frequently 2 = Occasionally 3 = Never Y = Yes N = No

FIG 33-7, cont'd
Food allergy questionnaire.

FINALE

We have no disagreements with the methods of testing or treatment used by anyone. Most of our work is patterned after that in other offices. However, we also have had noqualms about changing a technique that does work for us. The course that we have presented is simply a compilation of what we have learned, *by trial and error,* to be the best method of testing and treatment possible for our patients.

If you become involved in allergy work, we sincerely hope that the contents of this course, plus the knowledge gleaned from minds much more experienced than ours, can be taken and instructed to your own patients and their needs and to your type of practice.

REFERENCES

1. Dixon HS: Otolaryngologic Plain Film Radiography, with an Emphasis on the Temporal Bone—How To Do It. Am *J Otolaryngol* 3:, 1982.

34

Pharmacologic Management of Allergic Rhinitis

Helen F. Krause, M.D., F.A.C.S.

Allergy has been described as a great masquerader because it mimics many diseases. Frequently it is mistaken for infection. Also, allergy often involves not just the nose but may manifest itself as chronic fatigue, recurrent otitis media, asthma, skin problems including eczema and urticaria, headaches, gastrointestinal disturbances, or neurologic and musculoskeletal complaints. It may also predispose to recurrent upper respiratory infection.

For those of you not entirely familiar with allergy, it is a state of altered reactivity, that is, hypersensitivity acquired through exposure to a substance foreign to that person's body.

Over 40 million people in the United States have some form of allergy. About 25 million have what they call hay fever. It accounts for about 20% of all primary care visits but is often undiagnosed or treated incorrectly. The National Disease and Therapeutic Index found in 1985 of 1,370,000 visits surveyed, the average otolaryngologist saw 241 patients per year with allergic rhinitis. Of course, general otolaryngologists see more because some, such as head and neck surgeons, rarely see any. This figure has gradually risen each year, especially if we include most of the cases added recently called chronic rhinitis, many of which are probably due to undiagnosed allergy.

DIAGNOSIS OF ALLERGIC RHINITIS

The approach to identifying an allergic patient is having a high index of suspicion. The general and specific ENT allergy history and physical examinations are important. There are a number of differential diagnoses to consider. There may be infection of the upper respiratory tract or hormonal problems such as thyroid disease that must be considered. There may be nutritional deficiencies, cystic fibrosis, anemia, and even iatrogenic disorders.

There are a number of important factors that can influence the expression and severity of the allergy symptoms. The family history of allergy is important as is the actual sensitivity to individual allergens. The presence of infection can influence symptoms as can metabolic changes seen in puberty and pregnancy, stress, active and passive cigarette smoking, and chronic exposure to allergens, as well as exposure to chemicals and foods to which a patient may be allergic. Birth in a certain season appears to be important, related to maturing of the immune system.

In the nose, chronic allergic postnasal drainage must be differentiated from that of vasomotor rhinitis and other nonallergic types of rhinitis. Recurrent or persistent upper respiratory tract infections may suggest underlying allergy. These infections result from edema, the chronic obstruction predisposing to secondary infections. Patients may develop nasal, choanal, or sinus polyposis or recurrent sinusitis.

Allergic symptoms may be transient and mild, requiring no testing and minimal or no treatment, or they may be constant and overwhelming requiring extensive evaluation and the use of a variety of therapeutic modalities. These symptoms may vary both in severity and frequency and they may occur only seasonally or be perennial, that is, all year.

Allergies occur in a genetically predisposed person being stimulated by a foreign protein called an antigen or an allergen entering the body—usually by way of the respiratory tract. Allergens also occasionally enter through the skin, the gastrointestinal tract, other mucus membranes such as the conjunctiva, by injection, and today even by transplantation. The antigens involved are inhalants primarily, but foods and chemicals may also cause allergic symptoms. Occupational allergies are being recognized more frequently also. Latex allergy is more frequently seen now with the use of latex gloves by so many health professionals and others, such as the police.

These allergies begin when antigen in the nose stimulates B lymphocytes to become plasma cells; these then form IgE—a specific antibody which attaches to tissue mast

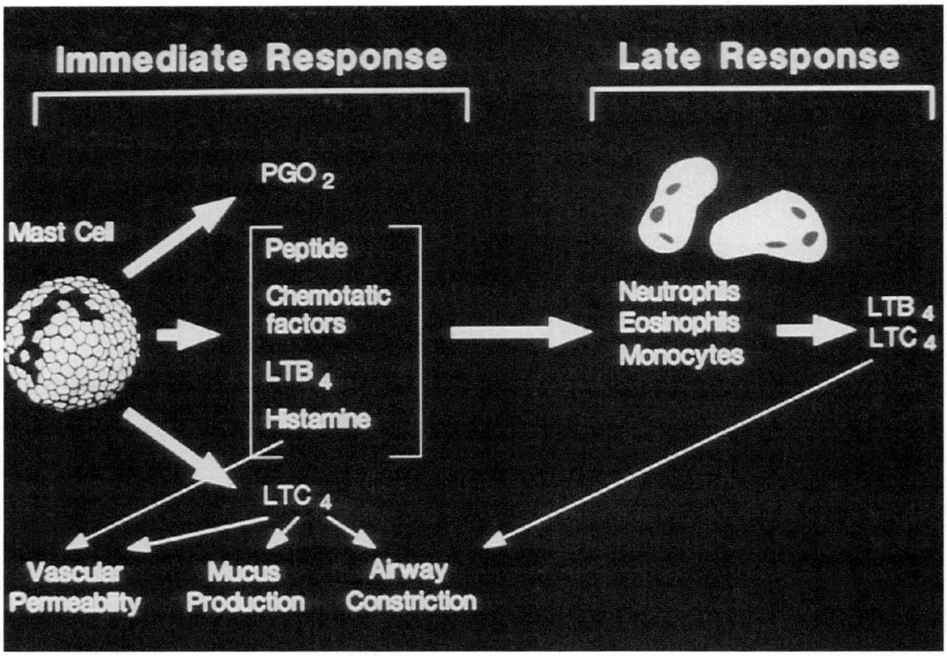

FIG 34-1
The immediate allergic response includes mucosal edema, increased secretions, sneezing, and itching. The inflammatory late response produces marked nasal congestion. (From Krause HF: Diagnostic Patterns in Otolarygic Allergy Symptoms. In *Otolaryngic Allergy and Immunology,* 1989, WB Saunders.)

cells. On repeat exposure, the mast cells are then stimulated by the antigen-IgE antibody complex to degranulate, releasing histamine and other chemicals which act on the nasal mucosa, the lungs, eyes, and skin to produce symptoms. This is very simplified. We now know that other chemical factors are involved and it is these which may produce immediate and late allergic responses.

The nose can produce only certain symptoms no matter what the etiology (Fig. 34-1). The immediate symptoms occurring rapidly include mucosal swelling due to vascular engorgement and tissue edema leading to mild congestion. Rhinorrhea and postnasal drainage are due to increased goblet cell activity and tissue transudation. Sneezing and itching are due to neurogenic reflex stimulation. The late reaction produces marked congestion which occurs several hours after initial exposure to the antigen with no further exposure being necessary. It is a cellular inflammatory reaction which is often more severe than the early reaction. Understanding these reactions and the chemicals producing them becomes important in determining drug therapy. Some pharmacotherapeutic agents will benefit the immediate response only; others will stop or protect against the late reaction.

There are several general body features of allergy to recognize: fatigue is one of the most common complaints which often goes unrecognized. Pruritus, i.e., itching which may be general or of a specific body part, is also common. There may be variations in the severity of the symptoms, when these symptoms occur, as well as frequent susceptibility to upper respiratory tract infection. There are also certain personality characteristics (the type "A") which are described as being typical of allergic patients. They have many concerns about their bodies and are very aware of their symptoms. Allergy patients often have mood swings and variations of energy levels. Many will say that they have frequent emotional and energy ups and downs.

Allergic patients have a number of visible characteristics.[25,35]

The allergic salute may eventually become the linea nasalis—these and mouth and nasal grimacing are all done to relieve the nasal itching. There may be gingival hypertrophy from mouth breathing and dental staining from antibiotic treatment of frequent and early childhood infections. The nares may become chronically irritated. The nasal mucosa may be swollen, pale, or, at times, appear nearly normal. Allergic shiners and Dennie's lines are often seen. Both are due to chronic vascular congestion. The discoloration is secondary to hemosiderin tissue staining. There may also be eyelid edema, conjunctival irritation, and tearing.

In infants and children facial eczema and mouth breathing may be due to food allergy, especially milk. Angioedema is occasionally seen of the lips and eyes—often due to food allergies. Nasal polyps may develop and headaches of a vacuum type may be intense.

The picture of typical adenoid facies (Fig. 34-2) may be seen in children with large tonsils and adenoids or with less

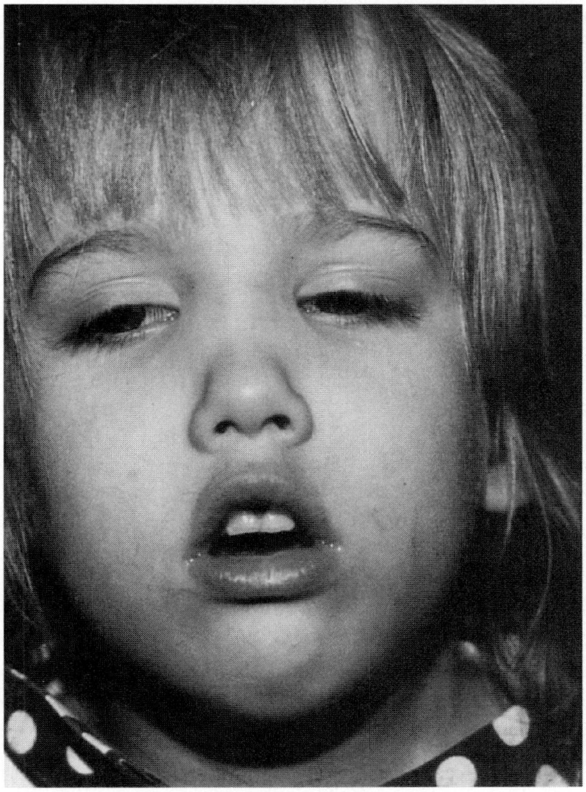

FIG 34-2
Typical "adenoid" facies in a patient with obstructing adenoids or "allergic" facies in a child with small adenoids but chronic nasal obstruction due to allergic rhinitis.[25]

lymphoid hypertrophy but with upper airway obstruction due to allergic nasal edema—this may really be allergic facies. These children usually develop associated high arched palates and may develop acute and even chronic secretory otitis media with secondary infection.

The individual expression of allergy is genetically determined but environmentally influenced. For example, if a patient is predisposed to ragweed allergy but lives on the West Coast, symptoms will not be present until moving to the eastern or central parts of the United States.

MANAGEMENT OF ALLERGIC RHINITIS

With mild transient symptoms, specific antigen avoidance or low dose drug therapy may be adequate. With persistent seasonal or perennial symptoms, a variety of drugs or specific immunotherapy and, occasionally, even surgery may be necessary.

The first step in management is to identify which allergens (or antigens) are important to determine if this is truly allergic disease. The antigens responsible may be identified by an extensive history and physical examination; then, as necessary, testing either by skin tests or a variety of in vitro techniques will identify the specific antigens involved.

Elimination Techniques

- Keep the environment as dust and mold free as possible, especially the bedroom.
- Dehumidify damp homes and, if necessary, use special mold preventatives.
- Replace potentially allergenic pillows, quilts, clothing, furniture, and carpeting with nonallergic products and wash them frequently.
- Cover mattress and pillows with plastic or barrier cloth and treat carpeting to kill mites.
- Ventilate areas conducive to mold formation, such as crawl spaces, and avoid mold sources.
- Use air conditioners and high-quality air cleaners.
- Avoid window fans that pull pollen into the house.
- Avoid being outside in high pollen seasons and protect from exposure to high levels, e.g., on warm windy days or as grass is being cut.
- Plan vacations to avoid the worst local exposure to inhalant allergies.
- Animals should be eliminated or contact avoided.
- Restrict animal movement in the house.
- Wash cats monthly.
- Eliminate sources of insects indoors and outdoors.
- Avoid gardening, lightly colored clothes, and perfume in areas of insects.
- Avoid chemical exposure to insecticides, strong cleaning agents and perfumes, and exposure when chemicals are being sprayed for fertilizer, weed, or insect control.
- Avoid environmental irritants such as tobacco smoke and highly perfumed or chemically treated materials which may act as environmental irritants, such as formaldehyde.
- Avoid known food allergies and additives by diet control.

Elimination techniques

Elimination of the offending allergen or avoidance of contact is the first line of defense.[18,19] The home environment and, as much as possible, the school or work place should be managed to decrease allergen exposure. Avoidance recommendations should be provided to the patient. The simplest way is to have handouts prepared (box above).

House dust, dust mites, and molds are always present.

The environment should by kept as free from these as possible. It is important to try to keep at least one room, usually the bedroom, as allergy free as possible. Pollen avoidance is difficult. The pollens should not be brought into the house. The allergic patient should try not to be outside when the pollens to which he is allergic are blowing at high levels.

Animals and insects are a problem. The patient who is allergic to his favorite pet will often get rid of the doctor before getting rid of the pet but must be cautioned about

Drug Additives

Binders	Colorings
Emulsifiers	Preservatives
Flavorings	Sulfites

exposure and treated with immunotherapy if necessary. If animals must be kept, contact must be avoided and the air flow of dander inhibited. Cats are less antigenic if washed once a month. Cockroaches and their debris have become recognized as a very significant problem, as have fire ants, honey bees, wasps, etc.

Patients who have food allergies or are chemically sensitive will be much improved if they learn to avoid those foods and materials which as allergens or irritants incite allergic symptoms. Even additives in medications can produce problems and may need to be recognized and eliminated. Patients may think they are having a drug reaction, but it may actually be a reaction to one of the multiple additives which most drugs contain (box above).

By eliminating sources of some of the major allergens and irritants, the total allergic load is reduced and some patients will need little or no further care. Other patients, however, will require pharmacotherapy.

Pharmacotherapy

Drug therapy for allergic rhinitis may be used to control the symptoms after they occur or to prevent symptom occurrence by short circuiting the reaction. Four groups of drugs are useful to treat allergic patients. Antihistamines are the most frequently used drugs for the treatment of allergic rhinitis. Decongestants, both oral and topical, are helpful, and corticosteroids may be important. Mast cell stabilizers may be used in the allergic nose, eyes, and lungs and orally for food allergy.

The choice of drug to use for allergic rhinitis and the duration of its use are determined by the symptom expression—for instance, is the primary symptom rhinorrhea or congestion or are both present? Patient age must be considered. Children and the elderly may react adversely to drugs safe in adulthood. Also, other medical problems the patient has and the drugs being used for those must be considered, such as beta blockers. Antihistamines help early allergy reactions. Steroids are effective primarily in the late response, cromolyn in both.

Antihistamines. Antihistamines are among the most common drugs used by patients—both over-the-counter and by prescription. Most antihistamines available for allergic management are H_1 antagonists primary activity of which is dose-related competitive binding of the H_1 receptors on the target cells. Some, especially the newer drugs, may also inhibit histamine release from degranulating mast cells and basophils, probably by stabilization of the cell membrane,

TABLE 34-1
Classic antihistamines

Classification	Generic name	Trade name
Ethanolamines	Diphenhydramine	Benadryl
	Clemastine	Tavist
Ethylenediamines	Tripelennamine	Pyribenzamine
Alkylamines	Chlorpheniramine	Chlortrimeton
	Brompheniramine	Dimetane
Piperazines	Hydroxyzine	Atarax
	Meclizine	Antivert
Phenothiazines	Promethazine	Phenergan
	Trimeprazine	Temaril
Piperidines	Cyproheptadine	Periactin

(From Woodward JK: Pharmacology of Antihistamines. In Journal Allergy of Clinical Immunology, vol. 86:606-612, 1990.)

and some will also prevent neurologic stimulation. Their primary action is to reduce symptoms of the immediate allergic response. Antihistamines usually relieve the itching sensation in the nose, throat, and eyes, and reflex sneezing, and they reduce the increased clear secretions in both the nose and the eyes.[6,51] They do not relieve severe congestion, which is primarily a late response. In general, the classic or older antihistamines (Table 34-1) have a rapid onset of action and reach peak plasma concentrations in 1 to 2 hours, with the effect lasting from 4 to 6 hours. It's important to understand the various classes, because, if a patient develops tolerance or side effects to one, switching to another class usually helps. Also some patients may tolerate one class better than another.

The classes most often used for allergic rhinitis are the ethanolamines and alkylamines. Ethanolamines are the oldest potent H_1 antagonists, often having strong sedative effects: e.g., diphenhydramine HCl (Benadryl) and clemastine furmarate (tavis)—now both are available over-the-counter. Ethylenediamines are effective H_1 blocking agents with possible sedative and gastrointestinal effects: e.g., tripelennamine HCl (Pyribenzamine). Alkylamines are the most frequently used H_1 antagonists with somewhat less sedation than the ethanolamines (for instance, chlorpheniramine maleate (Chlortrimeton and Teldrin), brompheniramine maleate (Dimetane), and dexchlorpheniramine maleate (Polarimine). These are often combined with various decongestants.

Piperazines have prolonged H_1 blocking activity but are not often used for respiratory symptom control. For example, hydroxyzine (Vistaril or Atarax) is used for its tranquilizing, antiemetic effects, and, by decreasing skin reactivity, it is very useful in chronic urticaria or acute itching rashes. Another drug in this class is meclizine (Antivert or Bonine) which is often used as an antivertigo or antimotion sickness drug. Phenothiazines are effective H_1 blockers but have exceptional sedative effects (e.g., promethazine (Phenergan) occasionally used for preoperative sedation. Trimeprazine tartrate is Temaril which has excellent antipruritic effects. Piperidines include the older drug, cyproheptadine, found in Periactin. This drug is effective for eczema but markedly sedating and is not used for allergic rhinitis.

The *Physician's Desk Reference* states that antihistamines should not be given to patients with asthma. However, antihistamines, except possibly promethazine, actually improve mild asthma and do not have bad effects on more severe asthma. In fact, some of the new antihistamines actually have specific bronchodilator effects. That problem is being addressed now and hopefully changes will be made soon.

Side effects of the older antihistamines may be significant.[7] CNS effects occur because they are lipophilic so they can cross the blood brain barrier and attach easily to H_1 receptors in the brain. Sedative effects result from the central inhibitory activity. The sedation may be transient, but there may also be psychomotor changes which go unrecognized when driving and writing.

There may also be significant anticholinergic effects, especially drying of mucous membranes of the upper and lower respiratory tracts. There may also be cardiac stimulation, blurred vision, and decreased gastrointestinal and urinary tract motility resulting in constipation and urinary retention, which is especially dangerous in the presence of prostatic hypertrophy. Impotence has also been described.

Other side effects of classic antihistamines may be adverse or may be used clinically. For example, some have antitremor effects, others antiemetic and antitussive benefits. Antivertigo benefits may be efficacious, while local anesthetic changes may also occur. There may be suppression of exocrine glands. Severe adverse effects rarely occur but should be considered if a patient develops unusual symptoms such as a blood dyscrasia, fever of undetermined etiology, toxic nephrosis, or topical sensitivity.

Drug interactions are especially important. Antihistamines may prolong the action of all CNS depressant drugs: MAO inhibitors, tricyclic drugs, alcohol, anti-Parkinson drugs, barbiturates, tranquilizers, and narcotics. Often overlooked, some antihistamines also react with oral contraceptives, progesterone, reserpine, and thiazide diuretics. They may also inhibit the action of anticoagulants. These are the adverse effects the newer antihistamines are being developed to avoid.

The new so-called nonsedating antihistamines are absorbed well when taken orally, are metabolized in the liver, and excreted renally or fecally. They are lipophobic, that is, less lipid soluble than the older ones so they do not cross the blood brain barrier easily. They have little affinity for H_1 brain receptors so they cause little sedation and few, if any, psychomotor changes. They also have little or no anticholinergic activity so they are safe for patients with glaucoma and prostatic hypertrophy. They also have few drug interactions. The half-lives of the new antihistamines vary so the dosage schedules also vary, but most are long acting. They are well distributed in the body and all except astemizole have a rapid onset of action. In general, their antihistamine activity is comparable to or possibly better than that of the classic antihistamines in the treatment of allergic rhinitis.[24,46,51]

Terfenadine, astemizole, loratadine, acrivastine, and ophthalmic levocabastine have been approved by the FDA. Cetirizine is awaiting FDA approval. A number of other preparations are in advanced research stages (Table 34-2).

Terfenadine, approved in 1985, is well known now.[24,46] When taken as 60 mg twice daily it produces rapid improvement in sneezing and rhinorrhea, a more gradual decrease in nasal and pharyngeal itching, but no changes in congestion. It has been released as Seldane-D combined with pseudoephedrine to help correct congestion when present, but it may now produce the same side effects and have the same contraindications as the other decongestants. Central nervous system effects of terfenadine occur in less than 6% of patients

Astemizole was approved in 1988.[45,46] It has the same general pharmacokinetic properties as the other new antihistamines Its onset of action, however, is slow. The dose is 10 mg once daily. Originally, for more rapid onset of benefits a loading dose was recommended, but this recommendation has been eliminated with the concern over possible cardiac alterations. Benefit starts usually within 3 or 4 days of the first dose. The inhibition of the urticarial response may persist for days or weeks. To some extent chronic allergic rhinitis is benefited by astemizole, but it is less popular than its use for urticaria. A small percent (3.6%) of patients gain weight while taking astemizole.

A new antihistamine approved in 1993 by the FDA is loratadine.[5] It has a very rapid onset of action and is effective for 18 to 24 hours with a dose of 10 mg daily. This drug has been found to significantly inhibit mast cell mediator release. There is little sedation and few, if any, psychomotor changes or CNS depressant drug interactions. No problem with electrocardiographic alterations has been reported yet.

Acrivastine has recently been approved by the FDA combined with the decongestant pseudoephedrine. It may be used up to 3 times a day and is somewhat more sedating than the other new antihistamines but has a very rapid onset of effect.[4]

Cetirizine is awaiting FDA approval. It is an active metabolite of hydroxyzine with all of the benefits but with little sedative effect.[7,43] It has a rapid onset of action; the metabolism is minimal so liver function is not of concern. Excretion is almost exclusively renal, so kidney function is very important. Because it is long acting, one daily dose of 10 mg is adequate, and it has shown no drug interaction or anticholinergic effects. Cetirizine appears to be slightly more sedating than placebo but equal to or less than most of the other second-generation antihistamines, the effect be-

TABLE 34-2
New nonsedating antihistamines

Classification	Generic name	Trade name	Dosage
Alkylamine	Acrivastine*	Semprex-D	8 mg up to 4 times daily prn (+ 60 mg of pseudoephedrine)
Piperazine	Cetirizine	Reactine Zyrtec	10 mg daily
Piperidine	Astemizole*	Hismanal	10 mg daily
	Ketotifen	Zaditen	2 mg twice daily
	Loratadine*	Claritin	10 mg daily
	Terfenadine*	Seldane	60 mg twice daily
	Ebastine		10 mg daily
Miscellaneous	Azelastine	Astelin	2 mg daily
	Oral		2 sprays per nostril daily or twice daily
	Nasal		
	Levocabastine	Livostin	1 drop each eye 4 times daily
	Ophthalmic*		2 sprays per nostril twice daily
	Nasal		

*FDA approved.

ing dose related. It may be the first drug to benefit both early and late allergy reactions.

Information about cardiac effects related to terfenadine and astemizole use has been available for several years.[40,49,54] Although there appears to be little drug interaction with these new antihistamines, there may be some potentially dangerous side effects. Torsades de pointes and other cardiac arrhythmias may occur with intentional overdoses of terfenadine or astemizole, if the metabolism is diminished by chronic liver disease or by drugs which may interfere with liver metabolism. These drugs require the cytochrome P 450 enzyme system for metabolism so there is competition producing a drug overdose and, possibly, cardiac abnormalities. Such drugs are the antifungal agents including ketoconozole and some macrolide antibiotics such as erythromycin. Possibly H_2 antagonists such a cimetadine may also compete. This cardiac problem does not appear to be of concern with loratadine because it does not block the delayed rectifier potassium channel as do terfenadine and astemizole at doses considerably higher than the usual clinical dose.[52]

Two very different drugs in the research stage are important to discuss because they will be the first topical, that is, intranasal, antihistamine preparations.

Azelastine is effective both orally and topically as an antiallergy and potentially an antiasthma drug.[15,38,44,48] It is an entirely new class of drug which inhibits the secretion of histamine and a number of other very important chemical mediators. Studies have shown that azelastine as a nasal spray is effective for seasonal allergic rhinitis. It is mildly sedating when taken orally. The only significant adverse findings so far reported are a dose-related taste alteration of dryness and metallic taste in 30% to 52% of patients. This is short lasting and occurs especially when liquids are taken.

Levocabastine used topically appears to be the most potent H_1 antagonist yet developed.[10,33,41] It is highly selective, has a very rapid onset of action, and prolonged activity in the nose and eyes. The ophthalmic form has been approved and found to be very useful. Dosage is usually one drop four times a day.

Ceterizine and these two topical antihistamines will set a new safe direction for antihistamine therapy.

A comparison of the pharmacologic profiles of both classic and new antihistamines indicate that all have essentially the same antihistaminic activity. The sedative effects are usually dose related. Although some patients complain of increased dryness, the new drugs appear to have little or no anticholinergic activity (Table 34-3).[51]

Decongestants. Decongestants may be used topically or orally to stimulate adrenergic receptors decreasing nasal edema (Table 34-4).* The most common ones used orally for allergic rhinitis are pseudoephedrine, phenylpropanolamine, and phenylephrine. These are often combined together, with an antihistamine, or the mucolytic, guiafenesin. There are a number of agents for topical use that are now mostly over-the-counter preparations. Epinephrine and cocaine are also decongestants but not commonly used strictly for decongestion in clinical practice.

Overuse of topical decongestants may produce rebound locally, referred to as chemical rhinitis or rhinitis medicamentosa. All decongestants, both oral and topical, may produce CNS stimulation and systemic vascular symptoms, including elevated blood and ocular pressures, urinary tract

*References 12, 16, 23, 24, 26.

TABLE 34-3
Pharmacologic profiles of nonsedating and classic antihistamines

	Pharmacologic property		
	Antihistaminic activity	**Sedative activity**	**Anticholinergic activity**
Nonsedating			
Terfenadine	+++	0	0
Astemizole	+++	0	0
Loratadine	+++	0/+*	0
Cetirizine	+++	0/+*	0
Mequitazine	+++	0/++	+/++
Classic			
Chlorpheniramine	+++	+/++*	+/++*
Diphenhydramine	+++	+++	++
Promethazine	+++	++	+/++
Clemastine	+++	+/++	++
Triprolidine			

Adapted from Woodward JK: Pharmacology of antihistamines. *Allergy Clin Immunol* 86:606-612, 1990.
0 = None, + = slight, ++ = moderate, +++ = marked.
*Dose dependent.

TABLE 34-4
Decongestants

Action	Drug
Stimulate adrenergic receptors	Pseudoephedrine (oral)
Sympathomimetic	Phenylpropanolamine (oral/topical)
Decrease nasal edema	Phenylephrine (oral)
	Ephedrine (oral/topical)
	Oxymetazoline (topical)
	Tetrahydrozoline (topical)
	Naphazoline (topical)
	Xylometazoline (topical)
	Epinephrine (systemic/topical)
	Cocaine (topical)

TABLE 34-5
Pharmacotherapy: corticosteroids

Characteristics	Uses
Versatile	Allergic and nonallergic respiratory disease
Anti-inflammatory	Late reaction
Systemic	Seasonal rhinitis
Topical	Rhinitis medicamentosa
	Aspirin sensitivity syndrome
	Pre- and postoperatively in allergic patients
	Allergic and nonallergic skin disorders

obstruction, and cardiac and gastrointestinal symptoms. They must be used cautiously at all times and avoided in patients with heart disease, hypertension, diabetes, glaucoma, prostate enlargement, hyperthyroidism, and peptic and possibly gastric ulcers. Oral decongestants will not produce rebound but their decongestant effect in the nose is variable. Some patients respond rapidly, others poorly, or some not at all. Beck et al have demonstrated that, in most medically controlled hypertensive patients, pseudoephedrine may be safely used for nasal congestion.[2]

All decongestants may react dangerously with MAO inhibitors, indomethacin, beta blockers and methyldopa, general anesthetics, digitalis, and possibly theophylline.

Corticosteroids. Corticosteroids are very versatile anti-inflammatory drugs available for systemic, oral, intramuscular, intravenous, and also topical use.[30] They have an important role in treating late reactions and in both allergic and nonallergic rhinitis. Systemic corticosteroids are used for the more difficult to manage problems. High-dose burst therapy may be indicated in severe seasonal allergic rhinitis, rhinitis medicamentosa, aspirin-sensitive patients, and pre- and postoperatively in markedly allergic patients (Table 34-5).

Intranasal corticosteroids have become perhaps the most important nasal medication.[31] They utilize the general effects of parenteral steroids for local responses in the nasal mucosa. Intranasal steroids are useful for both seasonal and perennial allergic rhinitis, after surgery for nasal polyposis to decrease recurrence, in aspirin-sensitive rhinosinusitis,

TABLE 34-6
Topical nasal steroids

Preparation	Delivery*	Dosage	Safety margin†	Days of Rx‡
Dexamethasone	FHP (170)	bid-tid	1+	14-28
Beclomethasone	FHP (200)	tid-qid	5	25-33
Beclomethasone aqueous	Pump (200)	bid	5	25-50
Flunisolide	Pump (200)	bid-tid	3.5	33-66
Triamcinolone	FHP (100)	Once daily	8	25

Adapted from Mabry RL: Corticosteroids in the management of upper respiratory allergy: the emerging role of steroid nasal sprays, *Otolaryngol Head Neck Surg* 107:855-60, 1992.
FHP, Fluorinated hydrocarbon propellant; *tid,* three times daily; *qid,* four times daily; *bid,* twice daily.
*Delivery system (pump or fluorinated hydrocarbon propellant); number of doses per container.
†Multiple of recommended maximum daily dose that results in significant risk of HPA suppression.
‡Number of days of therapy per container.

rhinitis medicamentosa, and some are "safe therapy" in pregnancy. Intranasal steroids available in the United States as of September 1994 are dexamethasone phosphate, beclomethasone diproprionate (aerosol and aqueous), flunisolide, triamcinolone acetonide, and budesonide. The most popular preparations in the United States are beclomethasone and triamcinolone. The absorption of dexamethasone is high, and since there may be alternation of the adrenal/pituitary axis it is rarely used now. There is minimal absorption of the other intranasal steroids, and any side effects of these drugs are usually transient. There is a lapse time of 3 to 7 days before these intranasal drugs are fully effective. They are available as aerosols with a variety of propellants and the aqueous pump spray form (Table 34-6).[31] Triamcinolone appears to be effective if used once a day (in doses of 220 or 440 μg) as an aerosol with virtually no side effects.[47]

The side effects of beclomethasone and flunisolide have been reported to be the development of atrophic rhinitis and rare septal perforations, especially with the earlier fluorinated hydrocarbon propellent type of aerosols. There is less problem with the aqueous formulas or the new so-called soft sprays. Flunisolide is dispensed with propylene glycol which stings, so it has lost much of its market. The company is trying to alter the preparation now by decreasing the propylene glycol and increasing the polyethylene glycol.[9]

Budesonide is the latest intranasal steroid to become available. It is an aerosol recommended for once-daily use in the United States, but requires four sprays each time. In Europe, it is used as two sprays twice daily. It appears to have little adverse reactions but is remarkably efficacious with a rapid onset of benefit.[1,53]

There are a number of other intranasal steroids not currently available in the United States which may well be available in the near future. Fluticasone is awaiting FDA approval. This will also be prescribed as a once-daily dose using two sprays on each side of the nose. Its onset of action is very rapid and has some benefit in relieving nasal-congestion as well as rhinorrhea.[5,8,29,50] Flucortin butyl esterase is a powdered form of intranasal steroid used with an apparatus called a Rhinolator. It appears to be as effective as the aerosol and pump sprays but less irritating.

Intranasal injection of steroids has been advocated by some otolaryngologists.[22] I find benefit from small-dose injections of steroid into nasal polyps. The drugs most often used are Decadron LA, Hydeltra TBA, and Aristocort. There may be a rapid decrease in polyp size. It may also be used postoperatively if there is recurrence of polyps. Occasionally I also recommend intraturbinate injections. A number of years ago there were reports of complications with steroid embolism by way of the ophthalmic artery to the eye or vascular spasm resulting in vision loss, both temporary and permanent (11 total, 6 permanent). However, if technically done properly this is not a problem, but it must be done with caution and thoughtfulness with topical decongestion and by superficial slow injection of a preparation with very small particle size, instilled primarily anteriorly and along the inferior border of the inferior turbinate.

Mast Cell Stabilizers. The final group of drugs available for the treatment of allergic rhinitis to discuss are mast cell stabilizers. Cromolyn sodium, the first identified, is available in a number of forms (Box on p. 393). The mechanism of action is not entirely clear, but it appears that cromolyn prevents the release of histamine and other mediators by stabilizing the mast cell wall and inhibiting the inflow of CA++ ions into the mast cell, preventing degranulation. It may also camouflage special receptors on the mast cells so that other cellular mechanisms, such as those producing the late reaction, do not occur. Cromolyn is the only drug available so far in this country that prevents both early and late allergic reactions. It is minimally metabolized and causes few side effects.[21]

Intranasally, cromolyn is most effective if used prior to a challenge such as mowing the lawn in a grass- or mold-sensitive patient or golfing in late August in a ragweed-sensitive patient or a grass-sensitive patient all year round in Texas. The problem with this excellent drug is the frequency of use at the beginning of treatment.

Mucolytics

Guiafenesin
Iodides
Nasal saline
Alkalol
Facial sauna
Rhinotherm
Virotherm*

*Not available in the United States.

Mast Cell Stabilizers

Cromolyn sodium	Nedocromil sodium
Intranasal (Nasalcrom)	Inhalation (Tilade)
Ophthalmic (Opticrom)	Intranasal (Tilarin [?])*
Inhalation (Intal)	Ophthalmic (Tilavist)*
Oral (Gastrocrom)	Ketotifen
Isospaglumic acid	Oral (Zaditen)*
Intranasal (N-acetyl-aspartyl-glutamate)*	

*Not FDA approved.

Cromolyn has been available as an ophthalmic preparation, and orally it has been approved for mastocytosis. The oral form has been found useful in some food-allergic patients.[50]

Nedocromil is a new mast cell stabilizer under study in the United States.[11,32,42] The dosage required will probably be less than that for nasalcrom which will improve patient compliance. It has been approved by the FDA for asthma. The intranasal product has not yet been released by the FDA. An ophthalmic preparation should also be available soon.

Other mast cell stabilizers are in the research stage.

In any form of intranasal therapy, steroids, or cromolyn, or the intranasal antihistamines when they become available, when the drug is first used, nasal edema may need to be adequately reduced by the use of oral decongestants, or occasionally, topical decongestants for the first 3 to 4 days to allow the intranasal medication to reach the affected respiratory mucosa. Remember to tell patients that these special intranasal drugs differ from the over-the-counter decongestant sprays and that chemical rhinitis will not occur from them.

Mucolytics. Mucolytics may also improve some symptoms of allergic rhinitis (box above). They are often combined with oral decongestants and cough preparations, especially the guiafenesin and iodide preparations. I find the most effective to be a daily dose of 2400 mg of guiafenesin in two divided doses. Mucolytics help thin the thick postnasal secretions, especially in perennial rhinitis, so it is cleared more readily.

Antiallergy Drugs

Anticholinergics
Ipratropium bromide nasal spray (Atrovent)
Atropine
Pentigetide (Pentyde)
Nasal solution
Capsaicin

Combining these with nasal saline or alkolol irrigations may increase clearing of the mucus as well as washing antigens from the nasal mucosa.

Warm moist air in various forms also appears soothing and aids in thinning secretions by providing additional moisture.[32,42] Utilizing these agents and techniques in patients with both seasonal and perennial rhinitis promotes improved nasal hygiene and often some of the uncomfortable symptoms.[13,17]

Miscellaneous antiallergy drugs. Another drug with antiallergy effects not yet available in the United States (box above) is ipratropium bromide nasal spray, an anticholinergic which improves the thin secretions of the immediate allergic reaction, cold exposure, and vasomotor rhinitis.[14,36,39]

Pentigetide as a nasal and ophthalmic solution is a very unique drug produced as a synthetic amino acid from the FC region of human IgE.[34] It has antiallergic and also anti-inflammatory properties. A capsaicin preparation (a product of chili peppers) is being studied as an antiallergy agent also. The calcium channel blocker, nifidepine, is also being evaluated.

Drug histories are of vital importance before drug therapy or skin testing is started, and patients must be cautioned to inform the allergist of any additional drugs prescribed by another physician while receiving pharmacotherapy or immunotherapy. With the influx of new drugs for nearly every disease, we must be cautious about cross-reactions and be on the alert for any changes that the patient reports.

Some patients respond well to one form of antiallergy medications but not to others. Therefore, if one is not effective, others should be tried. The use of the simplest form of therapy which will effectively relieve the symptoms is wisest.

Immunotherapy. If pharmacotherapy is inadequate the patient may need immunotherapy. Immunotherapy for allergy is a treatment technique of subcutaneous injections of increasing doses of allergens to which the patient is sensitive. It is antigen specific so the patient's sensitivities must be accurately determined and a starting point selected for each before any treatment vials are prepared. That is why the skin endpoint titration testing technique used by most otolaryngologists is so very important.[20]

Immunotherapy is usually reserved for those patients who have severe, prolonged, and, at times, disabling symptoms. It is also useful for those in whom elimination or avoidance is not possible and those whose drug management is inadequate or the side effects intolerable. It is also required when there is danger of anaphylaxis as with venom hypersensitivity. It is the only way to treat the underlying cause not just the symptoms.

The goal of immunotherapy is long-term symptom relief—hopefully for years or permanently. It should be safe, efficacious, and economical.[37]

Surgery. The final step in management of allergic rhinitis in some patients will be surgery. I strongly urge that the treatment of the allergic basis of the nasal disease be done initially or at least concurrently with elective surgery. If not, the pathology will return and the surgery will not have long-term success.[27] None of us as surgeons like to face that. Extensive discussion of the surgical procedures cannot be considered in this paper but it is important to illustrate just a few relations between allergy and surgery.

Some allergic patients have large tonsils and adenoids. We must be able to differentiate those who will improve with just allergy care. An 11-year-old boy had large obstructing adenoids. After 2 months of immunotherapy the obstruction was better and by 6 months the adenoids had shrunk so surgery was not necessary. Some patients may have large tonsils with few true bacterial infections but significant postnasal drainage that produces symptoms. In other cases, a tonsillectomy is truly necessary because of obstruction.

Allergy may be important in producing airway obstruction, malocclusion, and development of the long face syndrome. In a research study I completed several years ago, allergy was a vital factor in contributing to airway obstruction and secondary malocclusion and facial deformities.[27]

The study protocol involved the evaluation of: (1) the nasal anatomy—both tissue edema and structural deformities, (2) the size of the adenoids and tonsils and estimation of the degree of obstruction, (3) the evaluation of patients with significant allergic history, and (4) the diagnosis of structural deformities of the middle third of the face. (The age range was 4 to 16 years.) Of these 200 children, 58.5% had allergies alone or with some other factor associated, 38% had hypertrophic lymphoid tissue, and 21% had structural deformities, especially a deviated septum; 10% had microrhino dysplasia. Allergies were diagnosed by history, skin endpoint titration or modified RAST testing, diet diaries, and diet elimination and challenge.[28]

Twenty-four (12%) required nasal surgery, one having nasal polyps. Thirteen children in the study had had prior adenotonsillectomies but still had airway obstruction when seen, most often due to allergic edema of the nasal mucosa. Fifty-six (28%) of these children required tonsillectomies and/or adenoidectomies most often related to chronic recurrent infections, rarely from obstruction alone. Tonsillectomy is not an obsolete procedure.

Management of the airway was of significant importance in allowing for proper orthodontic procedures, including tolerance of appliances, prevention of relapse after completion of orthodontic treatment, and prevention of further development of the classic long face syndrome. Surgery alone would not solve many of these problems. Dana is a case in point. She had, at age 12, a typical long face syndrome and grotesque malocclusion. Allergy evaluation and treatment was started, followed by correction of her markedly deviated septum. These produced a normal airway. Within 9 months her malocclusion was well under way to being corrected and this was a much healthier and happier child, although stigmata of the long face syndrome do remain.

Other surgical problems in the allergic patient may include nasal polyps, sinusitis, and turbinate hyperplasia or hypertrophy. In the case of multiple, large polyps allergy control, including immunotherapy and pharmacotherapy is rarely effective. Systemic steroids or direct injection into the polyps may be of some benefit in reducing size but invariably the patients will require surgery. Polyps may become destructive if large enough. So, when the disease becomes extensive and conservative measures are not sufficient, surgery is necessary. If the problems are due to allergy, they will certainly recur unless the underlying disease is treated. Allergy management should precede the surgery except in threatening situations, such as orbital cellulitis or intracranial complications.

Lectures about sinusitis and its medical and surgical therapy are being presented frequently. Endoscopic sinus surgery is a "hot" subject and there is no time now to address all of its aspects. I will only caution sinus surgeons to consider the role allergy may play in producing chronic sinusitis or recurrences after surgical therapy. Early disease may be amenable to conservative therapy, but advanced disease will require surgery and continued medical management. I strongly advocate this approach.

Vocal cord edema may be due to allergy or develop after use of an endotracheal tube in an allergic patient with overreactive mucosa. Recurrent otitis media may have an allergic basis.

COMPLICATIONS OF SURGERY IN THE ALLERGIC PATIENT

Patients with allergies who undergo otolaryngic surgery may develop a number of complications, especially if the allergy is not under reasonable control. In the case of nasal or facial plastic surgery, the mucosa may be "twitchy"—that is overreactive with excessive and prolonged rhinorrhea and sneezing postoperatively. For example, there may be excessive bleeding and edema in the pharynx during a tonsillectomy. Surgery in the nose may result in subsequent thickening and uncontrolled scarring. There may be slow resolution of ecchymosis with tissue staining. Healing may be slow with prolonged tenderness. Adhesions or stenosis may develop. Sometimes there will be hyperplastic or metaplastic mucosal changes. Tape sensitivity and drug allergies, such as to betadine, must also be of concern, as well as allergy to suture material. If there is a history of allergy it should not be ignored.

In patients known to have allergy who undergo any type of surgery, the allergic symptoms should be under the best possible control for the safest anesthetic and postoperative care. Surgical risk and morbidity will be decreased and healing potential will be optimized.

If surgery must be done in allergic patients, especially in emergency situations, medications such as steroids, antibiotics, antihistamines, and decongestants should be used judiciously. Environmental controls may be needed as well as improved local hygiene. Surgical techniques should be done rapidly, but all tissues must be handled gently since they often overreact. Preferably, local anesthesia should be used along with vasoconstrictors. In the nose, packing should be inserted and removed carefully, and dressings should be firm and not hastily removed. Telfa packs and even Teflon splints in the nose may prevent adhesions and delayed bleeding. Immunotherapy must be continued after surgery. Many patients forget this and neglect the allergy care. They must be reminded that this is an ongoing disease and compliance with therapy encouraged.

Remember, allergy treatment cannot cure everything. Surgery cannot cure everything. We must understand the limitations of both the scalpel and the needle.

Not every otolaryngologist will want to actually include allergy treatment in his or her practice, but considering allergy as part of an otolaryngology practice will provide better diagnostic medicine, better understanding of the disease process, better ability to treat rhinitis patients, and, in general, better total patient care. There is also an economic factor. It is a great practice builder. So when patients ask us for care for nasal symptoms, do consider allergy in your differential diagnosis.

REFERENCES

1. al-Mohaimeid H: A parallel group comparison of budesonide and beclomethasone diproprionate for treatment of perennial allergic rhinitis in adults. *J Int Med Res* 21(2):67-73, 1993.
2. Beck RA, et al: Cardiovascular effects of pseudoephedrine in medically controlled hypersensitive patients. *Arch Int Med* 152:1242-45, 1992.
3. Bédard PM, et al: Onset of action of loratadine and placebo and other efficacy variables in patients with seasonal allergic rhinitis. *Clin Ther* 14:268-75, 1992.
4. Brogden RN, McTavish D: Acrivastine: a review of its pharmacological properties and therapeutic efficacy in allergic rhinitis, urticaria, and related disorders. *Drugs* 4:927-40, 1991.
5. Bryson HM, Faulds D: Intranasal fluticasone proprionate—review of its pharmacodynamic and pharmacokinetic properties; and therapeutic potential in allergic rhinitis [review]. *Drugs* 43:760-75, 1992.
6. Busse WW: Role of antihistamines in allergic disease, *Ann Allergy* 72:371-375, 1994.
7. Campoli-Richards DM, Buckley MMT, Fitton A: Cetirizine: a review of its pharmacological properties and clinical potential in allergic rhinitis, pollen-induced asthma, and chronic urticaria. *Drugs* 40:762-81, 1990.
8. Colovick MD, et al: Double-blind comparison of intranasal fluticasone proprionate 200 less g daily with 200 g twice daily in the treatment of patients with severe seasonal allergic rhinitis to ragweed. *Ann Allergy* 72:435-40, 1994.
9. Conley SF: Comparative trial of acceptability of beclomethasone diproprionate and a new formulation of flunisolide. *Ann Allergy* 72:529-32, 1994.
10. Dechant KL, Goa KL: Levocabastine: a review of its pharmacological properties and potential as a topical antihistamine in allergic rhinitis and conjunctivitis. *Drugs* 41:202-22, 1991.
11. Donnelly A, Casale TB: Nedocromil is rapidly effective in the therapy of seasonal allergic rhinitis. *J Allergy Clin Immunol* 91:997-1004, 1993.
12. Gardiner LJ: Decongestants, anticholinergics, and saline in allergic rhinitis management. *J Res Dis* 12(suppl 3):S29-S31, 1991.
13. Georgitis JW: Local hyperthermia and nasal irrigation for perennial allergic rhinitis: effect on symptoms and nasal airflow. *Ann Allergy* 71:385-389, 1993.
14. Georgitis JW: The anticholinergic treatment of allergic perennial rhinitis, *J Allergy Clin Immunol* 90:1071-1076, 1992.
15. Grossman J, et al: Double-blind assessment of azelastine in the treatment of perennial allergic rhinitis. *Ann Allergy* 73:141-46, 1994.
16. Hendeles L: Selecting a decongestant [review]. *Pharmacotherapy* 13:129S-34S. (Discussion 143S-146S, 1993.)
17. Johnston SL, et al: The effect of local hyperthermia on allergen-induced nasal congestion and mediator release. *J Allergy Clin Immunol* 92:850-856, 1993.
18. Keenan JP: General management of the allergic patient. In Krause HF editor: *Otolaryngic allergy and immunology.* Philadelphia, 1989, WB Saunders Co.
19. King HC: Approaching therapy of allergy. In *The otolaryngologist's guide to allergy.* New York, 1990, Thieme Medical Publishers, Inc.
20. King HC: Immunotherapy. In King HC: *An otolaryngologist's guide to allergy.* New York, 1990, Thieme Medical Publishers, Inc.
21. King HC: Mast cell stabilizers, *Otolaryngol Head Neck Surg* 107:841-844, 1992.
22. King HC, Mabry RL: Pharmacotherapeutic agents for the management of rhinosinusitis. In King HC, Mabry RL: *A practical guide to the management of nasal and sinus disorders,* New York, 1993, Thieme Medical Publishers, Inc.
23. Knight A: The role of decongestants in allergic rhinitis. *J Resp Dis* 13(suppl):S30-S33, 1992.
24. Krause HF: Antihistamines and decongestants. *Otolaryngol Head Neck Surg* 107:835-40, 1992.
25. Krause HF: Diagnostic patterns in otolaryngic allergy: symptoms. In Krause HF, editor: *Otolaryngic allergy and immunology,* Philadelphia, 1989, WB Saunders Co.
26. Krause HF: Pharmacotherapy for allergic nasal disease, *Curr Opinion Otolaryngol Head Neck Surg* 2:147-53, 1994.
27. Krause HF: Surgery and the allergic patient. In Krause HF, editor: *Otolaryngic allergy and immunology.* Philadelphia, 1989, WB Saunders Co.
28. Krause HF: Upper airway obstruction as a cause of dental and facial deformities. *Primary ENT* 3:2-8, 1987.
29. LaForce LF, et al: Fluticasone proprionate: an effective alternative treatment for seasonal rhinitis in adults and adolescents. *J Fam Prac* 38:145-152, 1994.

30. Mabry RL: Corticosteroids in rhinology. *Otolaryngol Head Neck Surg* 108:768-770, 1993.
31. Mabry RL: Corticosteroids in the management of upper respiratory allergy: the emerging role of steroid nasal sprays. *Otolaryngol Head Neck Surg* 107:855-60, 1992.
32. Mabry RL: Topical pharmacotherapy for allergic rhinitis: nedocromil [review]. *Am J Otolaryngol* 14:379-381, 1993.
33. Mabry RL: Topical pharmacotherapy for allergic rhinitis: new agents. *South Med J* 85:149-154, 1992.
34. Mansmann HC, et al: Pentigetide nasal solution: a multi center study evaluating efficacy and safety in patients with seasonal allergic rhinitis. *Ann Allergy* 62:409-415, 1991.
35. Marks MB: *Stigmata of respiratory tract allergies*. Kalamazoo, Michigan, 1977, Upjohn Co.
36. Meltzer EO: Intranasal anticholinergic therapy of rhinorrhea [review]. *J Allergy Clin Immunol* 90:1055-1064, 1992.
37. Meltzer EO: Today's approach to controlling allergic rhinitis *J Resp Dis* 13(6A suppl):S30-S39, 1992.
38. Meltzer EO, et al: Azelastine nasal spray in the management of seasonal allergic rhinitis. *Ann Allergy* 72:354-359, 1994.
39. Meltzer EO, et al: Ipratropium bromide aqueous nasal spray for patients with perennial allergic rhinitis: a study on its effect on their symptoms, quality of life and nasal cytology. *J Allergy Clin Immunol* 90:242-249, 1992.
40. Monahan BP, et al: Torsades de pointes occurring in association with terfenadine use, *JAMA* 264:2788-2790, 1990.
41. Naclario RM: The effect of antihistamines on the immediate allergic response: a comparative review. *Otolaryngol Head Neck Surgery* 108:723-730, 1993.
42. Parish RC, Miller LJ: Nedocromil sodium [review]. *Ann Pharma* 27:599-606, 1993.
43. Pierson WE. Cetirizine: a unique second-generation antihistamine for treatment of rhinitis and chronic urticaria. *Clin Ther* 13:92-99, 1991.
44. Rafferty P, et al: The in vivo potency and selectivity of azelastine as an H_1 histamine-receptor antagonist in human airways and skin. *J Allergy Clin Immunol* 82:1113-1138, 1988.
45. Richards DM, et al: Astemizole: a review of its pharmacodynamic properties and therapeutic efficacy. *Drugs* 28:38-61, 1984.
46. Simons FER, Simons KJ: Second-generation H_1-receptor antagonists. *Ann Allergy* 66:5-17, 1991.
47. Storms WW: Clinical experiences with triamcinolone in rhinitis. *J Resp Dis* 12:41-42, 1991.
48. Storms WW, et al: Effectiveness of azelastine nasal solution in seasonal allergic rhinitis. *ENT Journal* 73:382-394, 1994.
49. Tobin JR, et al: Astemizole-induced cardiac conduction disturbances in a child. *JAMA* 266:2737-2740, 1991.
50. van As A, et al: Once daily fluticasone proprionate is as effective for perennial rhinitis as twice daily beclomethasone diproprionate. *J Allergy Clin Immunol* 91:1146-1154, 1993.
51. Woodward JK: Pharmacology of antihistamines. *J Allergy Clin Immunol* 86:606-612, 1990.
52. Woosley R, Darrow WR: Analysis of potential adverse drug reactions—a case of mistaken identity. *Amer J Cardiol* 74:208-209, 1994. (letter.)
53. Wright RG, et al: A double blind comparison of intranasal budesonide 400 micrograms and 800 micrograms in perennial rhinitis. *Clin Otolarygol* 17:354-358, 1992.
54. Zipes DP: Q-T interval prolongation: etiology and relatives risks. In Antihistamine consensus conference (monograph), Health Learning Systems. Little Falls, NJ 1993, Temple University School of Medicine.

Part Nine

Practice Management

35

Giving Your Practice A Checkup

Karen Zupko, BSJ

HOW'S THE PRACTICE GOING?

When you're asked that question what is your reply? Are you one of those physicians who can deliver a positive and affirmative, "Great"! Or are you unsure? Maybe you feel like you've been working as hard as ever, but the financials do not look as good as they did last year. Or, maybe, you feel as though you are entering a demilitarized zone when you enter your office; the tension among staff is so thick. Something is wrong, but it is hard to say what it is exactly. There are symptoms of trouble but nothing you can really point to as the problem. In any case, perhaps it's time for your practice, just like your patients to have a check-up.

In our consulting work with otolaryngologists in solo, group, and academic practices, we frequently find that the initial malaise centers around people and financial issues. The diagnostic workup that follows will help you identify key issues. The treatment plan for each practice is necessarily different depending on the physician or physicians in the group, the administrator, and the degree of the pain the problem is causing.

Use the checklists below to help you identify where your practice can be improved. Let's start with business structure. Without a clearly defined structure for your practice and well-defined systems, there will be confusion and tension. A few of the issues requiring your consideration are outlined here:

1. Are the leadership and governance structures clear to the physicians and staff? Do they make sense?
2. Are reporting relationships well defined?
3. Do you hold business meetings in the mornings when everyone is fresh? Do you have an agenda? Do you start on time? How is consensus reached?
4. Whether solo or group, do you set aside time to plan for the coming year?
5. Have you outgrown your present method of handling the business side of the practice?

Karen Zupko is the president of the Chicago-based consulting firm which bears her name. Ms Zupko and her colleagues have assessed over 70 otolaryngology practices nationally. She is a frequent speaker at AAO-HNS programs, serves on the editorial board of Medical Economics Magazine, and is active in a number of health care organizations.

Many otolaryngologists do not think of their practices as a business. Today, it is necessary to give as much thought to practice administration as to clinical care. Thinking this way will sharpen your ability to make decisions in a reasonable period of time and reduce friction between partners, associates, and staff. For many practices, lack of attention to form impedes the ability to function. We'll talk about those issues later.

First, let's look at the aforementioned issues.

1. *If leadership and governance haven't grown as the practice has, this can be a big problem.* For example, is the practice still laboring under the rotating presidency? What serious business organization could have a new president or CEO each year? At least solo practices have the same hand at the helm from year to year. Group practices, however, often have a major change in president and policy each year. Not every group member is prepared to lead or is interested in doing so. Recognize this and set up terms of office. If yours is a large group, plan on training the younger members on practice administration and business through active, viable committees with specific responsibilities and budgetary accountability.
2. *Reporting relationships suffer when each physician has his or her own team.* Build loyalty to the practice instead of to the individual physician. If you

have an administrator, loosen up the reins and give him or her both the authority and responsibility to make decisions and run the business side of the practice.

3. *Late night meetings for physicians are sure to result in poor decisions.* Everyone is tired; a doctor's day starts early! Try morning meetings once a month. Your practice is your biggest and best investment; treat it as an asset. Insist on precirculated agendas and keep good minutes. Do not allow items to be tabled month after month; this institutionalizes inertia. Start on time and people will arrive on time. Look at your voting requirements. It might not be possible for everyone to agree on each and every item. It is necessary that everything comes to a vote—or should decisions less than the collective hourly rate of the physicians attending be decided by a committee or the president and administrator? There are no easy answers, but these are important questions to ask. The times require speedier action than that which many practices are accustomed. If you are in solo practice, it might be a good idea to meet collectively with your key advisors—accountant, attorney, banker, or insurance representative—at least twice a year and obtain their perspective and input on practice direction.
4. *Planning time is a must.* For one thing, it is impossible to do a budget if there is no plan! Will you be adding an associate, upgrading the computer system, facing the retirement of an partner—these changes are all predictable. And, then, you face some that are not: what would happen if a high-producing physician were struck with an illness? Does your practice have a transition plan? When do you make time to think strategically and formulate an action agenda? We suggest an annual weekend retreat with a moderator who can help you analyze the strengths, weaknesses, opportunities, and threats facing the practice. This excellent planning technique is known as a SWOT analysis.

   Bottom line: Organize yourself and plan. Change is a friend, not an enemy. The structure and systems of the practice must stretch and grow to succeed in today's environment.

BUSINESS SYSTEMS AND REPORTS

Without information you cannot manage your practice. It is often surprising how little many otolaryngologists know about their financial affairs. You should be able to answer "Yes" to the statements listed below.

1. *Our accountant specializes in physician practices and works with other high earning surgical specialists.* Because of the rapid changes in payment mechanisms to managed care and capitation, practices today require accountants who understand and are familiar with the nuances of the medical practice business. While your brother-in-law may be able to prepare your tax return, he might not be the best person to handle the practice accounting functions.
2. *The accountant or a representative visits the practice at least quarterly.*
3. *The practice receives a monthly income and expense statement which is understandable to the physician and useful as a management tool.* While most otolaryngologists receive such a statement, not all understand the document or find it helpful in making decisions about practice management. See if your accountant can spend time deciphering the statement with you and if he or she can point out key trends you should be tracking. Reformatting and defining more meaningful expense categories are often helpful and necessary steps.
4. *The practice has safeguards and audit controls in place.* There is no sense doing this after you have let the "creative bookkeeper" go. Be sure your practice numbered route slips—a clean audit trail and checks and balances in place. This is especially important if you have satellite offices. While the systems are in place at the main office, they often fail when physicians go away from "home plate" to see patients.
5. *We track charges, receivables, and write-offs by payor.* It is essential for you to know how each type of insurer is reimbursing you. Because categories are not clearly defined in the computer, many practices do not have the details. The gross numbers do not tell the story.

ACCOUNTS RECEIVABLE

1. *I know bills and claim forms go out monthly.* How do you know? Unless you regularly do a spot check of your surgery log against the computerized listing of patient accounts you cannot be sure. If you do not dictate on time, it is unlikely that all claims go out within 10 days of providing care, another factor we consider important. Smart physicians will also review the "unbilled" report that the computerized system can generate. Why are statements being suspended?
2. *The content of receivables has been analyzed and specific steps have been taken to correct errors.* On this point you are looking for a consistent pattern of amounts that appear in the 60-day and older category. Specifically, you should be concerned if there is a same amount that keeps appearing. For example, in one practice we found 16 charges of $2,750 and discovered these were all septorhinoplasties. This otolaryngologist insisted on operating without prior approval. Unfortunately, the insurance carriers were not paying as he told his patients they

would. This can be a costly error and create ill will among patients.

3. *The office staff makes a concerted effort to collect surgical prepayments for deductibles and copayments in advance.* Some otolaryngologists are not aware that many deductibles today exceed the charges for routine procedures, such as myringotomies. It is important that your staff verify the coverage and the deductible and provide the patient with detailed information about out of pocket costs. While doing so, we suggest that they ask for at least a portion of this money as a scheduling deposit, being sensitive to the patient's financial situation. Furthermore, the payment plan can be set up at this time.
4. *Our office tracks withholds on managed care plans accurately.* Because many plans keep 10% or 15% of the amount due you under their reimbursement schedule until six months after the year has ended, we feel that it is important that these "withholds" be tracked in the computer. Each managed care plan with a withhold should have a separate category. This will allow you to know monthly what is in the "withhold" accounts. Treat this money as a receivable, not as a "write off" as you do the difference between your charge and the plan reimbursement amount.

INSURANCE

1. *We have attended an AAO-HNS sponsored coding course this year.* Because of the extraordinary changes in CPT each year, especially for endoscopic sinus surgery, the otolaryngologist should attend the course. This will enable you to dictate operative reports more completely and thereby ensure better payment. Similarly, we recommend that all surgeons code their own cases.
2. *We bill electronically to carriers, including Medicare.* Electronically submitted claims get paid faster. Investigate implementing submission to as many carriers as possible. Ask your software vendor for help.
3. *Our office staff compares the payments shown on explanation of benefit forms with the claim form and the managed care company fee schedule.* Experience has shown that not all carriers pay according to the contractually agreed reimbursement schedule. Most computer systems allow you to load up to 100 fee schedules in the computer. You want an easy way to compare their payment with your charge and the allowable amount. Appeal when you are not paid according to the contract terms.
4. *Patients not seen within the last year are re-registered.* We live in a mobile society. It's important to have the patient's correct marital status, address, phone numbers, employer and insurance. Only an active registration process will guarantee that bills are sent to the right party the first time.

PERSONNEL

1. *Morale in the office is good.* If it is not, you and your patients will suffer. It is easy to be productive and cooperative when the organization by which you are employed values you, demonstrates that, and insists on cooperation and good service as standards It might be time for you to induce some of the disgruntled and moody staff members to find an environment that brings out their best selves. Check with your attorney first for state regulations and advice. On the other hand, maybe you need to first evaluate your own supervisory style. Or may be you have supervisors who need to understand that they are coaches, not wardens. In any case, this is a serious symptom and warrants an immediate intervention.
2. *We are sure we have the right number of people working in the practice, doing the right jobs.* Many practices are not sure and for good reason. Because the practice is "run like a family" they neglect to have job descriptions and performance reviews, and training is nonexistent. Nor is there any form of oversight. Many families are dysfunctional, as you know from reading the newspaper or tuning into daytime TV. Run your practice like a business, save the family feelings for home. Resist, too, the cookbook consulting formulas of three staff per physician. Unfortunately, these recipes do not take into account what the physician wants done, work quality standards, or the time expectations for completing projects. How many staff you need depends on your delegation style and the complexity of your practice.
3. *Our personnel policy manual is up to date.* Changes such as OSHA regulations, the American's Disability Act, and the heightened sensitivity with regard to sexual harassment all require that personnel manuals be "tuned up" in keeping with the times. You might use one of the computerized programs to help you craft a first draft. We still recommend that the practice attorney review the final product before distribution. Our group remembers reviewing one manual that referred to a pension plan that was nonexistent and a paragraph that said absolutely no overtime would be paid. These are all violations you will want to avoid.
4. *Written performance appraisals are done annually.* While you are checking with your lawyers about the policy manual, see if they agree with our recommendation about having documentation before terminating an employee. But this is only one reason for doing a yearly written review, and a negative one at that. Ideally, reviews are planned as an

event to help staff achieve higher levels of accomplishment. Replace the check-off form with a few more open-ended questions. And ask employees to participate in the review by evaluating themselves. Better yet, meet with your staff and set prospective goals on which agree. This is far preferable to the retrospective "scorecard" used by so many practices.

PATIENT RELATIONS

1. *We survey patient satisfaction each year.* It's a good idea to get feedback from your patients, especially since many managed care plans are now surveying plan members—better to learn of places to improve directly from your patients than a plan administrator. Waiting time is a number one complaint in our experience.
2. *The practice has a patient information booklet.* Every practice should. It is not advertising but rather a good way to help your established patients understand what you do, your hours and policies on appointment scheduling, prescription refills, and insurance. Written in a positive friendly tone, a patient information booklet will boost compliance. The AAO-HNS has an excellent assortment of pamphlets and videos you can use, making effective patient education easy to do.
3. *Service is one of the ways we differentiate our practice from competitors.* If you answered "yes" to this question, you undoubtedly interview carefully and train your staff in service skills and about practice operations before turning them loose on the phones or in the examination rooms. A practice that "walks this talk" will also have enough staff to handle the phones and all other functions without stressing them to the maximum.

That finishes the checkup. Consider this a Level II visit; it is not a comprehensive consultation. Hopefully, you found a few places where you can begin to improve your practice and correct deficiencies. May be you answered "yes" to each question and you feel better already about your practice. This does not mean that you are fine and that you do not have to think about systems, procedures, or administration. Because, as the saying goes, "Even if you are on the right track, you'll get hit if you just sit there." Seek out more information to use in your continuous quality improvement program.

If you are thinking that something still is not right, maybe it is time for a second opinion or a more thorough evaluation. Get the peace of mind you deserve and act now to remedy your situation.

There is a wonderful saying that we use in our office, "Remember your best competitive edge is your ability to manage change." That is because so few people are good at it or even willing to try. Improving or updating your practice will mean some disruption and commotion for the short run but will pay dividends in the long term. Make the commitment to change and improvement.

Index